MOLECULAR INTERRELATIONS
OF NUTRITION AND CANCER

The University of Texas
M. D. Anderson Hospital and Tumor Institute at Houston
34th Annual Symposium on Fundamental Cancer Research

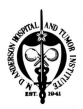

Published for
The University of Texas
M. D. Anderson Hospital and Tumor Institute at Houston
Houston, Texas, by Raven Press, New York

The University of Texas
M. D. Anderson Hospital and Tumor Institute at Houston
34th Annual Symposium on Fundamental Cancer Research

Molecular Interrelations
of Nutrition and Cancer

Edited by

Marilyn S. Arnott, Ph.D.

Department of Carcinogenetics
The University of Texas
M. D. Anderson Hospital
and Tumor Institute at Houston
Houston, Texas

Jan van Eys, M.D., Ph.D.

Department of Pediatrics
The University of Texas
M. D. Anderson Hospital
and Tumor Institute at Houston
Houston, Texas

Yeu-Ming Wang, Ph.D.

Department of Pediatrics
The University of Texas
M. D. Anderson Hospital
and Tumor Institute at Houston
Houston, Texas

Raven Press ■ New York

Raven Press, 1140 Avenue of the Americas, New York, New York 10036

Made in the United States of America

Library of Congress Cataloging in Publication Data

Symposium on Fundamental Cancer Research (34th: 1981:
    M. D. Anderson Hospital and Tumor Institute)
    Molecular interrelations of nutrition and cancer.

    Includes index.
    1. Cancer—Nutritional aspects—Congresses.
I. Arnott, Marilyn S.   II. Van Eys, Jan.   III. Wang,
Yeu-Ming.   IV. M. D. Anderson Hospital and Tumor
Institute.   V. Title.   [DNLM: 1. Diet—Adverse effects
—Congresses.   2. Neoplasms—Etiology—Congresses.
W3 SY5177 34th 1981m/QZ 202 S986 1981m]
RC261.A2S94 1981   616.99'407   81–23408
ISBN 0–89004–701–4   AACR2

This volume is a compilation of the proceedings of The University of Texas M. D. Anderson Hospital and Tumor Institute at Houston 34th Annual Symposium on Fundamental Cancer Research, held March 4–6, 1981, in Houston, Texas.

The material contained in this volume was submitted as previously unpublished material, except in the instances in which credit has been given to the source from which some of the illustrative material was derived.

Great care has been taken to maintain the accuracy of the information contained in the volume. However, the Editorial Staff, The University of Texas, and Raven Press cannot be held responsible for errors or for any consequences arising from the use of the information contained herein.

Preface

Thirty years after the 6th Annual Symposium on Fundamental Cancer Research, which was entitled "Nutritional Factors in Cancer Research," The University of Texas M. D. Anderson Hospital and Tumor Institute at Houston again focused on the subject of nutrition in the 34th Annual Symposium. The theme of the symposium was the link between nutrition and cancer in molecular terms.

The interaction of nutrition and cancer has been the focus of a number of other symposia and monographs in the past decade. The discussions were largely drawn from the influence of dietary factors, including contaminants, additives, fiber content, and alcohol consumption, on the causation and prevention of cancer. Unlike the present symposium, the earlier symposia were heavily therapy-oriented and usually discussed the nutritional consequences of therapy or the result of nutritional intervention or supplementation on the outcome of treatment and management of cancer.

The 34th Annual Symposium on Fundamental Cancer Research represented an attempt to determine whether there is an interrelation between the science of nutrition and the disease of cancer at a molecular level. Our plan was to examine this interrelation at three levels: cell-free systems, animals, and humans. Both macronutrients (carbohydrates and fat) and micronutrients (vitamins and minerals) were considered. The organization of the symposium was based on human cancer etiology and its extrapolation to the specifics of nutrition, immunity, and cancer.

What prevents us from effectively treating and preventing many cancers is a dearth of fundamental understanding of tumor cells and their environment in the human host. We know a great deal about nutritional biochemistry but not enough about the molecular biology of cancer to make a definitive correlation between the two. But there are many intriguing clues.

Among them are observations that incriminate dietary composition in the etiology of cancer. In addition, the diet is a vehicle for some carcinogens. Nutrients are needed in the human body in sufficient quantities to supply basic requirements. These basic requirements may also modify mutagenic or carcinogenic events. Nutrients are the elements that support a state of nitrogen and caloric equilibrium over a wide range of circumstances of varying metabolism and growth. Energy needs can be increased by diseases, including a number of malignancies.

Such concepts have been postulated to apply to humans, but very rarely has their applicability been firmly documented. Many interactions in tumor-bearing hosts have an impact on the utilization of macro- or micronutrients and the utilization of nutritionally supplied, but also endogenously synthesized, biosynthetic precursors. At the broad biological level, a mutual interrelation exists among nutrition, immunity, cancer, cancer therapy, and cancer prevention. In each case, the interrelation is a dialectic one. It is therefore impossible to simplify the interactions, for example, of nutrition, immunity, and cancer, into a single cause-and-effect relation. However, it is feasible to examine the mechanisms by which a defined nutrient affects the three processes and thus to examine their interaction in causation and prevention of cancer. Data so obtained will give insight into further approaches to nutritional modulation of the malignant process in the human host.

For this symposium, zinc was selected to model the effects of a single nutrient on cellular and animal systems. At the cellular level, it is certain that this nutrient modulates cellular growth, whether normal or malignant, and the manipulation of cellular growth can be easily understood on a molecular basis. Evidence suggests that certain other nutrients also modulate and inhibit cellular transformation induced by chemical reactions or physical stress.

To a degree, this information about the interrelation of nutrition and cancer at the cellular level can also be demonstrated in the whole-animal system. The symposium clearly presented the qualitative link between nutrients and cancer and the potential factors that affect this dependency. The translation of in vitro observations of this interrelation, however, is significantly hampered by the complexity of multicellular organization. The lack of a demonstrated quantitative relation between nutrition and cancer becomes especially obvious when either higher animals or humans are the experimental models. Furthermore, solid confirmation of the interrelation in vivo at the basic level is still needed, for example for the synthetic analog of vitamin A.

Ultimately, the question has to be answered for human beings. As yet, no controlled study pinpoints a specific nutrient, or nutrients in combination, as modifying, determining, or preventing cancer development.

Shortly after the symposium, we were pleased to discover that the National Cancer Institute generated two programs to initiate studies in model systems and in humans to construct the molecular interrelations of nutrients and cancer and to evaluate the roles of nutrients in cancer prevention. We strongly believe it will be much sooner than 30 years before we meet again to discuss and analyze the results obtained from such studies of nutrition and cancer.

Editors' Foreword

"Molecular Interrelations of Nutrition and Cancer" was the topic of the 34th Annual Symposium on Fundamental Cancer Research, held in Houston March 4–6, 1981. Interest in this timely topic was great because of its emphasis on the fundamental aspects of the interrelation.

As cochairmen, we acknowledge our appreciation to the many individuals who provided guidance and advice in all matters pertaining to this symposium and this volume. The symposium organizing committee members from The University of Texas M. D. Anderson Hospital and Tumor Institute at Houston were: Benjamin Drewinko, A. Clark Griffin, Guy R. Newell, and Antonio Orengo. The External Advisory Committee was composed of John J. Burn, Frank Chytil, William J. Darby, Robert A. Good, Seoras D. Morrison, Paul M. Newberne, Michael B. Sporn, and Takashi Sugimura.

Special thanks and appreciation are given to Frances Goff and her staff for the many functions that they expertly and carefully planned and conducted. We also give thanks to Beckman Instruments, Inc., Boehringer Mannheim Biochemicals, Delman Craft Company, Forma Scientific, Laboratory Data Control, Scimetrics, Inc., and Custom LC, Inc. for providing funds for the hospitality rooms in which speakers and guests could meet and discuss mutual interests. We are especially grateful to the National Cancer Institute and the Texas Division of the American Cancer Society for their continued support. We also thank The University of Texas Health Science Center at Houston Graduate School of Biomedical Sciences for its assistance. The Department of Scientific Publications and the Department of Public Information and Education aided invaluably in all matters pertaining to the information, announcements, and publications of the symposium. Walter J. Pagel of the Department of Scientific Publications edited and compiled the manuscripts into the monograph you are about to read.

Marilyn S. Arnott
Jan van Eys
Yeu-Ming Wang

Contents

x   CONTENTS

Energy Metabolism in Tumor Cells and Nutritional Sources of Calories

Nutritional Modulation of Cell Proliferation

Contributors

Alicja Andrejczuk
Department of Neoplastic Diseases
Mt. Sinai School of Medicine
New York, New York 10029

Hadara Arkin
Department of Neoplastic Diseases
Mt. Sinai School of Medicine
New York, New York 10029

Renato Baserga
Department of Pathology and Fels Research Institute
Temple University School of Medicine
Philadelphia, Pennsylvania 19140

William F. Benedict
Division of Hematology-Oncology
Childrens Hospital of Los Angeles
Los Angeles, California 90054

Ralph J. Bernacki
Cancer Drug Center
Roswell Park Memorial Institute
Buffalo, New York 14263

John S. Bertram
Cancer Drug Center
Roswell Park Memorial Institute
Buffalo, New York 14263

Carmia Borek
Radiological Research Laboratory
Cancer Center/Institute of Cancer Research
Columbia University College of Physicians & Surgeons
New York, New York 10032

W. Robert Bruce
Department of Medical Biophysics
University of Toronto
Toronto, Ontario, Canada

Elise A. Camelio
Department of Nutrition and Food Science
Massachusetts Institute of Technology
Cambridge, Massachusetts 02139

Ivan L. Cameron
Department of Anatomy
The University of Texas Health Science Center at San Antonio
San Antonio, Texas 78284

T. Colin Campbell
Nutrition and Cancer Program Project
Division of Nutritional Sciences
Cornell University
Ithaca, New York 14853

Kenneth K. Carroll
Department of Biochemistry
University of Western Ontario
London, Ontario, Canada N6A 5C1

J. Chowaniec
School of Pathology
Middlesex Hospital Medical School
London W1P 7LD, England

Frank Chytil
Department of Biochemistry
Vanderbilt University School of Medicine
Nashville, Tennessee 37232

William J. Darby
The Nutrition Foundation, Inc.
New York, New York 10017

Martha B. Davidson
Department of Biochemistry
University of Western Ontario
London, Ontario, Canada N6A 5C1

Noorbibi K. Day
Memorial Sloan-Kettering Cancer Center
New York, New York 10021

Krystyna Domanska-Janik
Cancer Drug Center
Roswell Park Memorial Institute
Buffalo, New York 14263

Gabriel Fernandes
Memorial Sloan-Kettering Cancer Center
New York, New York 10021

John D. Fernstrom
Department of Nutrition and Food Science
Massachusetts Institute of Technology
Cambridge, Massachusetts 02139

Norbel Galanti
Department of Pathology and Fels Research Institute
Temple University School of Medicine
Philadelphia, Pennsylvania 19140

Keyou Ge
Institute of Health
Chinese Academy of Medical Sciences
Beijing, China

C. A. Gleiser
Division of Veterinary Medicine and Surgery
The University of Texas M. D. Anderson Hospital and Tumor Institute at Houston
Houston, Texas 77030

Robert A. Good
Memorial Sloan-Kettering Cancer Center
New York, New York 10021

A. Clark Griffin
The University of Texas Science Park
Smithville, Texas 78957

A. Harvey
School of Pathology
Middlesex Hospital Medical School
London W1P 7LD, England

R. M. Hicks
School of Pathology
Middlesex Hospital Medical School
London W1P 7LD, England

Barbara W. Highison
United States Department of Agriculture
Science and Education Administration
Grand Forks Human Nutrition Research Center
Grand Forks, North Dakota 58202

James F. Holland
Department of Neoplastic Diseases
Mt. Sinai School of Medicine
New York, New York 10029

S. K. Howell
Department of Pediatrics
The University of Texas M. D. Anderson Hospital and Tumor Institute at Houston
Houston, Texas 77030

Gerald Jonak
Department of Pathology and Fels Research Institute
Temple University School of Medicine
Philadelphia, Pennsylvania 19140

Peter A. Jones
Division of Hematology-Oncology
Childrens Hospital of Los Angeles
Los Angeles, California 90054

Shoji Kawasaki
Department of Pathology and Fels Research Institute
Temple University School of Medicine
Philadelphia, Pennsylvania 19140

William R. Kidwell
Laboratory of Pathophysiology
National Cancer Institute
Bethesda, Maryland 20205

J. C. Kimball
Department of Pediatrics
The University of Texas M. D. Anderson Hospital and Tumor Institute at Houston
Houston, Texas 77030

Richard A. Knazek
Laboratory of Pathophysiology
National Cancer Institute
Bethesda, Maryland 20205

Tim R. Kramer
United States Department of Agriculture
Science and Education Administration
Grand Forks Human Nutrition Research Center
Grand Forks, North Dakota 58202

David Kritchevsky
The Wistar Institute of Anatomy and Biology
Philadelphia, Pennsylvania 19104

David H. Lawson
Division of Hematology and Oncology
Emory University School of Medicine
Atlanta, Georgia 30322

Wendell W. Leavitt
The Worcester Foundation for Experimental Biology
Shrewsbury, Massachusetts 01545

Mortimer B. Lipsett
Clinical Center
National Institutes of Health
Bethesda, Maryland 20205

Ilona Losonczy
Laboratory of Pathophysiology
National Cancer Institute
Bethesda, Maryland 20205

E. D. Massey
School of Pathology
Middlesex Hospital Medical School
London W1P 7LD, England

Taijiro Matsushima
Department of Molecular Oncology
Institute of Medical Science
University of Tokyo
Tokyo 108, Japan

Robert G. McConnell
Department of Nutrition and Food Science
Massachusetts Institute of Technology
Cambridge, Massachusetts 02139

Wallace L. McKeehan
W. Alton Jones Cell Science Center
Lake Placid, New York 12946

Theodore E. McNair
Department of Microbiology
University of Illinois
Urbana, Illinois 61801

Lawrence J. Mordan
Cancer Drug Center
Roswell Park Memorial Institute
Buffalo, New York 14263

Seoras D. Morrison
Laboratory of Pathophysiology
National Cancer Institute
Bethesda, Maryland 20205

Daniel W. Nixon
Division of Hematology and Oncology
Emory University School of Medicine
Atlanta, Georgia 30322

Takao Ohnuma
Department of Neoplastic Diseases
Mt. Sinai School of Medicine
New York, New York 10029

David E. Ong
Department of Biochemistry
Vanderbilt University School of Medicine
Nashville, Tennessee 37232

George M. Padilla
Department of Physiology
Duke University Medical Center
Durham, North Carolina 27710

John Roboz
Department of Neoplastic Diseases
Mt. Sinai School of Medicine
New York, New York 10029

Adrianne E. Rogers
Department of Nutrition and Food Science
Massachusetts Institute of Technology
Cambridge, Massachusetts 02139

Daniel Rudman
Clinical Research Facility
Department of Medicine
Emory University School of Medicine
Atlanta, Georgia 30322

Donald W. Salter
Department of Microbiology
University of Illinois
Urbana, Illinois 61801

J. Sato
Department of Pediatrics
The University of Texas M. D. Anderson Hospital and Tumor Institute at Houston
Houston, Texas 77030

Kenneth Soprano
Department of Pathology and Fels Research Institute
Temple University School of Medicine
Philadelphia, Pennsylvania 19140

T. P. Stein
Surgical Research Laboratories
Graduate Hospital
University of Pennsylvania
Philadelphia, Pennsylvania 19146

James J. Stragand
Department of Laboratory Medicine
The University of Texas M. D. Anderson
* Hospital and Tumor Institute at Hous-*
* ton*
Houston, Texas 77030

Takashi Sugimura
National Cancer Center Research Institute
Tokyo, Japan

Isao Takahashi
Department of Neoplastic Diseases
Mt. Sinai School of Medicine
New York, New York 10029

C. C. Tsai
Division of Veterinary Medicine and Sur-
* gery*
The University of Texas M. D. Anderson
* Hospital and Tumor Institute at Hous-*
* ton*
Houston, Texas 77030

Yoshihiro Tsutsui
Department of Pathology and Fels Re-
* search Institute*
Temple University School of Medicine
Philadelphia, Pennsylvania 19140

J. A. Turton
School of Pathology
Middlesex Hospital Medical School
London W1P 7LD, England

Jan van Eys
Department of Pediatrics
The University of Texas M. D. Anderson
* Hospital and Tumor Institute at Hous-*
* ton*
Houston, Texas 77030

Barbara K. Vonderhaar
Laboratory of Pathophysiology
National Cancer Institute
Bethesda, Maryland 20205

Y.-M. Wang
Department of Pediatrics
The University of Texas M. D. Anderson
* Hospital and Tumor Institute at Hous-*
* ton*
Houston, Texas 77030

Lee W. Wattenberg
Department of Laboratory Medicine and
* Pathology*
University of Minnesota Medical School
Minneapolis, Minnesota 55455

George Weber
Laboratory for Experimental Oncology
Indiana University School of Medicine
Indianapolis, Indiana 46223

Michael J. Weber
Department of Microbiology
University of Illinois
Urbana, Illinois 61801

Sidney Weinhouse
Fels Research Institute
Temple University School of Medicine
Philadelphia, Pennsylvania 19140

William C. Wetsel
Department of Nutrition and Food Science
Massachusetts Institute of Technology
Cambridge, Massachusetts 02139

Soon O. Yang
Department of Nutrition and Food Science
Massachusetts Institute of Technology
Cambridge, Massachusetts 02139

Bertner Memorial Award Lecture

Molecular Interrelations of Nutrition and Cancer,
edited by M. S. Arnott, J. van Eys, and Y.-M. Wang.
Raven Press, New York © 1982.

The Ernst W. Bertner Memorial Award Lecture: Tumor Initiators and Promoters Associated with Ordinary Foods

Takashi Sugimura

National Cancer Center Research Institute, Tsukiji 5-chome, Chuo-ku, Tokyo 104, Japan

The incidence of cancer of various organs differs greatly from country to country (Doll 1977, Segi and Kurihara 1962, Wynder and Gori 1977). Presently, the predominant form of cancer of the alimentary tract in Western countries is that of the large intestine, but in Japan, alimentary tract cancer still occurs most frequently in the stomach. Among immigrants from Japan to the United States, the incidence of stomach cancer is declining, while cases of cancer of the large intestine are increasing (Hirohata 1980). This is an example of how various environments influence, in different ways, the incidence of cancer in different organs.

Environments contain numerous factors possibly related to carcinogenesis. To a certain extent, human exposure to "carcinogens" is attributable to smoking, inhalation of air pollutants, drinking water contaminated with carcinogens, and contact with other "carcinogens" in the environment. However, the source of most of our contact with carcinogens is probably food. Carcinogenic factors responsible for the development of human cancer are sometimes clearly defined and limited, as in cases of occupational cancer and cancer due to accidental exposure to particular carcinogens. However, the causes of the majority of cancer cases remain ill defined and may lie in any of an unlimited number of factors. In such cases, although the number of factors involved may be large, the amount of each factor is actually very small. The effect of integrating these numerous factors results in the eventual development of the many kinds of cancer that commonly occur in humans.

The carcinogenic process comprises two steps, initiation and promotion, as revealed by Berenblum (1941). Initiation takes place when a change, such as mutation, occurs in chromosomal DNA. The changes brought about by this process persist for a long time. Many typical carcinogens are harmful to DNA, and mutagenic toward microbes and in vitro cultured mammalian cells, and they demonstrate an ability to produce chromosome aberrations, sistir chromatid exchanges, and unscheduled DNA synthesis in mammalian cells. These events are related to alterations of the primary structure of DNA, constituting the initiation of carcinogenesis, although the actual molecular mechanism involved is not clearly understood. What gene or genes in the host-cell genome are involved if somatic mutation is necessary for initiation? Are other, more drastic changes in chromosomal structure, such as transpositions and rearrangements of genes, more important than simple gene mutation (Cairns 1981)? These questions still remain to be answered. In practical terms, we are nevertheless able to detect carcinogenic factors in our environment that may cause DNA damage and mutation. This is why we continue to search for new mutagens in foods as possible carcinogens.

The second step in the carcinogenic process is promotion. Cancer cells cannot be developed from initiated cells alone; a promotion step, associated with cell multiplication, is required. Again, the actual molecular mechanisms of tumor promotion are not sufficiently understood, although various biological effects of promoters have been intensively investigated (Boutwell 1977, Hecker 1978, Weinstein et al. 1978).

Promoters include a variety of chemical compounds. The most common tumor promoter is 12-O-tetradecanoylphorbol-13-acetate (TPA), which can be isolated from croton oil found in the seeds of the croton plant (Hecker 1967, Van Duuren 1969). TPA is a rather specific promoter, which can bind with a specific receptor on a cell surface (Driedger and Blumberg 1980, Lee and Weinstein 1980). However, little is presently known about the mechanisms of promoter actions in commonly occurring forms of human cancers. Only evidence in experimental animals shows that saccharin is a promoter in urinary bladder carcinogenesis (Hicks et al. 1975), bile acid derivatives in colon carcinogenesis (Narisawa et al. 1974), and phenobarbital in hepatocarcinogenesis (Peraino et al. 1971). Tumor promoters present in ordinary foods should be more intensively studied.

Furthermore, it is important to understand various modulating factors in the carcinogenic process in order to understand the role played by food in the development of human cancer. The composition of foods has a great influence on the formation of carcinogens in the human body and on the metabolic conversion of carcinogens to their reactive form in the human body. Vitamin C inhibits the formation of nitrosamines (Bruce et al. 1979), and plant-origin flavonoids in foods may interfere with the metabolism of carcinogens in vivo (Nagase et al. 1964, Wattenberg et al. 1970). Modulation in the tumor-promotion step appears to be important in terms of preventing cancer as well. Substances related to vitamin A-retinoic acid, which are known to block tumor promotion, seem crucially important (Bollag 1971, Sporn et al. 1976). The fact that the incidence of cancer declines in those people who quit smoking should also be kept in mind. Cigarette tar is known to contain tumor promoters (Bock et al. 1971).

Less obvious factors in our environment have to be considered also. It is well documented that feeding human subjects charred beef induces P-450 cytochromes in the subjects' lymphoblasts (Conney et al. 1977). The composition of fatty acids in body lipid may be altered by that in food lipid. This alteration may change the properties of the cell surface, including those of the hormonal receptor or even those of the receptor for tumor promoters (Weinstein et al. 1980). Thus, hormonal conditions produced by a high calorie intake may be crucial for the development of cancer in endocrine-related organs.

A discussion of the ways in which molecular mechanisms relate to the mutually related topics of food, nutrition, and cancer induction would cover many important areas. However, this chapter will concentrate on recently discovered heterocyclic amines from pyrolysis products of amino acids, proteins, and proteinaceous foods. All were highly mutagenic and some have been proved to be carcinogenic in long-term animal tests. A new class of tumor promoter, indole alkaloid, also will be introduced in this chapter. This class includes teleocidin from *Streptomyces* and lyngbyatoxin from *Lyngbya,* a kind of seaweed. It is important to bear in mind the possibility that humans ingest TPA and indole alkaloid-type tumor promoters.

A SERIES OF NEW MUTAGENS PRODUCED DURING COOKING

The presence of a typical mutagen, benzo[a]pyrene, in cooked food was reported many years ago. Researchers have described aflatoxin contamination in some foods (Hsieh et al. 1977, Peers and Linsell 1973), and the presence of nitrosamines in foods processed in various ways has also been well documented (Kawabata et al. 1978, Preussmann et al. 1979, Tannenbaum et al. 1974). For a long time, the search for new carcinogens in food was hindered by the fact that animal tests for carcinogenicity require many animals and years to obtain clearly positive or negative results. Since most foods contain only a very limited amount of unknown carcinogens, experiments in which human food is given to animals may simply fail to prove the presence or absence of new carcinogens. To overcome this methodological stumbling block, we decided to use a mutation test to detect tumor initiators, that is, mutagens acting as carcinogens. The most convenient method for this purpose was the Ames method (Ames et al. 1975), which requires the use of *Salmonella typhimurium* and an S9 mix obtained from the livers of rats treated with polychlorinated biphenyls. We modified the Ames method slightly by adding a preincubation step (Sugimura and Nagao 1980). This made the Ames method more sensitive to some types of mutagens.

First, we observed that broiled sardines and broiled beef contained strong mutagenic potency to *Salmonella typhimurium* TA98 and TA100 (Sugimura et al. 1977b). Mutagenic activity was more clearly demonstrated with the metabolic activation system of S9 mix. The formation of mutagens under ordinary cooking conditions increased with the length of time required for cooking, as shown in Figures 1 and 2. Cooking sun-dried sardines for 5 to 7 minutes and hamburger 10 to 15 minutes yielded the best taste.

Sardines and beef consist mainly of proteins. Other foods may contain lipids and carbohydrates as major components. Sometimes nucleic acids also comprise a fairly large part of the food components. The charring of these components yielded mutagens, as shown in Table 1. Potent mutagenic activity was mainly

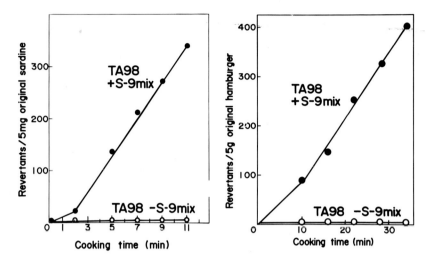

FIG. 1. Mutagenicity of broiled sardines at various cooking times.

FIG. 2. Mutagenicity of hamburger at various cooking times.

produced by pyrolyzing protein. The pyrolyzing of starch yielded weak direct-acting mutagen(s) toward *Salmonella typhimurium* TA100.

Since protein yielded the most potent mutagenic activity upon its pyrolysis, each amino acid and its related compounds were pyrolyzed. It was found that tryptophan, glutamic acid, creatine, creatinine, and others yielded mutagens (Nagao et al. 1977b). From tryptophan pyrolysate, two crystalline substances, 3-amino-1,4-dimethyl-5H-pyrido[4,3-b]indole (Trp-P-1) and 3-amino-1-methyl-5H-pyrido[4,3-b]indole (Trp-P-2), were isolated (Kosuge et al. 1978, Sugimura et al. 1977a). Their structures were determined by X-ray crystallography. Trp-P-1 and Trp-P-2 were chemically synthesized (Sugimura et al. 1980). Similarly, from glutamic acid pyrolysate, 2-amino-6-methyldipyrido[1,2-a:3′,2′-d]imidazole (Glu-P-1) and 2-aminodipyrido[1,2-a:3′,2′-d]imidazole (Glu-P-2) were isolated (Yamamoto et al. 1978). Their structures were determined by X-ray crystallography, and organic synthesis was successful.

2-Amino-5-phenylpyridine (Phe-P-1) (Sugimura et al. 1977a) and 3,4-cyclopentenopyrido[3,2-a]carbazole (Lys-P-1) (Wakabayashi et al. 1978) were isolated from pyrolysates of phenylalanine and lysine, respectively, for the first time. In pyrolysates of soybean globulin, the presence of 2-amino-9H-pyrido[2,3-b]indole (AαC) and 2-amino-3-methyl-9H-pyrido[2,3-b]indole (MeAαC) was demonstrated (Yoshida et al. 1978). From broiled sardines, very potent mutagens, 2-amino-3-methylimidazo[4,5-f]quinoline (IQ) (Kasai et al. 1980a,1980c) and 2-amino-3,4-dimethylimidazo[4,5-f]quinoline (MeIQ) (Kasai et al. 1980b,1980c), were isolated for the first time. Their structures were determined by data obtained with the 270 MHz ^{1}H-NMR spectrum, low- and high-resolution mass spectra, and chemical synthesis. The specific mutagenic activities of IQ and MeIQ were

TABLE 1. *Mutagenic activities of smoke condensates obtained by pyrolysis of biomacromolecules* *

| | TA100 | | TA98 | |
	+S9 mix	−S9 mix	+S9 mix	−S9 mix
Lysozyme	2319†	0	8311	0
Histone	1311	0	5012	0
DNA	170	0	278	0
RNA	0	0	83	0
Starch	70	338	0	0
Vegetable oil	85	0	0	0

* Adapted from Nagao et al. (1977a) and Sugimura et al. (1977b).
† Number of revertant colonies per milligram smoke condensate per plate.

highest among these heterocyclic amines, as shown in Table 2. More recently, 2-amino-3,8-dimethylimidazo[4,5-*f*]quinoxaline (MeIQx) was isolated from fried beef and identified for the first time (Kasai et al. 1981). IQ, MeIQ, and MeIQx were organic-chemically synthesized (Kasai et al. 1980a,1980b, 1981).

The specific mutagenic activities of all these mutagens (that is, those isolated from pyrolysates of amino acids and proteins, and from charred parts of proteinaceous foods) are given in Table 2, along with the full and abbreviated names and structure of each mutagen, its first source of isolation, and examples of other materials in which it is present. The range of variation in the specific mutagenic activities of these compounds was an order of magnitude 4. The specific mutagenic activity of MeIQ was 10,000 times greater than that of Phe-P-1.

The specific mutagenic activities of these compounds toward *Salmonella typhimurium* TA100 are given in Table 3, along with those of typical carcinogens, including aflatoxin B_1, 4-nitroquinoline 1-oxide, AF-2, dimethylnitrosamine, and *N*-methyl-*N'*-nitro-*N*-nitrosoguanidine. The specific mutagenic activities of some of these new compounds are higher than or comparable to those of aflatoxin B_1, 4-nitroquinoline 1-oxide, and AF-2. Whether S9 mix was needed and the optimum volume of S9 in the assay system depended on the chemicals being tested. The data for figures given in Tables 2 and 3 were obtained in our laboratory under the optimum conditions for each chemical.

The carcinogenicities of these new potent mutagens are being examined in long-term in vivo animal experiments. We have finished all histological examinations in the course of experiments in which Trp-P-1 and Trp-P-2 were fed to mice. Trp-P-1 and Trp-P-2 were found to be fairly stable during the preparation and storage of the pellet diet. They were also demonstrated to be clearly hepatocarcinogenic in mice, as shown in Table 4 (Matsukura et al. 1981). In a reversal of the tendency that holds true for most hepatocarcinogens, female animals proved to be more susceptible than males. Some hepatomas also metastasized to the lungs. The carcinogenic potentials of Trp-P-1 and Trp-P-2 were far less

TABLE 2. *Mutagens isolated from pyrolysates*

Full name (Abbreviation)	Structure	Source of isolation	Spec. Mut. Act. Revertants/μg TA98, +S9 mix	Present in
2-Amino-3,4-dimethyl-imidazo[4,5-*f*]quinoline (MeIQ)		Broiled sardine (Kasai et al. 1980b,c)	661,000	
2-Amino-3-methylimidazo-[4,5-*f*]quinoline (IQ)		Broiled sardine (Kasai et al. 1980a,c)	433,000	Fried beef (K. Wakabayashi, unpublished observation), heated beef extract (Spingarn et al. 1980)
2-Amino-3,8-dimethyl-imidazo [4,5-*f*]quinoxaline (MeIQx)		Fried beef (Kasai et al. 1981)	145,000	
3-Amino-1-methyl-5*H*-pyrido[4,3-*b*]indole (Trp-P-2)		Tryptophan pyroly-sate (Sugimura et al. 1977a)	104,000	Broiled sardine (Yamaizumi et al. 1980)
2-Amino-6-methyldipyrido-[1,2-*a*:3′,2′-*d*]imidazole (Glu-P-1)		Glutamic acid pyrolysate (Yama-moto et al. 1978)	49,000	
3-Amino-1,4-dimethyl-5*H*-pyrido[4,3-*b*]indole (Trp-P-1)		Tryptophan pyroly-sate (Sugimura et al. 1977a)	39,000	Broiled sardine (Yamaizumi et al. 1980), broiled beef (Yamaguchi et al. 1980b)
2-Aminodipyrido[1,2-*a*:3′,2′-*d*]imidazole (Glu-P-2)		Glutamic acid pyrolysate (Yama-moto et al. 1978)	1,900	Broiled dried-cuttlefish (Yamaguchi et al. 1980a)

Compound	Structure	Source		Occurrence
2-Amino-9*H*-pyrido[2,3-*b*]indole (AαC)		Soybean globulin pyrolysate (Yoshida et al. 1978)	300	Cigarette smoke (Yoshida and Matsumoto 1980, S. Sato, unpublished observation)
2-Amino-3-methyl-9*H*-pyrido[2,3-*b*]indole (MeAαC)		Soybean globulin pyrolysate (Yoshida et al. 1978)	200	Cigarette smoke (Yoshida and Matsumoto 1980, S. Sato, unpublished observation)
3,4-Cyclopentenopyrido[3,2-*a*]carbazole (Lys-P-1)		Lysine pyrolysate (Wakabayashi et al. 1978)	86	
2-Amino-5-phenylpyridine (Phe-P-1)		Phenylalanine pyrolysate (Sugimura et al. 1977a)	41	

TABLE 3. *Specific mutagenic activity of new mutagens and typical carcinogens toward* Salmonella typhimurium *TA100* *

	Revertants/μg
AF-2†	42,000
MeIQ‡	30,000
Aflatoxin B_1‡	28,000
MeIQ‡	14,000
4NQO†	9,900
IQ‡	7,000
Glu-P-1ƒ	3,200
Trp-P-2‡	1,800
Trp-P-1‡	1,700
Glu-P-2ƒ	1,200
MNNG†	870
B[a]P‡	660
MeAαC‖	120
Lys-P-1‖	99
Phe-P-1‖	23
AαC‖	20
DMN‖	0.23
DEN‖	0.15

* Adapted from Sugimura (1979) and Sugimura et al. (1980).
† Without S9 mix.
‡ 10 μl S9/plate.
ƒ 30 μl S9/plate.
‖ 150 μl S9/plate.
4NQO: 4-nitroquinoline 1-oxide; AF-2: 2-(2-furyl)-3-(5-nitro-2-furyl)acrylamide; DEN: diethylnitrosamine; DMN: dimethyl-nitrosamine; MNNG: *N*-methyl-*N'*-nitro-*N*-nitrosoguanidine.

than had been expected on the basis of their mutagenic potentials. This difference—between the expected and demonstrated carcinogenic potentials—may be partly due to the failure to take into account both the balance between activating and inactivating metabolic systems in vitro and the presence of various other inactivating mechanisms in vivo.

Trp-P-1, Trp-P-2, and Glu-P-1 were observed to be active in in vitro transformation of Syrian golden hamster cells (Takayama et al. 1977, 1979). Since Trp-P-1 and Trp-P-2 were the mutagens most intensively studied, information obtained about these two substances is given below.

Trp-P-1 and Trp-P-2 were activated into hydroxyamino derivatives by cytochrome P-448 (purified from the liver of rats treated with polychlorinated biphenyls or 3-methylcholanthrene), but not by P-450 (purified from the liver of rats treated with polychlorinated biphenyls or sodium phenobarbital) (Ishii et al. 1980). The *N*-hydroxyamino derivative of Trp-P-2 was isolated by high-performance liquid chromotography and showed direct-acting mutagenicity to-

TABLE 4. *Numbers of CDF₁ mice with hepatic tumors induced by Trp-P-1 and Trp-P-2**

Treatment	Sex	Effective no.	Hepato-cellular adenoma	Hepato-cellular carcinoma	Heman-gioma	Total (%)
Trp-P-1	Male	24	1	4	0	5 (21)
(0.02%)	Female	26	2	14	0	16 (62)
Trp-P-2	Male	25	1	3	0	4 (16)
(0.02%)	Female	24	0	22(2†)	0	22 (92)
Control	Male	25	0	0	1	1 (4)
	Female	24	0	0	0	0 (0)

* Adapted from Matsukura et al. (1981).
† Two mice had metastasis to the lung.

wards *Salmonella typhimurium* TA98 (Yamazoe et al. 1980). The *N*-hydroxy-amino derivative may be further acylated in bacterial cells to produce an ultimate reactant with DNA. Chemically synthesized acyl *N*-hydroxyamino compound reacted most strongly with DNA in vitro (Hashimoto et al. 1980b). The structure of one of the adducts of Trp-P-2 with a DNA base was determined to be 3-(C⁸-guanyl)amino-1-methyl-5*H*-pyrido[4,3-*b*]indole (Hashimoto et al. 1979). Similarly, the structure of one of the adducts of Glu-P-1 with a DNA base, namely, 2-(C⁸-guanyl)amino-6-methyldipyrido[1,2-*a*:3',2'-*d*]imidazole, was elucidated (Hashimoto et al. 1980a). The structures are shown in Figure 3.

Quantitative determination is very important for evaluating the hazards posed to humans by these mutagens. A method for quantifying these mutagens in food has not been standardized yet. As methods of partial purification, extraction with methanol or 1 N HC1, partition between alkaline water and dichlorometh-ane, silica gel column chromatography, and Sephadex LH-20 column chromatog-raphy were useful. Thin-layer chromatography and high-performance liquid chromotography were extremely effective means of further purification. Finally, gas chromatography/mass spectrography with multiple ion detection was and is being used for quantification of these new mutagens. A deuterium dilution technique using [²H₃]CH₃ derivatives as a standard sample made the procedure

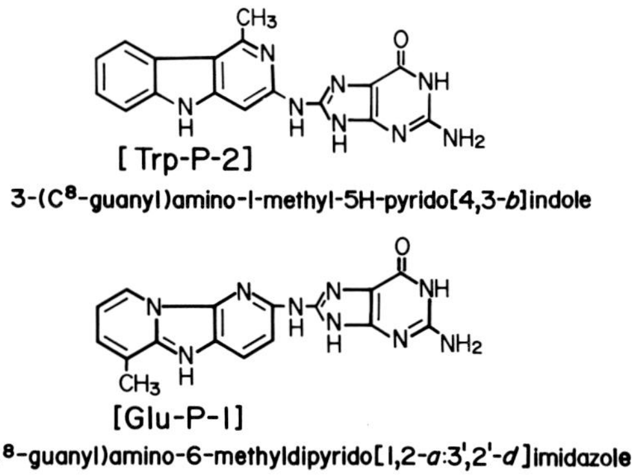

[Trp-P-2]

3-(C⁸-guanyl)amino-I-methyl-5H-pyrido[4,3-*b*]indole

[Glu-P-I]

2-(C⁸-guanyl)amino-6-methyldipyrido[I,2-*a*:3',2'-*d*]imidazole

FIG. 3. The structures of the adducts of Trp-P-2 and Glu-P-1 with a DNA base.

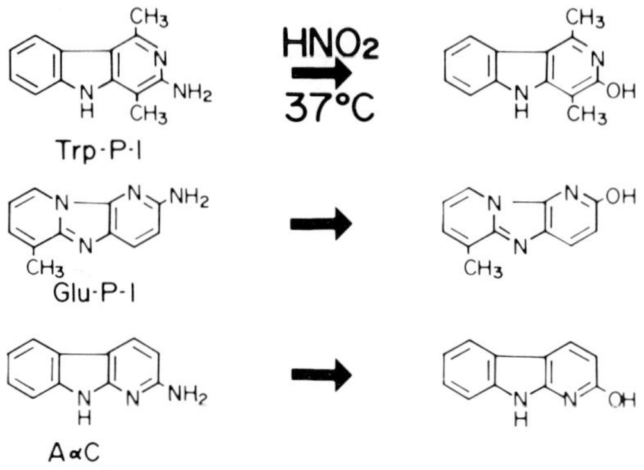

FIG. 4. Conversion of mutagens to nonmutagenic hydroxy compounds by nitrite.

simpler and more reproducible. Broiled sardines were found to contain 13.3 ng Trp-P-1, 13.1 ng Trp-P-2 (Yamaizumi et al. 1980), 158 ng IQ, and 72 ng MeIQ per gram (Z. Yamaizumi, unpublished observation). Broiled cuttlefish was found to contain 280 ng Glu-P-2 per gram of original material (Yamaguchi et al. 1980a). The IQ content of broiled beef accounts for only 10% of the total mutagenic activity in broiled beef (K. Wakabayashi, unpublished observation).

Information available on the actual content of these new mutagens indicates that their values might not be sufficiently high to warrant calling each component a risky substance for humans. Until the long-term in vivo animal experiments, using all these new mutagens on mice, rats, and hamsters, are finished, neither a positive nor a negative conclusion should be ventured.

These heterocyclic amines had interesting properties: they were quickly inactivated by a concentration of nitrite that can also be found in humans, under conditions of weak acidity (Tsuda et al. 1980). Deamination, as this reaction is known, produces a hydroxy compound, as shown in Figure 4. Peroxidase is known to activate some carcinogens to form a readily reactive form with DNA (Bartsch and Hecker 1971, Reigh et al. 1978). In the case of these heterocyclic amines, peroxidase (myeloperoxidase, lactoperoxidase, and horseradish peroxidase) and hydrogen peroxide inactivated these mutagens (Yamada et al. 1979). It is known that peroxidase is also present in intestinal epithelium. Furthermore, chlorinated water inactivated some heterocyclic amines very quickly (M. Tsuda, unpublished observation). Trp-P-2 completely lost its mutagenicity after incubation with tap water, but not after incubation with well water or distilled water.

NEW TUMOR PROMOTERS IN FOODS

The second phase of the carcinogenic process is the promotion step. 12-O-Tetradecanoylphorbol-13-acetate (TPA) was originally isolated from croton oil (Hecker 1967, Van Duuren 1969). Since then, detection of TPA in honey collected by bees has also been reported (E. Hecker, personal communication,

Upadhyay et al. 1980). Until now, TPA and its related diterpenes have been the only group of compounds capable of stimulating tumor promotion in mouse skin, in a two-step carcinogenesis experiment.

A connection between TPA-type tumor promoters and human cancer is suggested by the high incidence of nasopharyngeal cancer in an area of southern China where *Croton* plants grow (T. Hirayama and Y. Ito, in preparation). Croton oil, used in making a palm ointment to be applied to the nasal cavity, also may contribute to the incidence of nasopharyngeal cancer. Another case that points to this connection is that of the Curacao Islanders in the Caribbean (Weber and Hecker 1978). A high incidence of esophageal cancer was reported for this population, who were heavy drinkers of a peculiar, local tea. It has been suggested that the tea leaves contained a diterpene-type tumor promoter (Weber and Hecker 1978).

However, in spite of these findings, as well as the positive results obtained from experiments with mice and TPA-type tumor promoters, it has not yet been conclusively proved that exposure of humans to TPA-type tumor promoters necessarily carries serious consequences.

Currently, many experiments are being conducted to identify tumor promoters. Recently, the presence of a promoter substance in pickles from Linxian county in northern China has been reported (Cheng et al. 1980).

We have been looking for new tumor promoters in our environment, especially in our foods. During an examination of various spices and other foods, we had an opportunity to look at a compound, dihydroteleocidin B, which had been reported to cause skin irritation. Dihydroteleocidin B is a hydrogenated product of teleocidin, isolated from *Streptomyces* (Takashima and Sakai 1960). Teleocidin is an indole alkaloid and has a macrolide-type ring with a peptide bond, as shown in Figure 5.

One method we employed to search for new tumor promoters was to paint test substances on mouse skin and check them for induction of ornithine decarboxylase (ODC) activity. TPA induced the maximum value of ODC activity after 4 hours. Dihydroteleocidin B and teleocidin also induced the maximum value of ODC activity 4 hours after being applied to skin. The dose of dihydrotel-

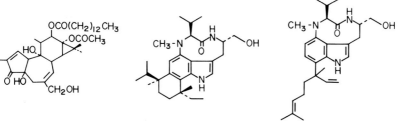

TPA   **Dihydroteleocidin B**   **Lyngbyatoxin A**

FIG. 5. The structures of TPA, dihydroteleocidin B, and lyngbyatoxin A.

eocidin B required to induce ODC was comparable to that of TPA (Fujiki et al. 1979).

In vivo long-term animal experiments on mouse skin were conducted with TPA and dihydroteleocidin B (Fujiki et al. 1981, Sugimura et al. 1981). A limited amount of 7,12-dimethylbenz[a]anthracene was administered followed by applications of TPA and dihydroteleocidin B. The results are given in Figure 6. It is evident that dihydroteleocidin B has a tumor-promoting activity in this system comparable to that of TPA. Almost all the biological activities demonstrated by TPA were demonstrated also by dihydroteleocidin B, as summarized in Table 5. It should be mentioned, too, that the concentration necessary to induce these biological activities was almost the same in both TPA and dihydroteleocidin B.

Lyngbya, a seaweed, produces lyngbyatoxin, which has a structure quite similar to that of teleocidin. Lyngbyatoxin induced ODC activity on mouse skin (Fujiki et al. 1981). It also demonstrated biological activity quite similar to that of TPA and teleocidin. In vivo long-term animal experiments are now being conducted. *Lyngbya,* which grows in Hawaii and Okinawa, and probably in many other tropical areas as well, has been claimed to contaminate the edible seaweed in a certain tropical area (R. E. Moore, personal communication). Since no solid evidence of the presence of this new class of tumor promoter in our food is available now, more intensive research into this possibility is necessary.

A method for discovering new promoters in food has not yet been fully established and standardized, and much greater efforts need to be made. Although we have found many initiators in foods, our progress has reached a bottleneck due to the lack of good methods, up to now, of identifying promoters in foods. The promoters that have been identified, such as those in *Streptomyces* fungi

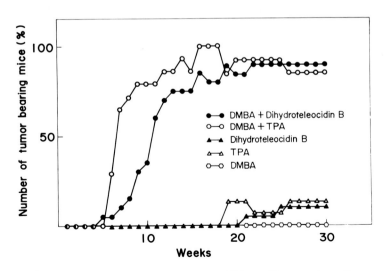

FIG. 6. Effects of dihydroteleocidin B and TPA on skin tumor formation.

TABLE 5. *TPA and dihydroteleocidin B have similar effects*

In Vivo Effect
1. In vivo ODC induction (Fujiki et al. 1979).
2. Retinoid inhibition of ODC induction (Fujiki et al. 1979).
3. Irritation of mouse ear test (Fujiki et al. 1979).
4. Induction of dark keratinocytes in mouse skin (M. Arai, unpublished observation).
5. Induction of hyperplasia and hyperkeratosis in mouse skin (Fujiki et al. 1981).
6. Tumor promotion in two-step carcinogenesis of mouse skin (Fujiki et al. 1981, Sugimura et al. 1981).

Membrane Effect
1. Cell adhesion of HL-60 cells (Fujiki et al. 1979).
2. Aggregation of NL-3 cells (Hoshino et al. 1980).
3. Increase in 2-deoxyglucose uptake (Umezawa et al. 1981).
4. Release of arachidonic acid (Umezawa et al. 1981).
5. Formation of prostaglandins (Umezawa et al. 1981, Sakamoto et al. 1981).
6. Release of choline (Sakamoto et al. 1981).
7. Inhibition of phorboid-receptor binding (Umezawa et al. 1981).
8. Inhibition of epidermal growth factor binding (Umezawa et al. 1981).
9. Production of superoxide anion radical (O_2^-) in human polymorphonuclear leukocytes (Goldstein et al. 1981).
10. Adaptation to allosteric site in phospholipase A_2 (J. R. Smythies, in preparation).

Differentiation Inhibition or Induction
1. Inhibition of induced differentiation (hemoglobin synthesis) in Friend erythroblastic leukemic cells (Fujiki et al. 1979).
2. Inhibition of induced melanogenesis in B16 melanoma cells (T. Sekiguchi, unpublished observation).
3. Inhibition of induced myogenesis in human myoblasts (I. B. Weinstein, personal communication).
4. Induction of differentiation of HL-60 cells (Nakayasu et al. 1981).
5. Amelanotic effect and morphological change of reconstituted cells (T. Sekiguchi unpublished observation).
6. Coincidence with TPA resistance in Friend erythroblastic leukemic cells (P. A. Marks, personal communication).

Transformation, Adenovirus and EB Virus
1. Increase in transformed foci after treatment with chemical carcinogen (Kakunaga et al. 1981).
2. Enhancement of colony formation of adenovirus-infected lymphocytes (I. B. Weinstein, personal communication).
3. Enhancement of colony formation of EBV-infected cord blood lymphocytes (Hoshino et al. 1981).
4. Enhancement of early antigen and viral capsid antigen production (Yamamoto 1981).

Others
1. Abnormal movements of nematode *(Caenorhabditis elegans)* (Y. Tabuse, in preparation).
2. Coincidence with TPA-resistant mutants of nematode *(C. elegans)* (Y. Tabuse, in preparation.)

and *Lyngbya* blue-green algae, belong to a class of plants that does not constitute human food. It is now necessary to reexamine contamination caused by typical promoters such as TPA and teleocidin in ordinary foods. Also, it is now more important than ever to intensify the search for other classes of tumor promoters.

COMPLEXITY OF PROBLEMS

Theoretical and practical means for identifying new tumor initiators in food are now available. In addition to hitherto known initiators, such as those found in food additives, pesticide residues, aromatic hydrocarbons, mycotoxins including aflatoxin B_1, and nitrosamines, we are now able to identify new potent heterocyclic amines produced by pyrolysis of protein and amino acids, and will continue to do so. New mycotoxins with initiating activities are also found. We will also be able to identify new nitrosamines, such as *N*-3-methylbutyl-*N*-1-methylacetonylnitrosamine found in moldy corn bread from Linxian county, where the incidence of esophageal cancer is high (Li et al. 1980).

We were able to obtain information on the carcinogenicity of these new mutagens, including the quantity of mutagenic substances in the local foods. However, in their daily lives, human beings are not exposed to a sole chemical, but to an integrated complex of many initiators. Although one might expect that the biological effectiveness of various chemicals could be determined by adding numerically the biological effectiveness for each chemical, the circumstances of the coexistence of these various chemicals may result in an actual biological effectiveness that is higher or lower than the sum of these numbers. It must be confessed that it is hard, at this moment, to evaluate the actual degree of risk of many tumor initiators found in human food for the development of cancer in humans.

A great deal of evidence confusing the relation of carcinogenicity to mutagenicity has been produced by investigations of flavonoids. Many flavonoids, especially quercetin and kaempferol, were proved to be mutagenic to *Salmonella typhimurium* TA98 and TA100 (Bjeldanes and Chang 1977, Brown et al. 1977, Sugimura et al. 1977c). Pamukcu et al. (1980) obtained positive carcinogenic results in experiments in which they fed quercetin to rats. Almost 80% of the rats developed either ileocecal tumors or urinary bladder tumors, both being malignant. On the other hand, experiments carried out by Japanese scientists, under the support of the Ministry of Health and Welfare, indicated almost no carcinogenicity in quercetin and its glycoside, rutin, after these had been fed to rats (Hirono et al. 1981), hamsters (K. Morino, in preparation), and mice (Saito et al. 1980, Sugimura 1979). The concentrations of quercetin used by Japanese scientists were much higher than that used by Pamukcu et al. (1980) and the durations of exposure were much longer. Although it is possible that this discrepancy is due to the particular strain of rats used by Pamukcu et al. (1980), a convincing explanation has still not been given.

It is crucially important to determine whether or not flavonoids are carcinogenic for two reasons: because quercetin is contained in many edible fruits and vegetables and because such a determination is necessary in order to assess the effectiveness of the microbial mutation test and other short-term tests for screening carcinogenic substances. For example, a can of orange juice contains about 50 mg of quercetin derivatives (Brown 1980). Is this amount significantly hazardous for humans? It has been proved that the mutagen found in sumac is kaempferol (Seino et al. 1978), those found in Japanese pickles are quercetin and isorhamnetin (Takahashi et al. 1979), that those found in dill weed are sulfates of quercetin and isorhamnetin (Fukuoka et al. 1980). Whenever we find mutagenicity in edible plants, vegetables, or fruits, the first thing to be considered is that it may be due to flavonoids. Sometimes flavonoids exist as glycosides; thus, the mutagenicity of tea is partly explained by flavonol glycosides. Fecalase, isolated from human feces, and hesperidinase, isolated from *Aspergillus niger,* were found to be capable of cleaving the glycosidic bonds (Tamura et al. 1980, Nagao et al. 1981a). This indicates that flavonoids and their glycosides are capable of producing mutation in vivo.

Quercetin, when applied to in vitro cultured mammalian cells, has been reported to be mutagenic (Amacher et al. 1980, Meltz and MacGregor 1981). Quercetin can also produce sister chromatid exchanges and chromosomal aberrations in cultured mammalian cells (Yoshida et al. 1980). It is difficult to understand why quercetin is not carcinogenic.

It was suggested that changes in genomes other than simple point mutations are more important to carcinogenic processes. For instance, enhancement of transposition was suggested to be a change more crucial to carcinogenesis than simple base modification followed by misrepair (Cairns 1981).

One class of mutagens was found in many cooked foods. This class includes mutagens found in a caramelization product (Bjeldanes and Chew 1979), pyrolyzed sugars (Nagao et al. 1977b), coffee (Aeschbacher and Würzner 1980, Nagao et al. 1979), and condensates of whisky and brandy (Loquet et al. 1981, Nagao et al. 1981b). The mutagens found in these items showed direct action toward *Salmonella typhimurium* TA100, without metabolic activation. The addition of S9 mix abolished the mutagenic potential in them. Since this type of mutagen is present in such a wide range of foods, its carcinogenic effect should be carefully examined. However, all attempts to purify these mutagens were unsuccessful. This failure may have been due to the fact that mutagenicity in these cases was due to the effect of combining a variety of compounds, although all the compounds may share the common reactive group to DNA. Without purification, the in vivo experiment becomes unpractical. Research in this area deserves more attention and greater efforts.

The situation concerning tumor promoters in foods is extremely complicated. TPA and dihydroteleocidin B are very specific tumor promoters. However, in the urinary bladder, saccharin and tryptophan and its metabolites act as tumor promoters (Cohen et al. 1979, Hicks et al. 1975). Bile acid derivatives may act as tumor promoters in colon carcinogenesis (Narisawa et al. 1974). Ethanol, which is ingested as an alcoholic beverage, may act as a tumor promoter in the esophagus and cardiac portion of the stomach (Lieber et al. 1979). A high concentration of sodium chloride in food and a high consumption of sodium chloride are related to a high incidence of stomach cancer (Sato et al. 1959). Sodium chloride may produce chronic gastritis, which, in turn, creates conditions under which tumor promotion can occur (Tatematsu et al. 1975). On the other hand, sodium chloride–induced chronic gastritis may result in "intestinaliza-tion," in which case the intestinal epithelium replaces the gastric epithelium (Stemmermann et al. 1977). This metaplasia weakens acidity, creating conditions that are probably more favorable to the production of mutagens and carcinogenic nitrosamines in the stomach (Stemmermann et al. 1980, Tannenbaum et al. 1977). Frequently, intestinal metaplasia is associated with gastric cancer (Matsu-kura et al. 1980). This is especially true of the differentiated type of adenocarci-noma, which is frequently surrounded by an intestinalized area. Intestinal meta-plasia may be either a precursor of cancer or a condition favorable to the development of endogenous mutagens/carcinogens.

Furthermore, nutrition, gross composition of diet, and total calorie intake are all factors that influence carcinogenesis in various organs through various channels (as described in the introduction).

PRACTICAL STEPS FOR PREVENTING CANCER IN TERMS OF NUTRITION, DIET, AND LIFE-STYLE

The National Cancer Center Research Institute, Japan, has made a list of mild recommendations for preventing cancer available to the general public. It is called "12 Tips for Preventing Cancer." These 12 points are, of course, based on scientific considerations, but the effectiveness and relative importance of each item are difficult to assess. Therefore, these recommendations were of-fered, not as hard and fast rules, but simply in the framework of suggestions with which everyone is urged to cooperate.

The 12 precautions are:

1. Keep your diet well balanced, in terms of both taste and nutrition.
2. Do not eat the same foods repeatedly and exclusively. Also exercise caution in taking the same medication over a long period.
3. Avoid excessive eating.
4. Avoid drinking too much alcohol.
5. Refrain from excessive smoking.
6. Take optimal daily doses of vitamins A, C, and E. Include a moderate amount of fibrous food ("roughage") in your diet.
7. Avoid excessive intake of salty food and do not drink too hot water, tea, and coffee.
8. Avoid eating too many "burnt" parts of food, such as you find in charcoal-grilled meat and fish.
9. Avoid moldy food which is not intentionally moldy, such as cheese.
10. Avoid excessive exposure to the sun.
11. Avoid overwork so that you do not lower your resistance to disease.
12. Bathe or shower frequently.

These recommendations are very tentative and will be revised later.

In addition to these things, which can be done by individuals, scientists have to intensify their research into initiators, promoters, and modulators in carcinogenesis. Although it is extremely difficult, the task of evaluating the relative risks posed by various environmental factors in regard to the development of cancer in humans must be done. Appropriate action by the regulatory agencies in charge of food and diet is of course essential. For instance, the control of contamination caused by aflatoxins and nitrosamine compounds that are already known to be carcinogenic and the regulation of artificial food additives should be strictly carried out. One problem is that no concrete evidence has been obtained on the actual cause of those forms of cancer that most commonly occur in humans. Scientists, regulatory agencies, and the general public need to cooperate closely in doing their best to institute and practice measures for the prevention of cancer.

ACKNOWLEDGMENTS

The works of our group cited were supported by Grants from the Ministry of Health and Welfare, the Ministry of Education, Science and Culture, Japan, the U.S.-Japan Medical Cooperative Program, the U.S.-Japan Cancer Research Cooperative Program, and the Princess Takamatsu Cancer Research Fund.

REFERENCES

Aeschbacher, H. U., and H. P. Würzner. 1980. An evaluation of instant and regular coffee in the Ames mutagenicity test. Toxicology Letters 5:139–145.

Amacher, D., S. C. Paillet, G. N. Turner, V. A. Ray, and D. S. Salsburg. 1980. Point mutations at the thymidine kinase locus in L5178Y mouse lymphoma cells. I. Test validation and interpretation. Mutat. Res. 72:447–474.

Ames, B. N., J. McCann, and E. Yamasaki. 1975. Methods for detecting carcinogens and mutagens with the *Salmonella*/mammalian-microsome mutagenicity test. Mutat. Res. 31:347–364.

Bartsch, H., and E. Hecker. 1971. On the metabolic activation of the carcinogen N-hydroxy-N-2-acetylaminofluorene. Biochim. Biophys. Acta 237:567–578.

Berenblum, I. 1941. The mechanism of carcinogenesis. Cancer Res. 1:807–814.

Bjeldanes, L. F., and G. W. Chang. 1977. Mutagenic activity of quercetin and related compounds. Science 197:577–578.

Bjeldanes, L. F., and H. Chew. 1979. Mutagenicity of 1,2-dicarbonyl compounds: Maltol, kojic acid, diacetyl and related substances. Mutat. Res. 67:367–371.

Bock, F. G., A. P. Swain, and R. L. Stedman. 1971. Composition studies on tobacco. XLIV. Tumor-promoting activity of subfractions of the weak acid fraction of cigarette smoke condensate. JNCI 47:425–436.

Bollag, W. 1971. Therapy of chemically induced skin tumors of mice with vitamin A palmitate and vitamin A acid. Experientia 27:90–92.

Boutwell, R. K. 1977. The role of the induction of ornithine decarboxylase in tumor promotion, *in* Origins of Human Cancer, Book B, H. H. Hiatt, J. D. Watson, and J. A. Winsten, eds. Cold Spring Harbor Laboratory, Cold Spring Harbor, New York, pp. 773–783.

Brown, J. P. 1980. A review of the genetic effects of naturally occurring flavonoids, anthraquinones and related compounds. Mutat. Res. 75:243–277.

Brown, J. P., R. J. Brown, and G. W. Roehm. 1977. The application of short term microbial mutagenicity tests in the identification and development of non-toxic, non-absorbable food additives, *in* Progress in Genetic Toxicology, D. Scott, B. A. Bridges, and F. H. Sobels, eds. Elsevier/North-Holland Biomedical Press, Amsterdam, pp. 185–190.

Bruce, W. R., A. J. Varghese, S. Wang, and P. Dion. 1979. The endogenous production of nitroso compounds in the colon and cancer at that site, *in* Naturally Occurring Carcinogens-Mutagens and Modulators of Carcinogenesis, E. C. Miller, J. A. Miller, I. Hirono, T. Sugimura, and S. Takayama, eds. Japan Scientific Societies Press, Tokyo, pp. 221–228.

Cairns, J. 1981. The origin of human cancers. Nature 289:353–357.

Cheng, S.-J., M. Sala, M. H. Li, M.-Y. Wang, J. Pot-Deprun, and Z. Chouroulinkov. 1980. Mutagenic, transforming and promoting effect of pickled vegetables from Linxian county China. Carcinogenesis 1:685–692.

Cohen, S. M., M. Arai, J. B. Jacobs, and G. H. Friedell. 1979. Promoting effect of saccharin and DL-tryptophan in urinary bladder carcinogenesis. Cancer Res. 39:1207–1217.

Conney, A. H., E. J. Pantuck, K.-C. Hsiao, R. Kuntzman, A. P. Alvares, and A. Kappas. 1977. Regulation of drug metabolism in man by environmental chemicals and diet. Fed. Proc. 36:1647–1652.

Doll, R. 1977. Strategy for detection of cancer hazards to man. Nature 265:589–596.

Driedger, P. E., and P. Blumberg. 1980. Specific binding of phorbol ester tumor promoters. Proc. Natl. Acad. Sci. USA 77:567–571.

Fujiki, H., M. Mori, M. Nakayasu, M. Terada, and T. Sugimura. 1979. A possible naturally occurring tumor promoter; teleocidin B from *Streptomyces*. Biochem. Biophys. Res. Commun. 90:976–983.

Fujiki, H., M. Mori, M. Nakayasu, M. Terada, T. Sugimura, and R. E. Moore. 1981. Indole alkaloids; dihydroteleocidin B, teleocidin and lyngbyatoxin A, as a new class of tumor promoters. Proc. Natl. Acad. Sci. USA 78:3872–3876.

Fukuoka, M., K. Yoshihira, S. Natori, K. Sakamoto, S. Iwahara, S. Hosaka, and I. Hirono. 1980. Characterization of mutagenic principles and carcinogenicity of dill weed and seeds. Journal of Pharmacobio-dynamics 3:236–244.

Goldstein, B. D., G. Witz, M. Amoruso, D. S. Stone, and W. Troll. 1981. Stimulation of human polymorphonuclear leukocyte super-oxide anion radical production by tumor promoters. Cancer Lett. 11:257–262.

Hashimoto, Y., K. Shudo, and T. Okamoto. 1979. Structural identification of a modified base in DNA covalently bound with mutagenic 3-amino-1-methyl-5*H*-pyrido[4,3-*b*]indole. Chem. Pharm. Bull. 27:1058–1060.

Hashimoto, Y., K. Shudo, and T. Okamoto. 1980a. Metabolic activation of a mutagen, 2-amino-6-methyldipyrido[1,2-*a*:3′,2′-*d*]-imidazole. Identification of 2-hydroxyamino-6-methyldipyrido-[1,2-*a*:3′,3′-*d*]imidazole and its reaction with DNA. Biochem. Biophys. Res. Commun. 92:971–976.

Hashimoto, Y., K. Shudo, and T. Okamoto. 1980b. Activation of a mutagen, 3-amino-1-methyl-5*H*-pyrido[4,3-*b*]indole. Identification of 3-hydroxyamino-1-methyl-5*H*-pyrido[4,3-*b*]indole and its reaction with DNA. Biophys. Biochem. Res. Commun. 96:355–362.

Hecker, E. 1967. Phorbol esters from croton oil, chemical nature and biological activities. Naturwissenschaften 54:282–284.

Hecker, E. 1978. Structure-activity relationships in diterpene esters irritant and cocarcinogenic to mouse skin, *in* Carcinogenesis, Mechanisms of Tumor Promotion and Cocarcinogenesis, Vol. 2, T. J. Slaga, A. Sirak, and R. K. Boutwell, eds. Raven Press, New York, pp. 11–48.

Hicks, R. M., J. St. J. Wakefield, and J. Chowaniec. 1975. Evaluation of a new model to detect bladder carcinogens or cocarcinogens; results obtained with saccharin, cyclamate and cyclophosphamide. Chem. Biol. Interact. 11:225–233.

Hirohata, T. 1980. Shift in cancer mortality from 1920 to 1970 among various ethnic groups in Hawaii, *in* Genetic and Environmental Factors in Experimental and Human Cancer, H. V. Gelboin, B. MacMahon, T. Matsushima, T. Sugimura, S. Takayama, and H. Takebe, eds. Japan Scientific Societies Press, Tokyo, pp. 341–350.

Hirono, I., I. Ueno, S. Hosaka, H. Takanashi, T. Matsushima, T. Sugimura, and S. Natori. 1981. Carcinogenicity examination of quercetin and rutin in ACI rats. Cancer Lett. 13:15–21.

Hoshino, H., M. Miwa, H. Fujiki, and T. Sugimura. 1980. Aggregation of human lymphoblastoid cells by tumor-promoting phorbol esters and dihydroteleocidin B. Biochem. Biophys. Res. Commun. 95:842–848.

Hoshino, H., M. Miwa, H. Fujiki, T. Sugimura, H. Yamamoto, T. Katsuki, and Y. Hinuma.

1981. Enhancement of Epstein-Barr virus-induced transformation of human lymphocytes by teleocidin. Cancer Lett. 13:275–280.

Hsieh, D. P., Z. A. Wong, J. J. Wong, C. Michans, and B. H. Rueber. 1977. Comparative metabolism of aflatoxin, in Mycotoxins in Human and Animal Health, J. V. Rodricks, C. W. Hesseltine, and M. A. Mehlman, eds. Pathotox, Park Forest South, Illinois, pp. 37–50.

Ishii, K., M. Ando, T. Kamataki, R. Kato, and M. Nagao. 1980. Metabolic activation of mutagenic tryptophan pyrolysis products (Trp-P-1 and Trp-P-2) by a purified cytochrome P-450-dependent monooxygenase system. Cancer Lett. 9:271–276.

Kakunaga, T., T. Hirakawa, H. Fujiki, and T. Sugimura. 1981. Extraordinary enhancement of chemically induced malignant transformation by a new chemical class of tumor promoter, dihydroteleocidin B. Proceedings of the American Association for Cancer Research, p. 72.

Kasai, H., S. Nishimura, K. Wakabayashi, M. Nagao, and T. Sugimura. 1980a. Chemical synthesis of 2-amino-3-methylimidazo [4,5-f]-quinoline (IQ), a potent mutagen isolated from broiled fish. Proceedings of the Japan Academy 56B:382–384.

Kasai, H., Z. Yamaizumi, T. Shiomi, S. Yokoyama, T. Miyagawa, K. Wakabayashi, M. Nagao, T. Sugimura, and S. Nishimura. 1981. Structure of a potent mutagen isolated from fried beef. Chem. Lett. pp. 485–488.

Kasai, H., Z. Yamaizumi, K. Wakabayashi, M. Nagao, T. Sugimura, S. Yokoyama, T. Miyazawa, and S. Nishimura. 1980b. Structure and chemical synthesis of Me-IQ, a potent mutagen isolated from broiled fish. Chem. Lett. pp. 1391–1394.

Kasai, H., Z. Yamaizumi, K. Wakabayashi, M. Nagao, T. Sugimura, S. Yokoyama, T. Miyazawa, N. E. Spingarn, J. H. Weisburger, and S. Nishimura. 1980c. Potent novel mutagens produced by broiling fish under normal conditions. Proceedings of the Japan Academy 56B:278–283.

Kawabata, T., H. Ohshima, and M. Ino. 1978. Occurrence of methyl-guanidine and agmatine, nitrosable guanidino compounds, in foods. J. Agric. Food Chem. 26:334–338.

Kosuge, T., K. Tsuji, K. Wakabayashi, T. Okamoto, K. Shudo, Y. Iitaka, A. Itai, T. Sugimura, T. Kawachi, M. Nagao, T. Yahagi, and Y. Seino. 1978. Isolation and structure studies of mutagenic principles in amino acid pyrolysates. Chem. Pharm. Bull. 26:611–619.

Lee, L-S., and I. B. Weinstein. 1980. Studies on the mechanism by which a tumor promoter inhibits binding of epidermal growth factor to cellular receptor. Carcinogenesis 1:669–679.

Li, M. H., S. H. Lu, C. Ji, Y. Wang, M. Wang, S. Cheng, and G. Tian. 1980. Experimental studies on the carcinogenicity of fungus-contaminated food from Linxian county, in Genetic and Environmental Factors in Experimental and Human Cancer, H. V. Gelboin, B. MacMahon, T. Matsushima, T. Sugimura, S. Takayama, and H. Takebe, eds. Japan Scientific Societies Press, Tokyo, pp. 139–148.

Lieber, C. S., H. K. Seitz, A. J. Garro, and T. M. Worner. 1979. Alcohol-related diseases and carcinogenesis. Cancer Res. 39:2863–2886.

Loquet, C., G. Toussaint, and J. Y. LeTalaer. 1981. Studies on mutagenic constituents of apple brandy and various alcoholic beverages collected in western France, a high incidence area for oesophageal cancer. Mutat. Res. 88:155–164.

Matsukura, N., T. Kawachi, K. Morino, H. Ohgaki, T. Sugimura, and S. Takayama. 1981. Carcinogenicity in mice of mutagenic compounds from a tryptophan pyrolysate. Science 213:346–347.

Matsukura, N., K. Suzuki, T. Kawachi, M. Aoyagi, T. Sugimura, H. Kitaoka, H. Numajiri, A. Shirota, M. Itabashi, and T. Hirota. 1980. Distribution of marker enzymes and mucin in intestinal metaplasia in human stomach and relation of complete and incomplete types of intestinal metaplasia to minute gastric carcinomas. JNCI 65:231–240.

Meltz, M. L., and J. T. MacGregor. 1981. Activity of the plant flavonol quercetin in the mouse lymphoma L5178Y TK$^{+/-}$ mutation, DNA single-strand break, and Balb/c 3T3 chemical transformation assays. Mutat. Res. 88:317–324.

Mirvish, S. S., and L. Wallcave. 1972. Ascorbate-nitrite reaction: Possible means of blocking the formation of carcinogenic N-nitroso compounds. Science 177:65–68.

Nagao, M., M. Honda, Y. Seino, T. Yahagi, T. Kawachi, and T. Sugimura. 1977a. Mutagenicities of protein pyrolysates. Cancer Lett. 2:335–340.

Nagao, M., N. Morita, T. Yahagi, M. Shimizu, M. Kuroyanagi, M. Fukuoka, K. Yoshihira, S. Natori, T. Fujino, and T. Sugimura. 1981a. Mutagenicities of 61 flavonoids and 11 related compounds. Environmental Mutagenesis 3:401–419.

Nagao, M., Y. Takahashi, K. Wakabayashi, and T. Sugimura. 1981b. Mutagenicity of alcoholic beverages. Mutat. Res. 88:147–154.

Nagao, M., Y. Takahashi, H. Yamanaka, and T. Sugimura. 1979. Mutagens in coffee and tea. Mutat. Res. 68:101–106.

Nagao, M., T. Yahagi, T. Kawachi, Y. Seino, M. Honda, N. Matsukura, T. Sugimura, K. Wakabayashi, K. Tsuji, and T. Kosuge. 1977b. Mutagens in foods, and especially pyrolysis products of protein, *in* Progress in Genetic Toxicology, D. Scott, B. A. Bridges, and F. H. Sobels, eds. Elsevier/North-Holland, Amsterdam, pp. 259–264.

Nagase, S., C. Fujimaki, and H. Isaka. 1964. Effect of administration of quercetin on the production of experimental liver cancers in rats fed *p*-dimethylaminoazobenzene. Proceedings of the Japanese Cancer Association, pp. 26–27.

Nakayasu, M., H. Fujiki, M. Mori, T. Sugimura, and R. E. Moore. 1981. Teleocidin, lyngbyatoxin A and their hydrogenated derivatives, possible tumor promoters, induce terminal differentiation in HL-60 cells. Cancer Lett. 12:271–277.

Narisawa, T., N. E. Magadia, J. H. Weisburger, and E. L. Wynder. 1974. Promoting effect of bile acids on colon carcinogenesis after intrarectal instillation of N-methyl-N'-nitro-N-nitrosoguanidine in rats. JNCI 53:1093–1097.

Pamukcu, A. M., S. Yalciner, J. F. Hatcher, and G. T. Bryan. 1980. Quercetin, a rat intestinal and bladder carcinogen present in bracken fern (*Pteridium aquilinum*). Cancer Res. 40:3468–3472.

Peers, F. G., and C. A. Linsell. 1973. Dietary aflatoxins and liver cancer—a population based study in Kenya. Br. J. Cancer 27:473–484.

Peraino, C., R. J. M. Fry, and E. Staffeldt. 1971. Reduction and enhancement by phenobarbital of hepatocarcinogenesis induced in the rat by 2-acetylaminofluorene. Cancer Res. 31:1506–1512.

Preussmann, R., B. Spiegelhalder, G. Eisenbrand, and C. Janzowski. 1979. N-Nitroso compounds in food, *in* Naturally Occurring Carcinogens-Mutagens and Modulators of Carcinogenesis, E. C. Miller, J. A. Miller, I. Hirono, T. Sugimura, and S. Takayama, eds. Japan Scientific Societies Press, Tokyo, pp. 185–194.

Reigh, D. L., M. Stuart, and R. A. Floyd. 1978. Activation of the carcinogen N-hydroxy-2-acetylaminofluorene by rat mammary peroxidase. Experientia 34:107–108.

Saito, D., A. Shirai, T. Matsushima, T. Sugimura, and I. Hirono. 1980. Test of carcinogenicity of quercetin, a widely distributed mutagen in food. Teratogenesis Carcinogenesis and Mutagenesis 1:213–221.

Sakamoto, H., M. Terada, H. Fujiki, M. Mori, M. Nakayasu, T. Sugimura, and I. B. Weinstein. 1981. Stimulation of prostaglandin production and choline turnover in HeLa cells by lyngbyatoxin A and dihydroteleocidin B. Biochem. Biophys. Res. Commun. 102:100–107.

Sato, T., T. Fukuyama, T. Suzuki, J. Takayanagi, T. Murakami, N. Shiotsuki, R. Tanaka, and R. Tsuji. 1959. Studies of the causation of gastric cancer. 2. The relation between gastric cancer mortality rate and salted food intake in several places in Japan. Bulletin of the Institute of Public Health 8:187–198.

Segi, M., and M. Kurihara. 1962. Cancer mortality for selected sites in 24 countries. No. 2 (1958–1959). Department of Public Health, Tohoku University School of Medicine, Sendai, Japan.

Seino, Y., M. Nagao, T. Yahagi, T. Sugimura, T. Yasuda, and S. Nishimura. 1978. Identification of a mutagenic substance in a spice, sumac, as quercetin. Mutat. Res. 58:225–229.

Spingarn, N. E., H. Kasai, L. L. Vuolo, S. Nishimura, Z. Yamaizumi, T. Sugimura, T. Matsushima, and J. H. Weisburger. 1980. Formation of mutagens in cooked foods. III. Isolation of a potent mutagen from beef. Cancer Lett. 9:177–183.

Sporn, M. B., N. M. Dunlop, D. L. Newton, and J. M. Smith. 1976. Prevention of chemical carcinogenesis by vitamin A and its synthetic analogs (retinoids). Fed. Proc. 35:1332–1338.

Stemmermann, G. N., W. Haenszel, and F. Locke. 1977. Epidemiologic pathology of gastric ulcer and gastric carcinoma among Japanese in Hawaii. JNCI 58:13–20.

Stemmermann, G. N., H. Mower, D. Ichinotsubo, L. Tomiyasu, M. Mandel, and A. Nomura. 1980. Mutagens in extracts of human gastric mucosa. JNCI 65:321–326.

Sugimura, T. 1979. Naturally occurring genotoxic carcinogens, *in* Naturally Occurring Carcinogens-Mutagens and Modulators of Carcinogenesis, E. C. Miller, J. A. Miller, I. Hirono, T. Sugimura, and S. Takayama, eds. Japan Scientific Societies Press, Tokyo, pp. 241–261.

Sugimura, T., H. Fujiki, M. Mori, M. Nakayasu, M. Terada, K. Umezawa, and R. E. Moore. 1981. Teleocidin: new naturally occurring tumor promoter, *in* Cocarcinogenesis and Biological Effects of Tumor Promoters, H. Hecker, ed. Raven Press, New York (in press).

Sugimura, T., T. Kawachi, M. Nagao, T. Yahagi, Y. Seino, T. Okamoto, K. Shudo, T. Kosuge, K. Tsuji, K. Wakabayashi, Y. Iitaka, and A. Itai. 1977a. Mutagenic principle(s) in tryptophan and phenylalanine pyrolysis products. Proceedings of the Japan Academy 53:58–61.

Sugimura, T., T. Kawachi, M. Nagao, M. Yamada, S. Takayama, N. Matsukura, and K. Wakabayashi. 1980. Genotoxic carcinogens and comutagens in tryptophan pyrolysate, *in* Biochemical and Medical Aspects of Tryptophan Metabolism, O. Hayaishi, T. Ishimura, and R. Kido, eds. Elsevier/North-Holland Biomedical Press, Amsterdam, pp. 297–310.

Sugimura, T., and M. Nagao. 1980. Modification of mutagenic activity, *in* Chemical Mutagens, Vol. 6, F. J. de Serres, and A. Hollaender, eds. Plenum Press, New York, pp. 41–60.

Sugimura, T., M. Nagao, T. Kawachi, M. Honda, T. Yahagi, Y. Seino, S. Sato, N. Matsukura, T. Matsushima, A. Shirai, M. Sawamura, and H. Matsumoto. 1977b. Mutagen-carcinogens in food, with special reference to highly mutagenic pyrolytic products in broiled foods, *in* Origins of Human Cancer, Book B, H. H. Hiatt, J. D. Watson, and J. A. Winsten, eds. Cold Spring Harbor Laboratories, Cold Spring Harbor, New York, pp. 1561–1567.

Sugimura, T., M. Nagao, T. Matsushima, T. Yahagi, Y. Seino, A. Shirai, M. Sawamura, S. Natori, K. Yoshihira, M. Fukuoka, and M. Kuroyanagi. 1977c. Mutagenicity of flavone derivatives. Proceedings of the Japan Academy 53:194–197.

Takahashi, Y., M. Nagao, T. Fujino, Z. Yamaizumi, and T. Sugimura. 1979. Mutagens in Japanese pickle identified as flavonoids. Mutat. Res. 68:117–123.

Takashima, M., and H. Sakai. 1960. A new toxic substance, teleocidin, produced by *Streptomyces.* Bulletin of the Agricultural Chemistry Society of Japan 24:647–651.

Takayama, S., T. Hirakawa, M. Tanaka, T. Kawachi, and T. Sugimura. 1979. *In vitro* transformation of hamster embryo cells with a glutamic acid pyrolysis product. Toxicology Letters 4:281–284.

Takayama, S., Y. Katoh, M. Tanaka, M. Nagao, K. Wakabayashi, and T. Sugimura. 1977. *In vitro* transformation of hamster embryo cells with tryptophan pyrolysis products. Proceedings of the Japan Academy 53B: 126–129.

Tamura, G., C. Gold, A. Ferro-Luzzi, and B. N. Ames. 1980. Fecalase: A model for activation of dietary glycosides to mutagens by intestinal flora. Proc. Natl. Acad. Sci. USA 77:4961–4965.

Tannenbaum, S. R., M. C. Archer, J. S. Wishnok, P. Correa, C. Cuello, and W. Haenszel. 1977. Nitrate and the etiology of gastric cancer, *in* Origins of Human Cancer, Book C, H. H. Hiatt, J. D. Watson, and J. A. Winsten, eds. Cold Spring Harbor Laboratory, Cold Spring Harbor, New York, pp. 1609–1625.

Tannenbaum, S. R., A. J. Sinskey, M. Weisman, and W. Bishop. 1974. Nitrite in human saliva. Its possible relation to nitrosamine formation. JNCI 53:79–84.

Tatematsu, M., M. Takahashi, S. Fukushima, M. Hananouchi, and T. Shirai. 1975. Effects in rats of sodium chloride on experimental gastric cancers induced by N-methyl-N'-nitro-N-nitroso-guanidine or 4-nitroquinoline 1-oxide. JNCI 55:101–105.

Tsuda, M., Y. Takahashi, M. Nagao, T. Hirayama, and T. Sugimura. 1980. Inactivation of mutagens from pyrolysates of tryptophan and glutamic acid by nitrite in acidic solution. Mutat. Res. 78:331–339.

Umezawa, K., I. B. Weinstein, A. Horowitz, H. Fujiki, T. Matsushima, and T. Sugimura. 1981. Similarity of teleocidin B and phorbol ester tumor promoters in effects on membrane receptors. Nature 290:411–412.

Upadhyay, R. R., S. Islampanah, and A. Davoodi. 1980. Presence of a tumor-promoting factor in honey. Gann 71:557–559.

Van Duuren, B. L. 1969. Tumor-promoting agents in two-stage carcinogenesis. Prog. Exp. Tumor Res. 11:31–68.

Wakabayashi, K., K. Tsuji, T. Kosuge, K. Takeda, K. Yamaguchi, K. Shudo, Y. Iitaka, T. Okamoto, T. Yahagi, M. Nagao, and T. Sugimura. 1978. Isolation and structure determination of a mutagenic substance in L-lysine pyrolysate. Proceedings of the Japan Academy 54:569–571.

Wattenberg, L. W., and J. L. Leong. 1970. Inhibition of the carcinogenic action of benzo(a)pyrene by flavones. Cancer Res. 30:1922–1925.

Weber, J., and E. Hecker. 1978. Cocarcinogens of the diterpene ester type from *Croton flavens L.* and esophageal cancer in Curacao. Experientia 34:679–682.

Weinstein, I. B., R. A. Mufson, L-S. Lee, P. B. Fisher, J. Laskin, A. D. Horowitz, and V. Ivanovic. 1980. Membrane and other biochemical effects of the phorbol esters and their relevance to tumor promotion, *in* Carcinogenesis: Fundamental Mechanisms and Environmental Effect, B. Pullman, P. O. P. Ts'o, and H. V. Gelboin. Reidel Publishing Co., Amsterdam, pp. 543–563.

Weinstein, I. B., M. Wigler, P. B. Fisher, E. Sisskin, and C. Pietropaolo. 1978. Cell culture studies on the biological effects of tumor promoters, *in* Carcinogenesis, Mechanisms of Tumor Promotion and Cocarcinogenesis, Vol. 2. Raven Press, New York, pp. 313–333.

Wynder, E. L., and G. B. Gori. 1977. The contribution of the environment to cancer incidence: An epidemiologic exercise. JNCI 58:825–832.

Yamada, M., M. Tsuda, M. Nagao, M. Mori, and T. Sugimura. 1979. Degradation of mutagens from pyrolysates of tryptophan, glutamic acid and globulin by myeloperoxidase. Biochem. Biophys. Res. Commun. 90:769–776.

Yamaguchi, K., K. Shudo, T. Okamoto, T. Sugimura, and T. Kosuge. 1980a. Presence of 2-aminodipyrido[1,2-*a*:3',2'-*d*]imidazole in broiled cuttlefish. Gann 71:743–744.

Yamaguchi, K., K. Shudo, T. Okamoto, T. Sugimura, and T. Kosuge. 1980b. Presence of 3-amino-1,4-dimethyl-5*H*-pyrido[4,3-*b*]indole in broiled beef. Gann 71:745–746.

Yamaizumi, Z., T. Shiomi, H. Kasai, S. Nishimura, Y. Takahashi, M. Nagao, and T. Sugimura. 1980. Detection of potent mutagens, Trp-P-1 and Trp-P-2, in broiled fish. Cancer Lett. 9:75–83.

Yamamoto, H., T. Katsuki, Y. Hinuma, H. Hoshino, M. Miwa, H. Fujiki, and T. Sugimura. 1981. Induction of Epstein-Barr virus by a new tumor promoter, teleocidin, compared to induction by TPA. Int. J. Cancer 28:125–129.

Yamamoto, T., K. Tsuji, T. Kosuge, T. Okamoto, K. Shudo, K. Takeda, Y. Iitaka, K. Yamaguchi, Y. Seino, T. Yahagi, M. Nagao, and T. Sugimura. 1978. Isolation and structure determination of mutagenic substances in L-glutamic acid pyrolysate. Proceedings of the Japan Academy 54B:248–250.

Yamazoe, Y., K. Ishii, T. Kamataki, R. Kato, and T. Sugimura. 1980. Isolation and characterization of active metabolities of tryptophan-pyrolysate mutagen, Trp-P-2, formed by rat liver microsomes. Chem.-Biol. Interact. 30:125–138.

Yoshida, D., and T. Matsumoto. 1980. Amino-α-carbolines as mutagenic agents in cigarette smoke condensate. Cancer Lett. 10:141–149.

Yoshida, D., T. Matsumoto, R. Yoshimura, and T. Matsuzaki. 1978. Mutagenicity of amino-α-carbolines in pyrolysis products of soy bean globulin. Biochem. Biophys. Res. Commun. 83:915–920.

Yoshida, M., M. Sasaki, K. Sugimura, and T. Kawachi. 1980. Cytogenetic effects of quercetin on cultured mammalian cells. Proceedings of the Japan Academy 56:443–447.

Nutritional Components in the Etiology of Cancer

Molecular Interrelations of Nutrition and Cancer,
edited by M. S. Arnott, J. van Eys, and Y.-M. Wang.
Raven Press, New York © 1982.

Nutrition, Diet, and Cancer: Concepts and Policy

William J. Darby

The Nutrition Foundation, Inc. New York, New York 10017

Only studies of nutrition and cancer at the molecular level can generate the scientific information essential for assessment and sound interpretation of the true significance of many hypotheses that too often are stated as established theory. It is refreshing to participate in a conference on nutrition and cancer that does not have, as a major theme, controversial regulatory topics stemming from the common practice of premature extrapolation of fragmentary information into policy through political action. During this symposium details of numerous fundamental concepts pertaining to nutrition and cancer will be updated. Many of these will bear on the question of diet as a "risk factor" in cancer.

RISK FACTORS

The nutritional concept of diet or nutriture ("state of nutrition") as risk factors in chronic diseases is not new. The earliest recognition of this relationship was in association with obesity—in fact, Hippocrates' Aphorism 44 reads (Adams 1849): "Persons who are naturally very fat are apt to die earlier than those who are slender."

A much later example was that interesting observation in 1829 by William Wadd, Esq., Surgeon Extraordinary to the King, etc., etc., etc.:

While we congratulate ourselves on the diminution of mortality, which has accompanied the improvements in the condition of society, our pleasure is alloyed by the reflection, that considerable deduction is to be made in our estimate, according to the mercantile phrase, of profit and loss, by the increase of a set of diseases, which are to be attributed to the augmentation of national wealth, with its concomitants, luxury and high living.

Thus, instead of finding the annual bills of mortality announcing in the deadly list, plague, pestilence, and famine—not forgetting the small pox—we read gout, appoplexy, palsy, and even obesity, and a host of minor evils connected with repletion. . . .

As a result of experimental and epidemiologic studies of diet and cardiovascular disease(s), diet and longevity, diet and diseases of later life (including cancer), the concept of dietary risk factors has become well recognized. Nevertheless, a majority of the postulated dietary risk factors remain as unproved scientific hypotheses. They stem from epidemiologic associations of a disease or diseases with some broad figures, or even impressions, concerning patterns of eating by groups or national food disappearance figures with reported mortality from cancer. Association of mortality or morbidity statistics with such dietary descriptions cannot be interpreted as indicating causation. This type of epidemiologic evidence should not serve as the basis for food policy or dietary change until appropriate supportive evidence of other types is sufficient to verify the hypothesized relationship.

Progress during the past decade is such that several of these hypothesized relationships can now be put into some focus. How firm or definitive is the evidence?

DIET AND CANCER

In *Healthy People: The Surgeon General's Report. . .,* (Surgeon General 1979) it is stated under "Diet and Cancer":

The association between diet and cancer is more tenuous than between diet and heart disease.

Because populations with different dietary patterns have differing cancer rates—and emmigrants assuming the patterns of their adopted country soon also assume new cancer rates—there has been much research into the possible diet-cancer association.

Studies in human populations have suggested a number of possibilities: that high consumption of animal protein may be linked to colon cancer; that low consumption of fiber from plant sources may also be linked to colon cancer; that high consumption of fats, both saturated and unsaturated, may be linked to colon cancer and to hormone-related cancers of the ovary and prostate. *All of these possibilities need further investigation.*

M. J. Hill (1981) of the Central Public Health Laboratory, London, recently examined the evidence concerning dietary fat and human cancer and concluded that: "Claims regarding the role of diet are more notable for the messianic certainty of their proponents than for the strength of the evidence in their favour; dietary fat is not an exception to this."

FIBER

A working party of the Royal College of Physicians has assessed the current state of knowledge concerning medical aspects of dietary fiber. Their report, published in 1980, considered *inter alia* cancer of the large bowel and states that there are four main theories:

. . . high fat intake, high meat intake, high cholesterol intake, and low-residue or low-fibre intake. The fat and meat hypotheses have achieved wide currency but there are conflicts in the evidence.

Three mechanisms might possibly link fibre-depleted foods and cancer of the large bowel. Firstly, at a given rate of carcinogen production, small stools with little fibrous matrix and a low water content will have a higher concentration of a carcinogen than large dilute stools. Secondly, slow transit of the colonic contents may allow greater bacterial formation of carcinogen. Nevertheless, other factors, such as pH and oxido-reduction potential, may be more important. Slow transit may also allow greater contact with the colonic mucosa. Thirdly, high-energy (calorie) intake seems to increase the sensitivity of many animal tissues to carcinogens. Obese people are probably more prone to cancer in general and to large bowel cancer in particular.

The evidence that longstanding constipation predisposes to large bowel cancer is suggestive rather than strong. . . .

Few studies have looked specifically at the intake of fibre-containing foods.

The report concludes:

There are reasonable grounds for the statement that, in genetically susceptible persons, large bowel cancer could be favoured by a fibre-depleted diet, but other explanations for the commonness of this cancer in Westernized countries are possible. Definite conclusions must await the identification of the carcinogen(s) and the study of environmental factors on its production. A high-fibre diet in the sense of one based on unprocessed starch foods would also be low in fat, cholesterol, and animal protein and would be protective against large bowel cancer by all current theories.

J. H. Cummings (1981) reviewed 11 epidemiologic studies in which reference to fiber-containing foods had been made. He noted that only in two studies was fiber intake of relevant populations measured, and stated that: "Over all . . . epidemiological studies of fibre and large bowel cancer are not conclusive."

He reviewed 8 case control studies of patients with cancer of the large bowel, 10 recent animal investigations, and other examinations of this proposed relationship, and concluded: "From none of these sources is there conclusive evidence that fibre will prevent large bowel cancer, although neither is there evidence that fibre is not involved. . . ."

It should be noted that diet of the types claimed to be cancer risk factors are those associated with what William Wadd termed "augmentation of national wealth, with its concomitants, luxury and high living," and as we soon shall see, improved longevity and national well-being.

DIET AND CANCER OF THE BREAST

B. E. Henderson et al. (1977) addressed the hormonal basis of breast cancer and its possible relation to diet. They wrote:

. . . we conclude that the familial risk of breast cancer is associated with elevated levels of several hormones, including prolactin, progesterone, and estrogen. . . .

The mechanism(s) producing these levels is obscure. There are at least two, not mutually exclusive, possible explanations: (1) increased secretion and (2) decreased metabolic clearance. . . .

Increased secretion of hormones is probably related to the factors affecting the onset of menarche. Menarche appears to be determined by the attainment of a critical body weight and body composition. . . . The effect of increased consumption of total calories and fat is to lower the age at menarche and perhaps to provide the milieu where there is subsequently hypersecretion of several pituitary and gonadal steroids. . . .

Other observations on breast cancer epidemiology are consistent with this concept of a generalized elevation of hormone levels. Increased body weight has been associated both with increased estrogen excretion . . . and with increased risk of breast cancer. Dietary changes leading to an earlier age at menarche and the associated hormonal changes provide an explanation for the pattern of change in rate of breast cancer in the immigrant Japanese population. Presumably these women adopted the typical American diet early in life and then assumed the rates associated with that diet. Variations in diet probably explain at least part of the increased risk of breast cancer among higher socioeconomic classes as well. . . .

These concepts of the nutriture-diet-cancer interrelationships well illustrate the complexity of the considerations and the tenuous state of our knowledge. As a nutritionist, I am unwilling to propose broad dietary changes on the basis of such evidence, in view of the present state of good nutritional health of the population.

CURRENT HEALTH STATUS

The Report of the Surgeon General (1979) referred to earlier opens:

The health of the American people has never been better. . . .
Since 1900, the death rate in the United States has been reduced from 17 per 1,000 persons per year to less than 9 per 1,000. . . . In 1977, a record low of 14 infant deaths per 1,000 live births was achieved. . . . A baby born in this country today can be expected to live more than 73 years on the average, while a baby born in 1900 could be expected to live only 47 years. . . . Deaths due to heart disease decreased in the United States by 22 percent between 1968 and 1977. . . .
Nearly all the gains against the once great killers . . . have come as a result of improvements in sanitation, housing, nutrition and immunization.

This report further emphasizes that continuing improved health promotion often requires but modest lifestyle changes to substantially reduce risk for several diseases.

Similarly, the most recently published age-adjusted cancer mortality figures (Silverberg 1981) show a decreasing (especially in the female) or stable rate for cancer of most sites except the lung.

These facts belie the statement frequently made in the media and in political situations warning that we are suffering an epidemic of cancer due to the quality of the American diet.

FOOD AND CARCINOGENS

Despite the millions of dollars and man-centuries of research and testing of food and ingredients (including additives) for carcinogenic properties, there is a striking paucity of evidence for any existing meaningful public health problem due to dietary carcinogens. Only limited evidence is available indicating the carcinogenicity in man of that powerful liver carcinogen, aflatoxin. The cycad nut is of restricted use so that the metabolite of cycasin can be incriminated in but relatively few cases of a food-induced cancer. Both of these carcinogens are naturally occurring. As for the question of food additives and cancer so widely discussed in the public media, the situation has very recently been succinctly summarized by F. A. Fairweather and C. A. Swan (1981):

There have been few instances where the carcinogenic potential of a food additive has been clearly determined in animal experiments and on these occasions the additive has been immediately withdrawn. . . . There have been no documented cases of food additives causing cancer in man. Needless to say there have probably been countless potential food additives which, when tested for carcinogenicity, would have exhibited a consumer risk that the manufacturers decided against marketing. . . .

The safety-in-use of food additives is closely monitored in the U.K. and other countries worldwide, and with the present laws the consumer is well protected against any deleterious effects of food additives. . . .

A relationship of alcoholic beverages to cancer of the mouth, pharynx, and esophogus has long been recognized. It remains uncertain whether the responsible agent is alcohol itself or some of the more than 400 congeners that have been identified in distilled liquors and liqueurs, somewhat less in wines, and still less in beers. Pure alcohol has not been found to be a carcinogen in experimental animals.

It should be noted that tobacco is a far-better established risk factor in cancer of these sites, and its concurrent use with alcoholic beverages greatly increases the risk (see Tuyns 1979).

Linsell and Peers (1977) conclude that: "A review of the evaluation of known chemical carcinogens and their potential risks to man indicates a depressing lack of human data, and it is difficult to discover the type and standard of the information needed before legislative action or other steps to prevent exposure are evoked."

And, significantly, J. W. Berg (1981) is of the opinion that: "Hypotheses generated by surveys of geographic patterns tend to remain merely speculative . . . (and) . . . that consideration of only the carcinogen to the neglect of cell susceptibility and accessibility, is a major block to fully understanding and exploiting the world-wide variations in cancer incidence."

I believe that this gives us some clear directions for productive research and its support.

NUTRITION IN TREATMENT OF CANCER

Progress in developing methodology for both acute and long-term nutritional support of the patient with cancer has been great during this decade. But to discuss this in any detail in Houston, Texas, would be "bringing coals to Newcastle." The establishment of nutrition support teams in medical centers and hospitals throughout the nation and abroad speak for the medical profession's judgment of such support as a modern imperative.

While we have not yet resolved the problem of ultimate cancer cachexia, there is much evidence of the enormous benefit of proper nutritional support to vast numbers of patients. The benefits reported include improvement in response to therapy and shortening of periods of hospitalization. Home maintenance of patients who otherwise would require continuous institutional care provides a quality of life for the patient that was not our privilege to provide 15 to 20 years ago.

Much remains to be developed in this broad area of nutritional management and cancer—not only in determination of requirements, improvement of technology, and other developmental efforts, but elucidation of metabolic information, of concepts of cellular nature and of organ function, of drug-nutrient interrelationships, and much more.

Without belaboring this important point further, nutrition in the management and treatment of patients, in my judgment, continues to deserve intensive research attention and support for research. Parenthetically, it is the research on basic concepts and improved therapy that I judge should have priority. Frankly, I am impatient with those who wish *solely* to compare the course of individuals receiving one or another modification of support through counting their hospital days. Such information should incidentally accrue as the consequence of good records and patient care.

QUALITY OF LIFE

Let me return briefly to the concept of quality of life. Abraham Maslow (1949) holds that man evolves through the five levels: survival, security, belongingness, esteem, and self-actualization.

Patients may well so progress! The stage of self-actualization is that attained when all basic needs are fulfilled—needs embracing affection, respect, self-esteem, belongingness, love, status, independence. It is to restore the patient to this level that we should strive, and I maintain that such is worthy of research investment, fully as worthy as to maintain him at the level of survival. Research in nutrition and cancer has contributed greatly to our progress toward attainment of the level of self-actualization for the cancer patient. Support for such research should continue to have high priority.

NEED FOR NUTRITION EDUCATION

To apply our current knowledge of nutrition to the full benefit of patients with cancer and to extend the research along profitable routes requires a continuing supply of young, broadly educated research personnel. It also requires that knowledge of nutrition be possessed widely by members of the medical and scientific community.

These needs were the subject of consideration at an intensive workshop at the NIH in June 1979. The recommendations of the assembled group are well summarized in *Nutrition and Cancer* (Darby 1980), and especially in the tabulated 35 specific recommendations for several levels of training that need expansion. It is to be hoped that policy and politics will permit the fulfillment of these needs.

"PREVENTION IS AN IDEA WHOSE TIME HAS COME"

In the report to the Surgeon General (1979), "prevention is an idea whose time has come" is quoted. In that report, the Surgeon General called for a reexamination of our priorities for national spending. None can quarrel with his thesis that: (1) prevention saves lives; (2) prevention improves the quality of life (for those who remain well); and (3) prevention saves dollars (for those who remain well).

In support of this thesis, the enormous effectiveness of medical science in conquering infectious, parasitic, and deficiency diseases is cited. Note that here scientists were dealing with *specific* causes and effects, not with nonspecific risk factors and unknown causes, as is the case of nutrition and cancer. Furthermore, there are those who argue that some cancer is unavoidable as a consequence of age attainment.

I again raise the question, therefore: Is it not of great importance that we keep before us with highest priority the concept of improving, through nutrition, the well-being of the patient who develops cancer? And of providing support for the requisite educational and research programs to do so?

This, in parallel with the furtherance of the basic research to promote fundamental understanding of the processes of the molecular interpretations of nutrition and cancer, will best serve to optimize our prevention and treatment of cancer insofar as can be accomplished by diet and nutrition. Nutrition cannot be expected to eradicate cancer.

REFERENCES

Adams, F., translator. 1849. The Genuine Works of Hippocrates, Sydenham Society, London.

Berg, J. 1980. The role of epidemiology in the nutritional aspects of cancer. Nutrition and Cancer 2:13–16.

Cummings, J. H. 1981. Dietary fibre and large bowel cancer. Proc. Nutr. Soc. 40:7–14.

Darby, W. J., chairman. 1980. Proceedings of a Workshop on Physician Education in Cancer Nutrition. Nutrition and Cancer 2:9–58.

Fairweather, F. A., and C. A. Swann. 1981. Food additives and cancer. Proc. Nutr. Soc. 40:21–30.

Henderson, B. E., M. C. Pike, V. R. Gerkins, and J. T. Casagrande. 1977. The hormonal basis of breast cancer: Elevated plasma levels of estrogen, prolactin, and progesterone, *in* Origins of Human Cancer, Book A: Incidence of Cancer in Humans, H. H. Hiatt, J. D. Watson, and J. A. Winsten, eds. Cold Spring Harbor Laboratory, Cold Spring Harbor, New York, pp. 77–86.

Hill, M. J. 1981. Dietary fat and human cancer. Proc. Nutr. Soc. 40:15–19.

Linsell, C. A., and F. G. Peers. 1977. Field studies on liver cell cancer, *in* Origins of Human Cancer, Book A: Incidence of Cancer in Humans, H. H. Hiatt, J. D. Watson, and J. A. Winsten, eds. Cold Spring Harbor Laboratory, Cold Spring Harbor, New York, pp. 549–556.

Maslow, A. H. 1949. *in* Moral Problems in Contemporary Society: Essays in Humanistic Ethics, P. Kurtz, ed. Prentice Hall, Englewood Cliffs, New Jersey.

Royal College of Physicians. 1980. Medical Aspects of Dietary Fibre: Summary of a Report of The Royal College of Physicians of London. Pitman Medical, London, 175 pp.

Silverberg, E. 1981. Cancer statistics, 1981. CA 31:13–28.

Surgeon General. 1979. Healthy People: The Surgeon General's Report on Health Promotion and Disease Prevention—1979. U.S. Government Printing Office, Washington, D.C.

Tuyns, A. J. 1972. Cancer and alcoholic beverages, *in* Fermented Food Beverages in Nutrition, A Nutrition Foundation Monograph, C. F. Gastineau, W. J. Darby, and T. B. Turner, eds. Academic Press, Inc., New York, pp. 427–437.

Wadd, W. 1829. Comments on Corpulency; Lineaments of Leanness: Mems on Diet and Dietetics. John Evers & Co., London.

Molecular Interrelations of Nutrition and Cancer,
edited by M. S. Arnott, J. van Eys, and Y.-M. Wang.
Raven Press, New York © 1982.

Mechanisms of Conversion of Food Components to Mutagens and Carcinogens

Taijiro Matsushima

Department of Molecular Oncology, Institute of Medical Science, University of Tokyo, Shirokanedai 4-chome, Minato-ku, Tokyo 108, Japan

There are many mutagens in food, some of which occur naturally and some of which are synthetic. The former include mutagens existing in vegetables and fruits, such as flavonoids and pyrrolizidine alkaloids, and mycotoxins, produced by fungi, such as aflatoxin B_1. The latter include food additives and pesticide contaminants. Nitrosamines are also produced by reactions between naturally occurring substances in food such as secondary amines and artificially added nitrite.

The mutagenic potencies of the mutagens produced during cooking and storage are the highest. The principal mechanisms of formation of these mutagens are pyrolysis reactions at higher temperature and the Maillard reaction–browning reaction at lower temperature. This chapter concerns the relation between the structures of newly found heterocyclic amines produced by pyrolysis and the structures of the precursors. Recent information on mutagen formation by the Maillard reaction–browning reaction is also reviewed. In addition, recent results on the formation of mutagens from methylguanidine derivatives and ribose are described.

MUTAGENS PRODUCED BY PYROLYSIS FROM AMINO ACIDS, PROTEIN, AND PROTEINACEOUS FOOD

Mutagens are formed from amino acids, proteins, and proteinaceous food by pyrolysis involving a radical reaction at higher temperature. In the case of pyrolysis of single amino acids, the relation of the precursor amino acids and the mutagens formed can be discussed. New mutagens formed in these pyrolysis reactions have been isolated and the structures established; namely, 3-amino-1,4-dimethyl-5*H*-pyrido[4,3-*b*]indole (Trp-P-1) and 3-amino-1-methyl-5*H*-pyrido[4,3-*b*]indole (Trp-P-2) from tryptophan (Sugimura et al. 1977), 2-amino-6-methyldipyrido[1,2-*a:* 3′,2′-*d*]imidazole (Glu-P-1) and 2-aminodipyrido[1,2-*a:* 3′,2′-*d*]imidazole (Glu-P-2) from glutamic acid (Yamamoto et al. 1978), 3,4-cyclopentenopyrido[3,2-*a*]carbazole (Lys-P-1) from lysine (Wakabayashi et al. 1978) and 2-amino-5-phenylpyridine (Phe-P-1) from phenylalanine (Sugimura et al. 1977).

Two of these five potent mutagens, Trp-P-1 and Trp-P-2, have an indole structure as a part of a pyridoindole structure, namely a γ-carboline structure. Very likely the original indole nucleus of the tryptophan molecule remains in the structure of Trp-P-1 and Trp-P-2. Phe-P-1, aminophenyl pyridine, retains part of the structure of phenylalanine (Figure 1).

Pyrolysis reactions produce many reactive fragments by radical reactions, and these fragments condense to form new heterocyclic structures. Such reactions can explain the formation of the entire molecules of Glu-P-1 and Glu-P-2, dipyridoimidazole compounds. The formation of Lys-P-1, cyclopentenocarbazole, from lysine is also of this type (Figure 1).

Trp-P-1 and Trp-P-2 are found in pyrolysates of casein and gluten (Uyeta et al. 1979) and in broiled sardine (Yamaizumi et al. 1980) and beef (Yamaguchi et al. 1980). 2-Amino-α-carbolines, 2-amino-$9H$-pyrido[2,3-b]indole (AαC) and 2-amino-3-methyl-$9H$-pyrido[2,3-b]indole (MeAαC) were isolated from soybean globulin (Yoshida et al. 1978). However, it is uncertain whether the indole

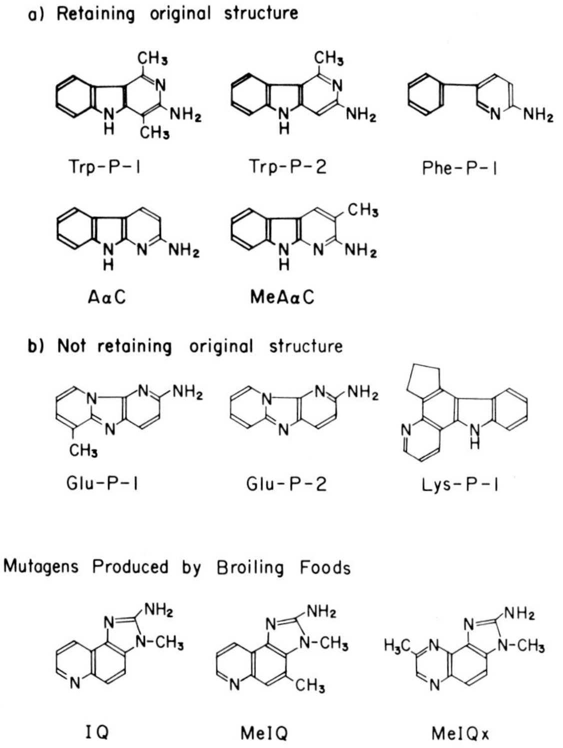

FIG. 1. Structures of mutagens produced by pyrolysis of amino acids, protein, and proteinaceous food.

moieties of Trp-P-1, Trp-P-2, AαC, and MeAαC originate from tryptophan molecules in peptide chains of protein or from fragments of other amino acids.

Three aminoimidazole derivatives were isolated as very potent mutagens from broiled food: 2-amino-3-methylimidazo[4,5-*f*]quinoline (IQ) and 2-amino-3,4-dimethylimidazo[4,5-*f*]quinoline (MeIQ) were isolated from broiled sardine (Kasai et al. 1980a, 1980b) and 2-amino-3,8-dimethylimidazo[4,5-*f*]quinoxaline (MeIQx) was isolated from fried beef (Kasai et al. 1981). These three compounds have a common structure, 2-amino-3-methylimidazole. The precursors of these mutagens in sardine and beef are not known, although methylguanidine is one possibility.

MUTAGENS PRODUCED BY THE BROWNING REACTION

Another mechanism of formation of mutagens during cooking and storage of foods is the Maillard reaction to yield amino-carbonyl compounds, followed by Amadori rearrangement and the browning reaction.

Several examples of this reaction could be cited, but the specific mutagenic activities of the products are all rather low. This reaction occurs at a lower temperature than the pyrolysis reaction and even proceeds at room temperature.

A direct-acting mutagen toward *Salmonella typhimurium* TA100 was produced by boiling an aqueous solution of lysine and glucose, but the structure of this mutagen has not yet been identified (Shinohara et al. 1980). A mutagen that required metabolic activation for activity toward *S. typhimurium* TA98 was produced by heating solutions of sugars, such as arabinose, glucose, rhamnose, and xylose, with ammonia at 100°C (Spingarn and Garvie 1979). Pyrazine and its derivatives are produced by the reaction of amino acids and hexoses and are flavor compounds in cooked and roasted foods. Pyrazine and 2-methyl-, 2-ethyl-, 2,5-dimethyl-, and 2,6-dimethyl-pyrazine were not mutagenic to *S. typhimurium* TA100, TA98, or TA1537, but induced chromosome aberrations in cultured Chinese hamster ovary cells (Stich et al. 1980).

Two mutagens, 1-(2-furyl)-pyrido[3,4-*b*]indole and 1-(2-furyl)-pyrido[3,4-*b*]indole-3-carboxylic acid, were isolated from a reaction mixture of tryptophan and ascorbic acid at room temperature. These were weakly mutagenic to *S. typhimurium* TA100 with metabolic activation but were not mutagenic to TA98 (Kanamori et al. 1980).

Many different types of mutagens should be formed from various amino groups and various reducing sugars, but present knowledge of the chemical nature of mutagens is very limited.

MODEL EXPERIMENTS ON MUTAGEN FORMATION FROM METHYLGUANINE DERIVATIVES AND RIBOSE

IQ, MeIQ, and MeIQx have a common structure, 2-amino-imidazole. Therefore, a model of mutagen formation from imidazole or guanidine derivatives was made by heating them with an equimolar amount of ribose at 200°C for 60 min. Ribose was selected because ribose and glucose are the main free sugars in fish meat (Jones 1958). Fine powders of the mixtures were heated in a hot aluminum block (dry-bath) in a test-tube attached to a condensor. The resulting tar was dissolved in dimethylsulfoxide and tested for mutagenicity. Mutagenicity was detected only with *S. typhimurium* TA98 and with metabolic activation. As shown in Table 1, 1-methyl-histidine and ribose yielded slight mutagenic activity, but histidine and 3-methyl-histidine and ribose did not produce any mutagenic substance. Arginine and N^G-methyl-arginine produced weak mutagens

TABLE 1. *Mutagen formation from imidazole or guanidine derivatives and ribose by heating at 200°C*

		Mutagenicity (His$^+$/μmol)
Histidine		0
1-Methyl-histidine		31
3-Methyl-histidine		0
Arginine		14
N^G-Methyl-arginine		33
Guanidine		0
Methyl-guanidine		306
Creatine		290
Creatinine		330

Imidazoles or guanidine derivatives were heated at 200°C for 60 min with an equimolar amount of D-ribose. The resulting tar was dissolved in dimethylsulfoxide and its mutagenicity was tested on *S. typhimurium* TA98 with S9 mix with preincubation at 30°C for 30 min (Matsushima et al. 1980).

when heated with ribose. Of the guanidine derivatives investigated, guanidine itself did not show any mutagenicity after heating with ribose, but methylguanidine yielded strong mutagenicity. Creatine and creatinine also yielded strong mutagenicities after heating with ribose at 200°C. All the compounds that yielded mutagens had a methylguanidine structure.

Figure 2 shows the temperature dependence of mutagen formation from methylguanidine, creatinine, and creatine heated with an equimolar amount of ribose at the indicated temperatures for 60 min. Methylguanidine plus ribose yielded a mutagenic substance and the optimum temperature for its formation was 175°C. Creatinine or creatine with ribose yielded the most mutagen at 225°C. Creatinine produced stronger mutagenicity than creatine. Guanidine did not produce any mutagenicity under these conditions. Without sugar, none of these compounds produce any mutagenic substance on heating to as high as 250°C.

Table 2 shows the formation of mutagenic substances on heating melthylguanidine derivatives with various sugars. Ribose was the most efficient precursor of mutagens under these conditions, glucose was less effective, and galactose and fructose were much less effective. Again, these sugars alone did not produce any mutagenicity toward *S. typhimurium* TA98 on heating under these conditions.

Figure 3 shows the time dependence of mutagen formation from an equimolar

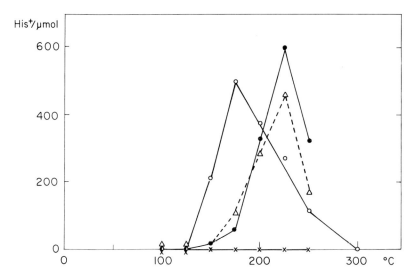

FIG. 2. Temperature dependency of mutagen formation from guanidine derivatives and ribose by heating. Equimolar mixtures of guanidine (—x—), methylguanidine (— ○ —), creatine (— △ —), or creatinine (— ● —) and ribose were heated at different temperatures for 60 min. The resulting tar was dissolved in dimethylsulfoxide and its mutagenicity was measured using *S. typhimurium* TA98 with an in vitro metabolic activation system (S9 mix prepared from the liver of a rat pretreated with phenobarbital and 5,6-benzoflavone [Matsushima et al. 1976]).

TABLE 2. *Mutagen formation from guanidine derivatives and sugars*

Guanidine	Sugar	Heating Conditions	Mutagenicity (His$^+$/μmol)
Methylguanidine	Ribose	175°C	269
	Glucose	60 min	169
	Fructose		36
	Galactose		102
	(none)		0
Creatine	Ribose	175°C	108
	Glucose	60 min	81
	Fructose		100
	Galactose		73
	(none)		0
Creatinine	Ribose	225°C	255
	Glucose	60 min	227
	Fructose		124
	Galactose		181
	(none)		0
(none)	Ribose	175°C	0
	Glucose	60 min	0
	Fructose		0
	Galactose		0

Samples of 1 mmol of guanidine derivatives and sugars were heated. The resulting tar was dissolved in dimethylsulfoxide and its mutagenicity was tested on *S. typhimurium* TA98 with S9 mix.

mixture of creatinine and ribose at 225°C. Mutagenic substances were produced very quickly, reaching a maximum within 10–20 min and remaining at this level until 60 min. Yoshida and Okamoto (1980) found that a mutagen was formed on heating creatine and glucose, optimum conditions being 2-hour heating at 150°C.

Creatine and creatinine are present in fish and animal meat and produced potent mutagenicity on heating in the presence of sugars at about 200°C, which is a usual temperature for cooking.

DISCUSSION

There are many reports on the formation of mutagens during cooking of food. Two main types of reactions are involved in their formation, a pyrolysis reaction and the Maillard reaction. Since cooking procedures range widely from mild heating to strong heating, the formation of mutagens during cooking may be due to both types of reactions. In contrast, the formation of mutagens under mild conditions during storage of food probably mainly results from a Maillard type reaction.

Mutagens found in coffee and tea (Nagao et al. 1979) and in whiskey and

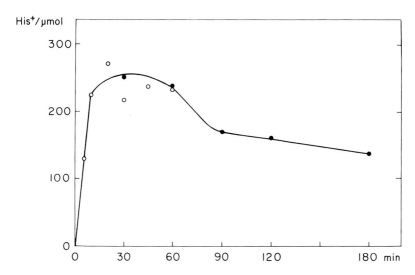

FIG. 3. Time-course of mutagen formation from creatinine and ribose. An equimolar mixture of creatinine and ribose was heated at 225°C for 5 min to 60 min (○) and 30 min to 180 min (●). The resulting tar was dissolved in dimethylsulfoxide and its mutagenicity was measured using *S. typhimurium* TA98 with S9 mix.

brandies (Nagao et al. 1981) may be partly formed by a pyrolysis reaction and Maillard reaction. Pyrolysis reactions are known to produce various carcinogenic aromatic hydrocarbons, including benzo(a)pyrene. Some new heterocyclic amines that are found in the charred parts of food and that are very strongly mutagenic have recently been shown to be carcinogenic. Many mutagens were produced by the Maillard reaction, but information on their structures is still very limited. The carcinogenicity of mutagens formed by the Maillard reaction has not been reported. Further intensive studies on the structures and biological activities of these mutagens are very important in assessing human risk from them.

ACKNOWLEDGMENTS

This work was supported in part by Grants from the Ministry of Education, Science, and Culture, the Ministry of Health and Welfare, Japan, the U.S.-Japan Cooperative Medical Science Program, the Princess Takamatsu Cancer Research Fund, and the Society for Promotion of Cancer Research.

REFERENCES

Jones, N. R. 1958. The estimation of free sugars in skeletal muscle of codling *(Gadus callarias)* and herring *(Clupea harengus)*. Biochem. J. 68:704–708.

Kanamori, H., K. Morimoto, N. Kinae, and I. Tomita. 1980. The formation of the mutagenic substances in the reaction between L-ascorbic acid and L-tryptophan. Chem. Pharm. Bull. 28:3143–3144.

Kasai, H., S. Nishimura, K. Wakabayashi, M. Nagao, and T. Sugimura. 1980a. Chemical synthesis of 2-amino-3-methylimidazo[4,5-*f*]quinoline (IQ), a potent mutagen isolated from broiled fish. Proceedings of the Japan Academy 56B:382–384.

Kasai, H., Z. Yamaizumi, K. Wakabayashi, M. Nagao, T. Sugimura, S. Yokoyama, T. Miyazawa, and S. Nishimura. 1980b. Structure and chemical synthesis of Me-IQ, a potent mutagen isolated from broiled fish. Chemistry Letters, pp. 1391–1394.

Kasai, H., Z. Yamaizumi, T. Shiomi, S. Yokoyama, T. Miyagawa, K. Wakabayashi, M. Nagao, T. Sugimura, and S. Nishimura. 1981. Structure of a potent mutagen isolated from fried beef. Chemistry Letters, pp. 485–488.

Matsushima, T., M. Sawamura, K. Hara, and T. Sugimura. 1976. A safe substitute for polychlorinated biphenyls as an inducer of metabolic activation system, *in* In Vitro Metabolic Activation in Mutagenesis Testing, F. J. de Serres, J. R. Fouts, J. R. Bend, and R. M. Philpot, eds. Elsevier/North-Holland Biochemical Press, Amsterdam, pp. 85–88.

Matsushima, T., T. Sugimura, M. Nagao, T. Yahagi, A. Shirai, and M. Sawamura. 1980. Factors modulating mutagenicity in microbial tests, *in* Short-Term Test System for Detecting Carcinogens, K. H. Norpoth and R. C. Garner, eds. Springer-Verlag, Berlin, Heidelberg, New York, pp. 271–285.

Nagao, M., Y. Takahashi, H. Yamanaka, and T. Sugimura. 1979. Mutagens in coffee and tea. Mutat. Res. 68:101–106.

Nagao, M., Y. Takahashi, K. Wakabayashi, and T. Sugimura. 1981. Mutagenicity of alcoholic beverages. Mutat. Res. 88:147–154.

Shinohara, K., R.-T. Wu, N. Jahan, M. Tanaka, N. Morinaga, H. Murakami, and H. Omura. 1980. Mutagenicity of the browning mixtures by amino-carbonyl reactions on *Salmonella typhimurium* TA100. Agricultural and Biological Chemistry 44:671–672.

Spingarn, N. E., and C. T. Garvie. 1979. Formation of mutagens in sugar-ammonia model systems. J. Agric. Food Chem. 27:1319–1321.

Stich, H. F., W. Stich, M. P. Rosin, and W. D. Powrie. 1980. Mutagenic activity of pyrazine derivatives: A comparative study with *Salmonella typhimurium, Saccaromyces cerevisiae* and Chinese hamster ovary cells. Food Cosmet. Toxicol. 18:581–584.

Sugimura, T., T. Kawachi, M. Nagao, T. Yahagi, Y. Seino, T. Okamoto, K. Shudo, T. Kosuge, K. Tsuji, K. Wakabayashi, Y. Iitaka, and A. Itai. 1977. Mutagenic principle(s) in tryptophan and phenylalanine pyrolysis products. Proceedings of the Japan Academy 53:58–61.

Uyeta, M., T. Kanada, M. Mazaki, S. Taue, and S. Takahashi. 1979. Assaying mutagenicity of food pyrolysis products using the Ames test, *in* Naturally Occurring Carcinogens-Mutagens and Modulators of Carcinogenesis, E. C. Miller, J. A. Miller, I. Hirono, T. Sugimura, and S. Takayama, eds. Japan Scientific Societies Press, Tokyo, pp. 169–176.

Wakabayashi, K., K. Tsuji, T. Kosuge, K. Tanaka, K. Yamaguchi, K. Shudo, Y. Iitaka, T. Okamoto, T. Yahagi, M. Nagao, and T. Sugimura. 1978. Isolation and structure determination of a mutagenic substance in L-lysine pyrolysate. Proceedings of the Japan Academy 54:569–571.

Yamaguchi, K., K. Shudo, T. Okamoto, T. Sugimura, and T. Kosuge. 1980. Presence of 3-amino-1,4-dimethyl-5*H*-pyrido[4,3-*b*]indole in broiled beef. Gann 71:745–746.

Yamaizumi, A., T. Shiomi, H. Kasai, S. Nishimura, Y. Takahashi, M. Nagao, and T. Sugimura. 1980. Detection of potent mutagens, Trp-P-1 and Trp-P-2, in broiled fish. Cancer Lett. 9:75–83.

Yamamoto, T., K. Tsuji, T. Kosuge, T. Okamoto, K. Shudo, K. Takeda, Y. Iitaka, K. Yamaguchi, Y. Seino, T. Yahagi, M. Nagao, and T. Sugimura. 1978. Isolation and structure determination of mutagenic substances in L-glutamic acid pyrolysate. Proceedings of the Japan Academy 54B:248–250.

Yoshida, D., T. Matsumoto, R. Yoshimura, and T. Matsuzaki. 1978. Mutagenicity of amino-α-carbolines in pyrolysis products of soy bean globulin. Biochem. Biophys. Res. Commun. 83:915–920.

Yoshida, D., and H. Okamoto. 1980. Formation of mutagens by heating creatine and glucose. Biochem. Biophys. Res. Commun. 96:844–847.

Molecular Interrelations of Nutrition and Cancer,
edited by M. S. Arnott, J. van Eys, and Y.-M. Wang.
Raven Press, New York © 1982.

Inhibition of Chemical Carcinogens by Minor Dietary Components

Lee W. Wattenberg

Department of Laboratory Medicine and Pathology, University of Minnesota Medical School, Minneapolis, Minnesota 55455

A vast quantity of data has previously demonstrated the presence of many carcinogenic agents in the environment. To this hazard has now been added a number of suspect carcinogens in food. These latter compounds have been identified by Dr. Sugimura and his colleagues and others on the basis of mutagenic activity (Sugimura 1981, see pages 3 to 24 this volume, Matsushima 1981, see pages 35 to 42 this volume, Stich 1981). In addition to chemical hazards, it should be recalled that the most ubiquitous carcinogenic agent to which we are all exposed is ultraviolet light.

Organisms of all types survive by being able to defend themselves against noxious environmental influences. It therefore should be anticipated that substantial and effective protective systems would exist against carcinogenic agents. This is particularly so since these agents attack DNA, probably the most essential chemical of living organisms. The expected defenses exist. In mammalian species they are multiple and sequential and include early events such as barrier functions and, ultimately, repair systems. The total range, intricacies, and interrelationships of these defense systems are incompletely understood. Likewise the extent to which they can be altered to enhance the capacity of various species, including humans, to withstand successfully the impact of carcinogens in the environment is just beginning to be explored.

This chapter focuses primarily on one group of defense mechanisms, detoxification systems. A number of minor dietary components have been shown to have the capacity to inhibit chemical carcinogens. Most of these dietary constituents occur naturally; a few are food additives. These inhibitors enhance carcinogen detoxification. Five such groups will be discussed: phenols, indoles, coumarins, aromatic isothiocyanates, and methylated flavones. The levels of activity of detoxification enzymes in tissues of the major portals by which carcinogens enter the organism are very responsive to members of these five groups of inhibitory agents. Other tissues are responsive as well. Thus, the environment contains opposing forces, i.e., carcinogens and inhibitors of carcinogens. Their interplay will have an effect in determining whether neoplasia occurs.

The recognition of the existence of dietary inhibitors of carcinogenesis has led to two major lines of investigation. The first is directed toward an understanding of the impact that inhibitors in the environment now play in preventing neoplasia, and to the related issue of how such protective effects might be enhanced. The second line of investigation is directed at producing highly potent inhibitors that would have potential use in intervention studies for protecting individuals at high risk of neoplasia.

CLASSIFICATION OF INHIBITORS OF CARCINOGENESIS

During the last decade a substantial number of compounds have been found to inhibit carcinogenesis. The number and diversity of these chemicals offers the possibility that they can be exploited for their protective effects in man. Many inhibitors occur naturally in vegetables and other edible plant materials. Others are synthetic. Inhibitors of carcinogenesis in general can be divided into three categories. In the first are compounds that prevent the formation of carcinogens from precursor substances. Ascorbic acid and α-tocopherol have this mechanism of action. In the second category are compounds that inhibit by preventing carcinogenic agents from reaching or reacting with critical target sites in the host. These inhibitors are called "blocking agents," which is descriptive of their mechanism of action. A third category of inhibitors acts subsequent to exposures to carcinogenic agents. The most extensively investigated inhibitors of this class are the retinoids (Sporn and Newton 1980). A second group of agents in this category have in common the fact that they are protease inhibitors (Troll 1980), and a third are those with a capacity to inhibit prostaglandin synthesis. The most extensively studied compound of this type is indomethacin. Anti-inflammatory steroids also come under this heading. Recently, sodium cyanate was found to inhibit carcinogen-induced neoplasia of the mammary gland and large bowel when administered subsequent to carcinogen exposure. Several related compounds also have this property (Wattenberg 1981).

GENERAL ASPECTS OF THE MECHANISMS OF
INHIBITION BY BLOCKING AGENTS

As described above, blocking agents prevent carcinogens from reaching or reacting with critical target sites. An understanding of their mechanisms of action is based on the contributions of the Millers and others in the field of chemical carcinogenesis (Miller 1978). A vast amount of data has been accumulated that demonstrates that chemical carcinogens act via common mechanisms. The ultimate carcinogenic form of carcinogens is a positively charged electrophilic species. Some carcinogens, termed "direct acting," exist in this form or assume it in solution. Others require metabolic activation. An implication of the existence of these common features is that they offer the possibility of obtaining compounds that will inhibit a broad range of chemical carcinogens by affecting a common mechanism or mechanisms required for carcinogenesis. The reality of the existence of such inhibitors has been demonstrated with phenolic antioxidants, particularly butylated hydroxyanisole (BHA), which inhibit a substantial variety of chemical carcinogens (Wattenberg 1978b, 1980).

On the basis of the information described above, it is possible to place blocking agents into three groups according to the mechanism of action. One group acts simply by inhibiting the activation of a carcinogen to its ultimate carcinogenic form (Fiala et al. 1977). Inhibitors of this nature are effective only against carcinogens requiring activation. A second group of blocking agents is effective by virtue of inducing increases in carcinogen-detoxification systems. This group of inhibitors is of particular interest because they have the capacity to inhibit a wide range of carcinogens. The third group of blocking agents has the capacity to act by scavenging the reactive forms of carcinogens. Inhibitors of this type are potentially effective against a very broad spectrum of carcinogenic compounds. One subgroup of scavengers of particular interest with regard to the gastrointestinal tract are high–molecular weight compounds that are not absorbed from the gastrointestinal tract. These compounds would scavenge the reactive forms of carcinogens occurring within the lumen of the alimentary tract.

Blocking agents frequently induce multiple enzymatic alterations. Two categories of such inductive effects have been identified, and it is likely that others exist as well. For purposes of further consideration, the two categories are designated type A and type B (Figure 1). The subdivisions can be understood better by considering two classes of enzyme systems proposed by Williams (1971) for the metabolism of noxious xenobiotic compounds. The two classes are termed phase I and phase II reactions. Phase I reactions introduce a polar group into

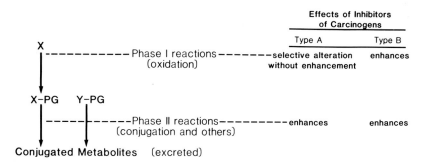

X -Xenobiotic compound lacking a polar group
X–PG -Metabolite of "X" containing a polar group
Y–PG -Xenobiotic compound containing a polar group

FIG. 1. Two categories of blocking agents enhancing a coordinated detoxification response. Butylated hydroxyanisole is an example of a type A inhibitor and β-naphthoflavone a type B inhibitor.

xenobiotic compounds. This type of reaction is most frequently carried out by the microsomal monooxygenase system. The introduction of a polar group into a xenobiotic compound provides a means by which a subsequent conjugation reaction can occur, leading to excretion. Phase II reactions, for the most part, are conjugating reactions such as formation of glucuronides, glutathione conjugates, and sulfates.

An example of a type A inhibitor is the phenolic antioxidant BHA. Coordinated detoxification reactions enhanced by BHA are shown in Figure 2. BHA is a food additive used to prevent oxidative spoilage of various dietary items. It inhibits a broad range of carcinogens under a variety of experimental conditions (Table 1). Studies of the mechanism of these inhibitions have shown that BHA produces a number of enzymatic alterations (Figure 2). Mice fed BHA for a period of 1 to 2 weeks under conditions used for carcinogen inhibition experiments show marked increases in glutathione S-transferase activity and tissue glutathione levels (Benson et al. 1978, 1979). The activity of UDP-glucuronyl transferase, a second important conjugating enzyme, is increased (Cha and Bueding 1979). BHA also causes an elevation in epoxide hydrolase activity (Benson et al. 1979, Cha et al. 1978).

An additional effect of BHA is its capacity to alter the microsomal mixed function oxidase system. This change is not accompanied by an increase in AHH activity. The alteration can be demonstrated by incubating BP with liver microsomes, cofactors required for mixed function oxidase activity, and added DNA. Under these conditions, reactive metabolites of BP bind to DNA. If liver microsomes from mice fed BHA are employed, binding of BP metabolites to DNA is approximately one-half that following incubation with control microsomes (Speier and Wattenberg 1975). High-pressure liquid chromatography (HPLC) studies of metabolites of BP occurring on incubation of BP with microsomes from mice fed BHA compared with controls likewise show changes. Two metabolic alterations are found that could result in inhibition of carcinogenesis. The first is a decrease in epoxidation of BP, which is an activation process,

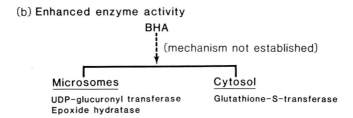

(a) Alteration in the microsomal monooxygenase system (occurs by two hours after BHA administration)

(b) Enhanced enzyme activity

BHA

(mechanism not established)

Microsomes   Cytosol
UDP-glucuronyl transferase   Glutathione-S-transferase
Epoxide hydratase

(c) Increased tissue levels of glutathione

FIG. 2. Coordinated response to a type A blocking agent.

TABLE 1. *Inhibition of carcinogen-induced neoplasia by BHA*

Carcinogen	Species	Site of neoplasm inhibited
Benzo(a)pyrene	Mouse	Lung (Wattenberg 1973)
Benzo(a)pyrene	Mouse	Forestomach (Wattenberg 1972a)
Benzo(a)pyrene-7,8-dihydrodiol	Mouse	Forestomach, lung, lymphoid tissue (Wattenberg et al. 1979)
7,12-Dimethylbenz(a)anthracene	Mouse	Lung (Wattenberg 1973)
7,12-Dimethylbenz(a)anthracene	Mouse	Forestomach (Wattenberg 1972a)
7,12-Dimethylbenz(a)anthracene	Mouse	Skin (Slaga and Bracken 1977)
7,12-Dimethylbenz(a)anthracene	Rat	Breast (Wattenberg 1972a)
7-Hydroxymethyl-12-methyl-benz(a)anthracene	Mouse	Lung (Wattenberg 1973)
Dibenz(a,h)anthracene	Mouse	Lung (Wattenberg 1973)
Diethylnitrosamine	Mouse	Lung (Wattenberg 1972b)
4-Nitroquinoline-N-oxide	Mouse	Lung (Wattenberg 1972b)
Uracil mustard	Mouse	Lung (Wattenberg 1973)
Urethane	Mouse	Lung (Wattenberg 1973)
Methylazoxymethanol acetate	Mouse	Large intestine (Wattenberg and Sparnins 1979)
trans-5-Amino-3-[2-(5-nitro-2-furyl)-vinyl]-1,2,4-oxadiazole	Mouse	Forestomach, lung, lymphoid tissue (E. Bueding, H. Dunsford, and P. Dolan, personal communication)

and the second is an increase in formation of 3-hydroxybenzo(a)pyrene, a metabolite of detoxification (Lam and Wattenberg 1977, Lam et al. 1980). Changes in microsomal metabolism of BP will occur within 2 hours after administration of BHA by oral intubation. At that time the microsomal metabolism of BP to metabolites binding to DNA has been reduced to one-half that found with microsomes from control animals, a reduction of the same order of magnitude as in mice fed BHA for a week or more (Speier et al. 1978). Changes in the BP metabolite pattern similar to those found after prolonged feeding occur 4 hours after a single dose of BHA, the earliest time interval studied. A point of importance is that no increase in the overall metabolism of BP, as determined by HPLC, occurs at any time after administration of BHA either by oral intubation or in the diet. Likewise, studies of BP metabolism determined by AHH activity do not show an increase.

Type B inhibitors induce increased microsomal monooxygenase activity. They also enhance the activity of major conjugating systems such as glutathione S-transferase and UDP-glucuronyl transferase. An increase in epoxide hydrolase activity also occurs. These inhibitors are complicated in that the microsomal monooxygenase system can both activate and detoxify chemical carcinogens. The classic example of this is with the aromatic amines. With these compounds, ring hydroxylation results in detoxification, whereas hydroxylation of the nitrogen is an activation reaction (Miller and Miller 1969). In most instances, when tested in experimental animal systems type B inhibitors have been found to inhibit chemical carcinogenesis (Wattenberg 1978a, 1978b). Presumably, the inductive effects on phase I and phase II systems enhance carcinogen detoxification overall. However, the fact that one constituent of the enzymes induced does enhance carcinogen activation makes it possible that conditions could exist in which an adverse effect occurs.

NATURALLY OCCURRING BLOCKING AGENTS IN THE DIET

Indoles

Indole-3-carbinol, 3,3'-diindolylmethane, and indole-3-acetonitrile occur in edible cruciferous vegetables such as Brussels sprouts, cabbage, cauliflower, and broccoli. These three indoles have been studied for their effects on benzo(a)pyrene (BP)- and 7,12-dimethylbenz(a)anthracene (DMBA)-induced neoplasia in rodents. When added to the diet, all three indoles inhibited BP-induced neoplasia of the forestomach. Their addition to the diet also inhibited BP-induced pulmonary adenoma formation. In other experiments, indole-3-carbinol and diindolylmethane inhibited DMBA-induced mammary tumor formation in female Sprague Dawley rats, but indole-3-acetonitrile was inactive in this experimental model (Wattenberg and Loub 1978). The original rationale for the use of the three indoles was based on their ability to alter microsomal mixed function oxidase activity. All three compounds induce increased activity of this system towards BP (designated AHH activity) and also with other substrates (Loub et al. 1975, Pantuck et al. 1976, 1979). In subsequent work, it has been found that all three indoles induce increased glutathione S-transferase activity.

Coumarins and Other Simple Lactones

The coumarins comprise an important group of natural products and are present in a variety of vegetables and fruits consumed by man (Späth 1937, Robinson 1963, Dean 1963). An initial report by Feuer et al. (1976) showed that DMBA-induced mammary tumor formation is inhibited by coumarin. Subsequently, this result was confirmed and further studies of the effects of three naturally occurring simple derivatives of coumarin have been carried out (Wattenberg et al. 1979). Additional compounds have also been investigated in order to obtain information about the relationships of chemical structure and inhibitory potency. In these studies, two animal test systems were used. The first was DMBA-induced mammary tumor formation in female Sprague Dawley rats and the second was BP-induced neoplasia of the forestomach in ICR/Ha mice. In the experiments with DMBA-mammary tumor formation, the effects of administration of coumarin and three of its derivatives, umbelliferone (7-hydroxy-coumarin), scopoletin (7-hydroxy-6-methoxycoumarin), and limettin (5,7-dimethoxycoumarin), were investigated. Coumarin was found to be a moderately potent inhibitor as demonstrated by a decrease in the number of animals bearing mammary neoplasms and the number of tumors per animal. Limettin was less effective and scopoletin had only a marginal inhibitory effect. Umbelliferone did not inhibit DMBA-induced neoplasia under the conditions employed (Wattenberg et al. 1979).

The same coumarins also have been studied to determine their capacities to inhibit BP-induced neoplasia of the mouse forestomach. Overall, the coumarins were less effective in this experimental model than in the rat mammary tumor experiments. Coumarin inhibited BP-induced neoplasia of the forestomach. Limettin, umbelliferone, and scopoletin were inactive. Several additional compounds have been studied for their effects on BP-induced neoplasia of the forestomach. Two five-membered benzolactones, 2-coumaranone and phthalide, were investigated, but neither was effective. Of four alicyclic lactones studied, only α-angelicalactone inhibited BP-induced neoplasia and was considerably more potent than coumarin. The other three, γ-valerolactone, L-ascorbic acid, and isocitric lactone, were without inhibitory effects (Wattenberg et al. 1979). Several structure-activity relationships are evident from data currently available. With the coumarins, increased polarity of substituents results in decreasing activity as inhibitors. For both the coumarins and the five-membered ring lactones studied, protic groups, such as hydroxy and carboxy groups, abolish the capacity to inhibit. While unsaturation in the lactone ring does not always lead to inhibitory activity, the presence of at least one double bond is essential. Thus, the property of inhibiting BP and DMBA is not a general characteristic of all coumarins and alicyclic lactones, but is restricted to those with specific structural features.

The mechanism or mechanisms by which the coumarins and α-angelicalactone cause inhibition of DMBA- or BP-induced neoplasia has not been established. Coumarin and α-angelicalactone, both of which are potent inhibitors of BP-induced neoplasia of the forestomach, are potent inducers of increased glutathione S-transferase activity. In contrast, umbelliferone and γ-valerolactone, which are inactive as inhibitors of BP-induced neoplasia of the forestomach, do not induce increased activity of this enzyme (Sparnins and Wattenberg 1981). Whether induction of increased glutathione S-transferase is a correlative event or substantially involved in the mechanism of inhibition remains to be determined.

Aromatic Isothiocyanates

Benzyl isothiocyanate and phenethyl isothiocyanate occur in cruciferous plants. Some of these plants, such as Brussels sprouts, cabbage, cauliflower, and brocolli, are consumed by man. The two isothiocyanates have been studied for their inhibitory effects against BP and DMBA in animal models in which neoplasia was produced in three organs, i.e., forestomach, lung, and mammary gland. In addition to the naturally occurring isothiocyanates, several synthetic compounds also have been investigated, i.e., phenyl isothiocyanate, diphenylmethyl isothiocyanate, and allyl isothiocyanate.

Benzyl isothiocyanate, phenethyl isothiocyanate, and phenyl isothiocyanate inhibit DMBA-induced neoplasia of the mammary gland in female Sprague

Dawley rats. Inhibition occurs when the isothiocyanates are administered by oral intubation 4 hours prior to DMBA. Further work on the effects on inhibition of altering the time of administration of the isothiocyanate relative to that of the carcinogen has been carried out using benzyl isothiocyanate. Inhibition is obtained when this test compound is given 2 hours prior to DMBA. Inhibition is markedly diminished when the time interval is increased to 24 hours prior to DMBA, and no inhibition occurs if the isothiocyanate is given 4 hours after the DMBA (Wattenberg 1977).

Addition of benzyl isothiocyanate or phenethyl isothiocyanate to a diet containing DMBA inhibits neoplasia of the forestomach in ICR/Ha mice. Benzyl isothiocyanate also inhibits BP-induced neoplasia of the forestomach under comparable conditions. Other experiments have been carried out with isothiocyanates added to the diet but in which BP was given by oral intubation. In this regimen, it was again found that benzyl isothiocyanate inhibited BP-induced neoplasia of the forestomach. Phenyl isothiocyanate also inhibited neoplasia, but sodium thiocyanate was inactive.

Studies of the inhibition of pulmonary neoplasia have been carried out using two experimental systems. The first entailed addition of a carcinogen and the test substance to the diet of ICR/Ha mice. Benzyl isothiocyanate inhibits DMBA-induced neoplasia of the lung under these conditions (Wattenberg 1977). A second experimental model has been employed using female A/HeJ mice. The test substance was fed in the diet, which was continued through the entire period of carcinogen administrations. Nine days after the start of the diets, the first dose of carcinogen was administered by oral intubation. Two weeks later a second dose of carcinogen was given. Twenty-four weeks after the first dose of carcinogen, mice were sacrificed and pulmonary adenomas counted. With DMBA as the carcinogen, the inhibitory capacities of the following compounds were studied: benzyl isothiocyanate, phenethyl isothiocyanate, benzyl thiocyanate, diphenylmethyl thiocyanate, phenyl thiocyanate, and allyl isothiocyanate. Results, in parenthesis, are expressed as the ratio of tumor counts in the animals receiving the test substance divided by the controls. Inhibition ($P < 0.05$ in each case) was produced by benzyl isothiocyanate (0.52), phenethyl isothiocyanate (0.64), phenyl thiocyanate (0.56), and diphenylmethyl thiocyanate (0.32). In contrast, benzyl thiocyanate (0.82) and allyl isothiocyanate (1.2) were inactive as inhibitors.

The work described above has demonstrated that the two naturally occurring isothiocyanates, benzyl isothiocyanate and phenethyl isothiocyanate, inhibit polycyclic aromatic hydrocarbon–induced neoplasia at three target sites, breast, lung, and forestomach. Two of these target sites are remote from the portal of entry of the isothiocyanates. In the case of the forestomach, there is direct contact of inhibitor and target site. The mechanism of carcinogen inhibition by these compounds has not been established. However, benzyl isothiocyanate has been found to be a highly potent inducer of glutathione S-transferase activity (Sparnins and Wattenberg 1981). This inductive effect may play a role in the inhibitory capacities of the compound.

Flavones

The study of flavones as possible inhibitors of chemical carcinogens was undertaken as a result of data that showed that a number of inducers of increased microsomal mixed function oxidase activity inhibit chemical carcinogens (Wattenberg 1978a, 1978b). In initial work, several flavones were found to induce increased AHH activity when BP was used as the substrate (Wattenberg et al. 1968). Flavone itself is a moderately potent inducer. In the compounds studied, hydroxylation reduced inducing activity, but corresponding methoxy compounds were active. The vast majority of naturally occurring flavones are polyhydroxy derivatives, and a small number contain only methoxy groups. Two of these, tangeretin (5,6,7,8,4′-pentamethoxyflavone) and nobiletin (5,6,7,8,3′4′-hexamethoxyflavone), were active inducers of increased AHH activity.

An investigation of inhibition of BP-induced carcinogenesis was carried out with three flavones. The compounds chosen for study were β-naphthoflavone (5,6-benzoflavone), quercetin pentamethyl ether, and rutin (3,3′,4′,5,7-pentahydroxyflavone-3-rutinoside). β-Naphthoflavone, a synthetic compound, is the most potent flavone found thus far in terms of its capacity to induce increased AHH activity. Quercetin pentamethyl ether is a moderately potent inducer of increased AHH activity. This synthetic compound was used as a substitute for tangeretin, which could not be obtained in sufficient quantity for carcinogen-inhibition studies. Both compounds are pentamethoxy flavones with similar inducing capacities. Rutin is a naturally occurring compound with very weak AHH-inducing activity. The three flavones were added to the diet of A/HeJ mice that subsequently were challenged with BP given by oral intubation. β-Naphthoflavone caused almost total inhibition of pulmonary adenoma formation; quercetin pentamethyl ether reduced the number of these neoplasms by half. The number of adenomas present in animals fed rutin and the control diet was the same. Thus, the inhibitory effects on BP-induced neoplasia paralleled the potency of the three flavones in inducing increased AHH activity (Wattenberg and Leong 1970). β-Naphthoflavone has been recently shown to induce increased glutathione S-transferase activity. Comparable studies with the other flavones have not been reported. In further experiments in which the only flavone employed was β-naphthoflavone, it inhibited DMBA-induced mammary tumor formation in the rat and BP-initiated epidermal neoplasia in the mouse (Wattenberg and Leong 1968, 1970).

Phenols

Investigations of the inhibitory effects of butylated hydroxyanisole (BHA) have been carried out with a number of chemical carcinogens as described previously. This antioxidant is of interest in that it is widely employed as a food additive. Inhibition occurs under a variety of experimental conditions and with a broad range of carcinogens. Structure-activity studies have been carried out to ascertain the structural features of phenols that determine their inhibitory capacities. Included in this work were three naturally occurring phenols, o-hydroxycinnamic acid, 3,4-dihydroxycinnamic acid (caffeic acid), and 4-hydroxy-3-methoxycinnamic acid (ferulic acid). All three inhibited BP-induced neoplasia of the mouse forestomach (Wattenberg et al. 1980). These data are of interest in that a large number of phenols exist in plants, including those used as food by man.

INDUCTION OF INCREASED GLUTATHIONE S-TRANSFERASE ACTIVITY AS A PARAMETER FOR SELECTING PUTATIVE INHIBITORS OF CHEMICAL CARCINOGENESIS

Glutathione S-transferase has been studied extensively as a major detoxification system; it catalyzes the binding of a vast variety of electrophiles to the sulfhydryl group of glutathione (Jacoby 1978, Chasseaud 1979). Since the reactive ultimate carcinogenic forms of chemical carcinogens are electrophiles, glutathione S-transferase takes on considerable importance as a mechanism for carcinogen detoxification. Enhancement of the activity of this system could increase the capacity of the organism to withstand the neoplastic effects of chemical carcinogens.

The effects on glutathione S-transferase activity of a number of compounds previously investigated for their capacity to inhibit BP-induced neoplasia of the mouse forestomach have been determined. Five of the compounds studied caused increases in glutathione S-transferase activity of the forestomach of between 78% and 182%. The five compounds are p-methoxyphenol, 2-tert-butyl-4-hydroxyanisole, coumarin, α-angelicalactone, and benzyl isothiocyanate. Increases in acid-soluble sulfhydryl levels also were observed, except with benzyl isothiocyanate, but were of a lesser magnitude. All five chemicals inhibit BP-induced neoplasia of the forestomach. These data indicate that enhancement of the glutathione S-transferase activity by 75% or greater in the forestomach is associated with a reduced carcinogenic response of that organ to BP (Sparnins and Wattenberg 1981). The data also suggest that such enhancement might be used to identify compounds likely to inhibit BP and other carcinogens detoxified in a similar manner. Since inhibition of the action of carcinogens may involve mechanisms other than detoxification by glutathione S-transferase, the failure to increase glutathione S-transferase activity substantially does not rule out the possibility that a compound is an inhibitor.

The effects of the type of diet and of specific dietary constituents on glutathione S-transferase activity have been studied. The glutathione S-transferase activity is significantly higher in tissues of animals fed crude diets than with those fed purified diets. Diets containing large quantities of cruciferous vegetables induce increased glutathione S-transferase activity (Sparnins 1980). As an extension of the investigation of induction of increased glutathione S-transferase activity by plant materials, a number of different beans were studied. This work lead to the observation that green coffee beans are quite remarkable in the magnitude of induction of glutathione S-transferase that they produce. Consumption by mice of a diet containing green coffee beans enhances the glutathione S-transferase activity of liver sixfold and of small bowel mucosa sevenfold (Sparnins et al. 1981). Inducing activity is found with roasted coffee beans, commercial instant coffee, and instant decaffeinated coffee. It is considerably less than in the unprocessed green coffee beans, indicating that some destruction of inducing compounds has occurred. The constituents of green coffee beans active as inducers of increased glutathione S-transferase activity are extracted into nonpolar solvents. Studies aimed at their identification are in progress. Powdered black tea leaves in the diet also enhance glutathione S-transferase activity.

DISCUSSION

This chapter has dealt largely with one facet of the overall protective systems against chemical carcinogens, namely blocking agents occurring in food. There has now been identified a substantial number of dietary constituents having the capacity to inhibit the neoplastic effects of chemical carcinogens. Evidence indicating that dietary inhibitors of carcinogenesis do play a role in man is of three types: the nature of the inhibitory compounds, the mechanisms of inhibition, and epidemiological data.

The inhibitors found thus far are very diverse in chemical structure and are widely distributed in the environment. The chemical diversity makes it likely that other inhibitors exist that have not yet been identified. Diversity and wide distribution are factors enhancing the probability that inhibitors have an impact on man. The second type of supporting evidence is the nature of the mechanisms of inhibition. A considerable amount of data indicates that many inhibitors are effective by virtue of enhancing host detoxification systems. These systems have been discussed in previous sections. An important characteristic of the detoxification pathways is that their activities can be changed by xenobiotic compounds occurring in the environment (Wattenberg 1970, 1978b).

Epidemiological data support the likelihood that inhibitors in the environment protect against neoplasia. An apparent protective effect of consumption of vegetables against several common cancers, particularly those of the alimentary tract, has been found. Vegetables are a source of many inhibitors of chemical carcinogens since they contain phenols, coumarins, aromatic isothiocyanates, and indoles. Cruciferous vegetables such as cabbage, Brussels sprouts, and cauliflower are a particularly rich source of known inhibitors. One of the most dramatic epidemiological investigations was a case-control study by Saxon Graham and co-workers (1978), which showed an inverse correlation between the magnitude of consumption of cabbage and the occurrence of cancer of the colon. The relative risk in individuals with the highest consumption of cabbage as compared to those with little or no intake of this vegetable is about one-third. In a second study, an analysis of risk factors for lung cancer in Singapore Chinese has shown that the relative risk was less in those consuming mustard greens and kale regularly than in those who ate them infrequently (MacLennan et al. 1977). Several investigations have been published in which an inverse relationship has been found between magnitude of consumption of other vegetables, including lettuce, celery, and tomatoes, and cancer of the stomach or precursor lesions in that organ (Haenszel et al. 1972, 1976). The reduced incidence of cancer in Seventh-Day Adventists, a group with a vegetarian diet, is well documented and is in accord with the above (Phillips 1975).

The group of epidemiological studies cited are of interest because of the occurrence of inhibitors of chemical carcinogenesis in vegetables. However, the results of these studies cannot be considered conclusive. Investigations have not been carried out in man to determine whether the relatively high consumption of vegetables has actually enhanced the effectiveness of protective systems against chemical carcinogens in the individuals at risk in epidemiological studies carried out thus far. Obtaining quantitative data of this nature is critical for establishing firmly a relationship between dietary factors and risk. High intake of cruciferous vegetables has been shown to alter metabolism of xenobiotic compounds in man in work carried out under carefully controlled conditions (Pantuck et al. 1979). However, these investigations have been limited and require expansion.

ACKNOWLEDGMENTS

Investigations included in this presentation were supported by Public Health Service Grants CA-09599, CA-15638, CA-14146, and Contracts NO1-CP-05605 and NO1-CP-85613 from the National Cancer Institute.

REFERENCES

Benson, A. M., R. P. Batzinger, S. L. Ou, E. Bueding, Y. N. Cha, and P. Talalay. 1978. Elevation of hepatic glutathione S-transferase activities and protection against mutagenic metabolites by dietary antioxidants. Cancer Res. 12:4486–4495.

Benson, A. M., Y. N. Cha, E. Bueding, H. S. Heine, and P. Talalay. 1979. Elevation of extrahepatic glutathione S-transferase and epoxide hydratase activities by 2(3)-tert-butyl-4-hydroxyanisole. Cancer Res. 39:2971–2977.

Cha, Y. N., and E. Bueding. 1979. Effects of 2(3)-tert-butyl-4-hydroxyanisole administration on the activities of several hepatic microsomal and cytoplasmic enzymes in mice. Biochem. Pharmacol. 28:1917–1921.

Cha, Y. N., F. Martz, and E. Bueding. 1978. Enhancement of liver microsome epoxide hydratase activity in rodents by treatment with 2(3)-tert-butyl-4-hydroxyanisole. Cancer Res. 38:4496–4498.

Chasseaud, L. F. 1979. The role of glutathione and glutathione S-transferases in the metabolism of chemical carcinogens and other electrophilic agents. Adv. Cancer Res. 29:175–274.

Dean, F. M. 1963. Naturally Occurring Oxygen Ring Compounds. Butterworths, London, pp. 176–219.

Feuer, G., J. A. Kellen, and K. Kovacs. 1976. Suppression of 7,12-dimethylbenz(a)anthracene-induced breast carcinoma by coumarin in the rat. Oncology 33:35–39.

Fiala, E. S., G. Bobotas, C. Kulakis, L. W. Wattenberg, and J. H. Weisburger. 1977. The effects of disulfiram and related compounds on the in vivo metabolism of the colon carcinogen 1,2-dimethylhydrazine. Biochem. Pharmacol. 26:1763–1768.

Graham, S., H. Dayai, M. Swanson, A. Mittelman, and G. Wilkinson. 1978. Diet in the epidemiology of cancer of the colon and rectum. JNCI 61:709–714.

Haenszel, W., P. Correa, C. Cuello, N. Guzman, L. Burbano, H. Lores, and J. Munoz. 1976. Gastric cancer in Columbia: Case control epidemiological study of precursor lesions. JNCI 57:1021–1026.

Haenszel, W., M. Kurihara, M. Segi, and R. K. C. Lee. 1972. Stomach cancer among Japanese in Hawaii. JNCI 49:969–988.

Jakoby, W. B. 1978. The glutathione S-transferases: A group of multifunctional detoxification proteins. Adv. Enzymol. 46:383–414.

Lam, L. K. T., A. V. Fladmoe, J. B. Hochalter, and L. W. Wattenberg. 1980. Short-time interval effects of butylated hydroxyanisole on the metabolism of benzo(a)pyrene. Cancer Res. 40:2824–2828.

Lam, L. K. T., and L. W. Wattenberg. 1977. Effects of butylated hydroxyanisole on the metabolism of benzo(a)pyrene by mouse liver microsomes. JNCI 58:413–417.

Loub, W. D., L. W. Wattenberg, and D. W. Davis. 1975. Aryl hydrocarbon hydroxylase induction in rat tissues by naturally-occurring indoles of cruciferous plants. JNCI 54:985–988.

MacLennan, R., J. DaCosta, N. E. Day, C. H. Law, Y. K. Ng, and K. Shanmugaratnam. 1977. Risk factors for lung cancer in Singapore Chinese, a population with high female incidence rates. Int. J. Cancer 20:854–860.

Matsushima, T. 1982. Mechanisms of conversion of food components to mutagens and carcinogens, in Molecular Interrelations of Nutrition and Cancer (Proceedings of The University of Texas System Cancer Center 34th Annual Symposium on Fundamental Cancer Research, 1981), M. S. Arnott, J. van Eys, and Y.-M. Wang, eds. Raven Press, New York, pp. 35–42.

Miller, E. C. 1978. Some current perspectives on chemical carcinogenesis in human and experimental animals. Cancer Res. 38:1479–1496.

Miller, J. A., and E. C. Miller. 1969. The metabolic activation of carcinogenic aromatic amines and amides. Prog. Exp. Tumor Res. 11:273–301.

Pantuck, E. J., K. C. Hsiao, W. D. Loub, L. W. Wattenberg, R. Kuntzman, and A. H. Conney. 1976. Stimulatory effect of vegetables on intestinal drug metabolism in the rat. J. Pharm. Exper. Therap. 198:277–283.

Pantuck, E. J., C. B. Pantuck, W. A. Garland, B. Mins, L. W. Wattenberg, K. E. Anderson, A. Kappas, and A. H. Conney. 1979. Effects of dietary Brussels sprouts and cabbage on human drug metabolism. Clin. Pharmacol. Ther. 25:88–95.

Phillips, R.L. 1975. Role of life-style and dietary habits in risk of cancer among Seventh-Day Adventists. Cancer Res. 35:3513–3522.

Robinson, T. 1963. The Organic Constituents of Higher Plants. Burgess Publishing Co., Minneapolis, pp. 45–69.

Slaga, T. J., and W. M. Bracken. 1977. The effects of antioxidants on skin tumor initiation and aryl hydrocarbon hydroxylase. Cancer Res. 37:1631–1635.

Sparnins, V. L. 1980. Effects of dietary constituents on glutathione S-transferase activity. (Abstract) Proceedings of the American Association for Cancer Research 21:80.

Sparnins, V. L., L. K. T. Lam, and L. W. Wattenberg. 1981. Effects of coffee on glutathione S-transferase activity and 7,12-dimethylbenz(a)anthracene-induced neoplasia. (Abstract) Proceedings of the American Association for Cancer Research 22:114.

Sparnins, V. L., and L. W. Wattenberg. 1981. Enhancement of glutathione S-transferase activity of the mouse forestomach by inhibitors of benzo(a)pyrene-induced neoplasia of this anatomic site. JNCI 66:769–771.

Späth, E. 1937. Die naturlichen cumarine. Berichte der Deutschen Chemischen Gesellschaft 70:83–117.

Speier, J. L., L. K. T. Lam, and L. W. Wattenberg. 1978. Effects of administration to mice of butylated hydroxyanisole by oral intubation on benzo(a)pyrene-induced pulmonary adenoma formation and metabolism of benzo(a)pyrene. JNCI 60:605–609.

Speier, J. L., and L. W. Wattenberg. 1975. Alterations in microsomal metabolism of benzo(a)pyrene in mice fed butylated hydroxyanisole. JNCI 55:469–472.

Sporn, M.B., and D. L. Newton. 1980. Recent advances in the use of retinoids for cancer prevention, in Cancer: Achievements, Challenges and Prospects for the 1980's, J. H. Burchenal, ed. Grune and Stratton, New York, pp. 541–548.

Stich, H. F. 1981. Intake, formation and release of mutagens by man, in Carcinogens and Mutagen Formation in the Gastrointestinal Tract, R. Bruce and M. Lipkin, eds. Cold Spring Harbor Press, New York (in press).

Sugimura, T. 1982. Tumor initiators and promoters associated with ordinary foods, *in* Molecular Interrelations of Nutrition and Cancer (Proceedings of The University of Texas System Cancer Center 34th Annual Symposium on Fundamental Cancer Research, 1981), M. S. Arnott, J. van Eys, and Y.-M. Wang, eds. Raven Press, New York, pp. 3–24.

Troll, W. 1980. Blocking of tumor promotion by protease inhibitors, *in* Cancer: Achievements, Challenges and Prospects for the 1980's, J. H. Burchenal, ed. Grune and Stratton, New York, pp. 549–556.

Wattenberg, L. W. 1970. The role of the portal of entry in inhibition of tumorigenesis. Prog. Exp. Tumor Res. 14:89–104.

Wattenberg, L. W. 1972a. Inhibition of carcinogenic and toxic effects of polycyclic hydrocarbons by phenolic antioxidants and ethoxyquin. JNCI 48:1425–1430.

Wattenberg, L. W. 1972b. Inhibition of carcinogenic effects of diethylnitrosamine and 4-nitroquinoline-N-oxide by antioxidants. Fed. Proc. 31:633.

Wattenberg, L. W. 1973. Inhibition of chemical carcinogen-induced pulmonary neoplasia by butylated hydroxyanisole. JNCI 50:1541–1544.

Wattenberg, L. W. 1977. Inhibition of carcinogenic effects of polycyclic hydrocarbons by benzyl isothiocyanate and related compounds.

Wattenberg, L. W. 1978a. Inhibition of chemical carcinogenesis. JNCI 60:11–18.

Wattenberg, L. W. 1978b. Inhibitors of chemical carcinogens. Adv. Cancer Res. 26:197–226.

Wattenberg, L. W. 1980. Inhibitors of chemical carcinogens, *in* Cancer: Achievements, Challenges and Prospects for the 1980's, J. H. Burchenal, ed. Grune and Stratton, New York, pp. 517–539.

Wattenberg, L. W. 1981. Inhibition of carcinogen-induced neoplasia by sodium cyanate, *tert*-butyl isocyanate and benzyl isothiocyanate administered subsequent to carcinogen exposure. Cancer Res. 41:2991–2994.

Wattenberg, L. W., J. B. Coccia, and L. K. T. Lam. 1980. Inhibitory effects of phenolic compounds on benzo(a)pyrene-induced neoplasia. Cancer Res. 40:2820–2823.

Wattenberg, L. W., D. M. Jerina, L. K. T. Lam, and H. Yagi. 1979. Neoplastic effects of oral administration of (±)-trans-7,8-dihydrobenzo(a)pyrene and their inhibition by butylated hydroxyanisole. JNCI 62:1103–1106.

Wattenberg, L. W., L. K. T. Lam, and A. Fladmoe. 1979. Inhibition of chemical carcinogen-induced neoplasia by coumarins and α-angelicalactone. Cancer Res. 39:1651–1654.

Wattenberg, L. W., and J. L. Leong. 1968. Inhibition of the carcinogenic action of 7,12-dimethylbenz(a)anthracene by β-naphthoflavone. Proc. Soc. Exp. Biol. Med. 128:940–943.

Wattenberg, L. W., and J. L. Leong. 1970. Inhibition of the carcinogenic action of benzo(a)pyrene by flavones. Cancer Res. 30:1922–1925.

Wattenberg, L. W., and W. D. Loub. 1978. Inhibition of polycyclic hydrocarbon-induced neoplasia by naturally-occurring indoles. Cancer Res. 38:1410–1413.

Wattenberg, L. W., M. A. Page, and J. L. Leong. 1968. Induction of increased benzopyrene hydroxylase activity by flavones and related compounds. Cancer Res. 28:934–937.

Wattenberg, L. W., and V. L. Sparnins. 1979. Inhibitory effects of butylated hydroxyanisole on methylazoxymethanol acetate-induced neoplasia of the large intestine and on nicotinamide adenine dinucleotide-dependent alcohol dehydrogenase activity in mice. JNCI 63:219–222.

Williams, R. T. 1971. Pathways of drug metabolism, *in* Handbook of Experimental Pharmacology, vol. 28. Springer-Verlag, New York, pp. 226–249.

Molecular Interrelations of Nutrition and Cancer,
edited by M. S. Arnott, J. van Eys, and Y.-M. Wang.
Raven Press, New York © 1982.

On Early Measures of the Effects of Diet Change with Relation to Cancer Incidence

W. Robert Bruce

Department of Medical Biophysics, University of Toronto, and Ludwig Institute for Cancer Research, Toronto Branch, Toronto, Ontario, Canada

Although epidemiological evidence points to the importance of dietary factors in the causation of many cancers (Higginson 1977, Wynder and Gori 1977, Armstrong and Doll 1975), it is not obvious how this information should be used for cancer prevention. In the case of colon cancer, for instance, epidemiological evidence points to the risk of Western diets that are high in fat and meat and low in fiber. While it would be possible to test the effect of a vegetarian, low-fat, high-fiber diet on the incidence of colon cancer, a problem with such a test would be the expense; it would require 10 or more years to complete and it would require the help of many thousands of volunteers (Bruce et al. 1981). But a more serious problem with such a test would be that it would give only a yes or no answer; it would not lead to any further understanding of the defect in the Western diet or how it could be most simply corrected. Less cumbersome intervention studies are needed. They could be developed if we had a more complete understanding of the events that lead from diet to disease. They would make it possible to test many hypotheses rapidly and with fewer individuals. But before such intervention studies can be designed, it is necessary to define the key events that lie between diet and cancer.

The events that lie between diet and disease are of three different classes. The first are the chemical events. Presumably the diet leads, in some at present unknown way, to carcinogenic or promoting or toxic chemicals in the body. It should be possible to determine the nature of these chemicals and how they are related to diet. The second are the cellular events. The chemical events may lead to effects in cells—to mutations, to chromosome aberrations, to death, or to other unknown effects. It should be possible to determine how diet affects the genotype and phenotype of cells of the target organ. The third are the tissue events. The diet may lead to the development of polyps, ulcers, cysts, or other pathology that might be thought of as precursors to cancer itself. Again, it should be possible to determine whether diet has an effect on these precursor lesions long before the appearance of frank malignancy.

Over the past few years, we have developed a number of methods for assessing the effect of environment (diet) on chemical, cellular, and tissue events in the colon. These methods are by no means the only ones that have been studied (a recent meeting of the Large Bowel Cancer Program was replete with examples), but the methods do give a picture of the possibilities for less cumbersome intervention studies for cancer prevention.

CHEMICAL EVENTS

Most chemical studies relating diet and cancer start with an agent that is defined chemically and proceed to determine whether the agent is important from a biological point of view. The short-term assays for chemical carcinogens (McCann et al. 1975, IARC 1980) make it possible to start the other way around, with agents that are defined biologically, and to determine the chemical nature of the agent later. Thus, it is practical to start by screening the contents of the body fluids for agents that are putative carcinogens (Bruce et al. 1977, 1981) and to find how the concentration of these agents is affected by diet and is related to cancer before determining their structure.

We have examined the contents of the colon for compounds that are mutagenic, using the *Salmonella* test system (Bruce et al. 1977), and have found that many individuals have fecal mutagens. A frequent mutagen, one that is active on TA-100 without S-9 activation (Bruce et al. 1979), is present in about 40% of individuals consuming Western diets, but is found less frequently in the feces of Africans on such diets (Ehrich et al. 1979). Presumably, the frequency of the fecal mutagen reflects dietary differences between the populations.

In an effort to determine which dietary factors might be responsible for differences in the mutagen levels in the populations, we have carried out a number of diet studies both with individuals and groups (Bruce and Dion 1980, Dion and Bruce, manuscript in preparation) that have shown that ascorbic acid, α-tocopherol, and bran fiber reduce the level of these mutagens as measured in the mutagen assay. We do not know whether the result—a fourfold reduction of the mutagen active on TA-100—will be exceeded in longer studies or whether such a reduction will be observed with other mutagens. Nevertheless, the studies do show that the levels of mutagens in feces can be affected by diet.

It seems likely that cells of the colon are exposed to many carcinogens and that the structures of many of these compounds have not yet been imagined. There are probably many mutagens that arise from food, are generated in digestion, and are produced by the gut bacteria. Ascertaining the relationship of each of these to diet and to disease will take some time. Purifying and identifying each will take longer.

CELLULAR EVENTS

It may be possible to circumvent some of the complexity of chemical studies by examining cellular events in carcinogenesis. As the cellular events leading to cancer become defined it may become possible to study the effect of diet on these phenomena rather than on the carcinogens themselves.

We have recently described the feasibility of scoring for the genetic effects of colon carcinogens directly on colonic cells of the body (Goldberg and Bruce 1981). The micronucleus method, developed by Schmidt (1973) and Heddle (1973) for studies of bone marrow cells was applied to the colonic epithelium. In this method, the mutagenic event assessed is the chromosome aberration. A fraction of such aberrations result in chromosomes and chromosomal fragments failing to join the daughter cell nuclei and appearing as micronuclei. Preliminary experiments show that micronuclei may be seen in the cells of the colonic epithelium following an exposure to the colon carcinogen dimethylhydrazine. It remains to be seen whether this assay. or other assays for measuring the early cellular effects of a carcinogen, can be sufficiently sensitive to quantitate the damage occurring to human colonic cells from the Western diet. If these assays can be developed, they will be a great help in defining advantageous changes to our diet.

TISSUE EVENTS

Histological changes leading to malignancy could provide another important method for studying the link between diet and disease. For instance, adenomatous polyps are frequently seen in the colons of individuals consuming a Western diet (Correa 1978). They may be associated with carcinomas and, indeed, an adenocarcinoma sequence has been suggested (Muto et al. 1975). These observations make it feasible to use the appearance of colonic polyps as a measure of effectiveness of a dietary intervention. We have described such a study in which the intervention was ascorbic acid and α-tocopherol (Bruce et al. 1981). It is proceeding with few technical difficulties at 2 years and is being followed with studies of other dietary variables. As more information on earlier histological changes associated with the development of polyps become known, it may well be possible to use earlier precursors as end points in these diet studies.

Thus, while it could be difficult to carry out intervention studies that relate diet to cancer directly, these three examples show that it may be possible to relate diet to chemical, cellular, and tissue events that lead to cancer. Dietary factors may be related to the presence or absence of mutagens, to the appearance of chromosomal aberrations, and to the appearance of colonic polyps. Which of these events will it be most useful to follow? It is likely that these approaches will complement each other. A study that demonstrates a dietary change that leads to a reduction in colonic polyps would be of immediate relevance. But the result would only lead to a limited understanding of the mechanism of carcinogenesis. Studies of the chemical or cellular events would potentially lead to a better understanding of mechanism but they could be of less relevance. Clearly a range of talents and approaches are needed to understand the relationship between diet and cancer.

REFERENCES

Armstrong, B., and R. Doll. 1975. Environmental factors and cancer incidence and mortality in different countries with special reference to dietary practices. Int. J. Cancer, 15:617–631.

Bruce, W. R., and P. W. Dion. 1980. Studies relating to a fecal mutagen. Am. J. Clin. Nutr. 33:2511–2512.

Bruce, W. R., G. M. Eyssen, A. Ciampi, P. W. Dion, and N. Boyd. 1981. Strategies for dietary intervention studies in colon cancer. Cancer 47:1121–1125.

Bruce, W. R., A. J. Varghese, R. Furrer, and P. C. Land. 1977. A mutagen in human feces, *in* Origins of Human Cancer, H. H. Hiatt, J. D. Watson, and J. A. Winsten, eds. Cold Spring Harbor Laboratories, New York, pp. 1641–1644.

Bruce, W. R., A. J. Varghese, P. C. Land, and J. F. J. Krepinsky. 1981. Properties of a mutagen isolated from feces, *in* Gastrointestinal Cancer: Endogenous Factors, W. R. Bruce, P. Correa, M. Lipkin, and S. R. Tannenbaum, eds. Cold Spring Harbor Laboratories, Cold Spring Harbor, New York, pp. 227–234.

Bruce, W. R., A. J. Varghese, S. Wang, and P. Dion. 1979. The endogenous production of nitroso compounds in the colon and cancer at that site, *in* Naturally Occurring Carcinogens-Mutagens and Modulators of Carcinogenesis, E. C. Miller, J. A. Miller, I. Hirono, T. Sugimura, and S. Takayama, eds. Japan Science Society Press, Tokyo, pp. 221–228.

Correa, P. 1978. Epidemiology of polyps and cancer, *in* The Pathogenesis of Colorectal Cancer, B. C. Morson, ed. W. B. Saunders Company, Philadelphia, London, Toronto, pp. 126–152.

Ehrich, M., J. E. Aswell, R. L. Van Tassell, and T. D. Wilkins. 1979. Mutagens in the feces of 3 South-African populations at different levels of risk for colon cancer. Mutat. Res. 64:231–240.

Goldberg, M. T., and W. R. Bruce. 1981. A micronucleus test for colon mutagens. (Abstract) Environmental Mutagen Society, Annual Meeting, San Diego, p. 54.

Heddle, J. A. 1973. A rapid *in vivo* test for chromosomal damage. Mutat. Res. 18:187–190.

Higginson, J., and C. S. Muir, 1977. Determination de l'importance des factors environmentaux dans le cancer human: Role de l'epidemiologie. Bull. Cancer 64:365–384.

International Agency for Research on Cancer. 1980. Long-Term and Short-Term Screening Assays for Carcinogens: A Critical Appraisal, IARC Monographs, Supplement 2. IARC, Lyons, France.

McCann, J., E. Choi, E. Yamasaki, and B. N. Ames. 1975. Detection of carcinogens as mutagens in the *Salmonella*/microsome test: Assay of 300 chemicals. Proc. Natl. Acad. Sci. USA 72:5135–5139.

Muto, T., J. R. Bussey, and B. C. Morson. 1975. The evolution of cancer of the colon and rectum. Cancer 36:2251–2270.

Schmidt, W. 1973. Chemical mutagen testing in vivo somatic mammalian cell. Agents Actions 3:77–85.

Wynder, W. L., and G. B. Gori. 1977. Contribution of the environment to cancer incidence: An epidemiologic exercise. JNCI 58:825–832.

Molecular Interrelations of Nutrition and Cancer,
edited by M. S. Arnott, J. van Eys, and Y.-M. Wang.
Raven Press, New York © 1982.

Carcinogenesis of Endocrine-Related Human Cancers: Interactions of Diet and Nutrition with the Endocrine System

Mortimer B. Lipsett

Clinical Center, National Institutes of Health, Bethesda, Maryland

Epidemiologists have pointed out the significant associations of cancers of the breast, endometrium, and prostate with obesity and dietary habits (Armstrong and Doll 1975). The incidence of breast cancer has been correlated with ponderosity (DeWaard 1975), and endometrial cancer and obesity have similarly been associated (Wynder et al. 1966). The correlations internationally among incidence rates of breast, endometrial, and prostrate cancer (Berg 1975) strengthen the hypothesis that there is a common factor, environmentally determined, that promotes cancer in these organs.

When these associations have been examined closely with respect to dietary constituents, total fat in the diet has been shown to be higher in women with breast cancer (Miller et al. 1978, Carroll 1980). In prostatic cancer, the fat intake was positively correlated with mortality (Wynder et al. 1971) and a similar relation to incidence was suggested by Blair and Fraumeni (1978). It has been often stated that the fat content of the diet is only one index of such parameters as socioeconomic status, life style, protein intake, food additives, and others. Nevertheless, even with the many known and unknown factors that can be correlated with incidence rates of endocrine-related cancers, it is meaningful to look to those associations where there is independent biologic evidence for a cause and effect relationship.

Berenblum (1978) has summarized the possible types of promoter effects of hormones, and evidence for these effects in humans has been reviewed (Lipsett 1979). Since the effects of nutrition on hormonal levels are small, though appreciable, one would expect the greatest effect of diet to be apparent during periods of declining hormone secretion, that is, after the menopause in women and late in life in men. The direct relation of obesity to endometrial cancer can only be demonstrated for postmenopausal endometrial cancer; the evidence for breast and prostate cancer is less convincing.

Diet and nutritional status have the potential of affecting endocrine gland function in many ways. They can alter not only the secretory rate of those steroid hormones acting at endocrine-dependent tissues, but they may also affect the hormones that regulate steroid hormone secretion. The production of protein growth substances may be dependent on caloric intake. The rates and routes of metabolism of the steroid hormones are affected by nutritional status. Even the action of the hormones may be modified by diet, since both peptide and steroid hormone receptor capacity can vary with many types of stimuli. In the subsequent discussion, I shall attempt to bring together the roles of diet and nutritional status for those endocrine functions pertinent to the hormone-sensitive cancers rather than focusing on specific hormone-cancer relationships.

RECEPTORS

It is now well accepted that receptors for polypeptide hormones are not fixed in number but vary widely in response to many environmental states. Since prolactin has been shown to be the important hormone for the growth of the dimethylbenz(a)anthracene(DMBA)-induced rat mammary tumor, and hepatic prolactin receptors have been shown to vary with hormonal stimuli, it was necessary to examine prolactin receptors in mammary cancer. The prolactin receptor content of the DMBA rat mammary tumor was reduced in animals with uncontrolled diabetes and increased by insulin administration (Smith et al. 1977). Thus, a lipogenic hormone has the capacity to increase the action of prolactin and thereby further the growth of the DMBA rat mammary tumor. Unsaturated fats have been shown to increase prolactin receptor content of the DMBA tumor (K. K. Carroll, personal communication). Prolactin itself has been shown to modulate estrogen receptor content, although estrogen may not influence the growth of this tumor (Arafah et al. 1980). In the DMBA system, prolactin produced a fourfold increase in tumor estrogen receptors, whereas uterine cytosol receptors were unchanged (Vignon and Rochefort 1976). Additional studies in the same system (Arafah et al. 1980) confirmed that prolactin given after hypophysectomy maintained tumor estrogen receptors. Thus, the specificity of the action of prolactin on estrogen receptors, as well as the magnitude of the effect, suggest that in this tumor system the interactions between estrogen and prolactin receptors may be an important variable.

It should be pointed out that although the evidence is excellent that prolactin is the important growth-promoting hormone for the DMBA-induced rat mammary tumor, there is little reason to believe that prolactin has a similar role in human beings, since epidemiologic studies of populations with presumptive high plasma prolactin levels have not revealed any increase in risk (Lipsett 1979, Labarthe and O'Fallon 1980). However, in primates, growth hormone is a potent lactogen as shown by its effects in organ culture using α-lactalbumin synthesis as the index of potency (Kleinberg and Todd 1980). In human breast cancer, then, one should be examining the roles of growth hormone and growth hormone receptors as well as those of prolactin.

Insulin has had variable effects on the level of estrogen receptors, and these have varied with the cell system. Hilf and his collaborators have reported that estrogen receptor content in DMBA tumor cells decreased with diabetes, coincident with regression of the tumors (Hilf et al. 1978, Shafie and Hilf 1978). Insulin reversed this process. Of interest was the finding that in the diabetic rats, some tumors continued to grow and maintained their estrogen receptor levels, suggesting that other growth substances (see below) are significant for some tumors. In the human breast cancer cell line MCF-7, the numbers of estrogen receptor sites were threefold greater in cells grown in the absence of insulin (Butler et al. 1981). Further, the insulin-induced receptor decrease correlated with a decreased sensitivity to estrogens and antiestrogens. At this point in our knowledge, it is less significant that estrogen receptor content moved in different directions in response to insulin lack in different experimental systems; it is more important that they can vary with the metabolic state.

PROMOTER EFFECTS

Given these findings, it is necessary to examine the relevance of the changes in receptors produced by prolactin to the promoter effect of obesity or a high fat intake. Several groups have shown that a high fat diet increases the incidence of DMBA-induced mammary tumors (Chan and Cohen 1974) and that it increases the proestrous serum prolactin level in these rats (Chan et al. 1975). There is even a suggestion that similar dietary changes may increase serum prolactin in humans (Hill and Wynder 1976). As in rats, the increase was noted only over a relatively short period of time.

The role of prolactin in the DMBA-induced rat mammary tumor would seem to be that of a conditioning agent (Berenblum 1978) rather than of a preparative or permissive agent. This can be concluded because pregnancy, with its increased secretion of prolactin, inhibits the carcinogenic effect of DMBA (Dao 1969), and prolactin acts as a promoter only when given after DMBA (Welsch and Meites 1978). The hormone that stimulates growth of mammary duct epithelium is estradiol, and in women it is this hormone that can be linked with those known risk factors for breast cancer that increase the length of exposure to estrogen, such as early menarche, late menopause (MacMahon et al. 1973), and estrogen administration to ovariectomized or postmenopausal women (Hoover et al. 1976).

If it is accepted that hormones are promoters of carcinogenesis, then if a high-fat diet acts via the endocrine glands, the diet should have a promoter effect. Carroll and Khor (1970) examined the role of high- and low-fat diets on initiation or enhancement of the DMBA-induced mammary tumor. The high-fat diet was effective only after DMBA had been given; thus, initiation was unaffected and only promoter activity was seen. This is consistent with the fat-hormone-promoter hypothesis. Ip (1980) confirmed that fat acted preferentially at the promoter phase of carcinogenesis and that this occurred irrespective of the age of the animal; however, in contrast to the earlier findings, he noted that feeding a high-fat diet prior to administration of DMBA increased the rate of tumor induction. Ip suggested that the high-fat diet created a favorable milieu for the action of DMBA. Ip and co-workers (1980) also showed that a high-fat diet had an effect independent of prolactin levels. It is important to examine the effects of a high-fat diet on prolactin receptors, as a high-fat diet is not only an effective promoter of DMBA-induced mammary tumors but also acts similarly with another carcinogen in three different strains of rats (Chan and Dao 1981).

SECRETION AND PRODUCTION RATES

Steroid Hormones

Evidence has just been quoted that a high-fat diet augments prolactin secretion; obesity, per se, can affect hypothalamic function, thereby inducing a number of significant changes in the hormonal milieu. Massive obesity is associated with impaired regulation of prolactin and growth hormone secretion in humans (Kopelman et al. 1979). Possibly more significant than these observations, though, is the association of obesity with anovulatory menstrual cycles due to disturbed hypothalamic-pituitary regulation of gonadotropin secretion. Anovulation presents the hormonal picture of continuous estrogen effect unopposed by progesterone, since corpus luteum function does not occur. Premenopausal women with anovulatory cycles have a higher incidence of endometrial cancer; these data and the biology of the development of endometrial cancer have been reviewed recently (Lipsett 1979). In breast cancer, Korenman (1980) has suggested that an unopposed estrogen effect renders the breast epithelium more susceptible to the carcinogenic event and has marshalled the evidence for this. And, finally, decreasing age of menarche attributable to good nutrition (Frisch and MacArthur 1974) has increased the number of years of ovarian function and, *pari passu,* the incidence of breast cancer (Paffenbarger et al. 1980, Choi et al. 1978). The recent association of obesity with early menarche (Sherman et al. 1981) further strengthens the link to breast cancer.

Hormones are *secreted* by the endocrine glands and are *produced* in peripheral tissues by the metabolism of closely related precursors. This peripheral production is particularly significant for the estrogens in older men and in postmenopausal women. After menopause, the ovary ceases to secrete estrogens, and adrenal androstenedione becomes the major source of plasma estrone (MacDonald et al. 1978), the dominant plasma estrogen. Obese women convert androstenedione to estrone at an increased rate (MacDonald et al. 1978), and plasma estrone levels are directly correlated with the extent of obesity (Judd et al. 1980). Continued estrogen stimulation of the endometrium increases the risk of endometrial cancer (Lipsett 1979), and the data from surveys of women using estrogen after menopause support this. For breast cancer, too, prolonged estrogen usage has now been shown to increase the risk (Hoover et al. 1976), so that one may, with more confidence, assert the causal chain of obesity-increased plasma estrogen–increased breast cancer.

Men, too, convert androgens to estrogens at a higher rate as weight increases (Schneider et al. 1979, Kley et al. 1980). It may be an anomaly to think of the prostate gland as a target organ for estrogen, but classical estrogen receptors have been identified in the human prostate and in prostatic cancer (Murphy et al. 1980), and there is now evidence that estrogen regulates the level of androgen receptor (Moore et al. 1979). Thus, facilitation of estrogen production by obesity in older men can now theoretically be linked to enhanced stimulation of the prostate gland. However, Hill et al. (1980) reported that plasma estradiol and estrone levels are 20% higher in South African blacks than in North American blacks, a finding opposite to that predicted by obesity or fat intake. This may be accounted for, however, on the basis of increased peripheral aromatization of plasma androgen because of the higher incidence of liver disease in South African black males. Of interest were changes in plasma testosterone produced by dietary changes, even though a consistent pattern could not be discerned.

There is additional tenuous circumstantial evidence linking nutrition and prostatic cancer. The incidence of latent carcinoma is the same in American blacks and Nigerian blacks (Kovi and Heshmat 1972) and is the same in Japanese living in Japan and Hawaii (Akazaki and Stennerman 1973). However, in both studies there was a higher incidence of invasive cancer of the prostate in the United States. And in both cases, the high incidence groups had a relatively high fat intake.

Growth Stimulators

The production rate of at least one of a group of important growth stimulators is dependent on nutrition. Hepatic synthesis of somatomedin is stimulated by caloric intake even though growth hormone secretion is suppressed (Phillips and Vassipoulou-Sellin 1980). Although somatomedin synthesis is only one mechanism by which growth hormone exerts its effects, it may be of particular significance to the genesis of many cancers. The somatomedins and other peptide growth substances have the capacity to accelerate the progress of a cell through the cell cycle. There is increasing evidence that susceptibility to carcinogenesis requires a large proliferative compartment (Coyama et al. 1978, Russo and Russo 1980), and the regulation of those growth substances that induce mitotic activity must be significant in carcinogenesis. There are many candidates other than the somatomedins: pituitary factors other than the known pituitary hormones, epidermal growth factor (Rudland et al. 1980), and other growth factors (Ptashne et al. 1979, Rudland et al. 1980). The demonstrated effect of nutrition on hepatic production of somatomedin should prompt a search for dietary influences on the production of other growth factors.

ROUTES OF METABOLISM

The route of metabolism of steroid hormones may be altered by diet. The hepatic mixed function oxidases that metabolize carcinogens also use steroids as substrates, and this oxidative metabolism of the estrogens may either enhance or decrease total estrogenic activity. Low fat (Campbell and Hayes 1974) or low protein (Nerurkar et al. 1978) can decrease the activity of the P-450 enzyme systems.

The main routes of metabolism of estradiol and estrone occur via 2-hydroxylation to the catechol estrogens and 16α-hydroxylation to estriol. Estriol is an active estrogen, with about 25% of the uterotropic potency of estradiol. The other principal metabolite, 2-hydroxyestrone, is a very weak estrogen. Nutritional status (Fishman et al. 1975, Fishman and Bradlow 1977) is a determinant of the distribution of metabolites, obesity favoring estriol production. Thus, obesity contributes in still another way to increasing the total estrogen load.

The physical state of a steroid hormone in plasma may be altered in obesity. This occurs in the following way: obesity has been shown to reduce the plasma level of sex steroid–binding globulin (Glass et al. 1977, Nisker et al. 1980), a protein that has a high affinity for testosterone and estradiol. Thus, obesity simultaneously increases the production of estradiol and estrone and decreases the fraction of the estradiol bound to protein. The increased frequency of obesity in women with endometrial cancer can thus result in higher overall levels of free estradiol (Davidson et al. 1981).

URINARY STEROIDS

The endocrinology of cancer in humans began with the study of steroid hormone metabolites in urine. It was assumed that the amounts of metabolites were accurate reflections of hormone secretion. This assumption has often been shown to be incorrect; for example, 6β-hydroxycortisol depends on the activity of the hepatic mixed function oxidases; urinary dehydroepiandrosterone excretion decreases with fasting, but plasma levels are unchanged; the amount of urinary estriol bears no relation to plasma estriol levels; the ratio of catechol estrogens to estriol in the urine depends on obesity, thyroid status, and other factors. Thus, unless a direct relationship between a urinary metabolite of a steroid hormone and either the plasma level or production rate can be proved, urinary levels of steroids may offer only a clue, and often a misleading one, with respect to the hormonal internal milieu. Urinary levels of steroids may have empirical value since the extent of cancer or particular cancers may alter steroid metabolism.

REFERENCES

Akazaki, K., and G. N. Stennerman. 1973. Comparative study of latent carcinoma of the prostate among Japanese in Japan and Hawaii. J. Natl. Cancer Inst. 50:1137–1144.

Arafah, B. M., A. Manni, and O. H. Pearson. 1980. Effect of hypophysectomy and hormone replacement on hormone receptor levels and the growth of 7,12-dimethylbenz(a)anthracene-induced mammary tumors in the rat. Endocrinology 107:1364–1369.

Armstrong, B., and R. Doll. 1975. Environmental factors and cancer incidence and mortality in different countries with special reference to dietary practices. Int. J. Cancer 15:617–631.

Berenblum, I. 1978. Established principles and unresolved problems in carcinogenesis. J. Natl. Cancer Inst. 60:723–726.

Berg, J. W. 1975. Can nutrition explain the pattern of international epidemiology of hormone-dependent cancers? Cancer Res. 35:3345–3350.

Blair, A., and J. F. Fraumeni. 1978. Geographic patterns of prostate cancer in the United States. J. Natl. Cancer Inst. 61:1379–1384.

Butler, W. B., W. H. Kelsey, and N. Goran. 1981. Effects of serum and insulin on the sensitivity of the human breast cancer cell line MCF-7 to estrogen and antiestrogens. Cancer Res. 41:82–88.

Campbell, T. C., and J. R. Hayes. 1974. Role of nutrition in the drug metabolizing enzyme system. Pharmacol. Rev. 26:171–197.

Carroll, K. K. 1980. Lipids and carcinogenesis. J. Environ. Pathol. Toxicol. 3:253–271.

Carroll, K. K., and H. T. Khor. 1970. Effects of dietary fat and dose level of 7,12-dimethylbenz(a)anthracene on mammary tumor incidence in rats. Cancer Res. 30:2260–2264.

Chan, P. C., and L. A. Cohen. 1974. Effect of dietary fat, antiestrogen and antiprolactin on the development of mammary tumors in rats. J. Natl. Cancer Inst. 52:25–30.

Chan, P. C., and T. L. Dao. 1981. Enhancement of mammary carcinogenesis by a high-fat diet in Fischer, Long-Evans and Sprague-Dawley rats. Cancer Res. 41:164–167.

Chan, P. C., F. Didato, and L. A. Cohen. 1975. High dietary fat, elevation of rat serum prolactin and mammary cancer. Proc. Soc. Exp. Biol. Med. 149:133–135.

Choi, N. W., G. R. Howe, A. B. Miller, V. Matthews, R. W. Morgan, L. Munan, J. D. Burch, J. Feather, M. Jain, and A. Kelly. 1978. An epidemiologic study of breast cancer. Am. J. Epidemiol. 107:510–521.

Coyama, E., H. Tsuda, D. S. R. Sarma, and E. Farber. 1978. Initiation of chemical carcinogenesis requires cell proliferation. Nature 275:60–62.

Dao, T. L. 1969. Studies on mechanisms of carcinogenesis in the mammary gland. Prog. Exp. Tumor Res. 11:235–261.

Davidson, B. J., J. C. Gambone, L. D. Lagasse, T. W. Castaldo, G. L. Hammond, P. K. Siiteri, and H. L. Judd. 1981. Free estradiol in postmenopausal women with and without endometrial cancer. J. Clin. Endocrinol. Metab. 52:404–408.

DeWaard, F. 1975. Breast cancer incidence and nutritional status with particular reference to body weight and height. Cancer Res. 35:3351–3356.

Fishman, J., R. M. Boyar, and L. Hellman. 1975. Influence of body weight on estradiol metabolism in young women. J. Clin. Endocrinol. Metab. 41:989–991.

Fishman, J., and H. L. Bradlow. 1977. Effect of malnutrition on the metabolism of sex hormones in man. Clin. Pharmacol. Ther. 22:721–728.

Frisch, R. E., and J. W. MacArthur. 1974. Menstrual cycles: Fatness as a determinant of minimum weight for height necessary for their maintenance or onset. Science 185:949–951.

Glass, A. R., R. S. Swerdloff, G. A. Bray, W. T. Dahms, and R. L. Atkinson. 1977. Low serum testosterone and sex-hormone-binding globulin in massively obese men. J. Clin. Endocrinol. Metab. 45:1211–1219.

Hilf, R., P. J. Hissin, and S. M. Shafie. 1978. Regulatory interrelationships for insulin and estrogen action in mammary tumors. Cancer Res. 38:4076–4085.

Hill, P., and E. L. Wynder. 1976. Diet and prolactin release. Lancet 2:806–807.

Hill, P., E. L. Wynder, H. Garnes, and A. R. P. Walker. 1980. Environmental factors, hormone status and prostatic cancer. Prev. Med. 9:657–666.

Hoover, R. A., L. A. Gray, P. Cole, and B. MacMahon. 1976. Menopausal estrogens and breast cancer. N. Engl. J. Med. 295:401–405.

Ip, C. 1980. Ability of dietary fat to overcome the resistance of mature female rats to 7,12-dimethylbenz(a)anthracene-induced mammary tumorigenesis. Cancer Res. 40:2785–2789.

Ip, C., P. Yip, and L. L. Bernardis. 1980. The role of prolactin in the promotion of dimethylbenz(a)anthracene-induced mammary tumors by dietary fat. Cancer Res. 40:374–378.

Judd, H. L., B. J. Davidson, A. M. Frumar, I. M. Shamonki, L. D. Lagasse, and S. C. Ballon. 1980. Serum androgens and estrogens in postmenopausal women with and without endometrial cancer. Am. J. Obstet. Gynecol. 136:859–871.

Kleinberg, D. L., and J. Todd. 1980. Evidence that human growth hormone is a potent lactogen in primates. J. Clin. Endocrinol. Metab. 51:1009–1013.

Kley, H. K., T. Deselaers, H. Peerenboom, and H. L. Krüskemper. 1980. Enhanced conversion of androstenedione to estrogens in obese males. J. Clin. Endocrinol. Metab. 51:1128–1132.

Kopelman, P. G., T. R. E. Pilkington, N. White, and S. L. Jeffcoate. 1979. Impaired hypothalamic control of prolactin secretion in obesity. Lancet 1:747–749.

Korenman, S. G. 1980. The endocrinology of breast cancer. Cancer 46:874–878.

Kovi, J., and M. Y. Heshmat. 1972. Incidence of cancer in Negroes in Washington, D.C. and selected African cities. Am. J. Epidemiol. 96:401–413.

Labarthe, D. R., and W. M. O'Fallon. 1980. Reserpine and breast cancer. J.A.M.A. 243:2304–2310.

Lipsett, M. B. 1979. Interaction of drugs, hormones and nutrition in the causes of cancer. Cancer 43:1967–1981.

MacDonald, P. C., C. D. Edman, D. L. Hemsell, J. C. Porter, and P. K. Siiteri. 1978. Effect of obesity on conversion of plasma androstenedione to estrone in postmenopausal women with and without endometrial cancer. Am. J. Obstet. Gynecol. 130:448–455.

MacMahon, B., P. Cole, and J. Brown. 1973. Etiology of human breast cancer. A review. J. Natl. Cancer Inst. 50:21–42.

Miller, A. B., A. Kelly, N. W. Choi, V. Matthews, R. W. Morgan, L. Munan, J. D. Barch, J. Feather, G. R. Howe, and M. Jain. 1978. A study of diet and breast cancer. Am. J. Epidemiol. 107:499–509.

Moore, R. J., J. M. Gazak, and J. D. Wilson. 1979. Regulation of cytoplasmic dihydrotestosterone-binding in dog prostate by 17β-estradiol. J. Clin. Invest. 63:351–357.

Murphy, J. B., R. C. Emmott, L. L. Hicks, and P. C. Walsh. 1980. Estrogen receptors in the human prostate, seminal vesicle, epididymis, testis, and genital skin: A marker for estrogen-responsive tissues? J. Clin. Endocrinol. Metab. 50:938–948.

Nerurkar, L. S., J. R. Hayes, and T. C. Campbell. 1978. The reconstruction of hepatic microsomal mixed function oxidase activity with fractions derived from weanling rats fed different levels of proteins. J. Nutr. 108:678–686.

Nisker, J. A., G. L. Hammond, B. J. Davison, A. M. Frumar, N. K. Takaki, H. L. Judd, and P. K. Siiteri. 1980. Serum sex hormone binding globulin capacity and the percentage of free estradiol in postmenopausal women with and without endometrial carcinoma. Am. J. Obstet. Gynecol. 138:637–642.

Paffenbarger, R. S., Jr., J. B. Kampert, and H. G. Chang. 1980. Characteristics that predict risk of breast cancer before and after the menopause. Am. J. Epidemiol. 112:258–268.

Phillips, L. S., and R. Vassipoulou-Sellin. 1980. Somatomedins. N. Engl. J. Med. 302:438–446.

Ptashne, K., H. W. Hsueh, and F. E. Stockdale. 1979. Partial purification and characterization of mammary stimulating factor, a protein which promotes proliferation of mammary epithelium. Biochemistry 18:3533–3539.

Rudland, P. S., D. C. Bennett, and M. J. Warburton. 1980. Growth and differentiation of cultured rat mammary epithelial cells, in Progress in Cancer Research and Therapy, Vol. 14, Hormones and Cancer, S. Iacobelli, R. B. J. King, H. R. Lindner, and M. E. Lippman, eds. Raven Press, New York, pp. 255–269.

Russo, J., and I. H. Russo. 1980. Influence of differentiation and cell kinetics on the susceptibility of the rat mammary gland to carcinogenesis. Cancer Res. 40:2677–2687.

Schneider, G., M. A. Kirschner, R. Berkowitz, and N. H. Ertel. 1979. Increased estrogen production in obese men. J. Clin. Endocrinol. Metab. 48:633–638.

Shafie, S. M., and R. Hilf. 1978. Relationship between insulin and estrogen binding to growth response in 7,12-dimethylbenz(a)anthracene-induced rat mammary tumors. Cancer Res. 38:759–764.

Sherman, B., R. Wallace, J. Bean, and L. Schlabaugh. 1981. Relationship of body weight to menarcheal and menopausal age: Implications for breast cancer risk. J. Clin. Endocrinol. Metab. 52:488–493.

Smith, R. D., R. Hilf, and A. E. Senior. 1977. Prolactin binding to 7,12-dimethylbenz(a)anthracene-induced mammary tumors in liver and diabetic rats. Cancer Res. 37:4070–4074.

Vignon, R., and H. Rochefort. 1976. Regulation of estrogen receptors in ovarian-dependent rat mammary tumors. I. Effects of castration and prolactin. Endocrinology 98:722–729.

Welsch, C. W., and J. Meites. 1978. Prolactin and mammary carcinogenesis, *in* Progress in Cancer Research and Therapy, Vol. 9, Endocrine Control in Neoplasia, R. K. Sharma and W. E. Criss, eds. Raven Press, New York, pp. 71–92.

Wynder, E. L., G. C. Escher, and N. Mantel. 1966. An epidemiological investigation of cancer of the endometrium. Cancer 19:489–520.

Wynder, E. L., K. Mabuchi, and W. E. Whitmore. 1971. Epidemiology of cancer of the prostate. Cancer 28:344–360.

Nutrition and Physiological Effects in the Cancer-Bearing Host

Molecular Interrelations of Nutrition and Cancer,
edited by M. S. Arnott, J. van Eys, and Y.-M. Wang.
Raven Press, New York © 1982.

The Influence of Nutrition on Development of Cancer Immunity and Resistance to Mesenchymal Diseases

Robert A. Good, Gabriel Fernandes, and Noorbibi K. Day

Memorial Sloan-Kettering Cancer Center, New York, New York 10021

McCay carried out a most important set of investigations in the middle and late 1930s which showed that dietary restriction of total food intake prolonged the life of rats (McCay et al. 1939, McCay 1942, 1952). These investigations were followed by those of Tannenbaum (1940, 1942) and others (Visscher et al. 1942, Carroll 1977), which showed that restriction of calories or fat intake inhibited development of mamary adenocarcinoma in mice and rats. Particularly mammary adenocarcinoma of C3H mice, shown to be caused by a viruslike factor transmitted in milk (Bittner 1936) and strongly under hormonal influence (Bittner 1952), was dramatically inhibited by dietary restriction (Tannenbaum 1942, Huseby et al. 1945).

Fernandes et al. (1976c) more recently picked up on these prior investigations and launched a series of investigations to dissect the influence of diet in cellular, immunologic, and molecular terms on development of cancers, particularly mammary cancer. We have found that restriction of calories from the time of weaning reduces the incidence of mammary adenocarcinoma in virgin female mice of the C3H/Bi strain from approximately 60–70% down to 0–5% (Fernandes et al. 1979b). In addition, restriction of calories without fat restriction is only minimally effective, whereas restriction of fat intake alone from the time of weaning reduces the frequency of breast cancer in C3H/Bi mice (Fernandes and Good 1980). The dietary restriction, although delaying slightly the time of onset of estrus, permits full development and regularity of the estrous cycle (Sarkar et al. 1980). Further, development of breast tissue occurs normally (Fernandes et al. 1979b, Sarkar et al. 1980). The ductular apparatus of the breast develops quite well, but fatty tissue of the breast is inhibited from developing, as are the precancerous glandular nodules and breast tumors. Efforts to quantify development and maturation of virus particles in the breast tissue have shown the latter to be arrested by the dietary manipulation (Fernandes and Good 1980).

In addition, we discovered that dietary restrictions that are effective in preventing the development of breast cancer inhibit formation of circulating antibodies directed against the envelope glycoprotein of the virus (Day et al. 1980) and inhibit formation of circulating immune complexes (CIC) in the blood, which develop in C3H/Bi mice with age prior to the development of breast cancer (N.K. Day, unpublished observations). Recent studies by Dong et al. (1981) have shown that CIC develop in C3H/Bi mice progressively as the animals age, prior to the development of breast cancer. When the breast cancer appears in the mice, levels of CIC, as measured by the standard assay with Raji cells, appear to fall. However, more detailed analyses show that this fall of CIC is only apparent. Circulating envelope glycoprotein, GP52, increases progressively in the circulation, and complexes continue to form, but their molecular composition changes. They cease to be able to fix complement and so become progressively unmeasurable by the Raji assay. The size of the CIC becomes smaller; presumably, as the complexes shift toward antigen excess, the total amount of CIC continues to increase if the CIC are measured by a method that does not depend upon the complement attached to the complex (Witkin et al. 1980). We found that dietary restriction inhibits the formation of all of the complexes. Thus, dietary restriction profoundly influences a fascinating set of molecular events while inhibiting the development of breast cancer in mice.

Another line of investigation has presented an opening inquiry into whether the influence of dietary intake of calories and fat on development of breast cancer in mice might operate through influences on prostaglandin metabolism. Karmali and co-workers (R.A. Karmali, N.H. Sarkar, E. Whittington, and R.A. Good, manuscript in preparation) have begun to study the influence of hormones on production of virus by cells of the mammary gland. In an initial study, they employed the GR cell system to study the influence of hormones on the production and maturation of the B-type virus particles. Several interesting influences have been uncovered in the initial investigations, showing that this line of investigation will be productive. It was shown that virus production by the GR cells in vitro requires adrenocorticosteroids and that prolactin augments the permissive influence of the adrenal hormones. That these influences were prostaglandin dependent was shown when they were inhibited by exposure of the cells to indomethacine.

Further, the inhibition of the hormonal influences by indomethacine was in turn overcome by exposing the cells in culture to purified prostaglandin $F_{2\alpha}$. It thus seems especially important to investigate further the influences of restriction of dietary fat and calories in preventing experimental mammary adenocarcinoma in mice in terms of influences on hormonal levels and hormonal metabolism. Particularly, the influences on prostaglandin metabolism of these dietary manipulations, which are effective in inhibiting development of breast cancer in mice, require intensive further investigation. Indeed, Calvano et al. (1981) have already been able to show that dietary calorie and fat restriction lowers levels of immunoreactive prostaglandins in lymphoid tissues.

Dietary influences on development of chemical carcinogen–induced malignancies have also been increasingly investigated in recent years. Wattenberg (1966,

1971) has shown that adding certain foods or chemicals to the diet can alter metabolism of chemical carcinogens and inhibit their effectiveness as cancer-producing agents. This line of inquiry, summarized elsewhere in this volume, promises an entire new science of cancer prevention (Wattenberg, see pages 43 to 56, this volume).

Inhibition of the development of chemical carcinogen–induced cancers or so-called spontaneous cancers by calorie restrictions have also been described (Tucker 1979, Clayson 1975). Tucker, for example, has reported that reduction of total food intake by 25% from the time of weaning can inhibit both chemical carcinogen–induced cancers and spontaneous cancers in both mice and rats. Whether the influence of these dietary manipulations operates via influences on the cancer itself, on metabolism or biochemical influences of chemical carcinogens, or on influences on the immunological systems, endocrinological mechanisms, prostaglandin metabolism, or some other bodily process will be determined only by subsequent systematic analyses. Suffice it for the present that diet can exert most powerful influences on whether or not cancer will occur in experimental animals.

Many of the influences of diet on cancer development in experimental animals require dietary restrictions. However, if dietary restrictions are imposed in humans, lack of conformity with restricting regimens is the rule. Further, nutritional disadvantages, as well as advantages, may result. Thus, fundamental knowledge of the mechanisms by which food restriction influences the occurrence of cancer in experimental systems becomes crucial. To develop approaches applicable to humans, alternatives to dietary restriction will have to be developed to achieve the influence or influences that the dietary restrictions so dramatically demonstrate.

Recent work by Schwartz (1979) and his colleagues demonstrates this approach. A group of investigators (Yen et al. 1977) recognized that, even though food was consumed in amounts identical to that of control mice, mice given the hormone dehydroepiandrosterone (DHEA) showed blunting of weight gain. Although not explained, the defect in weight gain was similar to that observed in mice fed a restricted diet that inhibited development of mammary adenocarcinoma. With these relationships in mind, Schwartz and his co-workers attempted to prevent development of mammary adenocarcinoma by administering DHEA to C3H mice (Schwartz 1979). They prevent, by this relatively simple endocrinological manipulation, the development of mammary adenocarcinoma. DHEA is now under intensive study in pharmacological perspective. Already, congeners of DHEA have been developed which, in certain analyses, may be 20 times or even 50 times more active than the parent compound.

This approach to prevention of breast cancer in mice and seeking an approach applicable to influencing breast cancer development in humans seems most interesting and deserves intensive pursuit.

Thus, it is already clear that dietary restriction can inhibit development of experimental viral oncogen–induced malignancies, chemical carcinogen–induced malignancies, and spontaneous malignancies. Dietary restriction, however, must be understood in fundamental molecular, cellular, endocrinological, or immunological perspective if these dramatic experimental observations are to be translated to practical application in man. Already, progress is being made in this direction.

Dietary manipulations that of themselves may be useful in addressing cancer are those in which a nutriment or dietary constituent may be added to the diet. One example is vitamin C. Vitamin C administration may provide a powerful approach to cancers of the gastrointestinal tract. Before the mid-1930s, stomach cancer was the most frequent cause of death from cancer in the U.S. Almost miraculously, in the mid-30s stomach cancer began to decline in frequency in the U.S., until, at present, it represents a cancer of relatively low frequency. When it occurs, however, it is still a highly lethal cancer, having essentially the same case fatality rate that it did in the early 1940s.

The dramatic decrease in deaths from this form of cancer and the increase in deaths from lung cancer represent the most dramatic change to occur in cancer incidence in modern medical history. There is little question that, if cigarette smoking could be stopped, most cases of lung cancer would gradually disappear. However, in spite of solid knowledge concerning the etiological role of cigarette smoking in pathogenesis of lung cancer, little progress has been made in decreasing the carcinogenic habit—the smoking of cigarettes. This would involve deprivation of something considered desirable by some, and it is not occurring, at least for the population in general.

In contradistinction to that pertaining for lung cancer is the situation with respect to stomach cancer. The case can be made that stomach cancer has been dramatically influenced by a dietary additive, vitamin C. The decline of stomach cancer in the U.S. began about 10–15 years following the advent of universal refrigeration and the introduction of widespread refrigerated shipping of food. These changes made possible the present American diet, which puts fresh fruits and vegetables on most American tables at almost every meal. This dietary change, coupled with promulgation of widespread use of vitamin C as a routine for children by pediatricians and general practitioners, may have led to the decline of stomach cancer.

By inhibiting the formation of nitrosamines high in the gastrointestinal tract, vitamin C may have led to the prevention of stomach cancer (Weisburger et al. 1977). This postulate can and should be tested in controlled studies in China and other areas of the Far East where stomach cancer is still rampant. In the Far East and in China in particular, stomach cancer continues to be the number 1 killing cancer. Further, over all of China the number 2 or number 3 killing cancer is esophageal cancer. Here too, formation of nitrosamines from dietary constituents by microbial catalysis of nitrosamine formation may be the crucial pathogenetic mechanism (Hsia et al. 1981). Administration of vitamin C alone or together with vitamin E to prevent this critical nitrosation and thus the formation of chemical carcinogens seems one reasonable approach to inhibition of both esophageal and stomach cancers. Surely this very safe and inexpensive nutriment, often in short supply in the regular diet in Eastern countries, could be tried as prophylaxis against one or two of the most common cancers in the world. Hopefully, if this approach is taken, the attempt at prophylaxis will be made in the form of a properly controlled clinical trial.

Recent studies by W. R. Bruce in Toronto have generated another set of observations (Bruce et al. 1977) that might be translated into an effective prophylactic approach to the most common cancer in America—colon cancer. Bruce discovered that feces and colon contents of persons on the usual American (or Canadian) diet frequently contain a somewhat labile N-nitroso compound— a nitrosamine—that he has shown to be mutagenic. This substance can be completely eliminated from the gut contents and feces if larger amounts of vitamin C (400–1000 mg/day) are taken as part of the diet. Vitamin E supplementation is also effective in inhibiting formation of this potential carcinogen. It is thought that, as oxidizing agents in sufficiently large amounts, these substances can inhibit the formation of the potential carcinogen that is usually produced by action of the microbial flora. If this is the case, prevention of polyp formation, abnormal differentiation of the gut epithelium, and cancer formation should follow appropriate nutritional therapy.

Perhaps trials to prevent cancer by these nutritional manipulations could be carried out in families with high frequencies of colon cancer. Alternatively, patients with primary immunodeficiencies who have high frequencies of cancer of the upper as well as lower GI tract and in whom action of microorganisms might be pathogenetically important, or even patients who have been subjected to partial or complete gastrectomy or vagal nerve operations for treatment of peptic ulcers, would be good subjects. GI cancers occur in very high frequency in these populations. Thus, it can be reasoned that sound dietary approaches to inhibition of cancers may be developed and that this line of inquiry can generate much important information in approaching several cancers of high frequency in different parts of the world.

NUTRITION AND IMMUNITY

The relation of immunity to nutritional state has received much attention in recent years. Indeed, considerable concern has focused on the immunodeficiencies associated with the protein-calorie (PC) malnutrition syndrome, which is widely distributed over the world (Kulapongs et al. 1977). In most settings, protein and PC malnutrition have regularly been associated with profound defects of cell-mediated immunities. By contrast, hyperglobulinemia and hypergammaglobulinemia, quite regularly found in these syndromes in most areas, have been taken as evidence of a relative sparing of humoral immunity during protein and PC malnutrition. The analysis of the influence of individual nutriments and of protein or PC malnutrition per se on immunological functions from studies of these syndromes under field conditions has been hampered by the complexity of nutritional deprivation in the field (Good 1977). In addition, children and adults suffering from protein or PC malnutrition syndrome regularly suffer also from infection and infestation, which themselves can exert substantial influence on immunological function (Good 1977).

The complexity of the situation has been brought into focus by the observations of several investigators that have suggested that protein or PC malnutrition may be associated with an increase in expression of certain cell-mediated immunities and even in the expression of certain forms of hypersensitivity in disease that occurs in malnourished children (Jose et al. 1970).

Because of these uncertainties and apparently conflicting findings, approximately 12 years ago we launched a systematic analysis of the influence of nutriments on immunologic functions under precisely controlled laboratory conditions (Jose and Good 1971, 1973a, 1973b, Jose et al. 1973, Cooper et al. 1974, 1975). We readily showed in several different systems that protein and PC restriction led to decreased antibody formation and decreased antibody-producing cellular responses in primary, secondary, and tertiary immune responses to a variety of antigens. Indeed, the degree of inhibition of humoral immune responses was quantitatively proportional to the amount of protein or PC restriction imposed. In surprising contrast, we discovered that both protein and PC restriction, up to the point of near-lethal deprivation, was associated with maintenance of vigor of the several cell-mediated immunities and, in some instances, actually increased strength of the cell-mediated immune phenomena. This relationship obtained in inbred mice of several strains, rats, guinea pigs (Kramer and Good 1978), and the few monkeys studied (Good et al. 1979). For example, guinea pigs fed a diet restricted to 9% or 6% protein had delayed allergic responses to BCG as large as those observed in guinea pigs fed a diet containing 27% protein. Similarly, allograft rejections of skin between mice and rats of strains disparate at the major histocompatibility locus was accelerated when chronic protein or PC restriction was imposed. Listed in Table 1 are the cell-mediated immunities found to be actually enhanced by protein and PC restriction.

When the dietary restriction of protein or PC became too profound, however, certain cell-mediated immunities also appeared to be enfeebled. With the delayed allergic skin test response in guinea pigs, this was shown not to be due to enfeeblement of immunity response but rather to inhibition of inflammatory response (Kramer and Good 1978). For example, guinea pigs chronically fed only 3% protein, which led to early death in 50% of the animals, showed

TABLE 1. *T-Cell immunity functions enhanced by dietary restrictions*

Tumor immunity
Allograft rejection
Delayed hypersensitivity
Production of migration inhibitory factor
Proliferative response to T-cell phytomitogens

---

inability to develop delayed allergy to simple protein antigen. These guinea pigs were not, however, unable to marshal T-cell-dependent immune response, because their lymphoid cells could be sensitized by minimum doses of antigen 10^3 times lower than that which would yield this cell-mediated immune response in well-fed guinea pigs. Thus, in all species of animals studied, until chronic protein or PC restriction was sufficiently profound to be life-threatening in a high proportion of animals, cell-mediated immunities were retained and even increased.

Zinc and Immunity

Thus, our research placed a paradox in sharp focus (Good et al. 1979). How could it be that protein and PC restriction in animals enhanced T-cell-mediated immunities, whereas T-cell-mediated immunities were quite regularly profoundly deficient in protein and PC malnutrition syndromes under field conditions? As is often the case, answers resolving the paradox, at least in part, came from study of experiments of nature. Two such experiments of nature were especially revealing.

These two included study of the A46 lethal mutant in Holstein-Friesian cattle (Andresen et al. 1974, Brummerstedt et al. 1971, 1974) and the often lethal disease known as acrodermatitis enteropathica (AE) in humans (Good et al. 1980). In both of these natural, genetically determined experiments of nature, severe T-cell or dual-system immunodeficiency is observed. In both of these highly lethal diseases, the single metabolic abnormality responsible for the skin lesions, increased susceptibility to infections, gastrointestinal malfunctions, central nervous system malfunction, and profound immunodeficiency turned out to be attributable to deficiencies of one nutriment, zinc (Good et al. 1979, Andresen et al. 1974, Moynahan and Barnes 1973, Fernandes et al. 1979a). Neither the A46 mutant cattle nor the patients with AE could absorb zinc normally from the gastrointestinal tract. The perfect and absolute cure for each of these diseases, including the immunodeficiency and other manifestations, was to take adequate amounts of zinc orally. Alternatively, injections of zinc also cure completely both of these terrible diseases. In both diseases, the thymus is small and poorly developed; T zones are depleted of cells, and T-cell-dependent immunologic function is grossly deficient. These lymphoid cellular deficits and immunologic functional deficits are also completely correctable by giving zinc in adequate amounts.

Simple chronic dietary restriction of zinc in mice produces deficiency of thymic hormone function, defects of all known T-cell functions, thymic involution that is not dependent on pituitary adrenal function, depletion of T cells in peripheral lymphoid tissues, and reversion of peripheral T lymphocytes to expression of thymic or prethymic characteristics, e.g., autologous rosetting (Good et al. 1979, Fernandes et al. 1979a, Scholen et al. 1979, Nash et al. 1979). Administration of zinc alone corrects these abnormalities. Dialysis of lymphocytes against

EDTA, which chelates divalent cations, prevents proliferative responses of T cells to phytomitogens, a state not corrected by restoring Ca^{++}, Mg^{++}, and Mn^{++}, but completely corrected by restoring Zn^{++} to the culture medium (Zanzonico et al. 1981). Thus, zinc was shown to be absolutely essential to development and function of the T lymphocytes.

It thus appeared that a possible resolution of the paradox posed by the differences between experimental results and field observations concerning protein and PC malnutrition was at hand. This interpretation was strengthened by observations indicating that serum levels of zinc and zinc excretion are low in persons expressing the protein or PC malnutrition syndrome. It is the study of Golden and co-workers (Golden et al. 1978, Golden and Golden 1979), however, that appears to have clinched this argument. These investigators found from studies in Jamaica that the profound cell-mediated immunodeficiencies seen in PC malnutrition could be corrected simply by administering the element zinc prior to correction of PC deficits. They further showed that application of zinc, even in one forearm only, in the form of an absorbable zinc ointment, corrected the defective expression of delayed allergy to tuberculin. Taken together, all of these findings argue strongly for the view that, in protein or PC malnutrition syndrome under field conditions, it is the regularly concomitant zinc deficiency that accounts for the T-cell immunodeficiency.

Zinc deficiency, of course, does not occur in chronic protein or PC restrictions under laboratory conditions because supplemental vitamins and minerals, including zinc, are given during the periods of dietary restriction. On the other hand, it seems quite possible to encounter the degree of protein or PC restriction that produces disease under field conditions without finding concomitant zinc deficiency sufficiently profound to impose deficits of T-cell-mediated immunological functions. One possible basis of the latter is that, in all immunological functions, the immune state depends upon clonal proliferation of the T and B cells involved in the immunologic process. Zinc is essential to the function of some 95 enzymes, among which are the very enzymes essential to cell proliferation, including the DNA and RNA polymerases and thymidine kinase (Vallee 1955, Prasad 1979). Further, Prasad has recently found that nucleoside phosphorylase, which is so essential to T-cell development, is a zinc-dependent enzyme (Prasad and Rabbani 1981).

With the establishment of the concept that zinc exerts profound influence on immunological functions, it became interesting to study the role of zinc deficiency in certain primary and secondary immunodeficiencies in man.

So-called total parenteral alimentation is quite regularly accompanied by zinc deficiency (Ota et al. 1978) if care is not taken to provide adequate zinc with the nutriment. Prasad, who first recognized the consequences of zinc deficiency in man, reported early that dietary zinc deficiency is associated with increased frequency of infection among zinc-deficient patients in Iran. In more contrived experiments, this investigator has tested the influence of moderate zinc restriction on a number of physiological parameters. From these studies, he showed that most significant defects of immunologic function are produced by zinc deficiency (Prasad et al. 1978). Cunningham-Rundles et al. (1979, 1981) have reported that zinc deficiency and thymic functional deficiency are sometimes present in sick patients who suffer from the common variable form of primary immunodeficiency. They showed further that administration of zinc can correct, to some degree, the cellular immunodeficiency in such patients.

Similarly, Garofalo et al. (1980, J. Garofalo, unpublished observations) showed that cellular immunodeficiency in some cancer patients is associated with apparent dietary deficiencies of zinc. In other cancer patients or patients with inflammatory manifestations, e.g., patients with Hodgkin's disease or lymphomas, low levels of zinc in the blood may be attributable to shifting of zinc from the circulatory compartment into the liver under the influence of interleukin II.

The Influence of Diet on Collagen or Mesenchymal Diseases

In the course of studying the influences of dietary restrictions on immunological function, we began to investigate the usefulness of NZB mice and the (NZB×NZW)F_1 hybrid as models of genetic propensity to develop autoimmunity. Fernandes et al. (1972, 1973) studied the influence of diet on reproduction, litter size, and expression of autoimmunity, especially of the NZB mice. The initial experiments revealed that mice given a diet high in protein and relatively low in fat reproduced less well but lived significantly longer lives than did mice fed a diet high in fat and lower in protein. This interesting influence was accompanied by very different expressions of the autoimmune hemolytic anemia, thymic size, and immunologic functions. Animals fed the lower protein, higher fat diet showed early thymic involution, more extensive splenomegaly, and earlier as well as greater manifestations of autoimmunity than the mice fed the diet higher in protein and lower in fat. Although the mice fed the protein-restricted diet showed profound immunologic involution, they did not live significantly longer than the mice fed a high-protein diet. These fascinating influences of diet on the development of mesenchymal disease led us to the next set of investigations, which demonstrated striking influences of diet on longevity, autoimmunity, renal disease, vascular disease, and mesenchymal disease in several strains of inbred mice prone to develop autoimmunity and mesenchymal disease.

Protein Restriction in NZB Mice

This lead was then pursued in NZB and later in B/W mice, by using more precisely defined diets. Initially, we studied the influence of diets of restricted protein composition in NZB mice (Fernandes et al. 1976b), in which protein was the single component varied in the diet. Mice fed a low-protein diet showed delayed onset of autoimmunity, delayed onset and decreased rate of thymic involution, inhibition of development of splenomegaly, slower tempo of development of autoimmunities, and slower and decreased involution of the lymphoid system, resulting in decreased immunodeficiencies with aging.

Calorie Restriction in B/W Mice

We studied the influence of restriction of several dietary components on life span, immunological involution with aging, thymic involution, formation of CIC with aging, development of autoantibodies, and development of renal disease in mice of the (B/W)F$_1$ hybrid strain (Fernandes et al. 1976a, 1978a). Mice of this strain show early in life a profound involution of immunologic function, development of numerous autoantibodies, and progressive renal disease based on immune complex deposition in a capillary distribution in the glomeruli. This entire complex of immunological events is dramatically delayed and inhibited from developing by reduction of total calorie intake from the time of weaning. Figure 1 shows the progressive involution of ability to mount a plaque-forming cell response as B/W mice age; it also shows sustained immunologic vigor reflected by an ability to mount the plaque-forming cell response to sheep red blood cells given parenterally to mice on the calorie-restricted diet. B/W mice fed a low-calorie diet from weaning lived at least twice as long as B/W mice fed a putatively normal calorie diet. Indeed, a few mice treated by calorie restriction from weaning lived three times as long as any of the mice on the normal calorie diet. Ability of the mice to produce antinuclear antibodies and anti-DNA antibodies was considerably reduced but not eliminated.

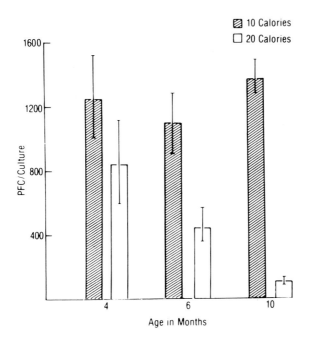

FIG. 1. Plaque-forming cell (PFC) response in vitro to sheep red blood cells of B/W mice fed 20 or 10 calories per day from age of weaning.

Recently, Izui et al. (1979) in Dixon's group found that immune complexes composed of complement and the gp70 of the Gross virus plus anti-gp70 develop in the blood of B/W mice. Further, the development and disposition of these complexes in a capillary distribution in the glomeruli correlates well with the development of progressive renal disease in these mice. In collaboration with this group of investigators, we have recently found that mice fed a low-calorie diet from weaning fail to develop both these autoantibodies and the immune complexes and do not have deposits of the complexes in a capillary distribution in the glomeruli. The glycoprotein gp70 is coded for in the genome of a virus but produced by nonmalignant cells, e.g., liver cells, in the B/W mice that bear the virus. Gardner et al. (1977) also found that dietary manipulation prevents the development of the mesenchymal disease in B/W mice but that this dietary manipulation does not inhibit the expression of the xenotrophic virus of Levy in these animals. In our studies with Izui et al. (Fernandes et al. 1981), we noted that the dietary calorie restriction in B/W mice, which inhibits almost entirely their expression of gp70 antigen and anti-gp70 antibody, does not inhibit production of albumin but does inhibit production of another glycoprotein, namely haptoglobin, which is also produced by liver cells. The increase of the level of CIC is strikingly depressed at six and less at nine months of age, but also in mice 12 and 14 months of age (Safai-Kutti et al. 1980, J. C. Cyong, G. Fernandes, H. Jyonouchi, N. K. Day and R. A. Good, manuscript in preparation).

One important question that derived from these experiments with dietary prevention of autoimmunity, immune complex formation, lupuslike renal disease, and inflammatory vascular disease in the B/W mice was whether or not delay of dietary restriction until autoimmunity and renal disease have set in might exert a beneficial influence. This question was clearly answered in the affirmative by the experiments of Friend et al. (1978). In these studies, we showed that when dietary restriction was delayed to 3, 4, or 5 months of age, instead of being imposed at weaning as in the initial experiments, clear inhibition of immunological abnormalities as well as inhibition of progression of renal disease was apparent.

Whereas restriction of calories inhibited the immunologic involution, development of autoimmunity, immune complex, and renal disease in B/W mice, no such dramatic influence was observed when protein was restricted in these mice. Fat, however, proved to be a critical variable, and restriction of dietary fat, coupled with calorie restriction, led to changes in immunity function and autoimmunity in these mice (G. Fernandes and R. A. Good, unpublished observation).

The Influences of Protein or Calorie Restriction in kd/kd Mutant Mice, which Develop Progressive Nephronophthisis

Lyon and Hulse (1971) discovered a new mutant strain of mice that appears to be autosomal recessive. The disease that develops in kd/kd mice is similar to nephronophthisis seen in man and is regularly fatal before the age of 6 months. We found that dietary protein restriction did not inhibit at all the development or progression of this renal disease, nor did it prevent the autoimmune hemolytic anemia that we had found to accompany its development. In striking contrast, both the renal disease and the accompanying autoimmunity were dramatically inhibited by dietary calorie restriction from the time of weaning (Fernandes et al. 1978b).

Zinc and Essential Fatty Acid Restriction in B/W Mice

Beach et al. (1981) have recently demonstrated that the development of auto-immunity and renal disease in B/W mice is strikingly inhibited by zinc restriction. They further found, in follow-up of the demonstration that zinc is crucial to thymic function and T-cell immunity, that this influence of zinc restriction was correlated with its influence on immunologic function in these mice.

In parallel studies, Hurd et al. (1981) showed that dietary restriction of essential fatty acids can also inhibit all of the critical variables and the development of renal lesions in B/W mice.

Atherosclerosis and Arteriosclerosis in B/W Mice

In an additional set of experiments with Fernandes (Fernandes and Good, 1980, G. Fernandes, D. R. Alonso, T. Tanaka, and R. A. Good, unpublished), we have discovered that the composition of the diet can profoundly influence the development of atheromatous lesions in the coronary arteries as well as in the aorta and large branches of the aorta in B/W mice. The lesions include inflammatory vasculitis and noninflammatory atheromatous lesions, some of which are free of lipid deposits. To develop these lesions with great frequency, the autoimmune-prone B/W mice must be fed diets high in calories and fats, or high in casein and low in soybean protein. Diets low in any of these components produce a much lower frequency of the lesions than do diets high in all these components. Further, the standard Purina laboratory chow diet, which is apparently relatively low in fat and high in fiber, does not produce such lesions in the B/W mice. The key seems to be that immunologic injury, coupled with high fat, especially unsaturated fat, produces the vascular lesions.

Although much further study is needed before the pathogenesis of these atherosclerotic and arteriosclerotic lesions that develop in B/W mice is understood, it already seems clear that diets high in saturated fats are particularly prone to produce such lesions. Thus, in inbred autoimmune-prone mice, genetic factors, immunological events (particularly immune complex formation), dietary fat, and dietary protein composition influence the development of atherosclerotic lesions. Similar dietary manipulations do not generally produce atherosclerotic lesions in long-lived autoimmune resistant mice. These provocative observations, which of course need much further study, suggest, in agreement with observations in patients receiving cardiac transplants (Bieber et al. 1970) and in experimental allergic reactions plus high lipid intake (Minick and Murphy 1973), that immunological processes—perhaps immune complex injury—may open the door to depositions of fatty substances derived from the diet during the pathogenesis of certain forms of atherosclerosis.

Protein-Calorie Restriction in MRL/lpr/lpr Mice

With the demonstration that dietary composition and calorie intake can exert profound effects on development and expression of immunological events and immunologically based pathological processes in autoimmunity-prone NZB and (NZB×NZW)F$_1$ mice, it became important to examine the influence of diet on the development of disease in other strains of mice prone to develop autoimmunity. In short, we discovered that MRL/lpr/lpr mice, which develop lymphoproliferative disease, profound immunodeficiencies, and autoimmunity-based diseases, are protected from all of the characteristic manifestations and permitted to live a long and vigorous life if their calorie intake is restricted from the time of weaning (Fernandes and Good 1979). This striking influence is currently being dissected from nutritional, immunologic, and pathogenetic perspectives.

Calorie Restriction in Humans with Mesenchymal Diseases

Results of attempts to extend the results with inbred mice to influence expression of lupus erythematosus by restricting food intake in patients with this disease have been interpreted as negative (Lockshin 1980). However, rather striking beneficial effects on the expression of rheumatoid arthritis and certain laboratory parameters accompanying rheumatoid arthritis (J. Palmblad, personal communication) that are associated with more profound dietary restrictions suggest that any negative interpretations of these observations be reserved until more data from more relevant experiments have been examined.

CONCLUSIONS

Thus, from the experimental laboratories, we and others have been able to generate observations that indicate that nutritional factors, including calories, fat, protein, vitamins, and minerals, can have profound influences on immunity functions, the development and manifestations of cancers, immunodeficiencies, autoimmunities, immune complexes, immune complex injuries, hyalinizing renal diseases, lymphoproliferative diseases, atherosclerosis and arteriosclerosis, and longevity. Progress is being made in defining these influences of diet in progressively fundamental terms, some of which may ultimately be translatable into approaches to the prevention of many presently highly lethal human diseases.

Certainly, definition of these influences of nutrition in molecular terms will broaden the potential usefulness of these laboratory and clinical observations.

ACKNOWLEDGMENTS

This work was aided by USPHSR grants CA-08748, AI-11843, NS-11457, AG-00541, AG-02247, and CA-29711 from the National Institutes of Health, by the Richard Molin Memorial Foundation, the Robert J., Jr. and Helen C. Kleberg Foundation, the Joseph and Helen Regenstein Foundation, the Neil A. McConnell Fund, the New Land Foundation, the Zelda R. Weintraub Cancer Fund, the Earl M. Coleman Laboratory, and the American Cancer Society (IM-185).

REFERENCES

Andresen, E., A. Basse, E. Brummerstedt, and T. Flagstad. 1974. Lethal trait A46 in cattle. Additional investigations. Nord. Vet. Med. 26:275–278.

Beach, R. S., M. E. Gershwin, and L. S. Hurley. 1981. Nutritional factors and autoimmunity. I. Immunopathology of zinc deprivation in New Zealand mice. J. Immunol. 126:1999–2006.

Bieber, C. P., E. B. Stinson, N. E. Shumway, R. Payne, and J. Kosek. 1970. Cardiac transplantation in man. VII. Cardiac allograft pathology. Circulation 41:753–772.

Bittner, J. J. 1936. Some possible effects of nursing on mammary gland tumor incidence in mice. Science 84:162.

Bittner, J. J. 1952. Studies on the inherited susceptibility and inherited hormonal influence in the genesis of mammary cancer in mice. Cancer Res. 12:594–601.

Bruce, W. R., A. J. Varghese, R. Furrer, and P. C. Land. 1977. A mutagen in the feces of normal humans, in Origins of Human Cancer, Book C, H. H. Hiatt, J. D. Watson, and J. A. Winsten, eds. Cold Spring Harbor Laboratory, Cold Spring Harbor, New York, pp. 1641–1646.

Brummerstedt, E., T. Flagstad, A. Basse, and E. Andresen. 1971. The effect of zinc on calves with hereditary thymus hypoplasia (lethal trait A46). Acta Pathol. Microbiol. Scand. (A) 79:686–687.

Brummerstedt, E., E. Anderson, A. Basse, and T. Flagstad. 1974. Lethal trait A46 in cattle. Immunological investigations. Nord. Vet. Med. 26:279–293.

Calvano, S. E., D. A. Mark, R. A. Good, and G. Fernandes. 1981. Age-related changes in lymphoid tissue content of prostaglandins in (NZB×NZW)F$_1$ mice (Abstract). Fed. Proc. 40:974.

Carroll, K. K. 1977. Dietary factors in hormone-dependent cancers, in Nutrition and Cancer, M. Winick, ed. John Wiley & Sons, New York, pp. 25–40.

Clayson, D. B. 1975. Nutrition and experimental carcinogenesis: A review. Cancer Res. 35:3292–3300.

Cooper, W. C., R. A. Good, and T. Mariani. 1974. Effects of protein insufficiency on immune responsiveness. Am. J. Clin. Nutr. 27:647–664.

Cooper, W. C., T. N. Mariani, and R. A. Good. 1975. The effects of protein deprivation on cell-mediated immunity. Birth Defects 11(1):223–228.

Cunningham-Rundles, C., S. Cunningham-Rundles, J. Garofalo, T. Iwata, G. Incefy, J. Twomey, and R. A. Good. 1979. Increased T lymphocyte function and thymopoietin following zinc repletion in man (abstract). Fed. Proc. 38:1222.

Cunningham-Rundles, C., S. Cunningham-Rundles, T. Iwata, G. Incefy, J. A. Garofalo, C. Menendez-Botet, W. Lewis, J. J. Twomey, and R. A. Good. 1981. Zinc deficiency, depressed thymic hormones and T lymphocyte dysfunction in patients with hypogammaglobulinemia. Clin. Immunol. Immunopathol. (in press).

Day, N. K., G. Fernandes, S. S. Witkin, E. S. Thomas, N. H. Sarkar, and R. A. Good. 1980. The effect of diet on autogenous immunity to mouse mammary tumor virus in C3H/Bi mice. Int. J. Cancer 26:813–818.

Dong, Z., S. S. Witkin, G. Fernandes, L. Poleshuck, V. Wahn, N. Sarkar, and R. A. Good. 1981. Comparative distribution of murine mammary tumor virus (MuMTV) antibody, antigen (gp52) and antigen-antibody complexes in sera of mammary tumor-bearing C3H/Bi mice (Abstract). Fed. Proc. 40:982.

Fernandes, G., and R. A. Good. 1979. Alterations of longevity and immune function of B/W and MRL/1 mice by restriction of dietary intake (Abstract). Fed. Proc. 38:1370.

Fernandes, G., and R. A. Good. 1980. Influence of diet on autoimmunity and longevity of B/W and MRL/1 mice, *in* International Congress of Immunology (4th, Paris), Abstracts, J. L. Preud'-homme and V. A. L. Hawken, eds. French Society of Immunology, Paris, Abstr. 14.1.07.

Fernandes, G., E. J. Yunis, J. Smith, and R. A. Good. 1972. Dietary influence on breeding behavior, hemolytic anemia, and longevity in NZB mice. Proc. Soc. Exp. Biol. Med. 139:1189–1196.

Fernandes, G., E. J. Yunis, D. G. Jose, and R. A. Good. 1973. Dietary influence on antinuclear antibodies and cell-mediated immunity in NZB mice. Int. Arch. Allergy Appl. Immunol. 44:770–782.

Fernandes, G., E. J. Yunis, and R. A. Good. 1976a. Influence of diet on survival of mice. Proc. Natl. Acad. Sci. USA 73:1279–1283.

Fernandes, G., E. J. Yunis, and R. A. Good. 1976b. Influence of protein restriction on immune functions in NZB mice. J. Immunol. 116:782–790.

Fernandes, G., E. J. Yunis, and R. A. Good. 1976c. Suppression of adenocarcinoma by the immuno-logical consequences of calorie restriction. Nature 263:504–507.

Fernandes, G., P. Friend, E. J. Yunis, and R. A. Good. 1978a. Influence of dietary restriction on immunologic function and renal disease in (NZB×NZW)F_1 mice. Proc. Natl. Acad. Sci. USA 75:1500–1504.

Fernandes, G., E. J. Yunis, M. Miranda, J. Smith, and R. A. Good. 1978b. Nutritional inhibition of genetically determined renal disease and autoimmunity with prolongation of life in *kdkd* mice. Proc. Natl. Acad. Sci. USA 75:2888–2892.

Fernandes, G., M. Nair, K. Onoe, T. Tanaka, R. Floyd, and R. A. Good. 1979a. Impairment of cell-mediated immunity functions by dietary zinc deficiency in mice. Proc. Natl. Acad. Sci. USA 76:457–461.

Fernandes, G., A. West, and R. A. Good. 1979b. Nutrition, immunity, and cancer—a review. Part III: Effects of diet on the diseases of aging. Clin. Bull. (MSKCC) 9:91–106.

Fernandes, G., S. Izui, N. K. Day, F. J. Dixon, and R. A. Good. 1981. Inhibition of retroviral gp-70-anti-gp70 immune complex formation and prolongation of life-span by dietary restriction in (NZB×NZW)F_1 mice (Abstract). Fed. Proc. 40:972.

Friend, P. S., G. Fernandes, R. A. Good, A. F. Michael, and E. J. Yunis. 1978. Dietary restrictions early and late: Effects on the nephropathy of the NZB×NZW mouse. Lab. Invest. 38:629–632.

Gardner, M. B., J. N. Ihle, R. J. Pillarisetty, N. Talal, and J. A. Levy. 1977. Type C virus expression and host response in diet-cured NZB/W mice. Nature 268:341.

Garofalo, J. A., E. Erlandson, E. W. Strong, M. Lesser, F. Gerold, R. Spiro, M. Schwartz, and R. A. Good. 1980. Serum zinc, serum copper and the Cu/Zn ratio in patients with epidermoid cancers of the head and neck. J. Surg. Oncol. 15:381–386.

Golden, B. E., and M. H. N. Golden. 1979. Plasma zinc and the clinical features of malnutrition. Am. J. Clin. Nutr. 32:2490–2494.

Golden, M. H. N., B. E. Golden, P. S. E. G. Harland, and A. A. Jackson. 1978. Zinc and immuno-competence in protein-energy malnutrition. Lancet 1:1226–1228.

Good, R. A. 1977. Biology of the cell-mediated immune response—a review, *in* Malnutrition and the Immune Response, R. M. Suskind, ed. Raven Press, New York, pp. 29–46.

Good, R. A., G. Fernandes, and A. West. 1979. Nutrition, immunity and cancer—a review. Part I. Influence of protein or protein-calorie malnutrition and zinc deficiency on immunity. Clin. Bull. (MSKCC) 9:3–12.

Good, R. A., A. West, and G. Fernandes. 1980. Nutritional modulation of immune responses. Fed. Proc. 39:3098–3104.

Hsia, C.-C., T.-T. Sun, Y.-Y. Wang, L. M. Anderson, D. Armstrong, and R. A. Good. 1981. Enhancement of formation of the esophageal carcinogen benzylmethylnitrosamine from its precursors by *Candida albicans*. Proc. Natl. Acad. Sci. USA 78:1878–1881.

Hurd, E. R., J. M. Johnston, J. R. Okita, P. C. MacDonald, M. Ziff, and J. N. Gilliam. 1981. Prevention of glumerulonephritis and prolonged survival in New Zealand black/New Zealand white F_1 hybrid mice fed an essential fatty acid-deficient diet. J. Clin. Invest. 67:476–485.

Huseby, R. A., Z. B. Ball, and M. B. Visscher. 1945. Further observations on influence of simple caloric restriction on mammary cancer incidence and related phenomena in C3H mice. Cancer Res. 5:40–46.

Izui, S., P. J. McConahey, A. N. Theofilopoulos, and F. J. Dixon. 1979. Association of circulating retroviral gp70-anti-gp70 immune complexes with murine systemic lupus erythematosus. J. Exp. Med. 149:1099–1116.

Jose, D. G., and R. A. Good. 1971. Absence of enhancing antibody in cell-mediated immunity to tumor heterografts in protein deficient rats. Nature 231:323–325.

Jose, D. G., and R. A. Good. 1973a. Quantitative effects of nutritional essential amino acid deficiency upon immune responses to tumors in mice. J. Exp. Med. 137:1–9.

Jose, D. G., and R. A. Good. 1973b. Quantitative effects of nutritional protein and calorie deficiency upon immune responses to tumors in mice. Cancer Res. 33:807–812.

Jose, D. G., J. S. Welch, and R. L. Doherty. 1970. Humoral and cellular immune responses to streptococci, influenza and other antigens in Australian aboriginal school children. Aust. Paediatr. J. 6:192–202.

Jose, D. G., O. Stutman, and R. A. Good. 1973. Long-term effects on immune function of early nutritional deprivation. Nature 214:57–58.

Kramer, T. R., and R. A. Good. 1978. Increased in vitro cell-mediated immunity in protein malnourished guinea pigs. Clin. Immunol. Immunopathol. 11:212–228.

Kulapongs, P., R. M. Suskind, V. Vithayasai, and R. E. Olson. 1977. In vitro cell-mediated immune response in Thai children with protein-calorie malnutrition, in Malnutrition and the Immune Response, R. M. Suskind, ed. Raven Press, New York, pp. 99–109.

Lockshin, M. D. 1980. Malnutrition does not ameliorate systemic lupus erythematosus. (Letter to the Editor) Arthritis Rheum. 23:132–133.

Lyon, M. F., and E. V. Hulse. 1971. An inherited kidney disease of mice resembling human nephronophthisis. J. Med. Genet. 8:41–48.

McCay, C. M. 1942. Nutrition, aging and longevity. Trans. Stud. Coll. Phys. Phila. 10:1–10.

McCay, C. M. 1952. Chemical aspects of aging and the effect of diet upon aging, in Cowdry's Problems of Aging, L. I. Lansin, ed. Williams & Wilkins, Baltimore, pp. 139–202.

McCay, C. M., L. A. Maynard, G. Sperling, and L. L. Barnes. 1939. Retarded growth, life span, ultimate body size and age changes in albino rats after feeding diets restricted in calories. J. Nutr. 18:1–13.

Minick, C. R. and G. E. Murphy. 1973. Experimental induction of atheroarteriosclerosis by the synergy of allergic injury to arteries and lipid-rich diet. II. Effect of repeatedly injected foreign proteins in rabbits fed a lipid-rich, cholesterol-poor diet. Am. J. Pathol. 73:265–300.

Moynahan, E. J., and P. M. Barnes. 1973. Zinc deficiency and a synthetic diet for lactose intolerance. Lancet 1:676.

Nash, L., T. Iwata, G. Fernandes, R. A. Good, and G. S. Incefy. 1979. Effect of zinc deficiency on autologous rosette-forming cells. Cell. Immunol. 48:238–243.

Ota, D. M., B. V. MacFayden, Jr., E. T. Gum, and S. J. Dudrick. 1978. Zinc and copper deficiencies in man during intravenous hyperalimentation, in Zinc and Copper in Clinical Medicine, K. M. Hambidge and B. L. Nichols, Jr., eds. Spectrum Publications, Inc., New York, pp. 99–112.

Prasad, A. S. 1979. Zinc in Human Nutrition. CRC Press, Boca Raton, Florida.

Prasad, A. S., and P. Rabbani. 1981. Nucleoside phosphorylase in zinc deficiency (Abstract). Clin. Res. 29:546A.

Prasad, A. S., P. Rabbani, A. Abbasii, E. Bowersox, and S. Fox. 1978. Experimental zinc deficiency in humans. Ann. Intern. Med. 89:483–490.

Safai-Kutti, S., G. Fernandes, Y. Wang, B. Safai, R. A. Good, and N. K. Day. 1980. Reduction of circulating immune complexes by calorie restriction in (NZB × NZW)F$_1$ mice. Clin. Immunol. Immunopathol. 15:293.

Sarkar, N. H., G. Fernandes, K. Karande, and R. A. Good. 1980. The effect of diet on the factors that influence the development of murine mammary cancer, in Proceedings of 12th Annual Meeting on Mammary Cancer in Experimental Animals and Man, Maastricht, Netherlands. Abstract.

Schloen, L. H., G. Fernandes, J. A. Garofalo, and R. A. Good. 1979. Nutrition, immunity, and cancer—a review. Part II. Zinc, immune function and cancer. Clin. Bull. (MSKCC) 9:63–74.

Schwartz, A. G. 1979. Inhibition of spontaneous breast cancer formation in female C3H (A^{vy}/a) mice by long-term treatment with dehydroepiandrosterone. Cancer Res. 39:1129–1132.

Tannenbaum, A. 1940. The initiation and growth of tumors. Introduction: I. Effects of underfeeding. Am. J. Cancer 38:335–350.

Tannenbaum, A. 1942. The genesis and growth of tumors. II. Effects of caloric restriction per se. Cancer Res. 2:460–467.

Tucker, M. J. 1979. The effect of long-term food restriction on tumors in rodents. Int. J. Cancer 23:803–807.

Vallee, B. L. 1955. Zinc and metalloenzymes. Adv. Protein Chem. 10:317–384.

Visscher, M. B., Z. B. Ball, R. H. Barnes, and I. Sivertsen. 1942. The influence of calorie restriction upon the incidence of spontaneous mammary carcinoma in mice. Surgery 11:48–55.

Wattenberg, L. W. 1966. Chemoprophylaxis of carcinogenesis: a review. Cancer Res. 26:1520–1526.

Wattenberg, L. W. 1971. The role of the portal of entry in inhibition of tumorigenesis. Progr. Exp. Tumor Res. 14:89–104.

Wattenberg, L. W. 1982. Inhibition of chemical carcinogens by minor dietary components, *in* Molecular Interrelations of Nutrition and Cancer (The University of Texas System Cancer Center 34th Annual Symposium on Fundamental Cancer Research), M. S. Arnott, J. van Eys, and Y.-M. Wang, eds. Raven Press, New York, pp. 43–56.

Weisburger, J. H., L. A. Cohen, and E. L. Wynder. 1977. On the etiology and metabolic epidemiology of the main human cancers, *in* Origins of Human Cancer, Book A, H. H. Hiatt, J. D. Watson, and J. A. Winsten, eds. Cold Spring Harbor Laboratory, Cold Spring Harbor, pp. 567–602.

Witkin, S. S., S. K. Shahani, S. Gupta, R. A. Good, and N. K. Day. 1980. Demonstration of IgG Fc receptors on spermatozoa and their utilization for the detection of circulating immune complexes in human serum. Clin. Exp. Immunol. 41:441–452.

Yen, T. T., J. V. Allan, D. V. Pearson, J. M. Acton, and M. M. Greenberg. 1977. Prevention of obesity in A^{vy}/a mice by dehydroepiandrosterone. Lipids 12:409–413.

Zanzonico, P., G. Fernandes, and R. A. Good. 1981. The differential sensitivity of T-cell and B-cell mitogenesis to in vitro zinc deficiency. Cell. Immunol. 60:202–211.

Molecular Interrelations of Nutrition and Cancer,
edited by M. S. Arnott, J. van Eys, and Y.-M. Wang.
Raven Press, New York © 1982.

Dietary Zinc Requirement for Concanavalin-A-Responsive Rat Spleen Lymphocytes

Tim R. Kramer and Barbara W. Highison

United States Department of Agriculture, Science and Education Administration, Grand Forks Human Nutrition Research Center, Grand Forks, North Dakota 58202

During recent years zinc has been demonstrated to be essential for the immunocompetence of man (Oleske et al. 1979, Pekarek et al. 1979) and animals (Pekarek et al. 1977, Gross et al. 1979, Fraker et al. 1977, 1978, Leucke et al. 1978, Luecke and Fraker 1979, DePasquale-Jordieu and Fraker 1979, Fernandes et al. 1979, Beach et al. 1980). Cell-mediated immune reactions, expressed as delayed hypersensitivity skin test reactions (Pekarek et al. 1979) and phytohemagglutinin (PHA)–induced in vitro lymphocyte proliferations (Oleske et al. 1979, Pekarek et al. 1979) are suppressed in man during zinc deprivation but corrected upon administration of zinc therapy. Several animal studies have demonstrated the suppressive effect of zinc deficiency on the thymus-derived lymphocyte (T-lymphocytes) division of the immune system (Pekarek et al. 1977, Gross et al. 1979, Luecke et al. 1978, Fraker et al. 1978, Fernandes et al. 1979).

Accepting these data, we decided to determine the dietary zinc requirement of young growing male rats as defined by immunocompetence of splenic T-lymphocytes. Earlier reports by Pekarek et al. (1977) and Gross et al. (1979) did not contain data on the concentration of dietary zinc that allowed for maximum proliferation of PHA- and concanavalin-A (Con-A)-responsive splenic T-lymphocytes. Pekarek et al. (1977) demonstrated depressed PHA-induced peripheral blood lymphocyte proliferation in young male Sprague-Dawley rats fed for 6 weeks a 20% egg-white protein diet that contained less than one part per million (ppm) of zinc. Gross et al. (1979) demonstrated depressed proliferation of PHA- and Con-A-induced splenic lymphocytes in young male Sprague-Dawley rats maintained for 4 weeks on a 30% EDTA-washed soybean protein diet containing 7 ppm of zinc as zinc carbonate. In those studies, dietary control levels of zinc were respectively (Pekarek et al. 1977, Gross et al. 1979) 50 and 60 ppm, which are considered above the dietary level of zinc required for normal growth of young Sprague-Dawley rats (Forbes and Yohe 1960, O'Dell et al. 1972). Therefore, to determine the dietary zinc requirement for maximum proliferation of Con-A-responsive splenic lymphocytes (SL) of young male rats, we fed weanling rats ad-libitum for 21 days a 20% egg-white protein diet that contained varying concentrations of one or more forms of zinc salt.

MATERIALS AND METHODS

Animals, Diets, and Experimental Design

Weanling (age, 21 days), outbred male Long-Evans (LE) and Holtzman Sprague-Dawley (SD) rats were purchased from Charles River Breeding Laboratories, Inc., Wilmington, MA.* Upon arrival they were placed in stainless steel cages and fed stock diet (Purina Rodent Laboratory Chow #5001, St. Louis, MO) with tap water for 72–96 hours. At age 28 days, the rats were matched by weight, placed in single, free-hanging stainless steel cages, and given free access to their designated test diets (Table 1) and deionized water. On day 21 of the dietary regimen, rats were weighed and on this and the next 4 days designated specimens were removed under ether anesthesia from an equal number of rats fed each of the test diets.

Spleen Lymphocyte Cultures

In plastic tissue culture dishes on ice, spleens were teased with sterile needles in Hanks' balanced salt solution (HBSS). The spleen lymphocytes (SL) were isolated from the spleen red cells by gradient centrifugation by use of the Ficoll-sodium metrizoate method of Böyum (1968). Briefly, 10 ml of the teased spleen cell suspension was placed on 4 ml of Ficoll-Hypaque (Histopaque, Sigma, St. Louis, MO) and centrifuged at room temperature at $400 \times g$ for 30 minutes. The isolated SL were washed three times with HBSS and viable (trypan blue exclusion) cell counts performed. The cells were cultured in RPMI-1640 (Gibco), L-glutamine (0.292 mg/ml), penicillin (100 units/ml), and streptomycin (100 μg/ml). Two hundred microliters of the cell suspension (2×10^5 cells/culture) was incubated per well in a flat-bottom Falcon Micro-Test plate (Micro-Test II, Falcon Plastics, Oxnard, CA) for 72 hours at 37°C in a 5% CO_2 95% humidified-air incubator.

Triplicate control (without inducer) cultures were evaluated for each SL sample, and triplicate test (with inducer) cultures were evaluated for each concentration of mitogen. Con-A was added to the test cultures at concentrations of 0.20, 0.39, 0.78, 1.56, 3.12, and 6.25 μg/2×10^5 cells. Twenty-four hours prior to termination of incubation, 1.0 μCi of ^{3}H-thymidine (methyl-^{3}H; 50–80 Ci/mmol; New England Nuclear, Boston, MA) was added to each culture. Following 24 hours of isotope labeling, the cultures were removed from the incubator and harvested with a Skatron multiple cell-culture harvester (Flow Laboratories, Inc., Rockville, MD). The cell culture fluid, cells, and distilled water rinses were collected on glass-fiber harvester filters (Flow Laboratories, Inc.). The filters were air-dried and placed in a toluene-based scintillation counting fluid

---

* Mention of a trademark or proprietary product does not constitute a guarantee or warranty of the product by the U.S. Department of Agriculture, and does not imply its approval to the exclusion of other products that may also be suitable.

TABLE 1. *Composition of basal diet**

Ingredient	Diets (μg zinc/g diet)				
	4	8	12	16	20
	g/kg diet				
Sucrose	631	627	623	619	615
Egg-white protein	200	200	200	200	200
Fibrous cellulose powder	50	50	50	50	50
Zinc-free salt mix	35	35	35	35	35
Vitamin mix	10	10	10	10	10
Biotin mix	10	10	10	10	10
Corn oil	60	60	60	60	60
Zinc mix	4	8	12	16	20

* Sucrose, Jack Frost, National Sugar Refining Co., Philadelphia, PA; egg-white protein, Teklad Mills division of ARS Sprague-Dawley, Madison, WI; fibrous cellulose powder, Whatman CF11, W. and R. Balston Ltd., London, England; zinc-free salt mix, AIN-76 mineral mix without zinc carbonate powder, Teklad Test Diets, Madison, WI; vitamin mix, Teklad (vitamin fortification mix) cat. no. 40060, Teklad Test Diets; Biotin mix, crystalline (15 mg Biotin in 1000 g corn starch), Grand Island Biological Co., Grand Island, NY; corn oil, Mazola, Best Foods, CPC International, Inc., Englewood Cliffs, NJ; zinc mix, zinc salts mixed with corn starch and designated amounts added to diets: zinc acetate: 3.35 g plus 996.65 g corn starch; zinc carbonate: 1.90 g plus 998.10 g corn starch; zinc sulfate: 4.40 g plus 995.60 g corn starch.

(Liquifluor, New England Nuclear). The scintillation vials were counted in a model Mark II Nuclear-Chicago liquid scintillation system.

Zinc Determinations

In the early experiments, plasma and freeze-dried organs were treated in a mixture of nitric acid, sulfuric acid, and hydrogen peroxide and then diluted with deionized water to volumes of 5, 50, and 100 ml for plasma, thymus, and liver, respectively. In subsequent experiments, serum instead of plasma was collected and was diluted 1:5 with deionized water. In all experiments, the femurs were first scraped free of muscle tissue, dried in a muffle oven at 450°C, and cooled, hydrochloric acid was added, and the mixture heated and diluted with deionized water. The zinc concentrations of the solutions were determined by atomic absorption spectrometry (Varian, Model 1250, Varian Techtron, Victoria, Australia) at 213.8 nm.

Statistics

Data were treated by analyses of variance followed by Scheffé contrasts. We have used Scheffé's recommendation that $P = 0.1$ be used as the point of significance (Scheffé 1959).

RESULTS AND DISCUSSION

The objective in three separate studies was to determine the dietary zinc requirement, when fed as acetate, carbonate, or sulfate, for maximum proliferation of Con-A-responsive SL of young male LE rats. In our animal facilities, the LE rat appears to experience fewer pulmonary infections under nutritional stress than do SD rats. For this reason, our initial studies were conducted with LE rats.

On day 21 of the dietary regimen, weight gain was significantly less (P < 0.01) for rats fed diets containing 4 ppm zinc in each salt form than for rats fed diets containing 8, 12, 16, and 20 ppm zinc (Table 2). With each zinc salt, weight gain did not significantly differ among rats fed 8–20 ppm zinc.

Growth has been used as the classic method to determine the dietary zinc requirement of young growing male albino rats (Forbes and Yohe 1960, O'Dell et al. 1972). Using a 15% egg-white protein diet, Forbes and Yohe (1960) demonstrated that young growing male SD rats require a dietary zinc level of 12.5 ppm for optimal growth. Using a 20% egg-white protein diet with three different zinc salts, we obtained normal levels of growth in young growing male nonalbino (LE strain) rats with diets containing 8 ppm zinc. It is unclear whether our lowered zinc requirement (8 vs 12 ppm) for normal growth response was due to our higher level of protein (20% vs 15%) in the basal diet, to other ingredients in the diet, to the difference in strain of rats studied, or to the weight of the rats at the time of initiation of the study.

Zinc levels in plasma and femur samples and total zinc amount in femur samples were significantly less in young male LE rats fed 4 and 8 ppm of each zinc salt than in rats fed the higher zinc levels (Tables 3, 4, and 5). Zinc levels in liver and thymus tissue did not differ significantly among rats fed the five concentrations of each zinc salt (Tables 6 and 7).

SL preparations from rats fed 4 and 8 ppm zinc, regardless of the zinc salt, did not display depressed levels of Con-A-induced ^{3}H-thymidine (^{3}H-TdR) incorporation (Figure 1). On the contrary, Con-A-stimulated SL from rats fed the 4 ppm zinc acetate diet displayed a significantly higher (P < 0.05) level of

TABLE 2. *Grams weight gain of Long-Evans strain rats**

Salt form of zinc	Range of mean initial wt. (g)	Diets (μg zinc/g diet)				
		4	8	12	16	20
Acetate	76–78	78 ± 11†,‡	132 ± 13	119 ± 16	127 ± 13	126 ± 16
Carbonate	80–82	88 ± 18	125 ± 12	130 ± 13	127 ± 13	128 ± 12
Sulfate	68–70	73 ± 17	111 ± 14	112 ± 14	108 ± 18	112 ± 18

* 21 days of diet.
† Mean ± standard deviation of 10 rats per diet.
‡ Rats fed 4 ppm zinc as each salt gained significantly less (P < 0.01) weight than did their counterparts fed 8–20 ppm.

TABLE 3. *Zinc in plasma of Long-Evans strain rats**

Salt form of zinc	Diets (μg zinc/g diet)				
	4	8	12	16	20
Acetate	22 ± 5†,[a]	72 ± 14[b]	100 ± 8[c]	95 ± 13[c]	112 ± 14[c]
Carbonate	37 ± 13[a]	107 ± 21[b]	141 ± 13[c]	152 ± 11[c]	147 ± 11[c]
Sulfate	46 ± 13[a]	125 ± 14[b]	157 ± 18[b,c]	170 ± 18[c]	185 ± 33[c]

* μg zinc/dl.
† Mean ± standard deviation of 6–10 rats per diet.
Values in the same horizontal row not followed by the same superscript letter are significantly different (P < 0.05).

TABLE 4. *Zinc in femur of Long-Evans strain rats**

Salt form of zinc	Diets (μg zinc/g diet)				
	4	8	12	16	20
Acetate	102 ± 5†,[a]	168 ± 6[b]	243 ± 12[c]	277 ± 8[d]	290 ± 20[d]
Carbonate	99 ± 6[a]	192 ± 15[b]	254 ± 11[c]	279 ± 7[c]	274 ± 9[c]
Sulfate	93 ± 6[a]	189 ± 27[b]	258 ± 7[c]	297 ± 12[c,d]	311 ± 28[d]

* μg zinc/g dry wt.
† Mean ± standard deviation of 4 rats per diet. Values in the same horizontal row not followed by the same superscript letter are significantly different (P < 0.05).

TABLE 5. *Total zinc in femur of Long-Evans strain rats**

Salt form of zinc	Diets (μg zinc/g diet)				
	4	8	12	16	20
Acetate	20 ± 2†,[a]	37 ± 2[b]	53 ± 5[c]	62 ± 9[c]	66 ± 6[c]
Carbonate	24 ± 4[a]	48 ± 2[b]	63 ± 3[c]	68 ± 5[c]	67 ± 7[c]
Sulfate	17 ± 1[a]	39 ± 6[b]	55 ± 8[c]	57 ± 4[c]	63 ± 4[c]

* Total μg zinc.
† Mean ± standard deviation of 4 rats per diet. Values in the same horizontal row not followed by the same superscript letter are significantly different (P < 0.05).

TABLE 6. *Zinc in liver of Long-Evans strain rats**

Salt form of zinc	Diets (μg zinc/g diet)				
	4	8	12	16	20
Acetate	75 ± 10†	78 ± 6	81 ± 6	80 ± 4	80 ± 8
Carbonate	78 ± 11	73 ± 7	75 ± 12	76 ± 2	90 ± 6
Sulfate	73 ± 8	86 ± 9	84 ± 10	90 ± 11	81 ± 6

* μg zinc/g dry wt.
† Mean ± standard deviation of 4–9 rats per diet.

TABLE 7. *Zinc in thymus of Long-Evans strain rats**

Salt form of zinc	Diets (µg zinc/g diet)				
	4	8	12	16	20
Acetate	90 ± 6†	91 ± 8	92 ± 1	94 ± 6	92 ± 4
Carbonate	104 ± 4	101 ± 4	101 ± 5	101 ± 11	101 ± 8
Sulfate	98 ± 8	96 ± 7	96 ± 5	98 ± 8	100 ± 5

* µg zinc/g dry wt.
† Mean ± standard deviation of 5–8 rats per diet.

[3]H-TdR incorporation than their counterparts fed 20 ppm zinc. For each zinc salt studied, the activity of Con-A-stimulated SL from rats fed 4 ppm zinc was equivalent to or greater than that from rats fed 20 ppm zinc.

Low zinc has been credited with impairing selected populations of lymphocytes while leaving other subpopulations functionally intact (Fraker et al. 1977, 1978, Fernandes et al. 1979). Our observation that Con-A induced significantly increased activity in SL from rats fed 4 ppm zinc acetate (Figure 1) suggests that lymphoid cell populations in the spleens of LE male rats may shift during states of low zinc nutrition.

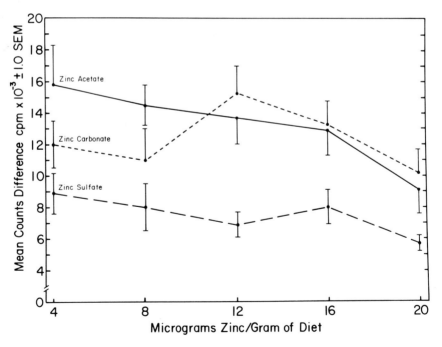

FIG. 1. Highest ^{3}H-thymidine incorporation by splenic lymphocytes from young male Long-Evans rats stimulated with multiple concentrations of concanavalin-A. See text for methods.

In addition to increased Con-A-induced SL proliferation in rats fed 4 ppm zinc, we noted that Con-A-stimulated SL from rats fed the five levels of each zinc salt displayed different levels of ^{3}H-TdR incorporation. Since each salt form of dietary zinc was studied separately, we could not determine whether these differences were due to the form of zinc salt or to variations within the immunological test used. But by studying the three zinc salts simultaneously we would be able to evaluate the effect of different zinc salts on the immunocompetence of young male LE rat SL responsive to Con-A stimulation.

Since we observed elevated Con-A-induced ^{3}H-TdR incorporation in SL of young male LE rats fed only 4 ppm zinc we decided to study in these rats: (1) the ability of a diet containing only 2 ppm zinc, when fed in a 20% eggwhite protein diet for 3 weeks, to maintain Con-A-responsive SL; and (2) if there exists a difference in the ability of three zinc salts to maintain Con-A-responsive SL. Therefore, weanling male LE rats were simultaneously fed ad-libitum for 21 days a 20% egg-white protein diet that contained one of three concentrations (2, 4, and 20 ppm zinc) of one of three different zinc salts (acetate, carbonate, and sulfate).

On day 21 of the dietary regimen, weight gain was significantly less (P < 0.05) for rats fed diets containing 2 or 4 ppm of zinc in the three salt forms than for rats fed diets containing 20 ppm zinc (Table 8). With all three zinc salts, weight gain was also significantly less (P < 0.05) for rats fed diets containing 2 ppm of zinc than for rats pair-fed 20 ppm or ad-libitum fed 4 ppm zinc.

The levels of zinc in serum and femur and total zinc in femur were significantly less (P < 0.01) in rats fed 2 ppm of each zinc salt than in rats pair-fed and ad-libitum fed 20 ppm zinc (Table 9). Levels of zinc in serum and femur samples and total zinc amount in femur samples were not significantly different in rats fed ad-libitum 2 and 4 ppm of each zinc salt and in rats pair-fed and ad-libitum fed 20 ppm zinc. One exception to this was the femur zinc concentrations in rats fed ad-libitum 2 and 4 ppm zinc carbonate.

Unlike the results of separate studies of the zinc salts, Con-A-induced SL of young male LE rats simultaneously fed similar levels of each zinc salt displayed

TABLE 8. *Grams weight gain of Long-Evans strain rats**

Salt form of zinc	Range of mean initial wt. (g)	Diets (μg zinc/g diet)			
		2	PF†	4	20
Acetate	66–68	32 ± 7‡,[a]	58 ± 20[b]	60 ± 8[b]	120 ± 18[c]
Carbonate	64–66	30 ± 6[a]	61 ± 14[b]	58 ± 10[b]	110 ± 8[c]
Sulfate	62–64	29 ± 6[a]	52 ± 19[b]	63 ± 12[b]	113 ± 16[c]

* On day 21 of dietary regimen.
†Pair-fed animals. Received 20 ppm zinc diet, pair-fed to rats fed 2 ppm zinc.
‡ Mean ± standard deviation of 10 rats per diet.
Values in the same horizontal row not followed by the same superscript letter are significantly different (P < 0.05).

TABLE 9. *Zinc in serum and femur of Long-Evans strain rats*

Specimen	N	Salt form of zinc	Diets (μg zinc/g diet)			
			2	PF*	4	20
Serum[†]	6	Acetate	48 ± 32[‡,a]	179 ± 21[b]	62 ± 25[a]	168 ± 23[b]
	6	Carbonate	34 ± 17[a]	174 ± 24[b]	65 ± 19[a]	199 ± 24[b]
	6	Sulfate	46 ± 32[a]	172 ± 25[b]	73 ± 25[c]	186 ± 19[b]
Femur[§]	4	Acetate	73 ± 9[a]	278 ± 25[b]	81 ± 10[a]	284 ± 24[b]
	4	Carbonate	65 ± 12[a]	287 ± 8[b]	89 ± 6[c]	292 ± 11[b]
	4	Sulfate	76 ± 10[a]	282 ± 16[b]	82 ± 12[a]	291 ± 9[b]
Femur[ǁ]	4	Acetate	11 ± 2[a]	47 ± 11[b]	13 ± 2[a]	61 ± 6[b]
	4	Carbonate	9 ± 2[a]	50 ± 7[b]	15 ± 1[a]	59 ± 5[b]
	4	Sulfate	11 ± 2[a]	47 ± 5[b]	13 ± 2[a]	61 ± 6[b]

* Pair-fed rats. Received 20 ppm zinc diet, pair-fed to rats fed 2 ppm zinc.
† μg zinc/dl.
‡ Mean ± standard deviation.
§ μg zinc/g dry wt.
ǁ Total μg zinc.
Values in the same horizontal row not followed by the same superscript letter are significantly different (P < 0.01).

equivalent levels of ^{3}H-TdR incorporation (Figure 2). As in our earlier studies, Con-A-stimulated SL from LE rats fed 4 ppm of each zinc salt displayed higher levels of ^{3}H-TdR incorporation than that of SL from their 20 ppm zinc counterparts. Con-A-stimulated SL preparations from rats fed 2 ppm of each zinc salt displayed lower levels of ^{3}H-TdR incorporation than those from rats fed 4 ppm zinc, but levels equivalent to those from rats fed 20 ppm zinc.

From these observations in young male LE rats plus our impression that LE rats display better resistance to pulmonary infections we decided to compare the dietary zinc requirement of young male LE and SD rats as defined by the immunocompetence of splenic T-lymphocytes. Therefore, to determine the dietary zinc requirement for maximum proliferation of Con-A-stimulated SL, we fed weanling rats of each strain ad-libitum for 21 days a 20% egg-white protein diet that contained one of five concentrations (4, 8, 12, 16, and 20 ppm) of zinc acetate.

On day 21 of the dietary regimen, weight gain was significantly less (P < 0.01) for both strains of rats fed 4 ppm zinc than for rats fed 8, 12, 16, or 20 ppm zinc acetate (Table 10). Weight gain did not significantly differ among rats fed the diets containing 8–20 ppm zinc. Weight gains were similar for both strains of rats at every level of dietary zinc.

The levels of zinc in serum and femur samples and the total amount of zinc in femur were significantly less in both strains of rats fed 4 and 8 ppm zinc than in rats fed the higher zinc levels (Table 11). Zinc levels in serum and femur samples and total amount of zinc in femur were similar for both strains of rats at every level of dietary zinc.

As in the studies reported above, Con-A-stimulated SL from young male

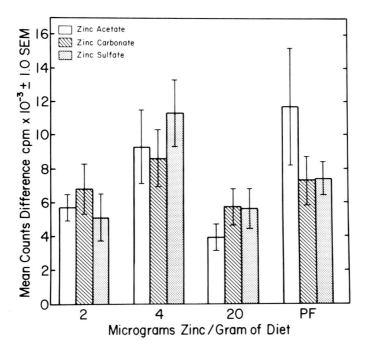

FIG. 2. Highest ^{3}H-thymidine incorporation by splenic lymphocytes from young male Long-Evans rats stimulated with multiple concentrations of concanavalin-A. See text for methods. PF, pair-fed rats. Received 20 ppm zinc diet, pair-fed to rats fed 2 ppm zinc.

LE rats fed 4 and 8 ppm zinc acetate displayed higher levels of ^{3}H-TdR incorporation than did their counterparts fed 12–20 ppm zinc (Figure 3). The peak Con-A-induced SL proliferation was displayed in LE rats fed 8 ppm zinc. In contrast to the LE rat, the peak Con-A-induced SL proliferation for young male SD rats was found in those fed 16 ppm zinc and the lowest was found in rats fed 4 and 8 ppm zinc. When the dietary zinc level was increased to 20 ppm, both

TABLE 10. *Grams weight gain of Long-Evans and Holtzman Sprague-Dawley rats**

Strain	Range of mean initial wt. (g)	Diets (μg zinc/g dry wt)				
		4	8	12	16	20
LE†	76–78	64 ± 10‡,§	110 ± 13	117 ± 16	113 ± 12	112 ± 10
SD‖	76–77	66 ± 12	116 ± 16	115 ± 19	110 ± 9	116 ± 18

* On day 21 of diet.
† Long-Evans [Crl:(LE)BR] strain rat.
‡ Mean ± standard deviation of 10 rats per diet.
§ Rats of each strain fed 4 ppm zinc gained significantly less (P < 0.01) weight than did their counterparts fed 8–20 ppm.
‖ Holtzman Sprague-Dawley [Crl:CD ®H(SD)BR] strain rat.

TABLE 11. *Levels of zinc in serum and femur of Long-Evans and Holtzman Sprague-Dawley rats*

Strain	Specimen	N	Diets (μg zinc/g diet)				
			4	8	12	16	20
LE*	Serum†	10	52 ± 20‡,ᵃ	113 ± 22ᵇ	155 ± 19ᶜ	153 ± 11ᶜ	158 ± 15ᶜ
SD§	Serum†	10	53 ± 21ᵃ	106 ± 17ᵇ	141 ± 22ᶜ	143 ± 14ᶜ	162 ± 11ᶜ
LE	Femurǁ	5	81 ± 5ᵃ	191 ± 18ᵇ	229 ± 16ᵇ	265 ± 9ᶜ	272 ± 11ᶜ
SD	Femurǁ	5	87 ± 15ᵃ	164 ± 10ᵇ	226 ± 20ᶜ	248 ± 12ᶜ	278 ± 10ᶜ
LE	Femur¶	5	15 ± 2ᵃ	43 ± 3ᵇ	52 ± 7ᵇ	59 ± 5ᶜ	62 ± 6ᶜ
SD	Femur¶	5	16 ± 3ᵃ	37 ± 3ᵇ	49 ± 3ᶜ	52 ± 9ᶜ·ᵈ	62 ± 6ᵈ

* Long-Evans [Crl:(LE)BR] strain rat.
† μg zinc/dl.
‡ Mean ± standard deviation.
§ Holtzman Sprague-Dawley [Crl:CD ®H(SD)BR] strain rat.
ǁ μg zinc/g dry wt.
¶ Total μg zinc.
Values in the same horizontal row not followed by the same superscript letter are significantly different ($P < 0.05$).

strains of rats displayed equivalent levels of Con-A-induced ^{3}H-TdR incorporation in SL.

SL from young male LE rats fed five levels of zinc required different doses of Con-A for induction of maximum incorporation of ^{3}H-TdR (Figure 4, top). Optimal Con-A doses for induction of maximum ^{3}H-TdR incorporation in 2 × 10^5 SL from young male LE rats was 3.12 μg for rats fed 4 ppm zinc, 1.56 μg for rats fed 8, 12, and 16 ppm zinc, and 0.78 μg for rats fed 20 ppm zinc

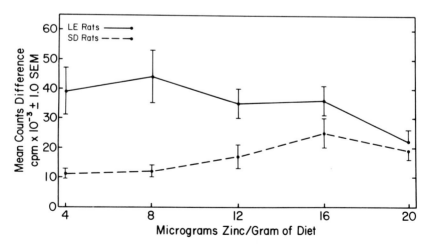

FIG. 3. Highest ^{3}H-thymidine incorporation by splenic lymphocytes from young male Long-Evans and Sprague-Dawley rats stimulated with multiple concentrations of concanavalin-A. See text for methods.

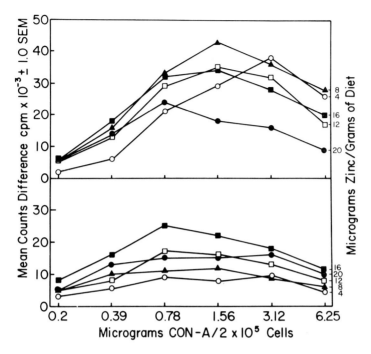

FIG. 4. ^{3}H-thymidine incorporation by splenic lymphocytes from young male Long-Evans (top) and Sprague-Dawley (bottom) rats stimulated with multiple concentrations of concanavalin-A. See text for methods.

(Figure 4, top). SL from SD rats fed the five levels of zinc did not require different doses of Con-A for induction of maximum incorporation of ^{3}H-TdR (Figure 4, bottom). These rats fed 4–20 ppm zinc required stimulation with 0.78 to 1.56 μg Con-A/2 $\times$ 10[5] SL for maximum incorporation of ^{3}H-TdR. From these results it appears that LE rats possess different subpopulations of Con-A-responsive SL, but SD rats do not. These subpopulations are evident when the LE rats are fed suboptimal levels of zinc.

The reason for this difference in Con-A-induced SL proliferation between SD and LE rats fed low levels of zinc is unclear. The rat spleen contains subpopulations of T-lymphocytes that differ in density and Con-A-induced activity (Rocha et al. 1979). It also contains adherent cells that influence the proliferation of Con-A-responsive lymphocytes induced in vitro (Folch and Waksman 1974, Webb and Brooks 1980).

The importance of the decrease in Con-A-induced splenic T-lymphocyte activity in SD rats fed low levels of zinc and the lack of decrease in LE rats is unclear. However, we think it is important to consider the following observations. First, we chose to study the effect of dietary zinc on the immune system of LE rats instead of SD rats because LE rats seem to develop fewer pulmonary infections. Second, Chan and Dao (1981) demonstrated that susceptibility to

N-nitrosomethylurea-induced mammary carcinogenesis was greatest in SD rats and least in LE rats when they were fed high-fat, low-fat, or nonpurified diets. We are not certain that their observed difference between SD and LE rats was influenced by the relative ability of these two strains of rats to produce adequate tumor immunity, but our work in animals fed low levels of zinc makes this a question of interest.

In conclusion, this report shows that in young male Long-Evans and Holtzman Sprague-Dawley rats fed a 20% egg-white protein diet ad-libitum for 21 days: (1) both strains of rats require 8 ppm zinc for normal growth; (2) both strains of rats require 12 ppm zinc to maintain normal zinc levels in the serum and total amount of zinc in the femur and 12–16 ppm zinc to maintain normal zinc levels in the femur; (3) Long-Evans rats require only 4 to 8 ppm zinc for maximum proliferation of Con-A-responsive spleen lymphocytes; (4) Sprague-Dawley rats require 16 ppm zinc for maximum proliferation of Con-A-responsive spleen lymphocytes; (5) Long-Evans rats appear to have subpopulations of Con-A-responsive spleen lymphocytes that are influenced by the amount of dietary zinc consumed, but Sprague-Dawley rats do not; and (6) for both strains of rats, decreased Con-A-induced splenic lymphocyte proliferation is displayed when the dietary level of zinc is increased above (20 ppm) that needed for normal growth (8 ppm), to maintain normal serum zinc levels (12 ppm), and to achieve maximum proliferation of Con-A-responsive spleen lymphocytes (8 and 16 ppm zinc for LE and SD rats, respectively).

ACKNOWLEDGMENTS

We thank LuAnn Johnson for statistical evaluation of the data, Jean Klava for preparation of the diets, and Elaine Johnson and Dr. Gary W. Evans for zinc analyses.

REFERENCES

Beach, R. S., M. E. Gershwin, R. K. Makishima, and L. S. Hurley. 1980. Impaired immunologic ontogeny in postnatal zinc deprivation. J. Nutr. 110:805–815.

Böyum, A. 1968. Separation of leukocytes from blood and bone marrow. Scand. J. Clin. Lab. Invest. 21 (Suppl. 97):7.

Chan, P. C., and T. L. Dao. 1981. Enhancement of mammary carcinogenesis by a high-fat diet in Fischer, Long-Evans, and Sprague-Dawley rats. Cancer Res. 41:164–167.

DePasquale-Jordieu, P., and P. J. Fraker. 1979. The role of corticosterone in the loss in immune function in the zinc-deficient A/J mouse. J. Nutr. 109:1847–1855.

Fernandes, G., M. Nair, K. Onoe, T. Tanaka, R. Floyd, and R. A. Good. 1979. Impairment of cell-mediated immunity functions by dietary zinc deficiency in mice. Proc. Natl. Acad. Sci. USA 76:457–461.

Folch, H., and B. H. Waksman. 1974. The splenic suppressor cell. I. Activity of thymus-dependent adherent cells: Changes with age and stress. J. Immunol. 113:127–139.

Forbes, R. M., and M. Yohe. 1960. Zinc requirement and balance studies with the rat. J. Nutr. 70:53–57.

Fraker, P. J., P. DePasquale-Jordieu, C. M. Zwickl, and R. W. Luecke. 1978. Regeneration of T-cell helper function in zinc-deficient adult mice. Proc. Natl. Acad. Sci. USA 75:5660–5664.

Fraker, P. J., S. M. Haas, and R. W. Luecke. 1977. Effect of zinc deficiency on the immune response of the young adult A/J mouse. J. Nutr. 107:1889–1895.

Gross, R. L., N. Osdin, L. Fong, and P. M. Newberne. 1979. I. Depressed immunological function in zinc-deprived rats as measured by mitogen response of spleen, thymus, and peripheral blood. Am. J. Clin. Nutr. 32:1260–1265.

Luecke, R. W., and P. J. Fraker. 1979. The effect of varying dietary zinc levels on growth and antibody-mediated response in two strains of mice. J. Nutr. 109:1373–1376.

Luecke, R. W., C. E. Simonel, and P. J. Fraker. 1978. The effect of restricted dietary intake on the antibody mediated response of the zinc deficient A/J mouse. J. Nutr. 108:881–887.

O'Dell, B. L., C. E. Burpo, and J. E. Savage. 1972. Evaluation of zinc availability in foodstuffs of plant and animal origin. J. Nutr. 102:653–660.

Oleske, J. M., M. L. Westphal, S. S. Starr, S. Shore, D. Gorden, J. Bogden, D. B. Coplen, and A. Nahmias. 1979. Zinc therapy of depressed cellular immunity in acrodermatitis enteropathica. Am. J. Dis. Child. 133:915–918.

Pekarek, R. S., A. M. Hoagland, and M. C. Powanda. 1977. Humoral and cellular immune responses in zinc deficient rats. Nutritional Reports International 16:267–276.

Pekarek, R. S., H. H. Sandstead, R. A. Jacob, and D. F. Barcome. 1979. Abnormal cellular immune responses during acquired zinc deficiency. Am. J. Clin. Nutr. 32:1466–1471.

Rocha, B., A. Freitas, and M. DeSousa. 1979. Characterization of rat spleen-cell population. I. Cell interactions in the regulation of in vitro response to concanavalin-A. Immunology 36:619–627.

Scheffé, H. 1959. The one-way layout. Multiple comparison, in The Analysis of Variance, H. Scheffé, ed. John Wiley & Sons, Inc., New York, 77 pp.

Webb, P. J., and C. G. Brooks. 1980. Macrophage-like suppressor cells in rats. I. Inhibition of natural macrophage-like suppressor cells by red blood cells. Cell. Immunol. 52:370–380.

Molecular Interrelations of Nutrition and Cancer,
edited by M. S. Arnott, J. van Eys, and Y.-M. Wang.
Raven Press, New York © 1982.

Biochemical Bases of the Differential Susceptibility of Malignant Immune Cells to Asparaginase and to Cytosine Arabinoside

Takao Ohnuma, Hadara Arkin, Isao Takahashi, Alicja
Andrejczuk, John Roboz, and James F. Holland

*Department of Neoplastic Diseases, Mt. Sinai School of Medicine,
New York, New York 10029*

During the past several years, increasing numbers of permanent human lymphocyte lines with normal and malignant characteristics have been described (Lozzio and Lozzio 1975, Minowada et al. 1972, 1977, Miyoshi et al. 1977, Schneider et al. 1977). Based on the expression of immunologic, cytogenetic, and enzymatic characteristics, subsets of lymphocyte lines have been identified. In view of the therapeutic and prognostic value of identifying subsets of acute lymphocytic leukemia (ALL) and chronic myelocytic leukemia (CML) in blastic crisis (Belpomme et al. 1977, Chessells et al. 1977, Sen and Borella 1975, Greaves and Lister 1981), the study of nutritional and pharmacologic effects on homogeneous subpopulations of human lymphocyte lines with different cell markers was undertaken. We hope to provide valuable in vitro models and thereby to establish useful guides in the treatment of malignant hematologic neoplasms.

Earlier studies in this laboratory revealed that two T-cell lines, MOLT-3 and RPMI-8402 (Table 1), required exogenous L-asparagine (Asn) for cell growth. They were both extremely sensitive to *Escherichia coli* asparaginase (Asnase) (Ohnuma et al. 1977). Recent study with another T-cell line, DND-41, revealed similar Asn dependence and high sensitivity to Asnase (Ohnuma, unpublished observation). In contrast, all four B-cell lines tested—RPMI-8422, RPMI-1788, B411-4, and B46M (Table 1)—were able to grow in medium devoid of Asn, and a high concentration of Asnase was required to inhibit B-cell growth. Thus, based on ID_{50} values (the drug concentration that produces 50% inhibition of cell growth by day 5) the differential sensitivity to Asnase was 800- to 2,000-fold.

Further studies revealed that T- and B-cells have differential sensitivity to cytosine arabinoside (ara-C) and 5-fluorouracil (5-FU) (Ohnuma et al. 1978). T-cells were 45–80 times more sensitive to ara-C, whereas human "normal" B-lymphocytes (RPMI-1788 and RPMI-8422) were 10–20 times more sensitive to 5-FU. When additional cell lines were studied, heterologous responses to 5-FU emerged (Ohnuma et al. 1980). Thus, two Burkitt's lymphoma cell lines

TABLE 1. Markers of human lymphocytic lines studied

Marker	T-cell lines			B-cell lines						
	MOLT-3 (T-ALL)*	RPMI-8402 (T-ALL)	DND-41 (T-ALL)	RPMI-8422 (T-ALL)	RPMI-1788 (Healthy donor)	B411-4 (Healthy donor)	B46M (BL)	DND-39A (BL)	BALM-2 (B-ALL)	BALL-1 (B-ALL)
E	+	–	+	–	–	–	–	–	–	–
EA	+	+	–	–	–	–	+	–	–	+
EAC	–	+	+	+	+	+	–	+	+	–
SmIg.	–	–	–	+	+	+	+	+	+	+
T-Ag	+	+	+	–	–	–	–	–	–	–
Ia-like	–	–	+	+	+	+	+	+	+	+
cALL	–	+	+	–	–	–	–	+	–	–
TdT	H	H	H	L	L	L	L	nd	L	L
EBV	–	–	–	+	+	+	+	–	+	–
Chr	A	A	A	A	N	N	A	A	A	A
MLC-S	–	–	–	+	+	+	+	+	+	+

* Origin of cell line.

ALL, acute lymphocytic leukemia; *BL,* Burkitt's lymphoma; *E,* sheep erythrocyte rosette; *EA,* rosette formed by bovine erythrocyte-IgG antibody complex; *EAC,* rosette formed by bovine erythrocyte-IgM antibody-complement complex; *SmIg,* cell surface membrane immunoglobulin; *T-Ag,* antigen specific to T-cells; *Ia-like,* human Ia-like p28,30 glycoprotein antigen; *cALL,* common ALL-associated antigen; *TdT,* terminal deoxynucleotidyl transferase (*H,* high activity 10–100 units/mg DNA; *L,* low activity ≤ 2 units/mg DNA); *EBV,* Epstein-Barr virus infection; *Chr,* chromosome; *A,* abnormal chromosome constitution; *N,* normal; *MLC-S,* stimulating capacity in mixed leukocyte culture assay; *nd,* not done. Modified from Minowada et al. (1980).

(B46M and DND-39A) were less sensitive than "normal" B-cells and fell within the T-cell range.

The observations of increased susceptibility of T-lymphocytes to Asnase and to ara-C appeared consistent with the clinical activity of these drugs against neoplastic diseases of T-cell lineage (see discussion in Ohnuma et al. 1978). Among the cell lines studied, only DND-41 originated in a patient who had been exposed to Asnase. Both Epstein-Barr virus–positive and –negative B-cells and both "benign" and "malignant" B-cells had similar insensitivity to Asnase. Therefore, the differential sensitivity observed was related only to the differences in phenotype.

We have now elucidated some of the biochemical bases of why T-cells are more sensitive to Asn depression and why B-cells are ara-C resistant.

ESTABLISHMENT AND CHARACTERIZATION OF L-ASPARAGINE–INDEPENDENT HUMAN T-CELL LINE MOLT-3/ASN

The human ALL cell line with T-cell characteristics, MOLT-3 (Minowada et al. 1972), and "normal" B-cell lines, RPMI-8422 and RPMI-1788 (see Minowada et al. 1980), have been maintained in our laboratory (Ohnuma et al. 1978) in culture flasks (#3013, Falcon Plastics, Oxnard, CA) containing RPMI-1640 medium (GIBCO, Grand Island, NY) with 10% heat-inactivated fetal calf serum (FCS) and antibiotics (penicillin 100 U/ml and streptomycin 100 μg/ml).

To establish the range of Asn concentrations required to maintain MOLT-3 cells, an aliquot of exponentially grown cell suspension was washed once and resuspended in RPMI-1640 medium devoid of Asn (GIBCO) containing 10% dialyzed FCS (GIBCO) at a final concentration of 2×10^5 cells/ml (suspension A). An additional aliquot of MOLT-3 cells was diluted with complete RPMI-1640 medium (Asn concentration 50 μg/ml) with 10% dialyzed FCS to a final concentration of 2×10^5 cells/ml (suspension B). Ten milliliters of cell suspension B were withdrawn and diluted with an equal volume of suspension A in a culture flask to yield an Asn concentration of half the original medium. Subsequent serial dilutions were made to yield final Asn concentrations of 12.5, 6.25, 3.125, 1.56, 0.78, and 0.39 μg/ml. Cell growth without feeding was observed daily for 7 days.

The results of this experiment are illustrated in Figure 1. The growth rate of MOLT-3 cells is clearly dependent on Asn concentration in the medium. MOLT-3 cells grew at the same rate as the control when the Asn concentration was reduced to 25% of that in the original medium (12.5 μg/ml). At lower concentrations of Asn in the medium, there was a progressive decrease in the growth rate, and at concentrations of less than 0.39 μg/ml, fewer viable MOLT-3 cells were found.

After the lowest concentrations of Asn at which cells were able to grow were determined (1.56 or 3.125 μg/ml), further cell growth was observed after periodic feeding with medium devoid of Asn but containing 10% dialyzed FCS.

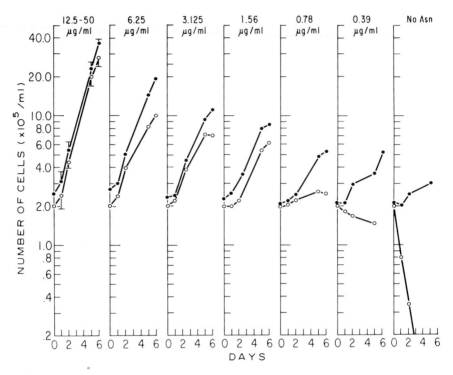

FIG. 1. Effects of different concentrations of asparagine (shown in the upper part of each graph) on the growth of MOLT-3 cells. Open circles, viable cell numbers; filled circles, total cell number (each point represents an average of duplicate experiments). Cell growth at asparagine concentrations of 12.5–50 µg/ml was essentially similar and the combined data from experiments with asparagine concentrations of 50, 25, and 12.5 µg/ml are shown as a single graph in the far left (each point represents the mean of three duplicate experiments with one SD).

Later, we simplified the establishment of Asn-independent MOLT-3 by growing the MOLT-3 cells for a week in a medium containing 25% of the Asn concentration in the original medium (12.5 µg/ml). Thereafter, the amount of Asn was successively reduced to approximately one-half the preceding Asn concentration by adding an equal volume of Asn-free RPMI-1640 medium with 10% dialyzed FCS once a week or biweekly. In 8 weeks the cells were able to grow vigorously in the Asn-free RPMI-1640 medium. These cells achieved a growth rate equal to that of the parent cell line (Figure 2) and were designated MOLT-3/Asn.

Asparagine Synthetase

Asparagine synthetase activity was measured by a method developed by Hakala (unpublished). Approximately 2×10^9 viable cells were pooled from 5 to 10 liters of cell suspension in logarithmic growth, collected by centrifugation for 10 minutes at $700 \times g$, washed twice with 0.15 M sodium chloride, and

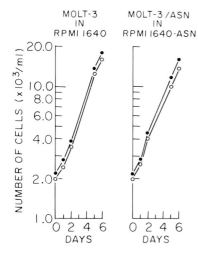

FIG. 2. Total (filled circles) and viable cell (open circles) growth of parent MOLT-3 cells in RPMI-1640 medium plus 10% FCS and MOLT-3/Asn in RPMI-1640 medium devoid of asparagine but with 10% dialyzed FCS.

frozen as a pellet at −75°C until assay. The cell pellets were homogenized in two parts of 50 mM Tris HCl-buffer, pH 7.4, containing 1 mM dithiothreitol and 0.5 mM ethylenediaminetetraacetic acid. The homogenate was centrifuged for 60 minutes at 105,000 × *g* and the supernatant dialyzed overnight at 4°C against 100 volumes of the same buffer, with two changes of the buffer. The reaction mixture consisted of 0.25 µCi ¹⁴C-L-aspartate (New England Nuclear Co., Boston, MA, specific activity, 50 mCi/mmol) in 4 mM of L-aspartate (Sigma Chemical Co., St. Louis, MO), 8 mM adenosine triphosphate (Sigma), 20 mM L-glutamine (Sigma), 4 mM $MgCl_2$, 50 mM Tris-HCl buffer, pH 7.6, and the crude cell extract in a total volume of 0.5 ml. The reaction mixture was incubated for 1, 2, 3, and 4 hours at 37°C, and the reaction stopped by adding 0.05 ml of 40% trichloroacetic acid (TCA). The TCA was removed by extraction with ether, and aliquots of the supernatant were analyzed for Asn formation by high-voltage paper electrophoresis (Horowitz et al. 1968). The enzyme activity was linear over an incubation time of 4 hours. Protein was measured by the method of Lowry et al. (1952).

Glutamic Oxaloacetic Transaminase

Enzyme activity of glutamic oxaloacetic transaminase was assayed by the method described by Babson et al. (1962) with a kit provided by Dow Diagnostics, Indianapolis, IN.

Asparaginase

Asnase was assayed by a method described by Meister et al. (1955) with the modification that the reaction mixture contained 0.1% FCS. Ammonia was determined by Russel's phenol hypochlorite reaction as modified by Konitzer

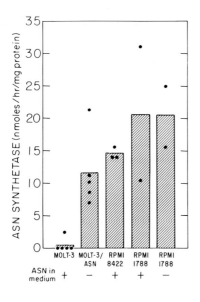

FIG. 3. Asparagine synthetase activity of MOLT-3, MOLT-3/Asn, RPMI-8422, and RPMI-1788. The + and − indicate presence or absence of asparagine in the RPMI-1640 medium, which contained 10% dialyzed FCS. The results of each experiment are shown as the filled circles, and the bars represent the average.

and Voigt. The details of this procedure have been described in our earlier communications (Ohnuma et al. 1967, 1972).

The Asn synthetase activities of MOLT-3, MOLT-3/Asn, RPMI-8422, and RPMI-1788 are illustrated in Figure 3. There was almost no Asn synthetase activity in the parent MOLT-3 cells. In contrast, the MOLT-3/Asn cells that had adapted to the Asn-free medium showed greatly increased Asn synthetase activity, approaching that of B-cells. Because of the endogenous Asnase (1.6 × 10⁻⁴ IU/mg protein) already present in MOLT-3/Asn cells and in the parent cells (1.4 × 10⁻⁴ IU/mg protein) (Table 2), the actual activity of Asn synthetase in MOLT-3/Asn is most probably higher. In the three enzyme systems measured—Asn synthetase, Asnase, and glutamic oxaloacetic transaminase—a marked increase in Asn synthetase was the only recognizable difference related to the adaptation of MOLT-3 cells to an Asn-free medium. This observation is consistent with the clinical observation that Asn resistance in patients with

TABLE 2. *Glutamic oxaloacetic transaminase and asparaginase activities of MOLT-3/Asn as compared to parent MOLT-3 and RPMI-1788 cell lines (average of 2 to 4 experiments)*

Cell line	Asn in the medium*	Glutamic oxaloacetic transaminase (units/ mg protein)	Asparaginase (iu/mg protein)
MOLT-3	+	0.20	1.4×10^{-4}
MOLT-3/Asn	−	0.19	1.6×10^{-4}
RPMI-1788	+	0.22	0.92×10^{-4}
RPMI-1788	−	0.26	not done

* Asn concentration, 50 μg/ml.

ALL is associated with an increase in Asn synthetase activity in ALL blasts (Haskell and Canellos 1969).

It is not clear whether the MOLT-3/Asn cell line represents a subpopulation of MOLT-3 cells insensitive to Asn deprivation or a mutation of the cells in the specific condition. The relative ease with which the new MOLT-3/Asn line was established and the lack of major cell death during the initial adaptation process support the possibility that the selecting procedure allowed an existing Asn-independent subpopulation to become established. It would require cloning experiments to prove this point. The present study establishes that an in vitro model of Asnase resistance in ALL is at hand.

BIOCHEMICAL BASES OF THE INSENSITIVITY OF HUMAN B-LYMPHOCYTES TO CYTOSINE ARABINOSIDE

Recently, such enzyme markers as terminal deoxynucleotidyl transferase (TdT), adenosine deaminase (ADA), and 5'-nucleotidase have been used as aids in subtyping leukemia and lymphoma (Coleman et al. 1978, Reaman et al. 1977; see also Anonymous 1977). ADA, an enzyme for purine metabolism, was found to be elevated in tissues with high lymphoid content, and the causal relationship between ADA deficiency and severe combined immunodeficiency has been explained (see Van der Weyden and Kelly 1976). Murine and human lymphocyte lines exposed to adenosine show decreased cell viability and proliferative activity. This toxic effect of adenosine was postulated to be secondary to an induced "pyrimidine starvation," as a depletion of the intracellular pyrimidine nucleotides occurred and the effect of adenosine could be circumvented by uridine (Green and Chan 1973). These observations led to speculation that immunodeficiency diseases associated with the absence of ADA might be the result of pyrimidine starvation of the cells in the lymphoid system (Green and Chan 1973, Ishii and Green 1973). In a study of established human lymphocyte lines, B-cells were found to have low ADA activity compared to that in T-cell lines (Tritsch and Minowada 1978). Uridine (Ur) administered in conjunction with a suboptimal dose of ara-C resulted in prolonged survival of mice bearing L1210 leukemia over that following administration of ara-C alone (Saslaw et al. 1968). In addition, uridine triphosphate (UTP) was reported to be a more effective phosphate donor than adenosine triphosphate for phosphorylation of ara-C when the latter nucleotide substrate level was low (Grindey et al. 1968, Kessel 1968). These reports suggested that differences in Ur metabolism between T- and B-cell lines contributed to their differential sensitivity to ara-C.

Effects of Uracil, Uridine, Deoxyuridine, and Tetrahydrouridine on Cell Growth Inhibition by Ara-C

In this experiment, six human lymphocyte lines were used: two T-cell lines (MOLT-3 and RPMI-8402) and four B-cell lines (RPMI-8422, BALM-2, DND-

39A, and BALL-1) (Table 1). Cells in stock culture were counted daily and used when they were in exponential growth phase. Cells at the initial concentration of 1.5×10^5/ml in culture tubes (#3033, Falcon) containing 10 ml of culture medium grew exponentially from day 0 to day 4.

The biological activity of ara-C (Upjohn, Kalamazoo, MI) was determined as follows: on day 0, 0.1 ml of ara-C solution at different concentrations was added to a 10-ml cell suspension, 1.5×10^5/ml, in culture tubes and incubated at 37°C for 3 days. On day 3, viable cells were counted on a hemocytometer, and the dose-response curve was drawn by calculating the viable cells as a percentage of the number in the control without ara-C. Viable cells were determined by trypan blue dye exclusion method. The influences of uracil (Sigma, diluted in phosphate-buffered saline, GIBCO, and sterilized by passing through 0.45 μm Millipore filter), Ur (Sigma), deoxyuridine (Sigma), and tetrahydrouridine (obtained from the National Cancer Institute, Bethesda, MD) on the biological activity of ara-C were determined by the comparison of dose-response curves in culture medium with or without the simultaneous addition of pyrimidines. All experiments were carried out in triplicate and repeated at least three times.

Dose-response curves of ara-C on each cell line are shown in Figure 4. The lower ara-C sensitivity of three B-cell lines (RPMI-8422, DND-39A, and BALM-2) than that of the two T-cell lines is in accord with our earlier observations

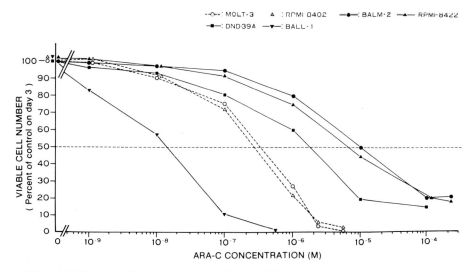

FIG. 4. Inhibition of cell growth of two T-cell lines (MOLT-3 and RPMI-8402) and four B-cell lines (RPMI-8422, DND-39A, BALM-2, and BALL-1) by ara-C. Culture tubes contained 1.5 × 10^5 cells/ml of RPMI-1640 medium with 10% FCS and different concentrations of ara-C. After 3 days, the viable cells were counted and plotted as a percentage of control without drug. Open symbols with broken lines, T-cells; closed symbols with solid lines, B-cells. Every point represents a mean of three to four repeated experiments in triplicate.

in which cells were exposed to ara-C for 5 days. An exceptional instance of very high sensitivity of BALL-1 to ara-C was recognized. Thus, based on ID_{50} (the drug concentration that produced 50% growth inhibition on day 3), with the exception of BALL-1, the differential sensitivity between T- and B-cells was 10- to 40-fold. (The exceptional ara-C sensitivity of the BALL-1 line will be discussed below.) Before the establishment of cell lines, all the patients from whom the cells were obtained, except for BALL-1 and BALM-2, had been treated with some antileukemic agents but had not received ara-C. BALL-1 and BALM-2 were established from patients before their treatment with antileukemic agents. It therefore appears that the differential susceptibility to ara-C presented here was not related to previous treatment with ara-C. Furthermore, although both RPMI-8402 and RPMI-8422 lines were derived from the same patient, Asn dependence as well as ara-C sensitivity differed.

Dose-response curves of ara-C in culture medium with the addition of 10^{-3} M Ur are shown in Figure 5. In the presence of Ur, the ara-C dose-response curve moved to the left, as the biological activity of ara-C in all six cell lines was potentiated by the Ur. Moreover, the sensitivity of the B-cell lines to ara-C, with the exception of BALL-1, was potentiated far more than that of the T-cell lines, so that on an ID_{50} basis the differential sensitivity between three B-cell lines (RPMI-8422, DND-39A, and BALM-2) and the two T-cell lines (MOLT-3 and RPMI-8402) was virtually nullified (Figure 6). The tails of the dose-response curves of the three B-cell lines in Figure 5 were higher than those of the T-cell lines, and ara-C could not produce more than 80% inhibition of cell growth after 3 days' exposure. This observation, together with the ability of ara-C to inhibit growth more effectively after 5 days' exposure (Ohnuma et

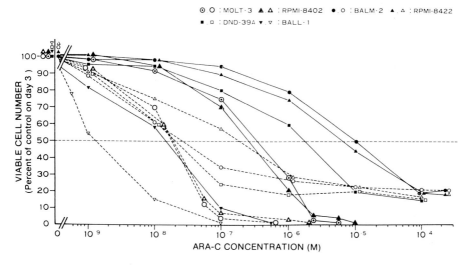

FIG. 5. Effects of uridine on cell growth inhibition by ara-C. Solid lines, medium without uridine (see Figure 4); broken lines, with 10^{-3} M uridine.

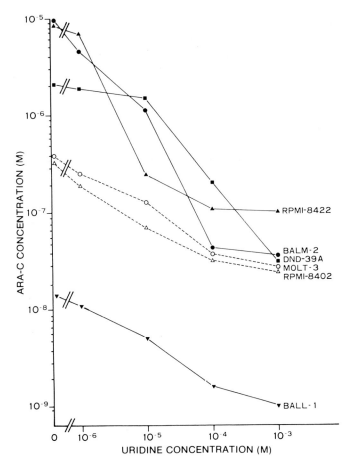

FIG. 6. Concentration-dependent potentiation by uridine of inhibitory effects of ara-C expressed as a shift of ID_{50}.

al. 1978), indicates two possibilities. Either these B-cell lines contain cells with a broader range of generation times and some of the cells were not in S-phase during the 3-day incubation period, or B-cells were more effectively blocked in their progression from G_1-phase to S-phase (Graham and Whitmore 1970).

Uracil at a concentration of 10^{-4} M showed no significant effects on the biological activity of ara-C, and the differential sensitivity among six cell lines was not changed (Figure 7), as was the case with deoxyuridine at the same concentration. In the presence of 10^{-4} M tetrahydrouridine, a pyrimidine nucleoside deaminase inhibitor (Camiener 1968), the biological activity of ara-C on all cell lines except BALL-1 was potentiated (Figure 8). The degree of potentiation in three B-cell lines (RPMI-8422, DND-39A, and BALM-2) was higher than in the two T-cell lines, and differential susceptibility to ara-C was reduced. The inability of tetrahydrouridine to shift ara-C dose-response curves

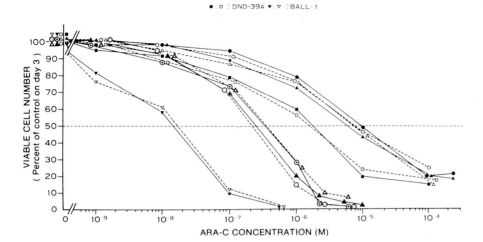

FIG. 7. Effects of uracil on cell growth inhibition by ara-C. Solid lines, medium without uracil (see Figure 4); broken lines, with 10^{-4} M uracil.

of BALL-1 suggests that BALL-1 has low deaminase activity. This in turn explains the high sensitivity of this cell line to ara-C.

Determination of Intracellular Cytosine Arabinoside Triphosphate (Ara-CTP)

In attempts to elucidate Ur's potentiation of the biological effects of ara-C, intracellular ara-CTP was measured. Protein-free cell extract was prepared as

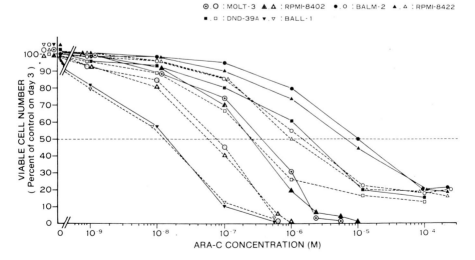

FIG. 8. Effects of tetrahydrouridine on the cell growth inhibition by ara-C. Solid lines, medium without tetrahydrouridine (see Figure 4); broken lines, with 10^{-4} M tetrahydrouridine.

described by Brenton et al. (1977). Briefly, aliquots of 10^7 cells were removed from stock cultures of the two T-cell lines (MOLT-3 and RPMI-8402) and three B-cell lines (BALM-2, RPMI-8422, and DND-39A), washed once, and resuspended in 10 ml of RPMI-1640 medium containing 10% FCS and 10^{-5} M ara-C with or without 10^{-4} M Ur. The cell suspension was incubated for 3 hours at 37°C. Cells were incubated simultaneously in medium that contained neither ara-C nor Ur to serve as control. The cells were washed twice with phosphate-buffered saline containing 5.5 mM glucose. One hundred microliters of 0.5 M perchloric acid was added to the cell pellet, which was stirred and then left in ice for 20 min. The milky substance was next centrifuged at 12,000 $\times g$ for 2 seconds (Eppendorf centrifuge #5412, Brinkmann Instruments, Westbury, NY), and the clear supernatant was neutralized with 12 μl of cold 4 M potassium hydroxide and 10 μl of 0.5 M sodium phosphate buffer, pH 7.4. They were mixed by centrifugation once, and 50 μl of supernatant was analyzed with a high-performance liquid chromatograph (Model 6000A solvent delivery system, Model 660 solvent programmer, and Model 450 variable wavelength detector, Waters Associates, Milford, MA) using xanthine diphosphate as an internal standard. Because it was found that nucleotides were unstable on prolonged storage at -20°C, the samples were analyzed on the same day they were prepared or after overnight refrigeration. A Partisil 10-SAX (What-

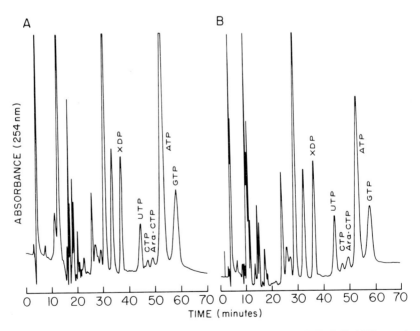

FIG. 9. High-performance liquid chromatographic separation of ara-CTP. Cells (10^7) were incubated in the medium containing 10^{-3} M ara-C with and without uridine, 10^{-4} M, at 37°C for 3 hours and protein-free cell extracts were assayed for nucleotide concentrations (see text for chromatographic conditions). Xanthine diphosphate, 1.5 nmoles, added as an internal standard. A, ara-C alone; B, ara-C plus uridine. Note increased ara-CTP peak in B.

man, Clifton, NJ) column was used. The column was eluted with a linear gradient (setting #6), starting with 0.007 M potassium phosphate buffer, pH 4.0, as the low-concentration eluent and 0.25 M potassium phosphate buffer/0.5 M potassium chloride, pH 4.5, as the high-concentration eluent; ambient temperature was used. The flow rate was 1.5 ml/min. The absorption at 254 nm was recorded with detection sensitivity of 0.02 a.u.f.s. Each peak was identified by comparing its retention time to that of known pure nucleotide standards. The concentration of ara-CTP was calculated from the peak height ratio of nucleotide to xanthine diphosphate, and the ratio was compared to those obtained when known concentrations of ara-CTP (Sigma) were added to protein-free extracts of the particular cell line studied. The detection limit for ara-CTP was 0.1 nmol/10^7 cells. Representative recordings are shown in Figure 9.

In the presence of Ur, there was a definite increase in ara-CTP peaks. The results, expressed as nmol/10^7 cells, ara-CTP/CTP or ara-CTP/GTP, are shown in Table 3. On whatever base used, there was a clear increase in ara-CTP in the presence of Ur. Ara-CTP increased by an average of 170% (data from RPMI-8422, in which ara-CTP could not be detected without Ur, are not included for the calculation). It was difficult to recognize any differences in the increase of ara-CTP between T- and B-cells.

Determination of Intracellular UTP and ATP Pools and UTP/ATP Ratio

After 3 hours of incubating 10^7 cells at 37°C with different concentrations of Ur, cell-free extracts were similarly prepared, and the intracellular UTP

TABLE 3. *Effects of Ara-C alone and Ara-C plus uridine on intracellular Ara-CTP*

	ara-CTP (nmol/10^7 cells)	ara-CTP/CTP	ara-CTP/GTP
T-cells			
MOLT-3			
ara-C alone	3.5	0.75	0.22
ara-C plus Ur	5.8 (166%)	0.63 (89%)	0.29 (132%)
RPMI-8402			
ara-C alone	1.0	0.42	0.066
ara-C plus Ur	2.2 (220%)	0.86 (205%)	0.13 (197%)
B-cells			
RPMI-8422			
ara-C alone	ud*	0	0
ara-C plus Ur	0.65	0.11	0.03
DND-39A			
ara-C alone	1.3	1.2	0.11
ara-C plus Ur	2.3 (177%)	1.7 (142%)	0.23 (209%)
BALM-2			
ara-C alone	0.2	0.18	0.02
ara-C plus Ur	0.5 (250%)	0.20 (111%)	0.03 (150%)

10^7 cells were incubated with 10^{-5} M ara-C with or without 10^{-4} M uridine for 3 hours and the protein-free cell extract was subjected to HPLC assay (see text).
  * Undetectable.

and ATP pools and UTP/ATP ratio were measured. The conditions for the high-performance liquid chromatographic assay were as follows: column, Parmaphase ABX (DuPont, Wilmington, DE); starting eluent, 0.001 M potassium phosphate buffer, pH 3.0; high-concentration eluent, 0.5 M potassium phosphate buffer, pH 3.4; flow rate 0.5 ml/min; concave gradient (setting #8); detection at 254 nm with sensitivity setting at 0.1 a.u.f.s. Concentrations of UTP and ATP were measured from peak heights and are expressed as nmol/10^7 cells (Table 4) or UTP/ATP ratio (Figure 10). The intracellular UTP pool for B-cells, 1.8 $\pm$ 0.6 (mean $\pm$ SD) nmol/10^7 cells, was 72% of that of T-cells (2.5 $\pm$ 0.5 nmol/10^7 cells). The intracellular ATP pool for B-cells (5.8 $\pm$ 2.4 nmol/10^7 cells) was 54% of that of T-cells (10.7 $\pm$ 4.1 nmol/10^7 cells). Incubation of cells with Ur resulted in a concentration-dependent increase in the intracellular pool for both T- and B-cell lines. The intracellular ATP pool was constant or tended to become lower with increasing Ur concentration for B-cell lines. When the increase in intracellular UTP was expressed as UTP/ATP ratio, that in BALM-2, RPMI-8422, DND-39A, and BALL-1 was far more than that in MOLT-3 and RPMI-8402 (Figure 10).

We interpret these findings as showing that ara-C resistance of certain B-cells is due to low intracellular UTP or ATP pools, or both, and that the potentiation of ara-C effects and progressive narrowing of the differential sensitivity to ara-C with increasing concentrations of Ur are the result of increased supply of UTP and concomitant increase in Ara-CTP. These observations and the interpretation are consistent with reports that ara-C phosphorylation is preferentially dependent on UTP as an energy source when the nucleotide level increases.

Our earlier work indicated that deoxycytidine kinase activity was not responsible for the differential sensitivity (Arkin et al. 1979). Reduced levels of deoxycyti-

TABLE 4. *Effects of uridine on intracellular UTP and ATP pools (results are shown as UTP/ ATP, nmol/10^7 cells)*

T-cells	Uridine added in the medium (M)	MOLT-3		RPMI-8402	
		Exp 1	Exp 2	Exp 1	Exp 2
	0	2.3/7.2	3.2/16.4	1.9/8.2	2.6/11.1
	10^{-5}	2.6/7.5	3.9/16.4	2.3/7.9	3.2/13.6
	10^{-4}	3.4/8.5	4.5/15.0	3.4/8.7	4.6/15.0
	10^{-3}	4.3/8.8	5.9/15.5	4.4/8.6	5.9/12.7

B-cells	Uridine added in the medium (M)	RPMI-8422	DND-39A	BALM-2		BALL-1	
		Exp 1	Exp 1	Exp 1	Exp 2	Exp 1	Exp 2
	0	0.9/1.8	1.9/7.7	1.7/4.3	2.3/6.6	2.6/8.5	1.4/6.0
	10^{-5}	nd*	1.9/7.0	2.3/4.5	3.0/5.4	7.1/7.5	2.0/4.7
	10^{-4}	1.6/2.0	3.5/6.5	2.3/3.3	4.7/6.3	8.1/6.2	4.3/4.7
	10^{-3}	nd*	4.6/5.8	2.7/2.6	6.7/7.0	12.1/5.7	7.4/5.1

* Not done.

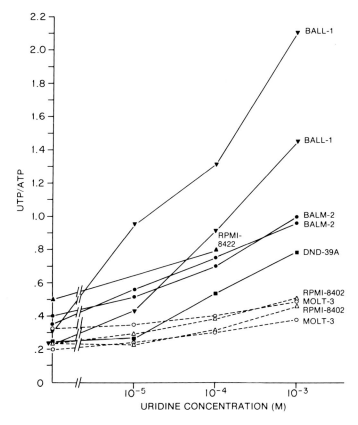

FIG. 10. Effects of uridine on intracellular UTP/ATP ratio. Cells (10^7) were incubated in the medium containing various concentrations of uridine at 37°C for 3 hours, and protein-free cell extracts were assayed for nucleotide concentrations by HPLC. (See text for chromatographic conditions.)

dine kinase, a larger pool of deoxycytidine nucleotides, a change in the affinity of ara-CTP, and increase in pyrimidine nucleoside deaminase have been described as mechanisms for acquired resistance to ara-C (Creasey 1975). Little is known, however, about the natural resistance of a tissue to ara-C, other than its relation to a slow cell cycle (Graham and Whitmore 1970). Our data strongly indicate that the natural resistance of certain tissue cell types to ara-C is due to low intracellular UTP or ATP pools, or both, and that this resistance can be overcome with the addition of Ur.

CONCLUSION

Human T-lymphocyte lines are Asn-dependent and sensitive to Asnase. We established an Asn-independent T-cell line, MOLT-3/Asn, and compared its enzymatic activities with the parent MOLT-3 line. The sensitivity of MOLT-3 cells to Asn depression was shown to be due to low levels of Asn synthetase.

Five of six human B-lymphocyte lines were shown to have a natural resistance to ara-C. This resistance was modified by the addition of Ur. B-cells were shown to have low intracellular pools of ATP and UTP. The addition of Ur resulted in an increase in intracellular UTP and ara-CTP pools for both T- and B-cells. For B-cells the addition of Ur resulted in a fourfold increase in the UTP/ATP ratio. In contrast, there was only a slight increase in the UTP/ATP ratio for T-cells. These results indicate that the natural ara-C resistance of B-cells is due to low levels of an energy source for conversion of ara-C to ara-CTP. The potentiation by Ur of the ara-C effect is associated with an increase in UTP, a likely energy source for the ara-C phosphorylation. Ara-C plus Ur may thus be considered worthy of exploration in therapy for certain ara-C-resistant neoplasms.

ACKNOWLEDGEMENT

We thank Dr. J. Minowada of the Roswell Park Memorial Institute, Buffalo, New York, for providing us with human lymphocyte lines used in this experiment. He also performed surface-marker analysis of DND-39A and DND-41 cell lines. This study was supported in part by US Public Health Service research grants CA 15936 and CA 25865 and by the United Leukemia Fund, Inc., New York, New York.

REFERENCES

Arkin, H., T. Ohnuma, G. Svet-Moldavsky, and J. F. Holland. 1979. Cytosine arabinoside and deoxycytidine combination in human T- and B-lymphocytes in culture (Abstract). Proc. Am. Assoc. Cancer Res. 20:162.

Anonymous. 1977. Enzyme markers in leukemia (editorial). Lancet 2:539–540.

Babson, A. L., P. O. Shapiro, P. A. R. Williams, and G. E. Phillips. 1962. The use of diazonium salt for determination of glutamic-oxaloacetic transaminase in serum. Clin. Chim. Acta 7:199–205.

Belpomme, D., G. Mathe, and A. J. S. Davis. 1977. Clinical significance and prognostic value of the T, B immunological classification of human primary acute lymphoid leukemias. Lancet 1:555–558.

Brenton, D. R., K. H. Astrin, M. K. Cruikshank, and E. Seegmiller. 1977. Measurement of free nucleotides in cultured human lymphoid cells using high pressure liquid chromatography. Biochem. Med. 17:231–247.

Camiener, G. W. 1968. Studies of the enzymatic deamination of ara-cytidine—V. Inhibition in vitro and in vivo by tetrahydrouridine and other reduced pyrimidine nucleosides. Biochem. Pharmacol. 17:1981–1991.

Chessells, J. M., R. M. Hardisty, N. J. Rapson, and M. F. Greaves. 1977. Acute lymphoblastic leukemia in children: classifications and prognosis. Lancet 2:1307–1309.

Coleman, S. M., M. F. Greenwood, J. J. Hutton, P. Holland, B. Lampkin, C. Krill, and J. E. Kastelic. 1978. Adenosine deaminase, terminal deoxynucleotidyl transferase (TdT), and cell surface markers in childhood acute leukemia. Blood 52:1125–1131.

Creasy, W. A. 1975. Arabinoside cytosine, in Antineoplastic and Immunosuppressive Agents, Part II, A. L. Sartorelli and D. G. Jones, eds. Springer-Verlag, New York, pp. 232–256.

Graham, F. L., and G. F. Whitmore. 1970. The effect of 1-β-D-arabinofuranosylcytosine on growth, viability and DNA synthesis of mouse L-cells. Cancer Res. 30:2627–2635.

Greaves, M. F., and T. A. Lister. 1981. Prognostic importance of immunologic markers in adult acute lymphoblastic leukemia. N. Engl. J. Med. 304:119–120.

Green, H., and T-S. Chan. 1973. Pyrimidine starvation induced by adenosine in fibroblasts and lymphoid cells: Role of adenosine deaminase. Science 182:836–837.

Grindey, G. B., L. D. Saslaw, and V. S. Waravdeker. 1968. Effects of uracil derivatives on phosphorylation of arabinosylcytosine. Mol. Pharmacol. 4:96–103.

Haskell, C. M., and G. P. Canellos. 1969. L-asparaginase resistance in human leukemia—asparagine synthetase. Biochem. Pharmacol. 18:2578–2580.

Horowitz, B., B. Madras, A. Meister, L. J. Old, L. A. Boyse, and E. Stocker. 1968. Asparagine synthetase activity of mouse leukemias. Science 160:533–535.

Ishii, K., and H. Green. 1973. Lethality of adenosine for cultured mammalian cells by interference with pyrimidine biosynthesis. J. Cell Sci. 13:429–439.

Kessel, D. 1968. Some observations on the phosphorylation of cytosine arabinoside. Mol. Pharmacol. 4:402–410.

Lowry, O. M., N. J. Rosebrough, A. L. Farr, R. J. Randall. 1952. Protein measurement with the Folin phenol reagent. J. Biol. Chem. 193:265–275.

Lozzio, C. B., and B. B. Lozzio. 1975. Human chronic myelogenous leukemic cell line with positive Philadelphia chromosome. Blood 45:321–334.

Meister, A., L. Levintow, R. E. Greenfield, and P. A. Abendschein. 1955. Hydrolysis and transfer reactions catalyzed by amidase preparations. J. Biol. Chem. 215:441–460.

Minowada, J., T. Ohnuma, and G. E. Moore. 1972. Rosette forming lymphoid cell lines. I. Establishment and evidence for origin of thymus-derived lymphocytes. J. Natl. Cancer Inst. 49:891–895.

Minowada, J., K. Sagawa, M. S. Lok, I. Kobonishi, S. Nakazawa, E. Tatsumi, T. Ohnuma, and N. Goldblum. 1980. A model of lymphoid-myeloid cell differentiation based on the study of marker profiles of 50 human leukemia-lymphoma cell lines, *in* International Symposium on New Trends in Human Immunology and Cancer Immunotherapy, B. Serrou and C. Rosenfeld, eds. Doin Publisher, Paris, pp. 188–199.

Minowada, J., T. Tsubota, M. F. Greaves, and T. R. Walters. 1977. A non-T, non-B human leukemia cell line (NALM-1): Establishment of the cell line and presence of leukemia associated antigens. J. Natl. Cancer Inst. 59:83–87.

Miyoshi, I., S. Hiraki, T. Tsubota, I. Kubonishi, Y. Matsuda, T. Nakayama, H. Kishimoto, and I. Kimura. 1977. Human B cell, T cell and null cell leukemic cell lines derived from acute lymphoblastic leukemias. Nature 267:843–844.

Ohnuma, T., H. Arkin, and J. F. Holland. 1980. Differences in chemotherapeutic susceptibility of human T-, B- and non-T/non-B lymphocytes in culture. Recent Results Cancer Res. 75:61–67.

Ohnuma, T., H. Arkin, J. Minowada, and J. F. Holland. 1978. Differential chemotherapeutic susceptibility of human T-lymphocytes and B-lymphocytes in culture. J. Natl. Cancer Inst. 60:749–752.

Ohnuma, T., F. Bergel, and R. C. Bray. 1967. Enzymes in cancer. Asparaginase from chicken liver. Biochem. J. 103:238–245.

Ohnuma, T., J. F. Holland, H. Arkin, and J. Minowada. 1977. L-asparagine requirements of human T-lymphocytes and B-lymphocytes in culture. J. Natl. Cancer Inst. 59:1061–1063.

Ohnuma, T., J. F. Holland, and P. Meyer. 1972. *Erwinia carotovora* asparaginase in patients with prior anaphylaxis to asparaginase from *E. coli.* Cancer 30:376–381.

Reaman, G. H., N. Levin, A. Muchmore, B. J. Holiman, and D. G. Poplack. 1977. Diminished lymphoblast 5'-nucleotidase activity in acute lymphoblastic leukemia with T-cell characteristics. N. Engl. J. Med. 300:1374–1377.

Saslaw, L. D., G. B. Grindey, and V. S. Waravdeker. 1968. Sparing action of uridine on the activity of arabinosylcytosine with normal and leukemic mice. Cancer Res. 28:11–20.

Schneider, U., H. Schwenk, and G. Bornkamm. 1977. Characterization of EBV-genome negative "null" and "T" cell lines derived from children with acute lymphoblastic leukemia and leukemic transformed non-Hodgkin's lymphoma. Int. J. Cancer 19:621–626.

Sen, L. and L. Borella. 1975. Clinical importance of lymphoblasts with T markers in childhood acute leukemia. N. Engl. J. Med. 292:828–832.

Tritsch, G., and J. Minowada. 1978. Differences in purine metabolizing enzyme activities in human leukemia T-cell, B-cell and null cell lines: Brief communication. J. Natl. Cancer Inst. 60:1301–1304.

Van der Weyden, M. B., and W. N. Kelley. 1976. Adenosine deaminase and immune function. Br. J. Haematol. 34:159–163.

Molecular Interrelations of Nutrition and Cancer,
edited by M. S. Arnott, J. van Eys, and Y.-M. Wang.
Raven Press, New York © 1982.

Control of Food Intake in the Experimental Cancerous Host

Seoras D. Morrison

Laboratory of Pathophysiology, National Cancer Institute, Bethesda, Maryland 20205

The central and definitive feature of the very complex syndrome known as cancer cachexia is progressive tissue depletion. This or any other tissue depletion can only arise from the metabolizable food intake of the organism falling short of the total metabolic cost. The existence of this shortfall of food intake can generally be reliably determined only by the existence of the resulting depletion. The food intake, to be deficient, does not necessarily decline absolutely: it may remain constant or even increase, but it must decline relative to metabolic cost. Ideally, the extent and progress of "decline" in food intake would be measured by its ratio to metabolic demand (Figure 1b).

In most experimental tumors that kill the host, there is cachexia and an absolutely declining food intake. Even in this simple situation, however, the interpretation is not straightforward. As the host is depleted, its metabolic demand falls so that the fraction of need represented by the declining food intake is greater than the quantitative decline would indicate. Contrarily, as the tumor grows, its maintenance cost and, usually, its daily accretion cost also grow so that the amount of food (nutrient) preempted by the tumor increases and the fraction of need represented by the ingested food available to the host is less than the total ingested food would indicate. These effects have to be evaluated and taken into account in order to assess the magnitude of the relative decline in food intake in order, in turn, to investigate the causes and mechanism of decline. A general picture of the course of cachexia, food intake, and some aspects of metabolic cost is shown in Figure 1 for three host/tumor organisms.[1]

In most normal, physiological processes, if food is freely available, food intake moves, eventually, to meet changes in metabolic cost. This occurs in (nonhibernating) exposure to cold (Brobeck 1960), change in motor activity (Mayer et al. 1954), change in caloric density of food (Adolph 1947), pregnancy and lactation (Slonaker 1925), and so on. There may be transient depletion or accretion, or change to a new stable level of tissue reserves, but, eventually, costs and

---

[1] Rat host/tumor organisms specifically cited here are: S-D/W256 (Walker 256 carcinosarcoma in Sprague-Dawley rats); S-D/4M (4M carcinoma in Sprague-Dawley rats); B/H5123 (Morris 5123 hepatoma in Buffalo rats); F/MCA-S (methylcholanthrene-originated sarcoma in Fischer 344 rats).

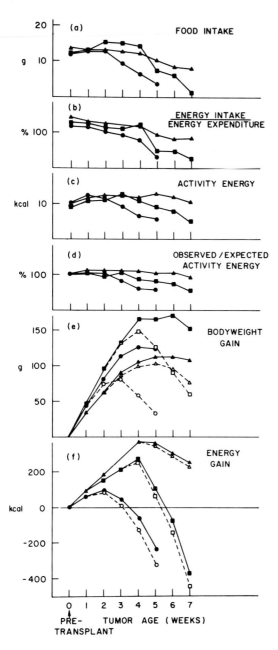

FIG. 1. Development of cachexia, including changes in food intake, in carcass weight and energy, and in motor activity, during growth of three different experimental, transplantable tumors in adult male rats. ●○ S-D/W256 organism; □■ S-D/4M organism; ▲△ B/H5123 organism. Solid symbols and lines are total organism (host plus tumor); open symbols and broken lines are host only. (Reproduced from Morrison 1973b.)

intake are brought back into balance. The problem of cachectic states is that the depletion and the imbalance between intake and cost are progressive.

There are three broad classes of change that might account for the progressive depletion. (1) The depletion might be a defense mechanism: the decline in food intake might be appropriate to the disease and advantageous to the host. (2)

Specific controls of feeding might be impaired by other systemic effects of the tumor. (3) Necessary conditions for feeding might be abolished by other systemic effects of the tumor.

DECLINE OF FOOD INTAKE AS A DEFENSE MECHANISM

For a response to disease, in this case decline of food intake, to be appropriate and defensive it is necessary that, on balance, it be advantageous. It must either improve chances of recovery or increase the span of survival. Some disease-induced anorexias do improve chances of recovery (Murray and Murray 1979). It seems patent that cachexia does not contribute to recovery from cancer—it does not lead to spontaneous regression of tumor—but its influence on span of survival is conjectural, is not at all self-evident, and has received no explicit consideration. Warren's assertion (1932) of starvation as a major cause of death in cancer patients has dominated cachexia research, and its tacit assumptions and implications have gone unquestioned.

What Warren and others saw is that many patients who die of cancer are starved (depleted) at death and show no other clearly identifiable cause of death. To justify his assertion, however, it would be necessary to show that if starvation were prevented the patient would, *in the absence of other treatment,* survive longer. To justify the possibility of cachexia being a defense mechanism, it would be necessary to show that the host in which cachexia is prevented dies sooner. This is obviously not a feasible line of investigation with human subjects. Neither has it been pursued in animal studies. But the fragmentary relevant data available, from artificial alimentation (Popp et al. 1981) and the existence of large energy reserves (Baillie et al. 1963), indicate that food input or energy reserves do not alter survival time substantially. It has been suggested, on the ground that tumor-bearing animals show a greater response than healthy ones to food novelty, that the host may mistakenly perceive disadvantage in feeding by relating the food eaten to the growing sense of being ill (Bernstein and Sigmundi 1980).

Although the question remains unresolved, there are trenchant arguments against cachexia being a defense mechanism. First, even if it modestly prolongs survival time, it is a miserably ineffective defense. Second, the host appears to invoke compensatory mechanisms that delay the appearance of cachexia and hypophagia (see later sections), and it is difficult to believe that the wisdom of the body could simultaneously invoke a defense mechanism and defend itself against the defense mechanism. All of these considerations refer only to the possible merits of nonfeeding or feeding in the absence of other treatment. It is possible and even likely that the unstarved host is better able to benefit from anticancer treatment than the starved one (Copeland et al. 1977).

FAILURE OF SPECIFIC FEEDING CONTROLS

Feeding is a behavior that must be integrated and operated by central nervous activity. The appropriate central nervous state that generates feeding behavior is set by inflow of information from the periphery concerning blood nutrient levels, nutrient reserves, liver function, gastrointestinal fill, rate of flow of nutrients across gut mucosa, core temperature, and rate of outward heat flow, and information from the environment concerning availability of food. The information is transmitted by both neural and humoral links. However, these are largely broad inferences drawn on the basis that feeding must logically be related to the consequences of food ingestion and on the basis of what variables can be technically measured. There is little precise knowledge of what variables are actually sensed by the organism, what vehicles are used to transmit the information to the brain, and what parts of the brain process the information.

Hypothalamic Function

A part of the brain definitely known to influence feeding is the central hypothalamus, operating as a component in the limbic circuit of the diencephalon (see, for example, Morgane and Jacobs 1969). The detailed knowledge of this area, its neurotransmitters and its relation to associated tracts, has expanded greatly in the last 10 or 15 years (see as examples Hernandez and Hoebl 1980, Stricker and Zigmond 1976). But the central evidence of its function in relation to feeding remains the earlier basic findings that destruction of one part, the ventromedial nucleus, produces hyperphagia and obesity (Brobeck et al. 1943) and destruction of the other part, the lateral area, produces total aphagia (Anand and Brobeck 1951). Recovery from the total aphagia, either spontaneously or after a period of artificial feeding, is characteristic of the lateral hypothalamic damage (Morrison and Mayer 1957, Teitelbaum and Epstein 1962), but residual deficits in feeding and drinking remain permanently after recovery from the acute aphagia (Epstein and Teitelbaum 1967, Stricker and Zigmond 1976). When tumors are grown in either of these hypothalamically damaged preparations, the course of tumor-induced cachectic depletion and decline of food intake is unaltered from that in intact animals (Baillie et al. 1965, Liebelt et al. 1971, Morrison 1968c). These studies were relatively crude, and no other central regions thought to influence feeding have been examined. Present evidence, then, gives no support for hypothalamic involvement in cancer anorexia, but application to the cancerous host of the more refined fractionating techniques now available (e.g., microtractotomy, local application of drugs, neurotransmitters, and neurotoxins) might allow a more confident conclusion on this point.

While the precise variables and hormones that control feeding are not known, there are a variety of stimuli and hormones that alter feeding in the healthy intact animal in reproducible and predictable ways. Many of these are independent, in the sense that they do not merely replace one another but produce responses that are additive or synergistic or antagonistic, and they can be regarded as reflecting independent control mechanisms. They include the feeding responses to change in caloric density of food (Adolph 1947), change in environ-

mental temperature (Brobeck 1960), exercise (Mayer et al. 1954), taste adulteration of food (Teitelbaum and Epstein 1962), and insulin and other hormones
(Mackay et al. 1940). Tumor-induced depression of the normal response to
these stimuli would indicate tumor-induced impairment of the specific feeding
control mechanisms.

It is important to distinguish between impairments that arise from the presence
of tumor and may potentially generate depletion, and those that are themselves
secondary to the developing depletion. In general, the appearance of impairment
of a response before there is any sign of depression of food intake or of depletion
is acceptable evidence that the impairment is primary. If the impairment pro-
gresses with tumor size and with depletion, its initial development may be
primary, but its final effect may be the result of positive feedback from the depletion.

Response to Change in Caloric Density of Food

Within limits (for the rat, between about 2 and 5 kcal/g), mammals respond
to change in metabolizable caloric density of food by altering bulk intake to
the extent that keeps metabolizable energy intake constant. Growth of Walker
256 in Sprague-Dawley rats (S-D/W256) reduces this response within the first
quarter of tumor life (time from implantation to death of host from tumor)
and completely abolishes it by the third quarter (Figure 2b) (Morrison 1972).
However, neither decline of food intake (Figure 2a) nor cachectic depletion is
detectable in this organism until the third quarter. This response is impaired,
and the impairment is primary and not dependent on advanced depletion, but
its extent increases with size of tumor. Since the impairment much precedes
any overt decline of intake it must be compensated, presumably by other as
yet unimpaired controls moving to different parts of their functional range.

The normal Buffalo strain of rat does not show this response to caloric dilution
(Figure 2b) (Morrison 1973c). When Morris 5123 hepatoma (B/H5123 organism)
is grown in this strain the normal zero response to 50% caloric dilution is
changed to a negative response and, eventually, feeding on the dilute diet is
totally inhibited (Figure 2b). However, the negative response does not appear
until tumor-induced decline in food intake is already detectable (Figure 2a).
In this case the impairment may be secondary to depletion.

Response to Reduced Environmental Temperature

The normal response of mammals to reduced environmental temperature is
an increase in food intake (Brobeck 1960). Stevenson and co-workers (1963)
showed that this response was at least qualitatively retained in S-D/W256 even
in an advanced cachectic state, but it was not possible to determine from the
data whether there was any quantitative impairment of the response. Because
the normal feeding response to cold is slow compared with the rapid increase

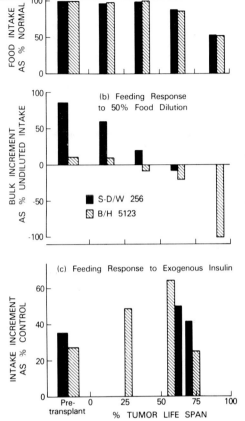

FIG. 2. The course of: a, decline of food intake; b, deterioration of response to caloric dilution; and c, response to exogenous insulin (1.5 U/100 g protamine zinc insulin) of S-D/W256 organism (solid blocks) and B/H5123 organism (hatched blocks). The growth of tumor is expressed as fractions of the life-span of the tumor (time from transplant to death of the host from the tumor).

in metabolic cost (to meet increased outward heat flow) there is an initial substantial cold-induced reduction of body weight. This complication must be added to the reduced host body weight due to cachectic depletion and the reduced availability of nutrient to the host due to tumor growth. When all these factors are taken into account, the cold-specific feeding response to cold of S-D hosts growing W256 is depressed by about 30% compared with normal rats at all reduced temperatures down to 5°C and is independent of tumor burden or extent of cachectic depletion (Morrison, manuscript in preparation). This response, then, is partially impaired by the simple presence of tumor, and the impairment is primary. Again, since this impairment appears well before overt hypophagia and cachexia, it must be compensated.

Both of these responses and the control mechanisms that they reflect appear to be normally independent of hypothalamic function (Carlisle and Stellar 1969, Epstein and Teitelbaum 1967).

Response to Exogenous Insulin

The two control mechanisms considered above act to maintain or restore balance between energy intake and cost. The increased food intake in response to exogenous insulin (Mackay et al. 1940) is a positive energy imbalance induced by an imposed hormonal imbalance that, in effect, increases the rate of sequestration (by lipogenesis) from the available pool of energy-yielding substrate. The influence of insulin on food intake is at least partly mediated by modification of glucose utilization by the central hypothalamus (Oomura 1976). This feeding response is not quantitatively impaired by the presence of even quite large tumors (Morrison 1973a), and there is some evidence that the response may be enhanced by the presence of tumor (Figure 2c). The enhancement may represent part of the compensatory process that the impairment of other responses seems to demand.

Palatability and Taste Perception

It is not certain that taste (and smell and other exteroceptive stimuli) represents a true control of food intake, although it can certainly influence it. Most experimental studies on taste, using taste adulteration of food, have been of very short duration and the changes found in food intake were probably transient. Idiopathic dysgeusias that have been described make life very miserable for the victims (Henkin 1977), but there is no clear evidence that they seriously affect food intake. They are related to zinc deficiency, which, when severe, produces cyclical hypophagia (Chesters and Quartermain 1970). However, food adulterated by bitter taste at a level that would produce no or only transient effect on food intake by intact rats depresses intake by rats with hypothalamic damage much more severely (Teitelbaum and Epstein 1962).

Both experimental and clinical studies have found altered taste perception, as measured by taste preference, in the presence of tumor (DeWys 1974). This consists of depressed perception of sweet and heightened perception of bitter. In the clinical studies, this dysgeusia did not appear until the patients were already cachectic and were being treated for their cancers. Objective response to therapy diminished the dysgeusia. In the experimental study (S-D/W256) the taste preference shift was not detected until 2 days before death from tumor. It seems possible, therefore, that this change is secondary to cachectic depletion. In a preliminary examination of this problem, S-D/W256 and B/H5123 organisms were given diets adulterated with quinine-HCl (bitter) for the 7-day period during which spontaneous hypophagia and cachexia first became detectable. A slight but significantly greater depression of food intake was seen in the tumor-bearing compared with tumor-free rats given similarly adulterated food (Morrison, unpublished work). Change in taste perception might, therefore, occur early enough to be primary rather than secondary to cachectic depletion. The adulteration levels used in this preliminary study were very high, and it is still not clear that the taste effect is an important contributor to tumor-induced hypophagia.

Response to Amino Acid Deficiency

Most nutritional deficiencies depress food intake. The anorexia induced by essential amino acid deficiency is regarded as the result of nitrogen utilization's being depressed to the level imposed by the limiting (deficient) amino acid. It is not clear whether this effect should be regarded as reflecting a specific control of food intake or as a necessary condition for feeding. The depression of food intake by this method has been reported to be mediated by the prepyriform cortex (Leung and Rogers 1971).

Rats were alternated between 2 days on a histidine-deficient diet and 3 days on a complete diet for a total of five cycles (days 10–35 of tumor growth). In the absence of tumor and before cachexia developed in rats growing W256, the food intake alternated in the expected way between deficient and complete diet. As tumor-induced cachexia developed, intake of the complete diet was depressed, but the additional deficiency-induced depression diminished and, eventually, vanished (Radcliffe and Morrison 1979). In another study (Radcliffe and Morrison 1980a), a diet deficient in both lysine and threonine depressed food intake of normal and of precachectic tumor-bearing rats, but did not further depress intake of rats already hypophagic because of tumors.

There are many possible explanations for these results. The simplest is that the hypophagic responses to cancer and to amino acid deficiency have a common central mediation (possibly the prepyriform cortex). By this view, the central area would respond to spurious signals, such as molecular fragments from the tumor (Theologides 1974). The central response capacity would be progressively occupied and, eventually, saturated by this spurious system, and excess capacity to respond to amino acid deficiency would be progressively reduced and, eventually, unavailable. No work has been done to test this or any other explanation.

An excess of tryptophan depresses food intake. However, this depression is added to the tumor-induced depression (Radcliffe and Morrison 1980b).

Compensation for Impaired Control Mechanisms

Since impairment of control mechanisms can be detected before there is any overt decline of food intake or cachexia, these impairments must be compensated. The apparent enhancement of response to insulin (Figure 2c) represents a possible compensatory mechanism, but the dependence of the mechanism on hypothalamic integrity and cachexia's apparent independence of the hypothalamus suggests that the mechanism is relatively unimportant.

Food intake can change by two modes: a change in total activity devoted to feeding or a change in the intensity or efficiency of feeding (the amount of food ingested per unit of feeding activity) (Morrison and Coffey 1973). In a study to establish which mode of feeding change is involved in cancerous anorexia, we (1976) found that total activity devoted to feeding started to fall immediately after transplant of tumor (W256, 4M, and H5123), but for the first two thirds of tumor life feeding efficiency increased so that food intake was maintained. Eventually, feeding efficiency plateaued or declined, and with the continued decline in feeding activity food intake declined, producing depletion (Figure 3). The breakdown of control of food intake starts early in tumor growth and is expressed as a reduction of feeding activity. For most of tumor life, however, it is behaviorally compensated by increased feeding efficiency.

Rats that have recovered from lateral hypothalamic damage show reduced feeding efficiency in the form of increased food scattering (Teitelbaum and Epstein 1962, Morrison 1968b). If lateral hypothalamic damage were also to result in depression of feeding efficiency as defined in the tumor studies, the tumor-induced increase in feeding efficiency might be disabled. Again, the effect would have to be deemed unimportant in practice.

Rats with lateral hypothalamic damage severe enough to have produced more than 2 days of total aphagia do show chronically increased feeding activity and decreased feeding efficiency after recovery from the acute aphagia. This

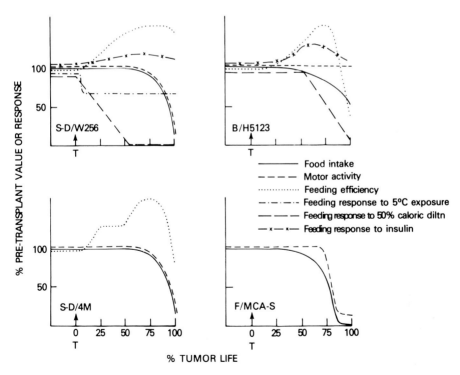

FIG. 3. Course of food intake and feeding-related functional impairments in four rat host/tumor organisms.

depression of feeding efficiency as a result of lateral hypothalamic damage does not, however, prevent a subsequent tumor-induced increase in efficiency in these rats (Morrison 1981). This behavioral compensation may thus be of practical importance, since it is mediated by an extrahypothalamic pathway.

NECESSARY CONDITIONS FOR FEEDING

In addition to specific controls that balance intake and cost, there are conditions that necessarily must be fulfilled if feeding is to take place at all and if the specific feeding controls are to have opportunity to operate. Obvious conditions are availability of food and nonspecific arousal: the animal has to be awake to be able to eat.

Feeding is a motor activity that, depending on physical ease of access to food and ease of mastication and deglutition, can engage a substantial motor energy cost (Morrison 1968a). Another necessary condition for feeding, therefore, is capacity for voluntary motor activity.

By using an animal calorimeter with suitably rapid response, it is possible to partition total daily energy expenditure into a compartment attributable to resting metabolism and a compartment attributable to all motor activity (Morrison 1968a). For normal rats in the environmental range of thermal neutrality the activity compartment accounts for about 25% of total energy expenditure. This fraction is not altered by food deprivation or body size (Morrison 1968a). Total energy cost of the S-D host growing W256 does not change more than would be expected from the change in body weight and food intake (until the terminal collapse), but the activity compartment of energy expenditure falls throughout the cachectic phase, with a corresponding increase in the rest compartment (Morrison 1971). When the activity compartment has fallen to about 10%, estimated to be the lower limit compatible with vital function, food intake is zero (Morrison 1971, 1973b). This diminution of the activity compartment to a value that represents effectively zero external motor activity has been found in three (S-D/W256, S-D/4M, F/MCA-S) of the four host/tumor organisms examined, but the detailed time relations and rates of depression vary (Figure 3). In these three organisms, also, the food intake eventually falls to or near zero. In the tumor-bearing organism that did not show depression and elimination of motor activity (B/H5123), food intake declined slowly through the second half of tumor growth but did not fall to zero (Figures 1 and 3).

Excision of the tumor (S-D/W256) immediately restored the activity compartment to normal (Morrison 1971). Prevention of cachectic depletion by total parenteral nutrition (F/MCA-S) did not prevent the depression and elimination of motor activity (Popp et al. 1981). The depression of motor activity, which can be regarded as the experimental analogue of the asthenia of clinical cancer, is thus a direct function of the tumor and is not secondary to cachectic starvation.

The cachectic process is often not examined until food intake has fallen to zero. It is important to recognize that it may not be possible to identify specific feeding impairments at that time, since all feeding may be disabled by constraint of motor activity. In principle, this could happen while all specific feeding controls are perfectly functional.

CONCLUSION

An attempt has been made here to define and to analyze the structure of cachectic depletion, which is the center from which many of the nutritional problems of cancer radiate. Since feeding and depletion are organismic phenomena, the analysis has been entirely at the organismic level. Optimum use of information at the subcellular and molecular level is dependent on a reasonably dense body of organismic information against which prediction can be tested.

The course of food intake and, as far as is at present known, of the impairments that potentially depress it are summarized in Figure 3 for four rat host/tumor organisms. When capacity for motor activity is constrained by tumor, food intake seems to be influenced more by this constraint than by specific feeding impairments. It seems likely that the wide variation observed in occurrence and extent of cachexia in clinical cancer (DeWys 1981) and in extent in experimental cancer is governed by the occurrence and timing of impairment of a variety of specific and nonspecific influences on food intake.

In principle, the differences in occurrence and extent of impairment among different feeding responses should allow, from the regions of coincidence and separation of the normal pathways, dissection of the particular components of feeding control that are impaired in cachectic hypophagia. Unfortunately, this requires a knowledge of the normal control pathways much more detailed than we possess. However, a reasonable, although admittedly speculative, start on functional dissection can be made. The hypothalamic independence of those responses so far found to be impaired and the hypothalamic dependence of the one response (to insulin) so far found to be unimpaired or enhanced corroborate the direct findings of hypothalamic independence of cancerous hypophagia and point to peripheral failure. On the other hand, the activation of an extrahypothalamic pathway for changes in feeding efficiency indicates that there is functional central involvement. This is also consonant with the paradoxical findings for amino acid deficiency. Peripherally, the quantitative and qualitative differences in impairment of response to change in caloric density of food and to change in environmental temperature suggest a common partial impairment dependent on tumor presence (e.g., impairment of response to depletion of lipid reserves) and a gastrointestinal impairment dependent on tumor burden (e.g., modification of liver function). Information on changes in pattern of feeding would make it possible to assess whether spurious satiety signals (reflected by smaller meals) or attenuated hunger signals (reflected by fewer meals) were the primary transmission error and would allow further dissection of peripheral deficits. Again, unfortunately, there is insufficient information on this point.

REFERENCES

Adolph, E. F. 1947. Urges to eat and drink in rats. Am. J. Physiol. 151:110–125.

Anand, B. K., and J. R. Brobeck. 1951. Hypothalamic control of food intake in rats and cats. Yale J. Biol. Med. 24:123–140.

Baillie, P., F. K. Millar, and A. W. Pratt. 1965. Food and water intakes and Walker tumor growth in rats with hypothalamic lesions. Am. J. Physiol. 209:293–300.

Bernstein, I. L., and R. A. Sigmundi. 1980. Tumor anorexia: a learned food aversion? Science 209:416–418.

Brobeck, J. R. 1960. Food and temperature. Recent Prog. Hor. Res. 16:439–466.

Brobeck, J. R., J. Tepperman, and C. N. H. Long. 1943. Experimental hypothalamic hyperphagia in the albino rat. Yale J. Biol. Med. 15:831–853.

Carlisle, H. J., and E. Stellar. 1969. Caloric regulation and food preference in normal, hyperphagic and aphagic rats. J. Comp. Physiol. Psychol. 69:107–114.

Chesters, J. K., and J. Quartermain. 1970. Effects of zinc deficiency on food intake and feeding patterns of rats. Br. J. Nutr. 42:1061–1069.

Copeland, E. M., J. M. Daly, and S. J. Dudrick. 1977. Nutrition as an adjunct to cancer treatment in the adult. Cancer Res. 37:2451–2456.

DeWys, W. D. 1974. Abnormalities of taste as a remote effect of a neoplasm. Ann. N.Y. Acad. Sci. 230:427–434.

DeWys, W. D. 1981. Clinical parameters related to anorexia. Cancer Treat. Rep. (in press).

Epstein, A. N., and P. Teitelbaum. 1967. Specific loss of the hypoglycemic control of feeding in recovered lateral rats. Am. J. Physiol. 213:1159–1167.

Henkin, R. I. 1977. New aspects in the control of food intake and appetite. Ann. N.Y. Acad. Sci. 300:321–334.

Hernandez, L., and B. G. Hoebl. 1980. Basic mechanisms of feeding and weight regulation, *in* Obesity, A. J. Stunkard, ed. W. B. Saunders, Philadelphia, pp. 25–47.

Leung, P. M.-B., and Q. R. Rogers. 1971. Importance of pre-pyriform cortex in food-intake response to amino acids. Am. J. Physiol. 221:929–935.

Liebelt, R. A., A. G. Liebelt, and H. M. Johnston. 1971. Lipid mobilization and food intake in experimentally obese mice bearing transplanted tumors. Proc. Soc. Exp. Biol. Med. 138:482–490.

Mackay, E. M., J. W. Callaway, and R. H. Barnes. 1940. Hyperalimentation in normal animals produced by protamine insulin. J. Nutr. 20:59–66.

Mayer, J., N. B. Marshall, J. J. Vitale, J. H. Christensen, M. B. Mashayekhi, and F. J. Stare. 1954. Exercise, food intake and bodyweight in normal rats and genetically obese adult mice. Am. J. Physiol. 177:544–548.

Morgane, P. J., and H. L. Jacobs. 1969. Hunger and satiety. World Rev. Nutr. Diet. 10:100–213.

Morrison, S. D. 1968a. The constancy of the energy expended by rats on spontaneous activity, and the distribution of activity between feeding and non-feeding. J. Physiol. (Lond.) 197:305–323.

Morrison, S. D. 1968b. The relationship of energy expenditure and spontaneous activity to the aphagia of rats with lesions in the lateral hypothalamus. J. Physiol. (Lond.) 197:325–343.

Morrison, S. D. 1968c. Effect of growth of a tumor on the regulation of water intake. JNCI 41:1241–1248.

Morrison, S. D. 1971. Partition of energy expenditure between host and tumor. Cancer Res. 31:98–107.

Morrison, S. D. 1972. Feeding response to change in absorbable food fraction during growth of Walker 256 carcinosarcoma. Cancer Res. 32:968–972.

Morrison, S. D. 1973a. Control of food intake during growth of a Walker 256 carcinosarcoma. Cancer Res. 33:526–528.

Morrison, S. D. 1973b. Limited capacity for motor activity as a cause for declining food intake in cancer. JNCI 51:1535–1539.

Morrison, S. D. 1973c. Differences between rat strains in metabolic activity and in control systems. Am. J. Physiol. 224:1305–1308.

Morrison, S. D. 1976. Generation and compensation of the cancer cachectic process by spontaneous modification of feeding behavior. Cancer Res. 36:228–233.

Morrison, S. D. 1981. Extra-hypothalamic mediation of changes in feeding behavior induced by growth of Walker 256 carcinosarcoma in rats. Cancer Res. 41:1710–1714.

Morrison, S. D., and N. F. Coffey. 1973. Feeding activity and feeding efficiency as distinct modes of change in food intake. J. Appl. Physiol. 34:268–270.

Morrison, S. D., and J. Mayer. 1957. Adipsia and aphagia in rats after lateral subthalamic lesions. Am. J. Physiol. 191:248–254.

Murray, M. J., and A. B. Murray. 1979. Anorexia of infection as a mechanism of host defense. Am. J. Clin. Nutr. 32:593–596.

Oomura, Y. 1976. Significance of glucose, insulin, and free fatty acid on the hypothalamic feeding and satiety neurons, *in* Hunger, Basic Mechanisms and Clinical Implications, D. Novin, W. Wyrwicka, and G. A. Bray, eds. Raven Press, New York, pp. 145–157.

Popp, M. B., S. D. Morrison, and M. F. Brennan. 1981. Total parenteral nutrition in a methylcholanthrene-induced rat sarcoma model. Cancer Treat. Rep. (in press).

Radcliffe, J. D., and S. D. Morrison. 1979. The effect of feeding a histidine-free diet on the food intake of normal and tumor-bearing rats. (Abstract) Fed. Proc. 38:1131.

Radcliffe, J. D., and S. D. Morrison. 1980a. Protein quality, food intake and growth in normal and Walker 256 carcinosarcoma-bearing rats. J. Nutr. 110:2182–2189.

Radcliffe, J. D., and S. D. Morrison. 1980b. Dietary tryptophan level, food intake and growth in normal and Walker 256 carcinosarcoma rats. Nutrition Reports International 22:563–569.

Slonaker, J. R. 1925. The effect of copulation, pregnancy, pseudo-pregnancy and lactation on the voluntary activity and food consumption of the albino rat. Am. J. Physiol. 71:362–394.

Stevenson, J. A. F., B. M. Box, and R. B. Wright. 1963. The effect of a cold environment on malignant anorexia. Can. J. Biochem. Physiol. 41:531–532.

Stricker, E. M., and M. J. Zigmond. 1976. Recovery of function after damage to central catecholamine-containing neurons: A neurochemical model for the lateral hypothalamic syndrome, *in* Progress in Psychobiology and Physiological Psychology, vol. 6. Academic Press, New York, pp. 121–188.

Teitelbaum, P., and A. N. Epstein. 1962. The lateral hypothalamic syndrome: Recovery of feeding and drinking after lateral hypothalamic lesions. Psychol. Rev. 69:74–90.

Theologides, A. 1974. The anorexia-cachexia syndrome: A new hypothesis. Ann. N.Y. Acad. Sci. 230:14–22.

Warren, S. 1932. The immediate causes of death in cancer. Am. J. Med. Sci. 194:610–615.

Molecular Interrelations of Nutrition and Cancer,
edited by M. S. Arnott, J. van Eys, and Y.-M. Wang.
Raven Press, New York © 1982.

Tumor-Induced Changes in the Host's Protein Metabolism

T. P. Stein

Surgical Research Laboratories, Graduate Hospital, and Department of Surgery, University of Pennsylvania, Philadelphia, Pennsylvania 19146

The average healthy, 50-year-old, 70-kg man contains about 12 kg protein and 17 kg fat. The 12 kg protein is evenly divided between muscle and nonmuscle protein (Cohn et al. 1980). He is likely to die if he loses 30% of his body protein; in contrast, if he loses 30% of his body fat, he may look thinner, but will still be able to function quite adequately (Cahill 1970). In this chapter we shall discuss: (1) why the maintenance of body protein metabolism is so important for survival, (2) how the presence of a tumor can lead to a loss of protein in the host, and (3) the potential role of nutritional intervention in preventing the loss of carcass protein by the host.

THE IMPORTANCE OF PROTEIN TURNOVER

Because of the central role of proteins in life-sustaining processes, one would expect alterations in protein metabolism to be devastating to an organism, but only in recent years have reliable methodologies become available to permit the meaningful investigation of these alterations in various disease states. Although not completely characterized, it now appears that abnormalities of protein metabolism are extremely common in most, if not all, life-threatening illnesses (e.g., cancer, trauma, sepsis, and shock) and that these alterations may in large part be responsible for the final common pathway for the deterioration and death of people with these disorders.

The human body is continuously synthesizing and degrading protein. An average healthy adult synthesizes 200–400 g of protein daily, of which half is visceral protein (enzymes, hormones, circulating proteins, etc.) and half skeletal muscle. There are also some proteins such as collagen and elastin which, although they comprise about 50% of the total body protein, have negligible turnover rates in adults. (Turnover is defined as the fraction of a given protein pool that is replaced per unit time.) Theoretical calculations (by totalling the amount of ATP required to make protein) and experimental determinations made during growth or repletion suggest that protein turnover and related processes may account for as much as 40% of the total resting energy expenditure. Teleologically, protein turnover must carry with it some significant advantage to justify this energy utilization, or evolutionary pressures would have selected a more energy-efficient alternative.

One theoretical advantage would be that rapid turnover serves to insure against the accumulation of damaged proteins. Although this is an attractive hypothesis, efforts to identify such damaged proteins have been consistently unsuccessful. Protein breakdown appears to be a random process. Newly synthesized proteins of a given species are as susceptible to degradation as older proteins. Of paramount importance in understanding this process was the recognition that the greater the importance of a protein in the regulation of metabolism (e.g., enzymes and hormones), the faster its rate of turnover (Schimke 1970, Goldberg and Dice 1974, Waterlow et al. 1978). In contrast, those proteins with no regulatory role, such as actin, myosin, or collagen, have very slow turnover rates.

The rapid turnover of regulatory enzymes provides a mechanism for metabolic control. There are three major mechanisms for the regulation of metabolic processes: hormone levels, substrate availability, and enzyme concentration. The importance of changes in enzyme levels is often underestimated. Consider the response of the enzymes that catalyze amino acid oxidation in the liver following a meal. These enzymes are not saturated at the concentration of substrate found in vivo, so that the rate of oxidation is proportional to the substrate concentration. Although substrate binding can be modulated within a limited range by hormonal means, and alterations in substrate concentration will produce changes in the rate of reaction (termed "fine control" by Krebs) more rapidly than will alterations in enzyme concentration, the major factor in adaptive control is appropriate changes in enzyme concentration. This is achieved primarily by altering the rate of enzyme breakdown. For example, the concentration of liver threonine deaminase varies 300-fold and that of ornithine amino-transferase 20-fold. In general, most enzyme concentrations have a 2- to 3-fold range, but such changes may be of great significance from a regulatory point of view. Rapid turnover insures a rapid response, given the appropriate stimulus (Hopkins et al. 1973, Krebs 1972, Waterlow et al. 1978).

Rapid protein turnover also enables a limited protein pool to be used with optimal efficiency. Liver protein, for example, consists mainly of some 600 different enzymes. The functional role of the liver is to maintain metabolic homeostasis by processing exogenous nutrients, by providing glucose and ketoacids for other tissues during fasting, and by detoxifying and excreting many waste products. The workload of the liver (and, therefore, the rate of liver protein synthesis) varies considerably with relation to meals, nutritional state, presence of stress or disease, and the rate of release of metabolic by-products from other tissues (Stein et al. 1981a). Rather than maintain optimal levels of all possible enzyme systems at all times, those that are not immediately needed are maintained at relatively low levels. As a result of rapid turnover rates, however, the concentration of an enzyme system can be rapidly increased in response to an appropriate stimulus, while other enzymes can simultaneously be rapidly degraded so that the total protein pool need not be expanded.

Such a state of dynamic protein turnover is not, however, without disadvantages. It is expensive in terms of energy and, to a lesser extent, amino acids. The reutilization of amino acids is not completely efficient. In general, the more rapid the turnover, the more amino acids lost and the more that must be replaced from the diet (Cahill 1970, Waterlow and Stephen 1966). If either amino acids or energy are limited in supply, the shifting from one metabolic pattern to another may be impaired. When the amount of available exogenous amino acid is insufficient, then amino acids must be diverted from some other endogenous metabolic role. In severe malnutrition or when amino acid demands are extremely high (e.g., in trauma, sepsis, or cancer), the body may be forced to choose between two important metabolic responses requiring protein synthesis, for example, synthesis of circulating proteins or wound healing.

The ability to heal a wound is more crucial to survival than the maintenance of muscle mass; thus, regulatory mechanisms divert amino acids from the muscle reservoir to protein synthesis within the wound (Moore and Brennan 1975). This ordering of biologic priorities permits the maintenance and even the expansion of protein compartments that are crucial to survival unless (1) there is serious malnutrition with protein depletion, (2) demands are exceptionally high because of an extreme insult, or (3) regulatory mechanisms are disordered.

Another example of a high priority system is the immune system. The total body protein pool is not large enough to contain adequate amounts of all possible immunoglobulins. Rather, they are maintained at low concentrations with rapid turnover rates so that levels can be changed rapidly by de novo synthesis in response to appropriate stimuli. Experimentally, it has been found that the lower the concentration of an immunoglobulin, the faster the rate of turnover and therefore the more rapidly the concentration can be increased (Waldman et al. 1970). Because adequate immune function is crucial to survival, maintenance of protein synthesis by the immune system has a high priority. In mild malnutrition, immune function remains relatively unimpaired (Parratt 1980). When malnutrition is sufficiently severe or demands are sufficiently high to compromise immune function, the prognosis becomes poorer.

In simple early starvation with or without a mild superimposed stress, nitrogen losses reflect primarily loss of muscle protein and are of little consequence. High priority pools (wound healing, immune function, circulating proteins) are maintained and survival is not threatened. When starvation (even short-term) is compounded, however, by a severe stress (such as a tumor, major surgery, trauma, or sepsis) alterations in protein metabolism may have a major impact on survival.

Thus, our current understanding of the role of protein turnover provides the rationale for why it is important to maintain protein homeostasis, but not why cancer patients waste away or how to prevent this from occurring.

PROTEIN METABOLISM IN THE HOST-TUMOR SYSTEM

Most studies of how a tumor affects protein metabolism in the host have been done with tumor-bearing animal models, usually rats or mice. What is seen is that the tumor grows while the host wastes away. The phenomenon has been described by Mider (1951, 1955) as the tumor functioning as a nitrogen and energy trap. However, the relevance of rodent tumor models to the human situation may not be quite so straightforward. It is not difficult to envisage that a 30-g tumor on a 200-g rat will kill the rat; the tumor comprises 15% of the rat's total body weight. But how does a 300-g tumor kill a 70,000-g man? After all, many men carry around 20–30 kgs (and more) of extra fat and adipose tissue for years.

There are a number of additional differences between human and animal tumor systems, not the least of which is that the human system is much harder to study than a closely controlled animal tumor model. Rodent studies usually involve studying a set of animals all carrying precisely the same tumor, and animals can be selected for the same size tumor. Rodent tumors are usually transplanted, and although the precise etiology of most human tumors is not known, they are not transplanted. Human tumors are highly variable and occur in an uncontrolled, heterogenous population. Furthermore, rat tumors are often studied after the tumor has been allowed to grow much larger without medical or surgical intervention than would a tumor on a patient. In spite of these caveats, much information relevant to the human situation can be learned from rodent tumor models.

As expected, the whole-body protein turnover rate is increased by the presence of a large tumor in a rat (Table 1). For the rats described in Table 2, the tumor was a transplantable, chemically induced adenocarcinoma, and all nutrients were given parenterally. What is significant about the increase, though, is that nearly all the increase is due to the tumor. There is also a slight increase in liver protein synthesis and protein content. On the other hand, skeletal muscle protein synthesis is reduced (Table 2). The turnover theory described above provides a logical explanation for these changes. The tumor has a high protein synthesis rate. In order to meet the added metabolic demands placed on it by

TABLE 1. *The effect of a tumor on the whole-body protein synthesis rate in a 180-g rat bearing a 20-cm³ tumor*

	Synthesis (mg N/kg body wt/day)	Breakdown (mg N/kg body wt/day)
Control rat	2863 ± 194	1931 ± 190
Tumor rat	3683 ± 213	2690 ± 197
% increase	22.4	28.2

Protein synthesis rates were determined by the method of Picou and Taylor Roberts, using ^{15}N-labeled glycine as the tracer.

TABLE 2. *Effect of 20-cm³ tumor (≈200 mg N) on liver and muscle protein metabolism in 200-g rat bearing transplanted adenocarcinoma*

Diet	Amino acids + Glucose		Starvation	
	Control	Tumor	Control	Tumor
Liver N content (mg N)	208 ± 27	201 ± 33	159 ± 16	193 ± 39*
Liver FSR (%/day)	16.6 ± 2.3	16.4 ± 1.8	17.7 ± 1.7	22.1 ± 4.1*
Muscle FSR (%/day)	5.2 ± 2.3	3.0 ± 1.2*	2.8 ± 1.0	3.1 ± 0.8
Tumor FSR (%/day)	—	28.6 ± 6.6	—	22.8 ± 3.0*

Comparison of the data with that given for the same rat-tumor system in Table 1 shows that the added protein synthesis from the tumor outweighs the decrease in muscle protein synthesis caused by the tumor. In the starved rats, the livers of the tumor-bearing rats are larger and have faster synthesis rates than the non-tumor-bearing control rats because of the combined added metabolic demands of the tumor plus adaptation to starvation.

* $p < 0.05$ vs control.
FSR = fractional protein synthesis rate. Data from Stein et al. (1976).

the tumor, the workload on the liver is increased, and this is manifested by both an increase in the liver fractional protein synthesis rate and its size. But, because nutritional intake was not increased correspondingly, there is a net shortage of energy and amino acids.

Since muscle is the lowest priority tissue, it is affected first. Muscle protein synthesis is reduced, thereby making available the energy that would have gone into muscle protein synthesis for use elsewhere (in this case by the tumor) and, by not reducing breakdown equally, providing a supply of amino acids. Eventually, muscle can supply no more energy and amino acids. There is some evidence to suggest that the next vulnerable tissue is lung (Stein et al. 1976). Hence, pulmonary complications (e.g., pneumonia) are frequently the immediate cause of death in cancer patients, secondary to starvation of the host, which, of course, is due to the insidious effects of the tumor on protein homeostasis (Warren 1932).

In man, the effect of the tumor on the host's protein metabolism is more complicated. Some cancer patients apparently have elevated whole-body protein synthesis rates in spite of their serious weight loss (Norton et al. 1980, Carmichael et al. 1980, Stein et al. 1981c). Yet the tumor size and its protein synthesis rate do not appear to be anywhere near large enough to account for the increased whole-body protein turnover. The suggestion was made by Carmichael et al. (1980) that the elevation of tumor burden is proportional to the the elevation in the whole-body protein synthesis rate. But the number of patients studied (11) was small, and there are problems in interpreting the data—as is also true for the other two published studies of protein turnover in cancer patients (Norton et al. 1980, Stein et al. 1981c). Nevertheless, it is clear from the combined results of all three studies that some cancer patients have anomalously high whole-body protein synthesis rates (Table 3).

It seems unlikely that the elevated synthesis rates found in some of the cancer patients are principally due to the excessive demand for nutrients of a very rapidly turning over tumor. This may have been the case for the rats described in Tables 1 and 2, which were studied after the tumors had become very large (20–25 cm³ on a 200 g rat). In this rat tumor system, the carcass maintains its weight until the tumor attains a size of 25–30 cm³, and then the rat enters the terminal phase, in which the tumor continues to grow, but now with a rapid loss of carcass nitrogen. This results in the death of the animal within a week (J. J. Steinberg and T. P. Stein, manuscript submitted).

If tumor-bearing rats are studied before the tumor size has become excessive (< 12 cm³), a parallel to the human situation is found. The carcass synthesis rate of rats bearing 10–12 cm³ tumors is double that of nontumor controls receiving the same amount of parenteral nutrition (T. P. Stein, unpublished results). (The advantage of feeding rats parenterally for this type of study is that it permits precise control of nutrient intake in the animals. It obviates the need for oral pair feeding, in which the diet is determined by how much the tumor-bearing animal will eat rather than what the experimenter wants to feed.) In that experiment, we also measured the absolute synthesis rate of the tumor by using a short (2 hour) ^{15}N-labeled glycine infusion (Stein et al. 1980b). The tumor fractional synthesis rate was about 80%/day, which is of the same order as visceral tissues (Garlick et al. 1973, 1976). This finding eliminates the hypothesis that the tumor exerts its effect on the host by having a disproportionately high protein turnover rate.

Measurement of relative human gastrointestinal tumor synthesis rates by a long (12–20 hours) infusion of ^{15}N-labeled glycine showed that the tumor synthesis rates were only about 40% higher than normal gastrointestinal tissues. This moderate increase cannot account for the twofold or more increase found in the whole-body rate, which indicates that, as in the rats with the "small" tumors, it is the host's tissue that has the anomalously high turnover rates (Stein 1978).

Thus, it appears likely that the tumor exerts its effects on the host by indirect means. There are several hypotheses that address the mechanisms by which

TABLE 3. *Whole-body protein synthesis rates (g protein/kg body wt/day) in tumor- and non-tumor-bearing adults*

Control, nontumor subjects	Tumor patients
2.9 ± 0.3*	4.3 ± 0.8
4.2 ± 0.5†	6.6 ± 0.5

* Data from Norton et al. (1980).
† Data from Stein et al. (1981b).

the tumor can cause increased Cori cycling, gluconeogenesis, wasting away of the host's body cell mass, and cachexia. (They are reviewed elsewhere in this volume by Morrison.) The discussion here will be limited to an analysis of how the tumor's protein metabolism could, by indirect means, cause all these effects (Stein et al. 1978b).

The host plus tumor requires more nutrients (amino acids, energy) than the host alone (Begg 1958, Goodlad 1964, Mider 1955). Unless the tumor causes a physical obstruction, the host is usually unaware of the presence of a tumor in its early stages, so nutritional input is not increased correspondingly. Eventually, competition for amino acids develops between the host and the tumor, with the tumor's needs being met preferentially. The resultant situation is the beginning of starvation of the host (Morrison 1978).

The tumor removes its complement of amino acids for protein synthesis plus any others that it requires in excess for its metabolic processes, leaving an amino acid imbalance. In man and animals, an amino acid imbalance causes cachexia (Harper et al. 1964). Furthermore, an unbalanced amino acid mixture is ineffective for protein synthesis; hence the excess is disposed of via oxidation and some gluconeogenesis. Gluconeogenesis is in turn partially regulated by substrate levels (Exton 1973, Krebs 1972), so the tumor-induced imbalance could provide additional driving force for the enhanced gluconeogenesis found in some cancer patients (Reichard et al. 1964, Holroyde et al. 1975, Waterhouse 1974, 1979).

We have recently obtained evidence suggesting that some of the tumor-induced alterations in host amino acid metabolism can be mitigated. After trauma or sepsis, supplemental administration of the three branch-chain amino acids (leucine, valine, and isoleucine) has a protein-sparing effect by decreasing net muscle breakdown (Blackburn et al. 1979, Freund et al. 1978). We have found a similar protein-sparing effect by the branch-chain amino acids in tumor-bearing rats (Table 4). The protein-sparing effect of a branch chain amino acid solution was determined in a rat tumor model. The preliminary results are summarized in Table 4. Although it appears from the table that rats given either of the two amino acid formulations are in positive nitrogen balance, the magnitude of positive balance may be more apparent than real. The errors inherent in rat nitrogen balance methodology are all unidirectional and tend to err in the direction of increased nitrogen retention. Nitrogen balance is the difference between intake and output, and it is very difficult to ensure that all excreted N has been collected. The N balance will be falsely biased towards the positive in direct proportion to the losses in the excreted N collection. Table 4 is therefore best interpreted as being indicative of relative changes in the nitrogen balance. The actual numbers for N retention may be overestimates, but the relative differences between groups are correct.

In the rats who received glucose but no amino acids, the host's net loss of nitrogen is given by the sum of nitrogen gained by the tumor plus that lost in the urine. The tumor gains 25 mg N/day during the 6 days of parenteral feeding

TABLE 1. *The protein-sparing effect of branch chain amino acids in tumor bearing rats**

	TPN Diet				
	bcaa	caa	No aa	Starvation	a/a
caa (N g/kg)	0	1.05	0	0	0
a/a (N g/day)	0	0	0	0	1.05
bcaa (N g/kg)	1.05	0	0	0	0
nonprotein cal (kcal/kg)	168	173	200	25	171
Tumor size (cm³)	19.4	20.3	12.4	19.9	22
N balance (mg N/rat/day)	47	37	−74	−91	−1

* 180–200 g female Lewis-Wistar rats bearing the AC-33 transplantable adenocarcinoma were fed parenterally one of four parenteral regimens for 4 or 6 days. Abbreviations: bcaa, branch chain amino acids; caa, a balanced solution of crystalline amino acids (Freamine II); aa, amino acids; ala, alanine. Data are taken from Stein et al. (1976), Buzby et al. (1980), and Stein and Steinberg (unpublished observations).

(Stein et al. 1976) and at least 74 mg N/day is lost in the urine, leading to the host losing a minimum of 100 mg N/day. Adding branch-chain amino acids to the glucose infusate converts the relative N balance value from a 74 mg/day loss to a 34 mg/day gain, whereas the nonspecific nitrogen effect with alanine is considerably less.

The tumor grows just as well with or without the branch-chain amino acids. Thus, the branch-chain amino acids have a protein-sparing effect of 34 − (− 74) = 108 mg N/day, and the nonspecific protein-sparing effect with alanine is only 75 mg N/day. Not unexpectedly, giving a balanced amino acid mixture with the glucose also has a protein-sparing effect. What is surprising is that the complete amino acid mixture is only slightly better than just the three branch-chain amino acids. The significant point about the data in Table 4 is that the branch-chain amino acids are almost as good as the complete amino acid mixture in maintaining nitrogen homeostasis relative to either starvation or amino acid deprivation.

There are a number of explanations for this effect. Two of them are described below. (1) The tumor has a disproportionately high demand for the branch-chain amino acids. Providing them exogenously reduces the need for muscle protein breakdown to supply the tumor with the branch-chain amino acids. There is a reason why a tumor might require a disproportionately greater amount of the branch-chain amino acids than of the other amino acids. These three amino acids have a dual metabolic role in tissues such as muscle, and, for this mechanism to be valid, in the tumor.

The three branch-chain amino acids can be considered to be simultaneously amino acids and ketone bodies. They share the same cofactors for catabolism as fatty acids and ketone bodies, and so can be utilized as a source of energy and for protein synthesis (Cahill 1976). Thus, the tumor's demands for the branch-chain amino acids may be much greater than its requirements for the other amino acids. In order to compensate for the irreversible loss of branch-chain amino acids via oxidation, either more protein will be needed from the diet, or more protein will have to be broken down to correct the deficit and provide enough of a balanced amino acid mixture for host protein synthesis. The excess amino acids from the additional protein breakdown will be in imbalance and so cannot be used for protein synthesis as efficiently as a well-balanced mixture. The source of the branch-chain amino acids is muscle because muscle consists largely of low-priority proteins. In tumor-bearing humans and rats, it is muscle that loses the greatest amount of protein.

In other words, according to this line of reasoning, Mider's description of the tumor functioning as a "nitrogen" trap should be modified to the tumor functioning as a sink for the branch-chain amino acids.

In the case of a rat in which the tumor comprises a considerable fraction of the total body weight, it is not difficult to envisage the tumor's requirements for the branch-chain amino acids causing a major distortion in the animal's protein metabolism. If it is assumed that human tumors partition the branch-chain amino acids between oxidation and incorporation into protein in the same proportion as muscle, then it can be shown by the following arguments that the irreversible loss of branch-chain keto acids to the tumor is likely to be very substantial in man, too.

Consider a 70-kg male with a 300-g tumor who has 6000 g skeletal muscle (Cohn et al. 1980). The relative human gastrointestinal tumor synthesis rates reported by Stein (1978) and Stein et al. (1980a) are minimal estimates, and even so are about 10 times the rates reported for skeletal muscle (Halliday and McKesan 1975). The tumor rates are underestimated because the assay used (continuous infusion of glycine for 12–20 hours) seriously underestimates the contribution of the rapidly turning over proteins (enzymes, etc.) in the tumor. Muscle, on the other hand, consists chiefly of the slowly turning over proteins, actin and myosin, and so the values obtained are likely to be close to the true rates. Thus, per gram of protein, the tumor oxidizes 10 times more branch-chain keto acids than muscle, or, expressed as a percentage of the total muscle branch chain amino acid oxidation, 50%. The calculation implies that a relatively small tumor has the same metabolic demands for the branch-chain amino acids as 3000 g muscle, which corresponds to 50% of the muscle in the body. To meet this large demand by the tumor for branch-chain amino acids would require the breakdown of a lot of muscle protein, with the residual amino acids providing the chronic imbalance necessary for the increased gluconeogenesis and appetite suppression.

For the second hypothesis, which we believe to be equally plausible, the argument is simpler, but the consequences the same. The tumor's demand is for glucose, a product of amino acid metabolism, rather than one or more specific amino acids per se. The tumor's demand for glucose is well known, but the body carries little in the way of carbohydrate reserves (glycogen). Consider what can happen if the combination of diet and glycogen hydrolysis are inadequate to supply the tumor and host with glucose. The only other source of glucose is gluconeogenesis from amino acids—chiefly the nonessential amino acids, with muscle being the provider. The residual amino acids will consist disproportionately of the essential amino acids, resulting in an imbalance. Again, the unbalanced mixture induces cachexia (Harper et al. 1964), leading to a decreased food intake, with the resultant vicious cycle of decreased intake causing increased net protein breakdown, which in turn decreases the appetite, leading to more net muscle protein breakdown. In this scenario, the branch-chain amino acids preserve muscle protein by directly acting on the muscle, whereas in the first proposed mechanism the branch-chain amino acids spare muscle protein by directly providing the tumor with substrate (keto acids). In summary, both mechanisms can result in an amino acid imbalance, but the relative physiological importance of each is yet to be determined.

There is another point to be considered that is common to both mechanisms. In other stress-induced protein losing enteropathies, such as trauma or sepsis, under conditions in which energy is not limiting, the loss of protein N from muscle does not seem to occur by a simple increase in the protein breakdown or reduction in the synthesis rate. Rather, synthesis and breakdown (i.e., turnover) are both increased, but synthesis is increased less than breakdown, hence the net loss of N (Birkhan et al. 1980, Kien et al. 1978, Moldauer et al. 1980, Stein et al. 1977). The observation that rats with smaller ($\simeq$ 10 cm^3) tumors have carcass protein synthesis rates about double that of control non-tumor-bearing rats is probably a manifestation of the same phenomenon.

NUTRITIONAL INTERVENTION

With the introduction of parenteral nutrition by Dudrick and his colleagues and the subsequent reawakening of interest in enteral nutrition, the means are now available to refeed and replete any malnourished patient. Most of the research has centered on the applicability of parenteral nutrition. During the last 5 years, the Diet, Nutrition and Cancer Program of the National Cancer Institute has sponsored a series of ongoing clinical trials to determine whether the primary benefit of nutritional intervention is to the tumor or the host. The discussion here will be limited to the effects of nutritional intervention on protein metabolism in the host-tumor system.

A major use of intravenous nutrition (IVN) is in repleting nutritionally depleted patients, but this application is of questionable value for the treatment of patients with malignant disease when it is not part of some other therapeutic program (e.g., chemotherapy or radiation therapy). It is suspected, although there is no conclusive evidence in man, that the primary benefit of IVN would be to the tumor, rather than the host. Numerous animal studies have shown

TABLE 5. *Effects of calorie source on tumor growth and host nitrogen balance**

Diet		Route	Description	Final tumor vol (cm^3)	Total N balance	Host N balance	Tumor N balance
I	Chow control	p.o.	Standard rat chow ad libitum	15.1	+476 ± 195	+220 ± 155	+254 ± 67
II	Starvation	—	No oral or I.V. nutrients	13.6	−454 ± 14	−668 ± 13	+215 ± 19
III	Carbohydrate	i.v.	18% dextrose	15.4	−512 ± 43	−704 ± 36	+193 ± 31
IV	Amino acids	i.v.	3% amino acids	19.1	+16 ± 24	−250 ± 28	+267 ± 18
V	Carbohydrate-based TPN	i.v.	18% dextrose + 3% amino acids	22.4	+388 ± 28	+49 ± 52	+339 ± 32
VI	Fat-based TPN	i.v.	6.4% fat emulsion + 3% amino acids	16.6†	+292 ± 36†	+90 ± 48	+201 ± 18†
VII	Carbohydrate/fat TPN	i.v.	3.2% fat, 9% dextrose, 3% amino acids	21.1	+448 ± 32	+104 ± 28	+343 ± 29

* 180–200 g female Lewis-Wistar rats were innoculated with the AC-33 transplantable mammary adenocarcinoma. After the tumors had attained a size of 3 ± 1 cm^3, the rats were randomized to one of the seven dietary regimens for 4 days. At the end of that period, the tumor volumes were measured, the animals were sacrificed, and their tumor and carcass N content measured. The P values were calculated by analysis of variance. Substitution of fat for glucose as the total nonprotein calorie source led to decreased tumor growth and increased host nitrogen retention (diets V vs VI). Data from Buzby et al. (1980).

† Diet V vs. Diet VI, $P < 0.002$.

that IVN increases the tumor growth rate (Cameron et al. 1977, Copeland et al. 1977, Steiger et al. 1975, Goodgame et al. 1979).

In man, in vivo, there is a preferential uptake of parenterally administered essential amino acids by the tumor during parenteral nutrition, which suggests that there is a benefit to the tumor from parenteral nutrition (Stein et al. 1981b). The problem of whether the benefit from IVN is to the tumor or the host is discussed in detail in the chapter by Larson. Nevertheless, certain observations can be made from the lack of definitive published data. Many cancer patients have been given total parenteral nutrition, but no spectacular remissions, increased survival times, or decreased survival times have been reported. It would seem, therefore, that any stimulatory effect on the tumor is small, which supports the current practice of using IVN as an adjunct (e.g., repleting debilitated patients so they can withstand surgery better, or as adjuvant therapy), but not giving IVN alone.

The other aspect of nutritional intervention of interest is the possibility of selectively nourishing the host. As is well known, tumors exhibit greater anaerobic utilization of glucose than most nonmalignant tissues. (The reasons for this are given in the chapter by Weinhouse.) Since lipid substrates cannot be oxidized anaerobically, it could be predicted that drastically reducing the availability of glucose to the tumor would reduce its growth rate. Replacing glucose with fat as the energy source should not affect host protein metabolism, as muscle and visceral protein can use lipid substrate or glucose equally well for energy.

Parenteral nutrition, with its totally synthetic mix of substrates, permits any combination of amino acids, fat, or carbohydrate to be given. When a tumor-bearing rat is given all of its calories parenterally as a fat emulsion instead of glucose, tumor growth is impaired as predicted, while the nitrogen retention by the host is as efficient as when glucose is the primary nonprotein calorie source (Table 5), because the host is better able to adapt to lipid substrates (Buzby et al. 1980). The study was not continued for long enough, however, to determine whether the regimen also had toxic effects on the host, or if the tumor, given time, could adapt to using lipids for energy.

Relatively little work has been done so far on tailoring an individual's nutrition to match his actual needs. Some success has been achieved in developing amino acid solutions specific for renal disease (low in nonessential amino acids) or for hepatic failure (low in nonessential and aromatic amino acids). The arguments in this review suggest that it may be possible to develop amino acid formulations (high in branch-chain amino acids) that minimize the debilitating effects of the tumor on the host by preventing excessive host-tissue protein breakdown.

ACKNOWLEDGMENTS

The work described in this chapter was supported by U.S. Public Health Service Grants Number AM 16658 and CA 18575.

REFERENCES

Begg, R. W. 1958. Tumor-host relations. Adv. Cancer Res. 5:1–54.

Birkhan, R. H., C. L. Long, D. Fitkins, J. W. Geiger, and W. S. Blakemore, 1980. Effects of major skeletal trauma on whole body protein turnover in man measured by L-(1, ^{14}C)-leucine. Surgery 88:294–300.

Blackburn, G. L., L. L. Moldauer, S. Usi, A. Bothe, Jr., S. J. D. O'Keefe, and B. R. Bistrian. 1979. Branch chain amino acid administration and metabolism during starvation, injury, and sepsis. Surgery 86:307–315.

Buzby, G. P., J. L. Mullen, T. P. Stein, E. E. Miller, C. L. Hobbs, and E. F. Rosato. 1980. Host-tumor interaction and nutrient supply. Cancer 45:2940–2948.

Cahill, G. F. 1970. Starvation in man. N. Engl. J. Med. 282:668–675.

Cahill, G. F. 1976. Protein and amino acid metabolism in man. Circ. Res. 38 (Suppl. I):109–114.

Cameron, I. L., W. J. Ackley, and W. Roger. 1977. Responses of hepatoma bearing rats to total parenteral hyperalimentation and to ad libitum feedings. J. Surg. Res. 23:189–195.

Carmichael, M. J., M. B. Clague, M. J. Keir, and I. D. A. Johnson. 1980. Whole body protein turnover, synthesis and breakdown in patients with colorectal carcinoma. Br. J. Surg. 67:736–739.

Cohn, S. H., D. Vartsky, S. Yasumura, A. Sawitsky, I. Zanzi, A. Vaswani, and K. J. Ellis. 1980. Compartmental body composition based on total body nitrogen, potassium and calcium. Am. J. Physiol. 239:E524–E530.

Copeland, E. M., B. V. MacFadyen, V. J. Lanzotti, and S. J. Dudrick. 1977. Intravenous hyperalimentation as an adjunct to cancer chemotherapy. Am. J. Surg. 129:167–173.

Exton, J. H. 1973. Gluconeogenesis. Metabolism 21:945–970.

Freund, H. R., J. A. Ryan, and J. E. Fischer. 1978. Amino acid derangements in patients with sepsis: Treatment with branch chain amino acid rich infusion. Ann. Surg. 188:423–431.

Garlick, P. J., D. J. Millward, and W. P. T. James. 1973. The diurnal response of muscle and liver protein synthesis in vivo in meal fed rats. Biochem. J. 136:935–945.

Garlick, P. J., J. C. Waterlow, and R. W. Swick. 1976. Measurement of protein turnover in rat liver. Analysis of the complex curve for decay of label in a mixture of proteins. Biochem. J. 156:657–667.

Goldberg, A. L., and J. F. Dice. 1974. Intracellular protein degradation in mammalian and bacterial cells. Ann. Rev. Biochem. 43:845–869.

Goodgame, J. T., S. F. Lowry, and M. J. Brennan. 1979. Nutritional manipulations and tumor growth. II. The effects of intravenous feeding. Am. J. Clin. Nutr. 32:2285–2294.

Goodlad, G. A. J. 1964. Protein metabolism and tumor growth, *in* Mammalian Protein Metabolism, Vol. 11, H. N. Munro and J. B. Allison, eds. Academic Press, New York, pp. 415–445.

Halliday, D., and R. O. McKesan. 1975. Measurement of muscle protein synthesis rate from serial muscle biopsies and total body protein turnover in man by continuous infusion of (L-α, 1-N) lysine. Clin. Sci. 49:581–590.

Harper, A. E., P. Leung, A. Yoshida, and Q. R. Rogers. 1964. Some new thoughts on amino acid imbalance. Fed. Proc. 23:1087–1093.

Holroyde, C. P., T. G. Gabuzda, R. C. Putnam, P. Pavle, and G. A. Reichard. 1975. Altered glucose metabolism in metastatic carcinoma. Cancer Res. 35:3710–3714.

Hopkins, H. A., R. I. Bonney, P. R. Walker, J. D. Yager, and V. R. Potter. 1973. Food and light as separate entrainment signals for rat liver enzymes. Adv. Enzyme Regul. 11:169–191.

Kien, C. L., V. R. Young, D. K. Rohrbaugh, and J. F. Burke. 1978. Increased rates of whole body protein synthesis and breakdown in children recovering from burns. Ann. Surg. 187:383–391.

Krebs, H. A. 1972. Some aspects of the regulation of fuel supply in omniverous animals. Adv. Enzyme Regul. 10:397–420.

Krebs, H. A., P. Lund, and M. Stubbs. 1976. Interrelations between gluneogenesis and urea synthesis. *in* Gluconeogenesis, Its Regulation in Mammalian Species, R. W. Hanson and M. A. Mehlman, eds. Wiley Interscience, New York, p. 269.

Mider, G. B. 1951. Some aspects of nitrogen and energy metabolism in cancerous subjects. A review. Cancer Res. 11:821–829.

Mider, G. B. 1955. Some tumour host relationships. Can. Cancer Conf. 1:120–137.

Moldauer, L. L., S. J. D. O'Keefe, A. Bothe, B. R. Bistrian, and G. L. Blackburn. 1980. In vivo demonstration of nitrogen sparing mechanism for glucose and amino acids in the injured rat. Metabolism 29:173–180.

Moore, F. D., and M. R. Brennan. 1975. Surgical injury: Body composition, protein metabolism and neuroendocrinology, in Manual of Surgical Nutrition, W. F. Ballinger, ed. W. B. Saunders, Philadelphia, pp. 169–222.

Morrison, S. D. 1978. Origins of anorexia in neoplastic disease. Am. J. Clin. Nutr. 31:1104–1107.

Norton, J. A., T. P. Stein, and M. F. Brennan. 1980. Whole body protein turnover studies in normal man and malnourished patients with and without cancer. Surg. Forum 31:94–97.

Parratt, D. 1980. Nutrition and immunity. Proc. Nutr. Soc. 39:133–140.

Reichard, G. A., N. F. Moury, H. J. Hochella, R. C. Putnam, and S. Weinhouse. 1964. Blood glucose replacement rates in human cancer patients. Cancer Res. 24:71–76.

Schimke, R. T. 1970. Regulation of protein degradation in mammalian tissues, in Mammalian Protein Metabolism, H. N. Munro, ed. Academic Press, New York, pp. 177–228.

Steiger, E., J. Oram-Smith, E. Miller, L. Kuo, and H. Vars. 1975. Effects of nutrition on tumor growth and tolerance to chemotherapy. J. Surg. Res. 18:455–461.

Stein, T. P. 1978. Cachexia, gluconeogenesis and progressive weight loss in cancer patients. J. Theor. Biol. 73:51–59.

Stein, T. P., G. P. Buzby, M. H. Gertner, W. C. Hargrove, M. J. Leskiw, and J. L. Mullen. 1980a. Effect of parenteral nutrition on protein synthesis and liver fat metabolism in man. Am. J. Physiol. 239:G280–G287.

Stein, T. P., G. P. Buzby, M. J. Leskiw, A. L. Giandomenico, and J. L. Mullen. 1981a. Protein and fat metabolism in rats during repletion with parenteral nutrition. J. Nutr. 111:154–165.

Stein, T. P., G. P. Buzby, M. J. Leskiw, and J. L. Mullen. 1981b. Parenteral nutrition and human gastrointestinal tumor protein metabolism. Cancer (in press).

Stein, T. P., G. P. Buzby, E. F. Rosato, and J. C. Mullen. 1981c. Effect of parenteral nutrition on protein synthesis in adult cancer patients. Am. J. Clin. Nutr. (in press).

Stein, T. P., M. J. Leskiw, G. P. Buzby, A. L. Giandomenico, H. W. Wallace, and J. L. Mullen. 1980b. Measurement of protein synthesis rates with ^{15}N glycine. Am. J. Physiol. 239:E294–E300.

Stein, T. P., M. J. Leskiw, J. C. Oram-Smith, and H. W. Wallace. 1977. Changes in protein synthesis after trauma. Importance of nutrition. Am. J. Physiol. 233:348–355.

Stein, T. P., J. L. Mullen, J. C. Oram-Smith, E. F. Rosato, H. W. Wallace, and W. C. Hargrove III. 1978. Relative rates of tumor, normal gut, liver and fibrinogen protein synthesis in man. Am. J. Physiol. 234:E648–E652.

Stein, T. P., J. C. Oram-Smith, M. J. Leskiw, H. W. Wallace, and E. E. Miller. 1976. Tumor-caused changes in host protein synthesis under different dietary situations. Cancer Res. 36:3936–3940.

Waldman, T. A., R. M. Blaese, and W. Strober. 1970. Physiological factors controlling immunoglobulin metabolism. in Plasma Protein Metabolism, M. A. Rothchild and T. A. Waldman, eds. Academic Press, New York, pp. 269–286.

Warren, S. 1932. The immediate cause of death in cancer. Am. J. Med. Sci. 184:610–616.

Waterhouse, C. 1974. How tumors affect host metabolism. Ann. N.Y. Acad. Sci. 230:86–93.

Waterhouse, C., N. Jeanpretre, and J. Keilson. 1979. Gluconeogenesis from alanine in patients with progressive malignant disease. Cancer Res. 39:1968–1972.

Waterlow, J. C., and J. M. Stephen. 1966. Adaptation of the rat to a low protein diet: Effect of a reduced protein intake on the pattern of incorporation of L-(^{14}C) lysine. Br. J. Nutr. 20:461–484.

Waterlow, J. C., P. J. Garlick, and D. J. Millward. 1978. Protein Turnover in Mammalian Tissues and in the Whole Body. North Holland Publishing Co., Amsterdam, Netherlands, pp. 1–14, 443–481.

Molecular Interrelations of Nutrition and Cancer,
edited by M. S. Arnott, J. van Eys, and Y.-M. Wang.
Raven Press, New York © 1982.

Mineral and Electrolyte Abnormalities in Patients with Advanced Cancer

David H. Lawson, Daniel W. Nixon, and Daniel Rudman*

*Division of Hematology and Oncology and the *Clinical Research Facility, Department of Medicine, Emory University School of Medicine, Atlanta, Georgia 30322*

The association between cancer and undernutrition has prompted intense interest in methods of improving the nutritional status of patients with malignant diseases. During the past 5 years, we have performed three sequential investigations designed to answer specific questions about cancer cachexia. In the first of these, we determined the prevalence of undernutrition in patients with advanced cancer as assessed by anthropometric measurements and by serum levels of albumin, transferrin, vitamins A, B_{12}, and C, folate, and thiamine. We then evaluated the relationship between these parameters and survival. In the second study, we compared the improvement in anthropometrics induced by hyperalimentation in patients with advanced cancer to that seen in undernourished patients with various nonneoplastic diseases. In this investigation, we also compared element retention in these two groups of patients by the metabolic balance technique. In the third study, we compared the survival of patients with advanced adenocarcinoma of the colon receiving 3 to 4 weeks of central venous hyperalimentation to that of similar patients not receiving vigorous nutritional support.

The metabolic balance studies performed during the second study revealed a high frequency of abnormalities of mineral and electrolyte metabolism in patients with advanced cancer and undernutrition. These deviations from the normal pattern are the focus of this report.

PREVALANCE OF UNDERNUTRITION IN PATIENTS WITH ADVANCED CANCER

During the summer of 1977, we assessed the degree of protein-calorie undernutrition in a series of 54 consecutive patients admitted to the medical oncology ward of Emory University Hospital (Nixon et al. 1980). These patients were not preselected for nutritional deficiencies. All had biopsy-proved carcinomas, and 93% had documented metastases. Most had been receiving chemotherapy for varying intervals prior to study. Thirty-six healthy subjects matched to patients by age and sex were also studied as controls.

Adipose mass was determined by measurement of the triceps skinfold (millimeters) (Butterworth and Blackburn 1975). This value and the midarm circumference were then converted to the midarm muscle area (square centimeters) (Jellife and Jellife 1971) to assess lean body mass. The ratio of the amount of creatinine excreted in 24 hours measured in milligrams to the height in centimeters (creatinine/height index) (Butterworth and Blackburn 1975) was also used to measure lean body mass. All three of these measurements were expressed as a percentage of the standard, with the standard defined as the average of values found in healthy subjects of ideal body weight. These were, for men and women respectively: triceps skinfold, 12.5 and 16.5 mm; midarm muscle area, 52 and 43 cm^2; and creatinine/height index, 9 and 6.2 mg/cm. Visceral (hepatic) nutritional function was examined by determining serum albumin levels.

As expected, undernutrition was very common in these patients (Table 1). Forty-two percent of the cancer patients had adipose stores that were less than 80% of standard, and 19% had stores less than 60% of standard. In contrast, only 3% of the controls had triceps skinfold measurements that were less than 80% of standard, and none had measurements less than 60% of standard. Midarm muscle area was decreased less often: 23% of the patients had measurements of less than 80% of standard, whereas 14% of controls had

TABLE 1. *Prevalence of undernutrition in hospitalized patients with advanced cancer*

	Percent of patients below standard	
Parameter	Control (normals)	Cancer
Triceps skinfold*		
<80% of standard	3	42
<60% of standard	0	19
Midarm muscle area*		
<80% of standard	14	23
Creatinine/height index*		
<80% of standard	28	88
<60% of standard	0	53
Serum albumin†		
≤ 3.5 g/dl	—	57
Serum transferrin†		
≤280 μg/dl	—	41
Thiamine†		
<1.6 μg/100 ml	—	4
Vitamin B_{12}†		
<330 pg/ml	—	4
Serum folate†		
<5 ng/ml	—	20
Vitamin C†		
<0.2 mg/100 ml	—	44
Vitamin A†		
<65 IU/100 ml	—	44

(Adapted from Nixon et al. 1980.)
* Assessed in patients not selected for weight loss.
† Assessed only in patients who had lost ≥ 6% of their premorbid weight.

measurements below this mark. The creatinine/height index was a much more sensitive indicator of lean body mass depletion than the midarm muscle area; 88% of the cancer patients had indices of less than 80% of standard and 53% had indices less than 60% of standard. Only 28% of controls had indices of less than 80% of standard, and none had less than 60% of standard. Lean body mass depletion as determined by decreased creatinine/height index was the most frequently noted nutritional abnormality in these patients.

During the fall of 1977 we completed the second phase of this study. Thirty additional patients were selected from among our hospitalized patients with advanced carcinoma on the basis of loss of at least 6% of premorbid weight. Serum levels of albumin, transferrin, thiamine, folate, vitamin A, vitamin B_{12}, and vitamin C were measured in these patients. The serum albumin level was less than 3.5 g/dl in 57%; serum transferrin levels were below normal in 41%. There was also a high prevalence of vitamin undernutrition in this group. Although only 4% had decreased serum thiamine or vitamin B_{12} levels, 20% were deficient in folate and 44% had subnormal vitamin A and vitamin C levels.

RELATIONSHIP BETWEEN NUTRITIONAL DEFICIENCIES AND SURVIVAL

We next determined the relationship between the indicators of nutritional deficiency and survival (Table 2) (Nixon et al. 1980). The patients described above were followed from the time of nutritional evaluation until death. The number dying within 70 days of study was compared in patients above and below selected levels of nutritional status. Degree of adipose mass depletion did not correlate significantly with mortality. Of 27 patients with triceps skinfold measurements less than or equal to 60% of standard, 12 died within 70 days of evaluation; 7 of 31 patients with triceps skinfold measurements greater than

TABLE 2. *Relationship between undernutrition and survival in patients with advanced cancer*

Parameter	Deaths within 70 days of study		
	Number	Percent	
Triceps skinfold			
$\leq$ 60% of standard	12/27	44	
$>$ 60% of standard	7/31	23	$p > 0.05$
Serum albumin			
$\leq$ 3.5 gm/dl	16/30	53	
$>$ 3.5 gm/dl	7/39	18	$p < 0.05$
Creatinine/height index			
$\leq$ 60% of standard	18/32	56	
$>$ 60% of standard	1/26	4	$p < 0.05$

(Adapted from Nixon et al. 1980.)

60% of standard died during this period (p $>$ 0.05). Decreased serum albumin levels, however, were significantly related to survival; 16 of 30 patients with levels less than or equal to 3.5 g/dl died during the 70-day follow-up period, compared to only 7 of 39 with higher levels (p $<$ 0.05). A creatinine/height index less than or equal to 60% of standard had the most ominous prognostic import: 18 of 32 patients with this degree of protein-calorie undernutrition died within 70 days of nutritional evaluation, compared to only 1 of 26 of their better-nourished counterparts (p $<$ 0.05).

COMPARISON OF RESPONSE TO VIGOROUS NUTRITIONAL SUPPORT OF CANCER AND NONCANCER PATIENTS

Improvement in Indicators of Undernutrition

Because of the association between indices of poor nutrition and decreased survival in patients with advanced cancer, we postulated that improvement in nutritional status might lead to increased longevity. There were reasons to believe, however, that nutrients provided to cancer patients might not be efficiently used to synthesize normal lean body mass. Animal studies have demonstrated that tumor growth is stimulated by increasing protein content of the diet (Babson 1954, Cameron and Rogers 1977, Daly et al. 1980, Steiger et al. 1975). Most of the nitrogen retained by animals bearing rapidly growing transplanted tumors is retained by malignant tissue rather than by normal host tissue (Sugimura et al. 1959). We therefore compared the effects of 3 to 4 weeks of parenteral or enteral hyperalimentation on body weight, triceps skinfold, creatinine/height index, midarm muscle area, and serum albumin level in undernourished cancer patients and in similarly underweight chronically ill noncancer subjects. Metabolic balance studies were also performed in these patients, as described in the next section.

For this study (Nixon et al. 1981a), we selected 15 patients with advanced carcinoma and severe undernutrition (both creatinine/height index and triceps skinfold measurements of less than 80% of standard). Ten of these patients had gastrointestinal cancer, three had squamous cell carcinomas of the head and neck, one had an adenocarcinoma of unknown primary site, and one had a squamous cell carcinoma of the lung. The mean age was 56 years; there were seven males and eight females. All but two had distant spread of disease.

Ten similarly undernourished noncancer patients referred to our Clinical Research Facility for nutritional support served as controls. Diagnoses in this group included: inflammatory bowel disease, two; anorexia of unknown cause, two; chronic pancreatitis, three; chronic obstructive pulmonary disease, one; anorexia nervosa, one; malabsorption of unknown cause, one. The average age of these patients was 47 years. There were six males and four females in this population.

Nine of the cancer patients and five of the noncancer patients received central venous hyperalimentation with a nutritionally complete formula by the method of Dudrick (Dudrick et al. 1977). Delivery of this solution was increased during the initial 72 hours of therapy to a final rate providing 30 to 35 calories and 0.2 to 0.3 grams of nitrogen per kilogram of body weight every 24 hours.

Six of the cancer patients and five of the noncancer patients received a commercially available complete liquid formula via 16-gauge nasogastric tube at a rate calculated to deliver 30 to 35 calories and 0.15 to 0.20 grams of nitrogen per kilogram body weight every 24 hours (Heymsfield et al. 1979). One of these patients required supplementation with peripheral venous hyperalimentation to achieve the desired protein-calorie intake; P-900, a 900-milliosmolar solution, was used (Isaacs et al. 1977).

Cancer patients received nutritional supplementation for 17 to 26 days; noncancer subjects received similar support for 21 to 28 days. Patients with cancer received one course of chemotherapy during the nutritional support period. Body weight, triceps skinfold, midarm muscle area, creatinine/height index, and serum albumin measurements at the beginning and end of the hyperalimentation period were compared (Table 3). Despite similar nitrogen retention, cancer patients as a group gained less weight than noncancer controls. For those receiving central hyperalimentation, the median change in body weight during the period of nutritional support was 5 kg for cancer patients and 8.5 kg for noncancer patients (p < 0.01). For enterally hyperalimented cancer patients, the median weight gain was 3.5 kg, compared with 9 kg for noncancer controls (p < 0.01). The enterally hyperalimented cancer patients had less improvement in creatinine/height index, midarm muscle area, and serum albumin concentration than did noncancer controls, but none of these differences attained statistical significance (p > 0.05). The centrally hyperalimented patients, however, showed

TABLE 3. *Comparison of improvement in nutritional indicators in response to either central venous or enteral hyperalimentation in noncancer controls and cancer patients*

Parameter	Improvement			
	Central venous hyperalimentation		Enteral hyperalimentation	
	Noncancer (n = 5)	Cancer (n = 9)	Noncancer (n = 5)	Cancer (n = 6)
Body weight (kg)	8.5	5	9	3.5
	(p < .01)		(p < .01)	
Serum albumin (g/dl)	0.5	0.1	0.3	0.0
	(p < .05)		(NS*)	
Creatinine/height index (% standard)	10	4	10	8
	(p < .05)		(NS)	
Midarm muscle area (% standard)	11	4	10.5	3
	(p < .05)		(NS)	
Triceps skinfold (% standard)	8	10	11	14.5
	(NS)		(NS)	

(Adapted from Nixon et al. 1981a.)
* NS = p > .05

significantly less (p < 0.05) improvement in serum albumin levels (+0.1 g/dl versus +0.5 g/dl), creatinine/height index (+4% of standard versus +10% of standard), and midarm muscle area (+4% of standard versus +11% of standard). There was no statistically significant difference between cancer and noncancer patients in repletion of adipose tissue as judged by improvements in triceps skinfold.

Metabolic Balance

Metabolic balance studies performed in the past in small numbers of patients with various malignancies have demonstrated abnormal mineral and electrolyte retention (Fenninger et al. 1953, Terepka and Waterhouse 1956, Watkin 1961). We therefore compared the daily balances of seven elements (nitrogen, phosphorus, potassium, sodium, chloride, calcium, magnesium) in the 15 cancer and 10 noncancer patients described above (Nixon et al. 1981a). These studies were performed in our Clinical Research Facility according to techniques previously described (Reifenstein et al. 1945, Rudman et al. 1975). The results presented are based on studies performed during the first 10 to 14 days of hyperalimentation in the cancer patients, during which time no chemotherapy was given, and on studies throughout the time of hyperalimentation in the noncancer patients. Data are daily balances (intake minus urinary and fecal excretion) expressed per 70 kg of body weight.

The noncancer patients responded to hyperalimentation as expected from previous reports (Table 4) (Reifenstein et al. 1945, Rudman et al. 1975). Average balances were strongly positive for all seven elements. There were no significant differences between elemental retention in patients receiving nutritional support via central vein and those receiving hyperalimentation via nasogastric tube.

Comparison of the centrally hyperalimented cancer patients with the non-

TABLE 4. *Comparison of metabolic balance data of noncancer and cancer patients undergoing either central venous or enteral hyperalimentation. (Data expressed as per 70 kg body weight: balances recorded on a per-day basis. Mean ± S.D.)*

Element	Central venous hyperalimentation		Enteral hyperalimentation	
	Noncancer	Cancer	Noncancer	Cancer
ΔNitrogen (g)	4.6 ± 1.8	5.1 ± 3.8*	5.3 ± 1.7	4.8 ± 1.5*
ΔPhosphorus (g)	0.27 ± 0.13	0.13 ± 0.19*	0.33 ± 0.19	0.07 ± 0.24*
ΔPotassium (mEq)	18.9 ± 6.5	18.7 ± 12.7*	15.2 ± 5.3	−3.1 ± 6.6†
ΔSodium (mEq)	23.4 ± 5.8	19.5 ± 7.4*	20.1 ± 8.7	−3.4 ± 14.8†
ΔChloride (mEq)	17.7 ± 4.9	12.6 ± 6.1*	13.2 ± 6.1	−5.5 ± 10.3†
ΔCalcium (g)	0.06 ± .16	−0.03 ± .20*	0.17 ± 0.25	0.09 ± 0.49*
ΔMagnesium (mEq)	11.9 ± 4.0	3.2 ± 5.9†	10.1 ± 7.5	−2.7 ± 8.1†

(Adapted from Nixon et al. 1981a.)
* p > .05, not significant.
† p < .01.

cancer patients revealed that, despite similar nitrogen retention, there were several differences in the balances of other elements. Although the average calcium balances in the two groups were not significantly different, calcium balance was negative in three of nine cancer patients and one of five noncancer patients. Magnesium balance was negative in three of the nine cancer patients and in none of the noncancer patients. Average magnesium retention was significantly less (p < 0.01) in the cancer patients than in the noncancer controls. There was also a marked variability in the metabolic balance data of the cancer patients as compared to the noncancer patients, as evidenced by the wider standard deviations.

There were also several differences in the metabolic balance data of the enterally hyperalimented cancer and noncancer patients. Despite similar nitrogen retention, balances of potassium, sodium, chloride, and magnesium were significantly lower (p < 0.01) in the cancer patients. Negative balances were uncommon in the noncancer patients but were frequently seen in the patients with malignant diseases; three of six patients were in negative balance for phosphorus, five of six were in negative balance for potassium, all six were in negative balance for chloride, and four of six were in negative balance for magnesium. Standard deviations were again wider in the cancer group than in controls. These negative balances resulted from excessive urinary excretion, not from augmented fecal loss.

The metabolic balances of cancer patients receiving enteral support and of those receiving parenteral nutritional support were also significantly different. Enterally hyperalimented patients retained significantly less (p < 0.05) phosphorus, potassium, sodium, chloride, and magnesium than their counterparts receiving nutritional support via central vein.

A comparison of all cancer patients receiving hyperalimentation with all noncancer patients receiving nutritional support revealed that although nitrogen retention was similar in patients with malignant and nonmalignant disease, the cancer patients retained significantly less magnesium (p < 0.01), phosphorus (p < 0.01), sodium (p < 0.03), and chloride (p < 0.02). The metabolism of these elements during hyperalimentation is thus clearly different in cancer patients than in malnourished patients with nonneoplastic diseases. The most striking of these differences was the abnormally low magnesium retention. Indeed, seven of the 15 patients with advanced cancer were in negative magnesium balance despite positive nitrogen balance. In contrast, none of the noncancer patients were in negative magnesium balance. Therefore, this ion was selected for closer analysis. For this purpose cancer patients with positive magnesium balance were compared with cancer patients with negative magnesium balance.

The Behavior of Magnesium

Examination of the clinical characteristics of these patients revealed no significant differences between those in positive magnesium balance and those exhibiting a net loss of this cation (Table 5). There was no association between any

TABLE 5. *Comparison of clinical data in cancer patients with positive and negative magnesium balances*

	Pos. Mg balance (n = 8)	Neg. Mg balance (n = 7)
Age (mean) (years)	55	57
Sex		
Male	5	2
Female	3	5
Diagnoses		
gastrointestinal cancer	5	5
squamous cell carcinoma of the head and neck	2	1
adenocarcinoma of unknown primary site	1	0
squamous cell carcinoma of the lung	0	1
Metastatic sites		
bone	4	0
liver	4	3
Degree of undernutrition as assessed by creatinine/height index		
$\geq 60 - 80\%$ of standard	4	3
$< 60\%$ of standard	4	4
Route of delivery of nutritional support		
central vein	6	3
nasogastric tube	2	4

one tumor type and negative magnesium balance. Magnesium loss was not accounted for by bone metastases; indeed, all four patients with bone metastases were in positive magnesium balance. Liver metastases were equally distributed between the two groups. There was also no association between degree of undernutrition as assessed by creatinine/height index and negative magnesium balance. However, all 15 cancer patients were severely undernourished according to the creatinine/height index (less than 80% of standard). Two of six enterally hyper-

TABLE 6. *Comparison of improvement in nutritional indicators in hyperalimented cancer patients in positive magnesium balance with those in negative magnesium balance (Mean ± S.D.)*

	Improvement	
Indicator (unit)	Pos. Mg balance group (n = 8)	Neg. Mg balance group (n = 7)
Body weight (kg)	4.6 ± 1.2	4.0 ± 1.6*
Creatinine/height index (% standard)	4.6 ± 3.9	7.0 ± 12.9
Triceps skinfold (% of standard)	10.9 ± 4.2	10.4 ± 10.1
Serum albumin (g/dl)	−0.06 ± 0.43	0.04 ± 0.39

* All differences were not statistically significant; $p > .05$.

TABLE 7. Comparison of metabolic balance studies in hyperalimented cancer patients in positive and negative magnesium balance

| Group | Element (mean ± S.D.) | | | | | | |
	N (g)	P (g)	K (mEq)	Na (mEq)	Cl (mEq)	Ca (g)	Mg (mEq)
Pos. Mg balance (n = 8)	+5.7 ± 3.5	+0.21 ± 0.17	+17.6 ± 16	+13.6 ± 16.9	+9.8 ± 14.6	+0.09 ± .22	+6.7 ± 2.9
Neg. Mg balance (n = 7)	+4.3 ± 1.6	+0.02 ± 0.15	+2.6 ± 9.4	+7.1 ± 11.8	+2.2 ± 7.9	−0.06 ± 0.42	−5.6 ± 4.1
(Significance)	(NS)	(p < 0.04)	(p < 0.05)	(NS)	(NS)	(NS)	

alimented patients were in positive magnesium balance, compared to six of nine patients receiving nutritional support via the central vein.

There was also no difference in degree of improvement in any of the parameters measured between patients in positive and negative magnesium balance (Table 6). Body weight increased 4.6 ± 1.2 kg in patients with positive magnesium balance, compared to 4.0 ± 1.6 kg in patients with negative magnesium balance. Lean body mass, as assessed by creatinine/height index, increased 4.6 ± 3.9% of standard in the patients with positive magnesium balance, and by 7.0 ± 12.9% of standard in the negative balance group. Triceps skinfold measurements also showed similar improvement in the two groups (10.9 ± 4.2% versus 10.4 ± 10.1% of standard), as did serum albumin concentration (−0.06 ± 0.43 g/dl versus 0.04 ± 0.39 g/dl). Similarly, there was no significant difference in survival between patients in negative magnesium balance (194 ± 111 days; range 33–348) and patients in positive magnesium balance (235 ± 181 days; range 26–527).

There were, however, differences in the metabolic balance profiles of the two groups of patients (Table 7). Patients in negative magnesium balance retained significantly less phosphorus (0.21 ± 0.17 g versus 0.02 ± .15 g; p < 0.04) and potassium (17.6 ± 16 mEq versus 2.6 ± 9.4 mEq; p < 0.05) than those in positive magnesium balance. There was no significant difference (p > 0.05) in retention of the other elements between the two groups.

The relationship between nitrogen, phosphorus, and calcium was abnormal in patients in either positive or negative magnesium balance. Reifenstein's equations relating nitrogen and calcium balance to phosphorus balance (Reifenstein et al. 1945) predicted a phosphorus balance of +0.43 g/70 kg body weight per day for the positive magnesium balance group; the observed balance was only +0.21 g. For the negative magnesium balance group, the predicted phosphorus balance was +0.26 g/70 kg body weight per day and the observed balance was +0.02 g. The relationship of potassium to nitrogen was closer to theoretical (Rudman et al. 1975) in the positive magnesium balance group (predicted nitrogen balance 6.5 g/70 kg body weight per day; observed 5.7 g) than in patients in negative magnesium balance (predicted nitrogen balance +.96 g/70 kg body weight per day; observed +4.3 g).

EFFECT OF CENTRAL VENOUS HYPERALIMENTATION ON SURVIVAL OF PATIENTS WITH ADVANCED ADENOCARCINOMA OF THE COLON

To test the hypothesis that vigorous nutritional support of patients with advanced malignancy might improve survival, we performed a third study involving only patients with advanced adenocarcinoma of the colon (Nixon et al. 1981b). Patients were first stratified on the basis of amount of weight loss (0–6%, >6–12%, and >12–24% of premorbid weight) and then randomly assigned to receive either chemotherapy plus ad lib feedings or identical chemotherapy plus

3 to 4 weeks (average, 24 days) of central venous hyperalimentation. Each study patient received hyperalimentation only once, and no control patient received intravenous nutritional support. Median survival of 20 patients receiving central venous hyperalimentation was only 79 days, compared to a median survival of 308 days in patients who did not receive nutritional support (p = 0.03). This difference was most marked in the patients who had lost the least weight (0–6% weight loss stratum), with hyperalimented patients surviving a median of 66 days, compared to 298 days for controls (p = 0.02). The differences in survival for the other two weight loss strata were not significant (p > 0.10); these median survivals were: ≥ 6–12% weight loss group, 96 vs 318 days; > 12–24% weight loss group, 123 vs 129 days.

Males and patients with liver metastases had especially poor survival in this series, and there were proportionately more of these in the hyperalimented group. When the survival data were adjusted for these variables, there was no longer any statistically significant difference in survival between the two groups.

DISCUSSION

Protein-calorie undernutrition is common in patients with advanced cancer. Lean body mass depletion as assessed by the creatinine/height index is especially frequent; furthermore, patients with an index of less than 60% of standard have a much shorter survival than patients with higher values.

These findings suggested that improvement in these indicators of lean body mass might result in increased survival. Since anorexia is such a common feature of the undernutrition seen in cancer, it was hoped that the nonvolitional provision of adequate nutrients might significantly improve the nutritional status, and hence the survival, of patients with advanced malignant diseases. Close examination of the response of these patients to central venous or enteral hyperalimentation revealed, however, less improvement in nutritional indicators than similarly treated noncancer controls, no improvement in survival, and marked abnormalities of mineral and electrolyte metabolism as assessed by the metabolic balance technique. This latter anomaly may represent either cause or effect of the abnormality that underlies the other two findings; therefore, it will be discussed in greater detail.

Undernourished adults with nonmalignant diseases have a characteristic pattern of response when nutritional support is begun (Reifenstein et al. 1945, Rudman et al. 1975). Five to 12 grams of nitrogen are usually retained per day. Simultaneously, the other elements that make up normal protoplasm (nitrogen, phosphorus, potassium, and magnesium), extracellular fluid (sodium and chloride), and bone (calcium, phosphorus, and magnesium) are also retained. The relative retention of these elements conforms to their relative concentrations in normal lean body mass, and reflects synthesis of this tissue. The undernourished noncancer patients in this series exhibited this characteristic response to hyperalimentation. Patients receiving central venous hyperalimentation retained nitrogen/phosphorus/potassium/sodium/chloride/calcium/magnesium in these ratios: 1/0.06/4.11/5.09/3.85/0.01/2.59. Enterally hyperalimented noncancer patients retained these elements in similar ratios: 1/.06/2.87/3.79/2.49/0.03/ 1.91. Nutritional indicators demonstrated that normal lean body mass was being synthesized.

In contrast to this normal response, cancer patients retained these elements in abnormal ratios. For the centrally hyperalimented patients, these values were: 1/0.03/3.67/3.86/2.47/−0.01/0.63. The enterally hyperalimented patients also demonstrated abnormal metabolic balances. The ratios of element retention in these patients were: 1/0.01/−0.65/−0.71/−1.15/0.02/−0.56. Since the components of lean body mass were not retained in ratios that conform to their concentration in normal tissue, it cannot be concluded that normal lean tissue is being synthesized by these patients. In these patients, nutritional indicators also indicated that synthesis of lean body tissue was less than expected.

Reifenstein and colleagues observed that the fixed ratios of nitrogen to phosphorus in normal protoplasm and of calcium to phosphorus in normal bone enable one to predict the balance of any one of these elements if the other two are known (Reifenstein et al. 1945). Application of this technique to the noncancer patients revealed a predicted phosphorus balance of +0.34 g/70 kg body weight per day for the centrally hyperalimented patients; this compares favorably with the observed balance of +0.27 g. For the enterally hyperalimented noncancer patients, these values were: predicted, +0.44 g; observed, +0.33 g. These relationships were distorted in the cancer subjects; for centrally hyperalimented patients the predicted phosphorus balance was +0.37 g/70 kg body weight per day compared to an observed balance of only +0.13 g. Predicted phosphorus balance in the enterally hyperalimented cancer patients was +0.37 g/70 kg body weight per day; the observed balance was only +0.07.

If these abnormal patterns of mineral and electrolyte retention are chronic, the inevitable result is that some compartments of lean body mass will have abnormal concentrations of these elements. In the case of magnesium, which is predominantly located in bone (60%), muscle (20%), and nonmuscle soft tissue (20%) (Aikawa 1978), chronic retention of a subnormal amount of magnesium relative to nitrogen would lead to subnormal concentrations of this ion in one or all of these compartments. Viewed differently, any of these compartments may be the source of the magnesium lost in patients who were in negative balance, with the result that over time the concentration of magnesium in this compartment would become abnormally low. The metabolic balance technique does not permit a determination of which of these compartments was the site of the abnormality in magnesium metabolism.

This anomalous retention of elements may play a causal role in the subnormal lean body mass synthesis noted in our cancer patients in response to hyperalimentation. We have previously shown that withholding any one of nitrogen, phosphorus, potassium, sodium, or chloride from the diet essentially blocks retention of the other elements and halts synthesis of protoplasm and extracellular fluid

(Rudman et al. 1975). Others have demonstrated that severe dietary restriction of magnesium effectively slows or halts protein synthesis in both host and tumor tissue (Young and Parsons 1977, Sugiura and Benedict 1935).

In summary, our studies have confirmed the prevalence and ominous prognostic import of undernutrition in patients with advanced cancer. Our studies do not, however, offer any support for vigorous nutritional therapy in these patients. Instead, we have found common mineral and electrolyte abnormalities that may cause, or merely reflect, what appears to be a partial block to the restoration of normal lean body tissue in persons with advanced cancer.

ACKNOWLEDGMENTS

The work in this manuscript was supported by: NIH Grants R01-CA-20997, 16255, and RR00039; NIH contract N01-CP-65802; the American Legion Gioia Osborne Cancer Research Fund; the State of Georgia Nutrition-Cancer Contract; and the Emory University Cancer Center.

REFERENCES

Aikawa, J. K. 1978. Biochemistry and physiology of magnesium. World Rev. Nutr. Diet 28:114–142.

Babson, A. L. 1954. Some host-tumor relationships with respect to nitrogen. Cancer Res. 14:89–93.

Butterworth, C. E., and G. L. Blackburn. 1975. Hospital malnutrition: How to assess the nutritional status of a patient. Nutr. Today 10:8–18.

Cameron, I. L., and W. Rogers. 1977. Total intravenous hyperalimentation and hydroxyurea chemotherapy in hepatoma-bearing rats. J. Surg. Res. 23:279–288.

Daly, J. M., H. M. Reynolds, B. J. Rowlands, S. J. Dudrick, and E. M. Copeland III. 1980. Tumor growth in experimental animals: Nutritional manipulation and chemotherapeutic response in the rat. Ann. Surg. 191:316–322.

Dudrick, S. J., B. V. MacFadyen, E. A. Souchon, D. M. Englert, and E. M. Copeland III. 1977. Parenteral nutrition techniques in cancer patients. Cancer Res. 37:2440–2450.

Fenninger, L. D., C. Waterhouse, and E. H. Keutmann. 1953. The interrelationship of nitrogen and phosphorus in patients with certain neoplastic diseases. Cancer 6:930–941.

Heymsfield, S. B., R. A. Bethel, J. D. Ansley, D. W. Nixon, and D. Rudman. 1979. Enteral hyperalimentation: An alternative to central venous hyperalimentation. Ann. Intern. Med. 90:63–71.

Isaacs, J. W., W. J. Millikan, J. Stackhouse, T. Hersh, and D. Rudman. 1977. Parenteral nutrition of adults with a 900 milliosmolar solution via peripheral veins. Am. J. Clin. Nutr. 30:552–559.

Jellife, D. B., and E. F. P. Jellife. 1971. Age-independent anthropometry. Am. J. Clin. Nutr. 24:1377–1379.

Nixon, D. W., S. B. Heymsfield, A. E. Cohen, M. H. Kutner, J. Ansley, D. H. Lawson, D. Rudman. 1980. Protein-calorie undernutrition in hospitalized cancer patients. Am. J. Med. 68:683–690.

Nixon, D. W., D. H. Lawson, M. Kutner, J. Ansley, M. Schwarz, S. Heymsfield, R. Chawla, T. H. Cartwright, and D. Rudman. 1981a. Hyperalimentation of the cancer patient with protein-calorie undernutrition. Cancer Res. 41:2038–2045.

Nixon, D. W., S. Moffitt, D. H. Lawson, J. Ansley, M. J. Lynn, M. H. Kutner, S. B. Heymsfield, M. Wesley, R. Chawla, and D. Rudman. 1981b. Total parenteral nutrition as an adjunct to chemotherapy of metastatic colorectal cancer. Cancer Treat. Rep. (in press).

Reifenstein, E. C., Jr., F. Albright, and S. L. Wells. 1945. The accumulation, interpretation and presentation of data pertaining to metabolic balances, notably those of calcium, phosphorus and nitrogen. J. Clin. Endocrinol. Metab. 5:367–395.

Rudman, D., W. J. Millikan, T. J. Richardson, T. J. Bixler II, J. Stackhouse, and W. K. McGarrity. 1975. Elemental balances during intravenous hyperalimentation of underweight adult subjects. J. Clin. Invest. 55:94–104.

Steiger, E., J. Oram-Smith, Jr., and E. Miller. 1975. Effects of nutrition on tumor growth and tolerance to chemotherapy. J. Surg. Res. 18:455–461.

Sugimura, T., S. M. Birnbaum, M. Winitz, and J. P. Greenstein. 1959. Quantitative nutritional studies with water-soluble, chemically defined diets. VII. Nitrogen balance in normal and tumor-bearing rats following forced feeding. Arch. Biochem. Biophys. 81:439–447.

Sugiura, K., and S. R. Benedict. 1935. The influence of magnesium on the growth of carcinoma, sarcoma and melanoma in animals. Am. J. Cancer 23:300–310.

Terepka, A. R., and C. Waterhouse. 1956. Metabolic observations during the forced feeding of patients with cancer. Am. J. Med. 20:225–248.

Watkin, D. M. 1961. Nitrogen balance as affected by neoplastic disease and its therapy. Am. J. Clin. Nutr. 9:446–459.

Young, G. A., and F. M. Parsons. 1977. The effects of dietary deficiencies of magnesium and potassium on the growth and chemistry of transplanted tumors and host tissues in the rat. Eur. J. Cancer 13:103–113.

Energy Metabolism in Tumor Cells and Nutritional Sources of Calories

Molecular Interrelations of Nutrition and Cancer,
edited by M. S. Arnott, J. van Eys, and Y.-M. Wang.
Raven Press, New York © 1982.

Changing Perceptions of Carbohydrate Metabolism in Tumors

Sidney Weinhouse

*Fels Research Institute, Temple University School of Medicine,
Philadelphia, Pennsylvania 19140*

Perhaps no better example can be found to illustrate the frustrations that have accompanied the quest for a solution to the cancer problem than the efforts to understand the neoplastic process in terms of aberrant carbohydrate metabolism. This subject has a colorful history; and while no clearcut definition has yet been reached, the past 60 years of experiment and argument [sometimes acrimonious (Warburg 1956a,b, 1966, Weinhouse 1956)] have illuminated many of the complexities of cellular metabolism that must underlie neoplastic behavior.

The focal point for this long-standing, unresolved question of whether deranged metabolism of glucose is central to the neoplastic process is the Warburg hypothesis (Warburg 1930). This hypothesis, propounded with evangelical fervor nearly 50 years ago by an illustrious scientist deservedly considered to be the father of modern biochemistry, so captured the imagination of the biological community that even up to the present day it has served as a guiding principle for several decades of studies toward the understanding and control of cancer. Although everyone has heard of the Warburg hypothesis, I suspect that few understand or appreciate its experimental basis. I will therefore undertake in this paper to review its experimental background and what I perceive to be its current status in the light of what we have learned about glucose metabolism during the past half century.[1]

THE WARBURG HYPOTHESIS AND ITS EXPERIMENTAL BACKGROUND

Utilizing the manometric procedures that bear his name and that for many years played a dominant role in studies of cellular physiology, Warburg in the early 1920s measured three parameters of glucose metabolism in tissue slices:

---

[1] The subject of this paper is too broad for complete bibliographic coverage. For the early history and subsequent discussions of the Warburg hypothesis and carbohydrate metabolism of tumors the reader is referred to the following reviews: Aisenberg (1961), Burk (1939), Greenstein (1954), Gregg (1972), Knox (1976), Schapira (1973), Shapot (1979), Warburg (1930), Weber (1977), Weinhouse (1955, 1972, 1976a), and Wenner (1975).

oxygen consumption and lactic acid production in the presence and absence of oxygen. He noted that slices of both normal and tumor tissues took up glucose and converted it to lactic acid, a process he termed glycolysis. He made the landmark observation that in normal tissues glycolysis occurred in the absence of oxygen, but was almost completely eliminated in the presence of oxygen. His physiologic insight led him to recognize this phenomenon as an important regulatory mechanism, even though at that time very little was known of the underlying biochemical reactions. He termed this the Pasteur effect, since he recognized its basic similarity to an observation by Pasteur 50 years earlier that when yeast was transferred from an anerobic to an aerobic environment, it ceased to convert glucose to ethanol. The Pasteur effect is still not totally understood, but it has served to stimulate a half century of discussion and speculation on the regulation of carbohydrate metabolism.

Warburg noted further that slices of both animal and human tumors also produced lactic acid and displayed a Pasteur effect, but anaerobic glycolysis was much higher in tumors and was only partially eliminated when tissues were incubated in oxygen. He thereupon reasoned that there was some defect in tumors in the capability of oxygen to reduce glycolysis. In his own words, taken from the preface of the English edition of his book (Warburg 1930), the Warburg hypothesis states:

Whilst, however, normal cells die if they glycolyze aerobically, the glycolyzing tumor cell . . . is . . . able to grow to an unlimited extent turning to account the chemical energy of the glycolysis.
Whether the respiration of the tumor cell is large or small, aerobic glycolysis is present in every case. The respiration is always disturbed, inasmuch as it is incapable of causing the disappearance of . . . glycolysis.

To understand the reasoning that generated this dogmatic pronouncement it is instructive to examine the experimental data on which it is based. These have been summarized in Table 1, taken from a review by Burk (1939) and from Warburg's monograph (Warburg 1930). They show that there is a wide

TABLE 1. *Experimental basis for the Warburg hypothesis**

		Lactate production		Pasteur	P.E.
	O_2 Uptake	Anaerobic	Aerobic	effect	O_2 uptake
14 Normal tissues	9.3	7.2	2.1	5.1	0.55
	(3–21)	(2–19)	(0–10)	(1–17)	
15 Animal tumors	11.8	25.6	14.0	11.6	0.98
	(5–20)	(14–35)	(5–25)	(6–18)	
13 Human tumors	5.3	20.5	13.3	7.2	1.35
	(2–6)	(13–29)	(5–19)	(3–11)	
11 Flexner Jobling	8.0	32.1	23.6	7.0	0.88
rat carcinomas	(4–13)	(27–37)	(19–28)	(3–9)	

* Data are condensed from Warburg (1930) and Burk (1939). Values are in Q notation, μliters equivalent/hr/mg dry wt. Ranges are in parentheses.

TABLE 2. *Evidence of normal respiration in tumors*

1. Oxygen uptake is quantitatively normal
2. Oxidative phosphorylation is quantitatively normal in tumor mitochondria
3. Mitochondria of tumors are structurally and functionally normal
4. Respiration in tumors is responsible for major formation of ATP
5. Glucose, fatty acids, and amino acids all contribute substantially
   to respiratory CO_2
6. The citric acid cycle operates normally as a terminal oxidation
   system
7. Tumor cells in culture require oxygen to survive

range of values for the three measurements and reveal clearly that there are no crucial quantitative differences between the normal and tumor tissue slices. Oxygen uptakes were all in overlapping ranges; and whereas there is indeed a higher anerobic glycolysis in tumors than in the normal tissues studied, there is no evidence of a diminished Pasteur effect in tumors. In fact, within the range of values observed, the Pasteur effect in tumors is somewhat greater. Thus the foundation stone of the Warburg hypothesis, that "respiration is always disburbed . . . ," is not borne out by his own experimental data. There is neither a quantitative diminution nor an inability of tumors to respond to oxygen by a decrease in glycolysis. If, as in the last column of Table 1, we express the Pasteur effect in terms of oxygen uptake, again we observe that, for all tissues, by and large each molecule of oxygen absorbed reduces lactic acid production by one-half molecule in normal tissues to one to one and one-half molecules in tumors. Logic would have been better served to say that the anerobic glycolysis of tumors is so high that a normal respiration and a normal or greater than normal Pasteur effect fails to eliminate it.[2]

Throughout a long lifetime, Warburg vigorously defended this hypothesis against a constantly rising tide of opposition (Warburg 1966). From our present vantage point, other defects are all too apparent. We know that normal cells do not die if they glycolyze aerobically, nor can tumor cells survive without oxygen (Gregg 1972). Erythrocytes, kidney medulla, intestinal mucosa, and retina glycolyze aerobically (Aisenberg 1961), and glycolysis in striated muscle during violent exercise exceeds by far that in the most highly glycolyzing tumor.

Despite efforts of many investigators to find some measure of support for a respiratory defect in tumors, the weight of evidence (Table 2) indicates that respiration is not diminished in tumors (Weinhouse 1951) and that tumor mitochondria utilize the same mechanisms to the same degree and in the same

---

[2] It is sometimes assumed erroneously that the Pasteur effect is merely the result of oxidation of the lactate that might otherwise accumulate. However, according to the equation $CH_3CHOHCOOH + 3\ O_2 \longrightarrow 3\ CO_2 + 3\ H_2O$ oxidation can only account for 0.33 mole of lactate per mole of O_2 consumed, whereas the Pasteur effect has a magnitude two to six times higher.

manner as do normal mitochondria in utilizing oxygen and coupling oxygen uptake with phosphorylation (Wenner 1975, Gregg 1972, Racker 1976). ATP is also generated by glycolysis, and one might wonder whether glycolytic ATP production has some special quality that favors cell proliferation or whether the high glycolysis adds significantly to the energy budget of the cancer cell. There is no evidence in experiment or theory for the former, and as for the latter, the ATP energy increment due to increased glycolysis is likely to be small compared with that provided by oxidative phosphorylation.

SUBSTRATE UTILIZATION FOR RESPIRATION

The Warburg hypothesis reflects the viewpoint of 50 years ago that all tissues except liver depend on glucose catabolism to support their energy requirements. We know now, however, that fatty acids are utilized as respiratory fuel for many tissues, including muscle and brain; and tumors are no exception. Isotope tracer studies demonstrated many years ago (Weinhouse 1955) that a variety of mouse and rat tumors can oxidize fatty acids to CO_2 in vitro and that dietary fatty acids ingested in vivo may serve also as respiratory fuel for tumors. Studies by Bloch-Frankenthal et al. (1965) and by Cederbaum and Rubin (1976) showed an inverse relationship between fatty acid oxidation and the extent of liver tumor dedifferentiation. Hepatic tumors, e.g., the Morris hepatomas, that are well differentiated, grow slowly, and have low glycolytic capability readily oxidize fatty acids to CO_2 and ketone bodies, whereas poorly differentiated, rapidly growing hepatic tumors have largely lost the ability to oxidize fatty acids, but have taken on the capability for high glycolytic activity (Weber et al. 1961, Elwood et al. 1963). These findings demonstrate that with hepatic tumors at least, high aerobic glycolysis is not necessarily a requirement for neoplasia, but rather is a consequence of a late stage of tumor dedifferentiation, in which glucose catabolism replaces that of fatty acids.

Tumors may also utilize amino acids as respiratory fuels (Lavietes and Coleman 1980, Reitzer et al. 1979), thus further discounting a rigid requirement for glycolysis as an energy source for tumor survival. A balanced viewpoint based on current knowledge would regard high aerobic glycolysis as a common feature of many tumors, but by no means a crucial factor for all tumors. Studies of the Morris hepatomas make it clear that even tumors that arise from a single cell source may vary greatly in their ability to utilize the various metabolic fuels, as well as in many other properties (Weinhouse 1972, Morris and Meranze 1975).

NEOPLASTIC CELLS IN CULTURE

Culture of tumors cells in vitro has broadened our perceptions of their nutritional and metabolic requirements but have added little to the significance of glycolysis to neoplasia. Like solid tumors, malignant cells in culture exhibit a

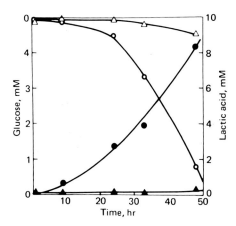

FIG. 1. Glucose utilization and lactic acid production in exponentially growing mutant DS 7 line and 023 parental line. Glucose utilization: mutant, △, parental ○; lactic acid: mutant, ▲, parental, ●. (Data taken from Figure 4, Pouysségur et al. 1980a, with permission of the National Academy of Sciences, U.S.A.)

wide range of respiration and anerobic and aerobic glycolysis. However, the differences between normal and transformed cells are not nearly so marked as with solid tumors, and in some instances there are no differences (Gregg 1972). Eagle showed many years ago (Eagle et al. 1958) that both normal and malignant cells grew as well on fructose or galactose, in which glycolysis was low, as they grew on glucose or mannose, in which glycolysis was high. Moreover, glycolysis with the latter sugars was as high in the normal as in the transformed cells. Glycolysis in cultured cells presumably may be determined not only by their malignancy but also by their growth rate and population density (Bissel et al. 1972).

In two important recent papers Pouysségur et al. (1980a,b) described a tumorigenic Chinese hamster fibroblast mutant, induced and selected by treatment with tritium-labeled 2-deoxyglucose. This clone, termed DS7, is devoid of phosphohexose isomerase, a glycolytic enzyme, and has only one-fifth the glucose transport rate of the parent line and only 7% of the rate of glycolysis in 5 mM glucose. As shown in Figure 1, almost no glucose was utilized, and virtually no lactic acid was produced by these cells; yet growth in the mutant strain was nearly as high as that of the parent. Despite a virtually complete loss in the ability to utilize glucose, these cells retained all of the malignant properties of the parent cells, including ability to grow in low serum concentration, anchorage independence, and the ability, when injected into nude mice, to produce tumors that retain the same glycolytic defect. These results leave no doubt of the independence of glycolysis from a tumorigenic phenotype.

FUNCTIONAL ROLE OF ISOZYME ALTERATIONS IN CARBOHYDRATE METABOLISM

Though we accept the view that high aerobic glycolysis is not intrinsic to the neoplastic process, it is still instructive to consider why it occurs in many tumors. This feature of the neoplastic process, as well as the closely related Pasteur effect, have been focal points for two generations of effort to understand how cellular metabolism is regulated. Unfortunately, as the problem is investigated in increasing depth, further complexities rather than solutions are revealed. In the next few paragraphs I would like to discuss findings that I feel shed some light on glycolytic regulation, and perhaps more importantly, may tell us something about the nature of the neoplastic process itself.

Almost 20 years ago, pioneering studies of Weber and others (1961) showed that the so-called minimum deviation Morris hepatomas (Morris and Meranze 1975) exhibited a wide range of phenotypic properties, including highly variable aerobic glycolysis. They thus were an advantageous experimental system for studies on control factors in glycolysis. Several years earlier, Markert (Markert and Möller 1959) demonstrated that enzymes commonly exist in multiple forms, having different primary structures and different chemical and kinetic properties. The term that he coined for this phenomenon, isozyme, has now become common in the biomedical vocabulary with the recognition that isozymes hold a key to cellular regulatory mechanisms. Schapira (Schapira et al. 1963, Schapira 1973) first demonstrated that the aldolase in certain experimental and human liver tumors differed from the enzyme of normal liver. The tumor form subsequently was identified with an isozyme present in normal nonhepatic tissues and fetal liver. At about that time, we demonstrated in studies of hepatic glucose metabolism that liver contained a major hexokinase isozyme that differed from other hexokinase isozymes (Weinhouse 1976b). It has a high Km for glucose, thereby explaining why the liver takes up glucose only in hyperglycemia, and it has the striking property of being under host dietary and endocrine control. We found, as shown in Figure 2, that this isozyme was retained in certain Morris hepatomas that were well differentiated, glycolyzed minimally, and grew slowly, but was lost from those hepatomas that were poorly differentiated, glycolyzed highly, and grew rapidly. More striking was our finding that this host-regulated

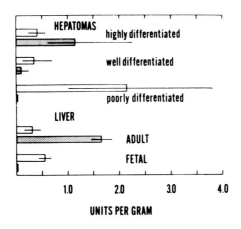

FIG. 2. Hexokinase isozymes in rat liver and hepatomas. Hexokinase(s) shown in open bars, glucokinase in shaded bars. (Reproduced from Shatton et al. 1969, with permission of *Cancer Research*.)

TABLE 3. *Enzymes expressing fetal forms in hepatomas**

Hexokinase	tRNA methylase
Aldolase	Thymidine kinase
Pyruvate kinase	Uridine kinase
Glycogen phosphorylase	DNA polymerase
α-Glycerophosphate dehydrogenase	Deoxycytidine deaminase
Alcohol dehydrogenase	Glucosamine 6-phosphate synthetase
Branched-chain amino acid amino-	Hexosaminidase
transferase	Alkaline phosphatase
Glutaminase	γ-Glutamyl peptidotransferase
Carbamyl phosphate synthetase	Plasminogen activators
Ornithine decarboxylase	Ribonucleotide reductase

* Adapted from Ibsen and Fishman 1979.

isozyme, kinetically geared for normal hepatic function, was replaced by a high activity of other isozymes of hexokinase, not under host regulation but geared for avid glucose utilization. This switch of isozyme composition clearly offers clues, not only to the high glycolysis of tumors, but also to a molecular basis for the lack of host control of cell proliferation. Our further exploration of isozyme alterations in these tumors was thus prompted. As a result of work from our own and other laboratories we recognize this now as a common phenomenon. A recent review (Ibsen and Fishman 1979) lists 21 instances in which, as shown in Table 3, normal hepatic isozymes are replaced by forms normally present in fetal liver. Among these are such key enzymes of carbohydrate metabolism as hexokinase, aldolase, pyruvate kinase, glycogen phosphorylase, α-glycerophosphate dehydrogenase, glucosamine 6-phosphate synthetase, and hexosaminidase. Since enzymes are the cellular machinery, it would follow that this wholesale replacement of isozymes geared for normal tissue function would have profound effects on tumor metabolism.

PYRUVATE KINASE AS A REGULATORY SITE FOR GLYCOLYSIS AND THE PASTEUR EFFECT

A key to the aerobic glycolysis of at least some tumors has emerged from the dramatic change observed in the activity and isozyme composition of pyruvate kinase (Farina et al. 1974). The typical pattern of isozyme alteration is similar to that observed for hexokinase. As shown in Figure 3, type I, the adult liver form, predominates in normal liver, but is accompanied by a low level of type III, the fetal form. Type I is highly regulated, is also under endocrine control, and is geared kinetically to function as a control site for gluconeogenesis (Friedmann et al. 1971). In well-differentiated hepatomas, the liver pattern is retained, but in rapidly growing, poorly differentiated, and highly glycolyzing hepatomas, the liver form is nearly entirely replaced by high activity of the fetal form.

As shown in Figure 4, pyruvate kinase has a special strategic role in glycolysis,

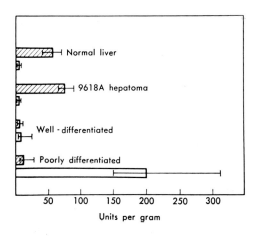

FIG. 3. Pyruvate kinase isozymes in rat liver and hepatomas. Type I, the normal adult liver form, is shown in the shaded bars and Type III, the fetal or tumor form, in open bars. (Reproduced from Weinhouse 1972, with permission of *Cancer Research.*)

because it requires ADP as a cosubstrate, and thus it competes for this nucleotide with the mitochondrial respiratory system. As a connecting link with oxidative phosphorylation through a common ADP requirement, it is obviously an attractive site for glycolytic-respiratory interaction.[3] Competition for ADP would lower glycolysis by oxygen, thereby accounting for the Pasteur effect, and a high fetal pyruvate kinase activity such as has been generally observed in highly glycolyzing tumors (Shonk et al. 1965) could account for the high aerobic and anerobic glycolysis accompanying normal respiration. Another phenomenon observed in highly glycolyzing tumors is the Crabtree effect, manifested by a lowered respiration in the presence of glucose. This is also consistent with preferential utilization by pyruvate kinase of ADP that would otherwise be utilized for oxidative phosphorylation.

To assess the extent and significance of competition for ADP we employed a model system in which the relative concentration of pyruvate kinase and mitochondria could be manipulated while maintaining a limiting steady production of ADP (Gosalvez et al. 1974). The results are shown in Figure 5. As shown in Figure 5A, oxygen uptake progressively decreased with increasing pyruvate kinase, a typical Crabtree effect that we attribute to increasingly successful competition for the ADP otherwise available for oxidative phosphorylation. Further evidence for this supposition is shown in Figure 5B, where pyruvate formation was increased with increasing pyruvate kinase, in parallel with the decreased O_2 uptake.

If the mitochondrial respiratory system was increased and the pyruvate kinase level held constant, respiration increased as shown in Figure 5C, and pyruvate formation decreased, as shown in Figure 5D.

---

[3] Lynen (1941) and Johnson (1941) suggested that the Pasteur effect could be mediated by competition for ADP and inorganic phosphate, but attention in more recent years has been directed to phosphofructokinase, whose participation in the Pasteur effect in muscle and brain is well documented.

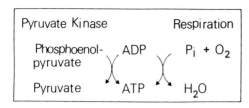

FIG. 4. Diagrammatic representation of the competition between pyruvate kinase and mitochondrial oxidative phosphorylation for the common substrate ADP.

All of the above-described effects were lost when oxidative phosphorylation was uncoupled from oxygen uptake by addition of 2,4-dinitrophenol or rotenone. Thus, the quasi-Pasteur and Crabtree effects observed in this isolated segment of the glycolytic system can clearly be attributed to competition for ADP. Further evidence for glycolytic regulation in intact tumor cells by interaction between pyruvate kinase and oxidative phosphorylation was obtained in a study of glycolysis in respiring Ehrlich ascites cells. When these cells were incubated aerobically with glucose, the addition of cysteine or phenylalanine, which are inhibitors of pyruvate kinase, lowered glycolysis and increased oxygen uptake (Gosalvez

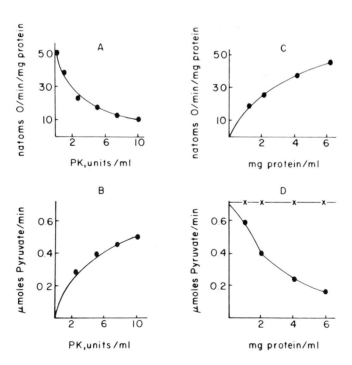

FIG. 5. Interaction of pyruvate kinase and mitochondrial respiration in a model system continuously regenerating ADP. A and B, pyruvate kinase varied and mitochondria held constant; C and D, mitochondria varied and pyruvate kinase held constant. (Reproduced from Gosalvez et al. 1975, with permission of the *European Journal of Biochemistry*.)

et al. 1975). This effect was also lost if oxidative phosphorylation was uncoupled by dinitrophenol.

Although we have focused on pyruvate kinase because of the marked switch of isozyme patterns in poorly differentiated, rapidly growing tumors, other sites should also be considered: for example, competitive interaction with oxidative phosphorylation can occur with triose phosphate dehydrogenase and 3-phosphoglycerate kinase. Phosphofructokinase has been implicated in the Pasteur effect of muscle and brain, but its role in tumors remains unresolved. A possible role of glucose transport in tumor glycolysis is the subject of a vast and also controversial literature (Parnes and Isselbacher 1978, Hatanaka 1974) and is discussed in the next chapter (see Weber, pages 183–190, this volume). Racker (private communication) has proposed that the high glycolysis of Ehrlich ascites cells may be due to a low efficiency of Na^+K^+-ATPase caused by the maintenance of this enzyme in phosphorylated form by a phosphorylation cascade catalyzed by protein kinases that are highly active in these cells. The problem of explaining the high aerobic glycolysis is thus not so much to discover a cause, but rather to choose among a multiplicity of sites in the complicated metabolic network of the cell.

GLUCOSE METABOLISM IN TUMOR-BEARING HOSTS

Studies of tissue metabolism in vitro, however elegant, can tell us only what can happen, not what does happen, in vivo. The whole animal, with its multiplicity of extracellular controls superimposed on intracellular controls, is therefore a "court of last resort" for validation of concepts based on the tissue slice, the isolated cell, or its subcellular components. Even before the Warburg era, aberrations of carbohydrate metabolism, in the form of abnormalities in blood glucose levels or glucose tolerance, were observed in human cancer (Stern and Willheim 1943, Shapot 1979); and arteriovenous differences in glucose and lactate in blood traversing tumors in experimental animals (Tadenuma et al. 1923; Cori and Cori 1925) demonstrated the utilization of glucose and production of lactic acid in vivo. Despite continuing effort during ensuing decades, however, there is still no clear indication that excessive glycolysis of tumors plays a significant role in the ultimately catastrophic effects of tumors on the host.

The dynamics of glucose metabolism are illustrated diagrammatically in Figure 6. The plasma glucose is replenished by dietary carbohydrate, which enters the liver to be converted in part to glycogen. Glucose provides the fuel for brain metabolism, and for muscle metabolism during periods of muscular activity. Lactic acid thus formed enters the blood and is transferred to the liver. During fasting or carbohydrate deprivation, the plasma glucose is replenished by gluconeogenesis, which occurs in accordance with need through hormonal mediation. The building blocks are the glucogenic amino acids originating either from the diet or protein breakdown and lactic acid arising from glycolysis in brain, muscle, and erythrocytes. The cyclic reconversion to glucose from lactic

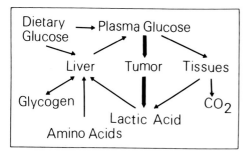

FIG. 6. Pathways of glucose utilization and synthesis in the tumor-bearing host.

acid arising via glycolysis is termed the Cori cycle. If glycolysis is unduly high in the tumor patient, the Cori cycle should be high.

A powerful homeostatic mechanism, mediated by diet and hormones, normally maintains the blood glucose concentration within well-defined limits. An excessive drain on the available glucose might be expected to disturb this system, with deleterious consequences to the host. However, the plasma glucose remains within normal limits, with only occasional exceptions, even in advanced human cancer (Reichard et al. 1964, Holroyde et al. 1975). The exceptions generally involve tumors of endocrine origin or those that secrete insulin or insulin-like polypeptides as a consequence of ectopic hormone secretion (Imura 1980), a bizarre but not uncommon feature of human cancer.

If excessive glycolysis occurs, it must be compensated for by enhanced gluconeogenesis. Increased ingestion of glucose probably plays a minor role, if any. Peculiarities in appetite are not unusual in cancer patients, but there is no undue craving for sugar. In fact, anorexia is a common symptom of advanced cancer.

How the cancer patient maintains a normal plasma glucose level in the face of a drain by high glycolytic activity was first studied in our laboratory by isotope tracer techniques (Reichard et al. 1964). By administering appropriately labeled glucose to human cancer patients, and by following the level and distribution of radioactivity in the plasma glucose over several hours, we were able to measure rates of glucose production and to estimate what proportion of the total glucose production came from glucose that had been converted to lactic acid and was reconverted in the liver to glucose, by the Cori cycle.

Results of the study are shown in Table 4. Ten normal subjects, with normal blood glucose values of 99 mg/100 ml, had a glucose turnover rate of 120 mg/kg/hr. Seventeen patients with cancer had normal mean blood glucose values of 104 mg/100 ml and a turnover rate of 131 mg/kg/hr, a value not significantly different from normal. These data do not disclose any major abnormality in the rate at which the cancer patient utilizes or synthesizes glucose. However, they do not include the contribution of the Cori cycle. To assess the magnitude of tumor glycolysis in vivo, tracer experiments were conducted to estimate the Cori cycle and its contribution to glucose turnover. Results are displayed in

TABLE 4. *Plasma glucose levels and turnover in normal humans and cancer patients**

	Subjects studied	
	10 Normal	17 Cancer
Plasma glucose		
mg/100 ml (range)	98 – 107	93 – 106
Net glucose turnover		
mg/kg/hr (mean ± S.D.)	120 ± 17	113 ± 29
	4 Normal	7 Cancer
Glucose recycled (Cory cycle)		
mg/kg/hr (mean ± S.D.)	26 ± 6	50 ± 20
Total glucose turnover		
mg/kg/hr (mean ± S.D.)	161 ± 23	192 ± 49

* Adapted from Reichard et al. 1964.

the lower portion of Table 4. In four normal subjects the total glucose turnover rate was 161 ± 23 mg/kg/hr, of which 26 ± 6 mg/kg/hr (16%) was contributed by the Cori cycle. In seven cancer patients, the total glucose turnover was 192 ± 49 mg/kg/hr, of which 50 ± 20 mg/kg/hr (26%) was contributed by the Cori cycle. These data indicate, within a rather wide range of variation, that more lactate was being converted to glucose in the cancer patient and that this difference was most likely attributable to tumor glycolysis. Similar experiments conducted subsequently by Holroyde et al. (1975, 1979) and by Waterhouse (1974) reveal Cori cycle rates two to four times normal and somewhat higher than normal blood lactate levels in cancer patients. Other parameters of glucose and lactate metabolism, such as pool size, space, conversion to CO_2, etc., were not outside normal values in cancer patients.

The observed rates of the Cori cycle in human cancer patients, which range between 50 and 100 mg glucose/kg/hr, are within the bounds that one might expect from usual ranges of tumor glycolytic activity observed in vitro. The aerobic glycolysis of tumors in vitro is approximately 0.5 μmole lactate/hr/ mg tissue dry weight. For a person weighing 60 kg, carrying a tumor with a dry weight of 100 g, we can calculate an aerobic tumor glycolysis in vivo of 4.5 g/hr or 76 mg/kg/hr. One can assume from these considerations that human tumors do indeed glycolyze in vivo at rates similar to those observed in vitro and that the homeostatic mechanism operating in normal humans to maintain the plasma glucose operates without substantial impairment in the cancer patient.

CONCLUDING COMMENTS

From our present perspective it seems fair to state that the Warburg hypothesis, however productive in stimulating decades of discussion and experiment, is at best a gross oversimplification and is unsupported even by Warburg's own experiments. Although its experimental foundation, namely, high aerobic glycolysis, has stood the test of time as a common feature of cancer, its importance as a necessary cause or consequence of neoplasia has been thoroughly eroded. It can now be perceived to be one end result, among many others, of a chain of alterations in sensitive regulatory mechanisms stemming from an initial impairment of the normally rigid control of gene expression operating in normal adult tissues. This phenomenon is a common thread interwoven throughout the whole fabric of cancer biology. It encompasses virtually all gene products; not only enzymes, the cellular machinery with which we are concerned here, but also a host of other proteins, including antigens, structural components of cell membranes, growth factors, and a large number of polypeptide hormones (Hall 1974, Imura 1980, Lehmann 1979, Weinhouse 1980). The repression of genes coding for normal adult proteins and the re-activation of genes (often fetal genes) that are normally repressed during or after embryonic development probably hold the key, not only to high glycolysis and other alterations of metabolism, but also to uncontrolled cell proliferation in cancer. The abnormality of gene regulation that gives rise to these properties also must be responsible for the tremendous diversity of tumors. Much of the confusion in cancer research is due to the unfortunate but understandable tendency to make generalizations based on limited tumor types. If after that statement I dare to generalize, it would be to say that while there are tumors that utilize glucose for metabolic fuel, others utilize fatty acids or amino acids, or all combinations. As yet there is no clear pattern of metabolism that defines the neoplastic state. It is a sobering reflection on the "state of the art" that the cancer cell still resists definition in terms of its cellular machinery. Our progress, if any, in the efforts of a half century to find unique metabolic and nutritional features of the neoplastic state consists first in recognizing the complexities of the problem and second in unlearning what is not true.

ACKNOWLEDGMENT

Work of the author described in this paper was supported by Grants CA-10916 and CA-12227 from the National Cancer Institute, U.S. Department of Health and Human Services, and Grant BC-74 from the American Cancer Society. Thanks are expressed to Harold P. Morris for long-continued collaboration and to Jennie B. Shatton and Albert Williams for constant help over many years.

REFERENCES

Aisenberg, A. C. 1961. The Glycolysis and Respiration of Tumors. Academic Press, London and New York.
Bissell, M. J., C. Hatie, and H. Rubin. 1972. Patterns of glucose metabolism in normal and virus-transformed chick cells in tissue culture. JNCI 49:555–565.
Bloch-Frankenthal, L., J. Langan, H. P. Morris, and S. Weinhouse. 1965. Fatty acid oxidation and ketogenesis in transplantable liver tumors. Cancer Res. 25:732–736.

Burk, D. 1939. A colloquial consideration of the Pasteur and neo-Pasteur effects. Cold Spring Harbor Symp. Quant. Biol. 7:420–459.

Cederbaum, A. I., and E. Rubin. 1976. Fatty acid oxidation, substrate shuttles and activities of the citric acid cycle in hepatocellular carcinomas of varying differentiations. Cancer Res. 36:2980–2987.

Cori, C. F., and G. T. Cori. 1925. The carbohydrate metabolism of tumors. II. Changes in the sugar, lactic acid, and CO_2-combining power of blood passing through a tumor. J. Biol. Chem. 65:397–405.

Eagle, H., S. Barban, M. Levy, and H. O. Schultz. 1958. The utilization of carbohydrates by human cell cultures. J. Biol. Chem. 233:551–558.

Elwood, J. C., Y. C. Lin, V. J. Cristofalo, and S. Weinhouse. 1963. Glucose utilization in homogenates of the Morris hepatoma 5123 and related tumors. Cancer Res. 23:906–913.

Farina, F., J. B. Shatton, H. P. Morris, and S. Weinhouse. 1974. Isozymes of pyruvate kinase in liver and hepatomas of the rat. Cancer Res. 34:1439–1436.

Friedmann, B., E. H. Goodman, Jr., H. L. Saunders, V. Kostos, and S. Weinhouse. 1971. Estimation of pyruvate recycling during gluconeogenesis in perfused rat liver. Arch. Biochem. Biophys. 143:566–578.

Gosalvez, M., L. Lopez-Alarcon, S. Garcia-Suarez, A. Montalvo, and S. Weinhouse. 1975. Stimulation of tumor-cell respiration by inhibitors of pyruvate kinase. Eur. J. Biochem. 55:315–321.

Gosalvez, M., J. Perez-Garcia, and S. Weinhouse. 1974. Competition for ADP between pyruvate kinase and mitochondrial oxidative phosphorylation as a control mechanism in glycolysis. Eur. J. Biochem. 46:133–140.

Greenstein, J. P. 1954. Biochemistry of Cancer, ed. 2. Academic Press, New York.

Gregg, C. T. 1972. Some aspects of the energy metabolism of mammalian cells, *in* Growth, Nutrition and Metabolism of Cells in Culture, vol. 1, V. J. Cristofalo and G. H. Rothblatt, eds. Academic Press, New York, pp. 83–136.

Hall, T. C. 1974. Paraneoplastic syndromes. Ann. N.Y. Acad. Sci. 230:1–557.

Hatanaka, M. 1974. Transport of sugars in tumor cell membranes. Biochim. Biophys. Acta 355:77–104.

Holroyde, C. P., R. D. Axelrod, C. L. Skutches, A. C. Huff, P. Paul, and G. A. Reichard. 1979. Lactate metabolism in patients with metastatic colorectal cancer. Cancer Res. 39:4900–4904.

Holroyde, C. P., T. P. Gabuzda, R. B. Putnam, P. Paul, and G. A. Reichard. 1975. Altered glucose metabolism in metastatic carcinoma. Cancer Res. 35:3710–3714.

Ibsen, K. H., and W. H. Fishman. 1979. Developmental gene expression in cancer. Biochim. Biophys. Acta 560:243–280.

Imura, H. 1980. Ectopic hormone production viewed as an abnormality of gene expression. Adv. Cancer Res. 33:39–75.

Johnson, M. J. 1941. The role of aerobic phosphorylation in the Pasteur effect. Science 94:200–202.

Knox, W. E. 1976. Enzyme Patterns in Fetal, Adult and Neoplastic Rat Tissues, ed. 2. S. Karger, Basel.

Lavieties, B. B., and P. S. Coleman. 1980. The role of lipid metabolism in neoplastic differentiation. J. Theor. Biol. 85:523–542.

Lehmann, F.-G., ed. 1979. Carcino-Embryonic Proteins. Chemistry, Biology, Clinical Applications (2 vols.). Elsevier, Amsterdam, New York, Oxford.

Lynen, F. 1941. The aerobic phosphate requirement of yeast: The Pasteur effect. Ann. Chem. 546:120–141.

Markert, C. K., and F. Möller. 1959. Multiple forms of enzymes: Tissue, ontogenetic and species-specific patterns. Proc. Natl. Acad. Sci. USA 45:753–763.

Morris, H. P., and D. R. Meranze. 1975. Induction and some characteristics of "minimal deviation" hepatomas. Recent Results Cancer Res. 44:104–114.

Parnes, J. R., and K. Isselbacher. 1978. Transport alterations in virus-transformed cells. Prog. Exp. Tumor Res. 22:79–122.

Pouysségur, J., A. Franchi, J.-C. Salomon, and P. Sylvestre. 1980a. Isolation of a hamster fibroblast mutant defective in hexose transport and aerobic glycolysis: Its use to dissect the malignant phenotype. Proc. Natl. Acad. Sci. USA 77:2698–2701.

Pouysségur, J., A. Franchi, and P. Sylvestre. 1980b. Relationship between increased aerobic glycolysis and DNA synthesis initiation studied using glycolytic mutant fibroblasts. Nature 287:445–447.

Racker, E. 1976. A New Look at Mechanisms in Bioenergetics. Academic Press, New York, San Francisco, London.

Reichard, G. A., N. F. Moury, N. J. Hochella, R. C. Putnam, and S. Weinhouse. 1964. Blood glucose replacement rates in human cancer patients. Cancer Res. 24:71–76.

Reitzer, L. J., B. M. Wice, and D. Kennell. 1979. Evidence that glutamine, not sugar, is the major energy source for HeLa cells. J. Biol. Chem. 254:2669–2676.

Schapira, F. 1973. Isozymes and cancer. Adv. Cancer Res. 18:77–153.

Schapira, F., J. C. Dreyfus, and G. Schapira. 1963. Anomaly of aldolase in primary liver cancer. Nature 200:995–997.

Shapot, V. S. 1979. On the multiform relationships between the tumor and the host. Adv. Cancer Res. 30:89–150.

Shatton, J. B., H. P. Morris, and S. Weinhouse. 1969. Kinetic, electrophoretic, and chromatographic studies on glucose-ATP phosphotransferases in rat liver and hepatomas. Cancer Res. 29:1161–1172.

Shonk, C. E., H. P. Morris, and G. E. Boxer. 1965. Patterns of glycolytic enzymes in rat liver and hepatoma. Cancer Res. 25:671–676.

Stern, K., and R. Willheim. 1943. Biochemistry of Malignant Tumors. Reference Press, Brooklyn.

Tadenuma, K., S. Hotta, and J. Homma. 1923. Der stoffwechsel verpflanzter tumoren. Biochemische Zeitschrift 137:536–541.

Warburg, O. 1930. The Metabolism of Tumors. Arnold Constable, London.

Warburg, O. 1956a. On the origin of cancer cells. Science 123:309–314.

Warburg, O. 1956b. On respiratory impairment in cancer cells. Science 124:269–270.

Warburg, O. 1966. Oxygen the creator of differentiation, in Current Aspects of Biochemical Energetics, N. O. Kaplan, and E. Kennedy, eds. Academic Press, London and New York, pp. 103–109.

Waterhouse, C. 1974. Lactate metabolism in patients with cancer. Cancer 33:66–71.

Weber, G. 1977. Enzymology of cancer cells. N. Engl. J. Med. 296:486–493, 541–551.

Weber, G., G. Banerjee, and H. P. Morris. 1961. Comparative biochemistry of hepatomas. I. Carbohydrate enzymes in Morris hepatoma 5123. Cancer Res. 21:933–937.

Weinhouse, S. 1951. Studies on the fate of isotopically labeled metabolites in the oxidative metabolism of tumors. Cancer Res. 11:585–591.

Weinhouse, S. 1955. Oxidative metabolism of neoplastic tissues. Adv. Cancer Res. 11:585–591.

Weinhouse, S. 1956. On respiratory impairment in cancer cells. Science 124:267–268.

Weinhouse, S. 1972. Glycolysis, respiration and anomalous gene expression in experimental hepatomas. Cancer Res. 32:2007–2016.

Weinhouse, S. 1976a. The Warburg hypothesis fifty years later. Guest editorial. Z. Krebsforschung, 87:115–126.

Weinhouse, S. 1976b. Regulation of glucokinase in liver. Curr. Top. Cell. Regul. 11:1–50.

Weinhouse, S. 1980. New dimensions in the biology of cancer. Cancer 45:2975–2980.

Wenner, C. E. 1975. Regulation of energy metabolism in normal and tumor tissues, in Cancer: A Comprehensive Treatise, F. F. Becker, ed., Vol. 3. Plenum Press, New York, pp. 103–109.

Molecular Interrelations of Nutrition and Cancer,
edited by M. S. Arnott, J. van Eys, and Y.-M. Wang.
Raven Press, New York © 1982.

Increased Glucose Transport in Malignant Cells: Analysis of Its Molecular Basis

Michael J. Weber, Donald W. Salter, and Theodore E. McNair

Department of Microbiology, University of Illinois, Urbana, Illinois 61801

Alterations in carbohydrate metabolism, notably, an increased rate of aerobic glycolysis, are frequently observed in malignant cells (Warburg 1930). These alterations in glycolysis are associated with, and may even be in part a consequence of, an increased rate of glucose transport across the cell membrane (Weber 1973, Bissell 1976). Over the past several years we have been investigating in detail the molecular basis for the increased glucose transport activity. A rigorous examination of the molecular biology of this alteration can set a firm foundation for investigation of the changes in cellular regulation that underlie malignancy as well as for examination of the role that the glycolytic and transport alterations play in the growth of the tumor in its host.

RESULTS

The Biological System

The system we chose for these investigations is chicken embryo cell cultures transformed by Rous sarcoma virus. The advantage of the system is that one can reproducibly obtain large quantities of primary malignant cells without being subject to the variability and limited availability of clinical material or spontaneous tumors, and without some of the artifacts that established cell lines and some transplantable tumors are subject to. In addition, temperature-conditional mutants in the transforming gene *(src)* are available (Vogt 1977) that allow one to "switch on" and "switch off" the transformed phenotype simply by changing the temperature at which infected cells are incubated.

Elevated Hexose Uptake is Transformation Specific

Uptake of many nutrients and ions changes with the growth state of the cell, being low in quiescent, density-inhibited cultures, and higher in rapidly proliferating cultures (Table 1). However, of the uptake systems examined, only hexose uptake was specifically increased by transformation, when comparison

TABLE 1. *Relative rates for nutrient uptake in density-inhibited, normal-growing, and transformed cells**

Nutrient	Density inhibited	Normal growing	Transformed
2-Deoxyglucose	1.0	6.8	23.9
3-0-Methylglucose	1.0	6.5	32.8
Uridine	1.0	4.0	3.4
Adenosine	1.0	2.1	Not determined
Thymidine	1.0	9.0	8.9
α-Aminoisobutyric acid†	1.0	4.5	4.5
Phosphate	1.0	1.9	1.8
Potassium	1.0	1.8	1.6

* Linear uptake rates into acid-soluble materials, essentially as described by Weber (1973), Nakamura and Weber (1979).

† In cultures deprived of amino acids, the rate of α-aminoisobutyric acid uptake can be increased in transformed, but not in normal, cultures. Thus, the "A" amino acid transport system displays a transformation-specific inducibility (Nakamura and Weber 1979).

was made with normal, uninfected cells growing at the same rate. Thus, the elevation in hexose uptake is not likely to be due to a generalized increase in membrane activity.

Increased Hexose Uptake Depends on *src*

Malignant transformation by Rous sarcoma virus depends on the activity of the *src* gene: viruses that carry deletions in *src* are capable of replication, but are unable to transform cultured cells or to cause tumors in vivo. Viruses with temperature-conditional lesions in *src* are hindered in their transforming and tumorigenic potential (Vogt 1977). We thus wished to determine whether increased uptake of glucose was dependent on the expression of the *src* gene. To do this, we took advantage of a temperature-conditional *src* mutant of Rous sarcoma virus (Martin 1970). This mutant is capable of replicating as well as wild-type virus, but at 41°C, the restrictive temperature, cells infected with this mutant are phenotypically normal and display a low rate of hexose uptake (Figure 1). On the other hand, cells infected with this mutant and incubated at 36°C, the permissive temperature, are phenotypically transformed and display a high hexose uptake rate. When infected cells are shifted from 41°C to 36°C, they quickly increase their hexose uptake rate, and conversely, when cells are shifted from the low permissive temperature to the restrictive temperature, their capacity to take up the sugar declines. By contrast, uninfected cells or cells infected with wild-type virus do not show this temperature sensitivity in their transport rate.

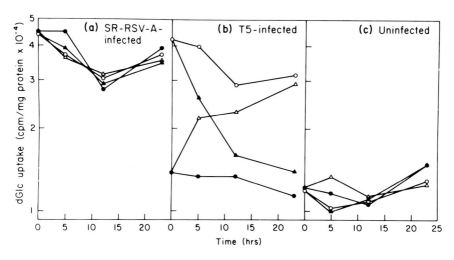

FIG. 1. Rate of [³H]-2-deoxyglucose uptake into cultures of chicken embryo cells infected with wild-type virus (a); with the temperature-conditional *src* mutant, T5 (b); or uninfected (c). Cultures held at 42°C (●——●) or at 36°C (○——○) or shifted from 42°C to 36°C (△——△) or from 36°C to 42°C (▲——▲). (Reproduced from Martin et al., 1971.)

Increased Hexose Uptake Requires Increased Transport

Because of the frequent reports that malignancy was associated with glycolytic alterations, it was important to determine whether the transport step *per se* was altered by viral transformation. Several approaches have been taken to examining this problem:

1. Uptake of 3-0-methylglucose, a nonmetabolizable glucose analog, is increased in transformed cells [Table 1; (Weber 1973)]. Since uptake of this analog measures only the transport step, this demonstrates that the transport rate is increased, independent of the effects of posttransport metabolism. The increased uptake of 3-0-methylglucose also occurs in 3T3 cells infected with polyoma virus (Eckhart and Weber 1974) and is an early event in the course of malignant transformation (Lang and Weber 1978).

2. Membrane vesicles prepared from transformed cells display elevated levels of hexose uptake (Inui et al. 1979, Zala and Perdue 1980).

3. Incubation of normal and transformed cultures with 75 mM glucose, a concentration sufficiently high to bypass much of the requirement for a membrane transport system, revealed only a 1.5- to 2-fold elevation in lactic acid production, considerably less than the 5-fold elevation of transport rate we generally see (Table 2). This modest elevation in glycolytic flux is consistent with the reports of others (Singh et al. 1974, 1978, Carroll et al. 1978).

Thus, it seems clear that the rate of transport of hexoses across the cell membrane is elevated in these transformed cells, and that the magnitude of

TABLE 2. *Lactate production and glucose utilization in normal and transformed cells*

Cell type	Lactate/cell/hr*	Glucose uptake†
tsNY68, 36°C	0.10	0.72
Normal cells, 36°C	0.06	0.12
tsNY68, 42°C	0.10	0.23
Normal cells, 42°C	0.08	0.09

* pmoles/cell/hr. Cells grown in 75 mM glucose. Lactate production measured after 24 hr growth. Note that there are significant temperature-dependent changes in lactate production in both normal and infected cells. However, lactate production is higher in tsNY68-infected cells than in normal cells, when both are held at 36°C (the permissive temperature for tsNY68 transformation). However, at 42°C, at which tsNY68-infected cells are phenotypically normal, the rate of lactate production is close to that shown by normal cells at 42°C.
† 2-deoxyglucose uptake rate, pmol/min/µg cell protein.

this elevation is transport is sufficient to account for most of the changes in glycolysis. Moreover, Bissell (1976) has reported that inhibition of glucose transport can restore altered glycolytic patterns to near normal. Thus, the weight of the evidence indicates that glucose transport is elevated in transformed cells, and that this elevation may well be necessary for at least part of the alterations in sugar metabolism that are associated with malignancy. However, it has not yet been determined with certainty whether significant alterations in glycolysis can occur independently of, or even prior to, the changes in transport rate.

Molecular Basis of Increased Transport Activity

We have characterized the hexose transport system of cultured chicken embryo fibroblasts in some detail, and found it to be a "facilitated diffusion" system (Weber 1973). Moreover, the K_m for transport appears to be unaffected by transformation, but the Vmax is increased (Weber 1973).

In theory, transformation could increase the transport rate by (1) inducing the synthesis of a new type of transporter, (2) increasing the activity of preexisting transporters either through an allosteric mechanism or by affecting their localization, or (3) increasing the number of glucose transporters in the cell membrane.

To distinguish between these possibilities, we used cytochalasin B, a potent inhibitor of glucose transport in chicken embryo cells (Salter and Weber 1979). In the case of the human erythrocyte glucose transporter, it has been demonstrated that cytochalasin B binds directly to the isolated transport protein (Baldwin et al. 1980). We thus felt that the amount of cytochalasin B binding to normal and transformed cells could be used to quantitate the number of transporters in these cells. Because cytochalasin B also binds with high affinity to

TABLE 3. *Hexose uptake and cytochalasin B binding to normal and transformed intact cells and membrane fractions*

Cells	Assay conditions	2-Deoxy-glucose uptake*	Cytochalasin B binding†		
			Intact cells	Membrane-enriched fraction	Purified membranes
Transformed	+D-Mannitol	8783	42.8	41.3 ± 2.1	89.2
	+D-Glucose	349	25.4	9.7 ± 0.6	19.4
	Glucose-specific‡	8434	17.4	31.6	69.8
Normal confluent	+D-Mannitol	1084	20.2	9.8 ± 0.4	18.0
	+D-Glucose	748	18.6	6.9 ± 0.3	11.6
	Glucose-specific‡	336	1.6	2.9	6.4

* pmol/mg protein/15 min.
† pmol/mg protein.
‡ Uptake or binding in the presence of D-mannitol minus uptake or binding in the presence of D-glucose.

D-Mannitol and D-glucose were present in the assay mixture at a final concentration of 182 mM for intact cells and membrane-enriched fractions and 200 mM for purified membranes. 2-Deoxyglucose uptake (45 µM), and cytochalasin B binding (91 nM for intact cells and membrane-enriched fractions and 112 nM for purified membranes) to intact cells and membrane fractions were performed as previously described (Salter and Weber 1979). Data for 2-deoxyglucose uptake and cytochalasin B binding to intact cells are the average of duplicate determinations from the same samples and the numbers are averages ± S.D. Data for purified membranes are single-point determinations.

cellular components not involved in glucose transport (e.g., the cytoskeleton) we determined the "glucose-specific" cytochalasin B binding, i.e., that portion of the high-affinity cytochalasin B binding that could be inhibited by D-glucose but not by L-glucose or mannitol. This glucose-specific binding presumably represents binding to the glucose transporter. As can be seen from the data in

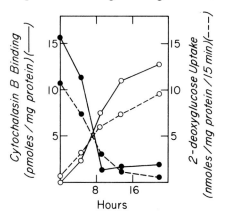

FIG. 2. Hexose uptake and glucose-specific cytochalasin B binding to cells infected with the temperature-conditional *src* mutant tsNY68 after shifting from 42°C to 36°C (o——o) or from 36°C to 42°C (●——●). (Reproduced from Salter and Weber 1979, with permission from the *Journal of Biological Chemistry*.)

Table 3, the amount of the glucose-specific cytochalasin B binding increases in transformed cells in proportion to the increase in the transport rate. Moreover, the glucose-specific cytochalasin B binding is enriched by purification of plasma membranes, as would be expected for a membrane transport protein. In addition, the kinetics with which the increase in glucose-specific cytochalasin B binding occurs during the process of transformation parallels closely the kinetics of increase in the glucose transport rate (Figure 2).

DISCUSSION

Based on the data just described, we can now begin to distinguish between the three possible ways by which transformation could bring about an increase in the hexose transport rate:

1. We do not believe that a new transport system is induced in transformed cells, since the half-saturation constants for 3-0-methylglucose and 2-deoxyglucose and the K_i for inhibition of transport by phlorizin or cytochalasin B were indistinguishable in normal and transformed cells (Weber 1973, Salter and Weber 1979). Thus, we believe that the increased transport rate is due to quantitative rather than qualitative changes in the glucose transporter.

2. Since the kinetic constants of the transporter were not affected by transformation, there is no reason to propose allosteric alteration of the transporter as the mechanism. There may, however, be a redistribution of the transporter between membrane fractions during transformation. It is worth noting that just such a redistribution has been shown to occur upon insulin stimulation of glucose transport in adipocytes (Suzuki and Kono 1980, Cushman and Wardzala 1980).

3. Since the amount of the glucose-specific cytochalasin B binding increases in transformed cells in direct proportion to the transport rate, it seems most probable that the increased glucose transport rate in transformed cells results from an increase in the number of transporters synthesized. This conclusion, of course, depends on the assumption that the cytochalasin B binding component is, in fact, the glucose transporter. Direct tests of this assumption are in progress.

Since the transformation-related increase in transport rate occurs even in the presence of actinomycin D, but is blocked by cycloheximide (Kawai and Hanafusa 1971, Kletzien and Perdue 1976) or enucleation (Beug et al. 1978), it seems possible that the *src* gene product is able to increase the synthesis of the glucose transport protein at a posttranscriptional level, e.g., by affecting transport or processing of mRNA. Experiments to examine this possibility directly are under way.

The work described in this chapter provides a firm biochemical basis for future investigations of the role that increased glucose transport plays in tumorigenicity. For example, we have isolated mutants of Rous sarcoma virus that are defective in their ability to induce an increased glucose transport rate (Anderson et al. 1981). Tumors formed in nude mice by cells infected with this mutant are smaller than normal (Kahn, Shin, and Weber, unpublished data), in agreement with results reported by Pouysségur et al. (1980), who found that a transformed cell mutant defective in glucose uptake and metabolism also forms slowly growing tumors. Thus, these findings, although preliminary, support the notion that the enhanced ability to utilize glucose, although not necessary for loss of growth control, may provide a selective advantage for the growth of tumors that are poorly vascularized and oxygen deficient (Warburg 1930).

ACKNOWLEDGMENTS

This work was supported by USPHS grants CA 12467 and CA 20410 (to MJW) and postdoctoral fellowship CA 05518 (to DWS).

REFERENCES

Anderson, D. D., R. P. Beckmann, E. H. Harms, K. Nakamura, and M. J. Weber. 1981. Biological properties of "partial" transformation mutants of Rous sarcoma virus and characterization of their pp60[src] kinase. J. Virol. 37:445–458.

Baldwin, J. M., G. E. Lienhard, and S. A. Baldwin. 1980. The monosaccharide transport system of the human erythrocyte. Orientation upon reconstitution. Biochim. Biophys. Acta 599:699–714.

Beug, H., M. Claviez, B. Jokusch, and T. Graf. 1978. Differential expression of Rous sarcoma virus specific transformation parameters in enucleated cells. Cell 14:843–856.

Bissell, M. 1976. Transport as a rate limiting step in glucose metabolism in virus-transformed cells: Studies with cytochalasin B. J. Cell. Physiol. 89:701–710.

Carroll, R. C., J. F. Ash, P. K. Vogt, and S. J. Singer. 1978. Reversion of transformed glycolysis to normal by inhibition of protein-synthesis in rat kidney cells infected with temperature-sensitive mutants of Rous sarcoma virus. Proc. Natl. Acad. Sci. USA 75:5015–5019.

Cushman, S. W., and L. J. Wardzala. 1980. Potential mechanism of insulin action on glucose transport in the isolated rat adipose cell. Apparent translocation of intracellular transport systems to the plasma membrane. J. Biol. Chem. 255:4758–4762.

Eckhart, W., and M. J. Weber. 1974. Uptake of 2-deoxyglucose by Balb/3T3 cells: Changes after polyoma infection. Virology 61:223–228.

Inui, K. I., D. E. Moller, L. G. Tillotson, and K. J. Isselbacher. 1979. Stereospecific hexose transport by membrane vesicles from mouse fibroblasts; Membrane vesicles retain increased hexose transport associated with viral transformation. Proc. Natl. Acad. Sci. USA 65:3972–3978.

Inui, K. I., L. G. Tillotson, and K. J. Isselbacher. 1980. Hexose and amino acid transport by chicken embryo fibroblasts infected with temperature-sensitive mutant of Rous sarcoma virus: Comparison of transport properties of whole cells and membrane vesicles. Biochim. Biophys. Acta 598:616–627.

Kawai, S. and H. Hanafusa. 1971. The effects of reciprocal changes of temperature on the transformed state of cells infected with a temperature-sensitive Rous sarcoma virus mutant. Virology 46:470–479.

Kletzien, R. F., and J. F. Perdue. 1976. Regulation of sugar transport in chick embryo fibroblasts and in fibroblasts transformed by a temperature-sensitive mutant of the Rous sarcoma virus. J. Cell. Physiol. 89:723–728.

Lang, D., and M. J. Weber. 1978. Increased membrane transport of 2-deoxyglucose and 3-0-methylglucose is an early event in the transformation of chick embryo fibroblasts by Rous sarcoma virus. J. Cell. Physiol. 94:315–320.

Martin, G. S. 1970. Rous sarcoma virus: A function required for the maintenance of the transformed state. 227:1021–1023.

Martin, G. S., S. Venuta, M. Weber, and H. Rubin. 1971. Temperature-dependent alterations in sugar transport in cells infected by a temperature-sensitive mutant of Rous sarcoma virus. Proc. Natl. Acad. Sci. USA 68:2739–2741.

Nakamura, K. D., and M. J. Weber. 1979. Amino acid transport in normal and Rous sarcoma virus-transformed chicken embryo fibroblasts. J. Cell. Physiol. 99:15–22.

Pouysségur, J., A. Franchi, J. C. Salomon, and P. Silvestre. 1980. Isolation of a Chinese hamster fibroblast mutant defective in hexose transport and aerobic glycolysis: Its use to dissect the malignant phenotype. Proc. Natl. Acad. Sci. USA 77:2698–2701.

Salter, D. W., and M. J. Weber. 1979. Glucose-specific cytochalasin B binding is increased in chicken embryo fibroblasts transformed by Rous sarcoma virus. J. Biol. Chem. 254:3554–3561.

Singh, V. N., M. Singh, J. T. August, and B. L. Horecker. 1974. Alterations in glucose metabolism in chick-embryo cells transformed by Rous sarcoma virus: Intracellular levels of glycolytic intermediates. Proc. Natl. Acad. Sci. USA 71:4129–4132.

Singh, M., V. N. Singh, J. T. August, and B. L. Horecker. 1978. Transport and phosphorylation of hexoses in normal and Rous sarcoma virus-transformed chick embryo fibroblasts. J. Cell. Physiol. 97:285–292.

Suzuki, K., and T. Kono. 1980. Evidence that insulin causes translocation of glucose transport activity to the plasma membrane from an intracellular storage site. Proc. Natl. Acad. Sci. USA 77:2542–2545.

Vogt, P. K. 1977. The genetics of RNA tumor viruses, in Comprehensive Virology, vol. 9, H. Fraenkel-Conrat and R. Wagner, eds. Plenum Press, New York, pp. 341–455.

Warburg, O. 1930. The Metabolism of Tumors. Constable, London.

Weber, M. J. 1973. Hexose transport in normal and in Rous sarcoma virus-transformed cells. J. Biol. Chem. 248:2978–2983.

Zala, C. M., and J. F. Perdue. 1980. Stereospecific D-glucose transport in mixed membrane and plasma membrane vesicles derived from cultured chick embryo fibroblasts. Biochim. Biophys. Acta 600:157–172.

Molecular Interrelations of Nutrition and Cancer,
edited by M. S. Arnott, J. van Eys, and Y.-M. Wang.
Raven Press, New York © 1982.

Differential Carbohydrate Metabolism in Tumor and Host

George Weber

*Laboratory for Experimental Oncology, Indiana University School of Medicine,
Indianapolis, Indiana 46223*

Identification of important differences between the metabolism of tumor and host may throw light on the often-observed malnutrition in cancer patients and may also provide targets for selective anticancer chemotherapy. The questions most frequently raised concern the etiology of this malnutrition and its effect on the course of treatment. There is also the hope that nutritional therapy would result in better resistance to infections and improved response to treatment, including chemotherapy (Copeland et al. 1979, Ota et al. 1977, Reynolds et al. 1980).

The mechanisms that may account, in part at least, for cancer cachexia include responses to surgery, radiation, or chemotherapy, hypothalamic dysfunction, abnormalities of smell and taste, and aversion to food. Other important factors that have been postulated are increased energy expenditure and competition of tumor and host for precursors and substrates (Burt and Brennan 1981).

Since the purpose of chemotherapy is to destroy cancer cells selectively without materially damaging the host, there is a major overlap in interest between the nutritionists who study tumor-host competition for substrates and the biochemical pharmacologists who investigate strategic differences in the pattern of substrate utilization, enzymology, and metabolism of normal and cancer cells. The purpose of this presentation is to analyze and integrate some of the current evidence regarding differences in carbohydrate metabolism at the molecular level between cancer cells and host cells.

MATERIALS AND METHODS

Biological Systems

The histological and growth properties and karyotype of the chemically induced, transplantable hepatomas and renal cell carcinomas of different growth rates in the rat have been outlined (Weber 1977a, 1977b). The source and properties of chemically induced, transplantable mouse colon adenocarcinomas have also been reported (Weber et al. 1978c). The properties of slow and rapidly proliferating human colon carcinoma xenografts grown in nude mice were cited in a recent work (Weber et al. 1981a). The selection of patients and the difficulties inherent in biochemical studies of human tumors and control tissues are outlined in a paper dealing with cases of renal cell carcinoma (Weber 1980) and in a current study of the biochemistry of primary human colon carcinoma (Weber et al. 1980a).

Biochemical Methods

The colorimetric, spectrophotometric, and isotopic methods for determination of the various key enzymes were those adapted in this laboratory for the various tissues of animals and humans (Weber, 1977a, 1977b, 1980, Weber et al. 1978c). Proteins were determined by the routine method (Lowry et al. 1951). The concentrations of ribonucleotides were determined by high-pressure liquid chromatography (Jackson et al. 1980) of samples obtained by application of the freeze-clamp method for neoplastic tissues (Weber et al. 1971). The techniques for assaying concentrations of deoxynucleoside triphosphates have been presented previously (Weber et al. 1980b).

Expression of Biochemical Results

Enzymic activities were calculated as specific activities in nanomoles per hour per milligram protein. The biochemical results were also expressed as percentages of the values in corresponding normal tissues of origin of the neoplasms. Results were subjected to statistical evaluation by means of the t test for small samples. Differences between means giving a probability of less than 5% were considered significant.

RESULTS AND DISCUSSION

The Main Functions of Carbohydrate and Pentose Phosphate Metabolism in the Liver

The main function of glycolysis (degradation of glucose) in conjunction with the Krebs cycle is to supply energy in the form of ATP. An additional function is to supply carbon skeletons for the production of various cell constituents, such as alanine, aspartate, glutamate, galactose, glucosamine, and acetyl-CoA. Precursors are also provided as glycerophosphates and free fatty acids for lipid biosynthesis.

The gluconeogenic pathway (pyruvate to glucose) opposes the glycolytic one. The function of gluconeogenesis is the production of glucose for the blood stream from noncarbohydrate sources. These precursors (L-alanine, lactate, glycerol) are brought by the blood stream into the liver, and through the final common path of gluconeogenesis in liver and kidney, they are converted to glucose. The triad of key glycolytic enzymes is opposed by a quartet of key gluconeogenic enzymes (Weber 1977a, 1977b).

The chief function of the pentose phosphate cycle is the production of reduced nicotinamide-adenine dinucleotide phosphate (NADPH) for use as a reducing agent in many biosynthetic steps and the supply of ribose-5-phosphate for the synthesis of RNA and DNA. Ribose-5-phosphate is utilized by phosphoribosyl-pyrophosphate (PRPP) synthetase for the production of PRPP. This important enzyme is the only source for de novo PRPP production. PRPP is utilized in both de novo and salvage pathways of purine and pyrimidine biosynthesis and is also an allosteric activator of the first and rate-limiting enzyme of de novo pyrimidine biosynthesis, carbamoyl phosphate synthetase II (glutamine hydrolyzing). There are striking differences in the concentrations of the various metabolites and in the activities of the key enzymes of the different pathways.

Orders of Magnitude of Concentrations of Metabolites and Activities of Key Enzymes in Liver

Freeze-clamp preparations were utilized to provide accurate information on the in vivo concentrations of carbohydrates, ribonucleotides, and deoxyribonucleoside triphosphates (the methods employed in this laboratory are cited in Materials and Methods).

Biochemical Pattern of Metabolites in Liver and Hepatomas

There are striking differences in the concentrations of metabolites of carbohydrate metabolism and of ribonucleotides and deoxyribonucleotides. The concentrations of fuels used in generation of energy, such as glucose and lipids, are among the highest. ATP occurs in millimolar concentrations, GTP and UTP are present in one tenth the concentration, and the pool of CTP is the lowest among the ribonucleotides. The concentrations of deoxynucleoside triphosphates are the very lowest in this comparison (Table 1). These differences are in line with the functions of the metabolites that are involved as fuels in energy production and utilization and that play a role in various metabolic activities. In contrast, the deoxynucleoside triphosphates primarily function in DNA repair and replication. The alterations in the concentrations of metabolites in rapidly growing hepatoma 3924A support this argument. There was an increase in the level of CTP, the only ribonucleotide whose concentration was elevated. The role of CTP in RNA and DNA biosynthesis and as a target of chemotherapy has been discussed elsewhere (Weber et al. 1980b, 1981b). The pools of deoxynucleoside triphosphates were enlarged 4.7- to 17.7-fold in the rapidly growing hepatoma 3924A (Jackson et al. 1980).

TABLE 1. *Biochemical pattern of liver cancer (nmol/g wet weight)*

Metabolites	Liver	Hepatoma 3924A % of liver
Glucose	9,340	11*
Total lipids	3,090	48*
Glutamate	1,810	227*
Pyruvate	127	43*
Lactate	2,590	290*
ATP	2,290	42*
GTP	371	87
UTP	303	85
CTP	51	406*
dATP	1.0	1,770*
dGTP	0.9	478*
dTTP	0.7	1,214*
dCTP	6.6	795*

* Significant difference ($p < 0.05$).

Orders of Magnitude of Liver Enzyme Activities from Glucose Utilization to DNA Synthesis

As Table 2 shows, when all enzymic activities are presented as specific activity, those of glycolysis and pentose production are represented by three- to five-digit numbers. Thus, they have the most powerful capacities among the enzymic steps in this table. The activities in the utilization of the pentose phosphates

TABLE 2. *Decrease in enzyme activities from glucose utilization to DNA synthesis*

Metabolic areas	Liver enzymes	Activity (nmol/hr/mg protein)
Carbohydrate catabolism	Hexokinase	200
	6-Phosphofructokinase	2,000
	Pyruvate kinase	40,000
Pentose production	G6P dehydrogenase	1,000
	Transaldolase	3,000
Pentose utilization	PRPP synthetase	100
Purine synthesis	Amidophosphoribosyltransferase	60
	IMP dehydrogenase	6
Pyrimidine synthesis	Carbamoyl-P synthetase II	9
	CTP synthetase	5
DNA synthesis	Thymidine kinase	2
	DNA polymerase	0.06
	Ribonucleotide reductase	0.03

G6P = glucose-6-phosphate, PRPP = phosphoribosylpyrophosphate.

are represented by three-digit numbers and those of the key enzymes of purine and pyrimidine de novo biosynthesis by one- or two-digit numbers. The activity of the rate-limiting enzyme of de novo DNA biosynthesis, ribonucleosidediphosphate reductase, is the lowest; the activity of the final enzyme of DNA biosynthesis, DNA polymerase, is the second lowest. The activities of these two enzymes are increased to the greatest extent in the rapidly growing hepatomas.

Enzymic Program of Carbohydrate Metabolism in Tumors

The enzymic activities of rapidly growing hepatoma 3683 and kidney tumor MK-3 are summarized in Table 3. The activities were calculated as specific activities and were expressed as percentages of the values in corresponding homologous normal tissue, i.e., liver for hepatoma and kidney cortex for renal cell carcinoma. In these chemically induced, transplantable hepatomas, the activities of the key glycolytic enzymes were markedly increased and those of the gluconeogenic ones were decreased. Since glycolysis and gluconeogenesis oppose each other, these reciprocal alterations are of interest. The only convenient system to utilize for testing whether such opposing changes also occur in other tissues is the renal cortex, which has a gluconeogenic activity comparable to that of the liver. The results in Table 3 indicate that in the chemically induced, transplantable MK-3 kidney tumor the activities of the glycolytic enzymes also increase and those of the gluconeogenic ones also decrease. The ratios of the activities of the opposing key enzymes of glycolysis and gluconeogenesis reveal the marked shift to glycolytic capacity in these tumors.

TABLE 3. *Specific activities of glycolytic and gluconeogenic enzymes in tumors**

Enzymes	E.C. no.	Control tissue %	Hepatoma 3683 (% of liver)	MK-3 kidney tumor (% of kidney)
Glycolysis				
Hexokinase	2.7.1.1	100	1,430	632
6-Phosphofructokinase	2.7.1.11	100	277	505
Pyruvate kinase	2.7.1.40	100	499	782
Gluconeogenesis				
Glucose-6-phosphatase	3.1.3.9	100	<1	10
Fructose-biphosphatase	3.1.3.11	100	<1	18
PEP carboxykinase	4.1.1.49	100	<1	
Pyruvate carboxylase	6.4.1.1	100	<1	
Ratios of activities				
Hexokinase/G6Pase		100	8,800	6,630
6-Phosphofructokinase/FBPase		100	6,463	2,862

* nmol/hr/mg protein.
PEP = phosphoenolpyruvate, G6Pase = glucose-6-phosphatase, FBPase = fructose-biphosphatase.

Increased Glycolysis and Decreased Gluconeogenesis in Hepatomas

Measurement of enzymic activities is helpful in gaining understanding of the pattern of gene expression and the capabilities relevant to the activity of the metabolic pathway in which the enzymes play a role. However, it is important to measure the actual activity of the overall metabolic pathway to test whether the enzymic indications correspond with the overall behavior of intermediary metabolism. Glycolysis (lactate production from glucose) and gluconeogenesis (glucose production from pyruvate) were measured in slices of liver and hepatomas. The results indicated that in the slowly growing hepatomas aerobic glycolysis was in the range of that of normal liver, and it increased in parallel with the increase in tumor growth rate (Weber 1961). In contrast, gluconeogenesis decreased with tumor proliferative rates (Ashmore et al. 1958, Weber 1961, Sweeney et al. 1963). These observations confirm the enzymic indications.

Warburg (1956) believed that increased aerobic glycolysis was a common property of all tumors. It is assumed that he reached this conclusion because the tumors he had access to were rapidly growing neoplasms, since inbred strains of animals were not in use in his day. The availability of inbred strains of rats made it possible to transplant very slowly growing, well-differentiated, chemically induced hepatocellular carcinomas (Morris and Wagner 1968). In such slowly growing hepatomas it was discovered in this laboratory that glycolysis was not increased, but was in the normal range (Weber 1961, Weber et al. 1961, Sweeney et al. 1963). Similar results were reported subsequently and independently by Aisenberg and Morris (1961) and Lin et al. (1962). In a series of transplantable hepatomas of different growth rates, it was first observed in the Laboratory for Experimental Oncology that glycolysis increased with the rise in tumor growth rates (Weber 1961). Warburg's concept of the role of respiration and glycolysis in cancer cells was critically examined by Weinhouse in 1955 and also in his chapter in this monograph (Weinhouse 1982, pages 167–181, this volume). The role of carbohydrate metabolism and particularly of glycolysis and its relationship to transformation and progression were the subjects of a critical inquiry by Weber (1968). The increased glycolytic activity observed only in intermediate and rapidly growing tumors is in good agreement with the rise in activity of the key enzymes of glycolysis and the decrease in activity of the key gluconeogenic ones.

Enzymic Program of Pentose Phosphate Metabolism in Tumors

In pentose phosphate synthesis in cancer cells, the most important enzymes are those directly involved in the channeling of the hexose monophosphates into pentose biosynthesis. Thus, fructose-6-phosphate is routed into pentose production by the rate-limiting enzyme of the direct oxidative pathway, glucose-6-phosphate dehydrogenase, and fructose-6-phosphate is channeled by transaldolase. An examination of the behavior of the activities of glucose-6-phosphate

TABLE 4. *Glucose-6-phosphate dehydrogenase, 6-phosphogluconate dehydrogenase, transaldolase, and transketolase specific activities in hepatomas of different growth rates*

Tissues	Growth rate (months)	Protein	Oxidative pathway		Nonoxidative pathway	
			Glucose-6-phosphate dehydrogenase	6-Phosphogluconate dehydrogenase	Transaldolase	Transketolase
Normal control liver		100	100	100	100	100
Hepatomas						
66	13	79*	1262*	300*	284*	167*
47C	8	74*	727*	392*	228*	169*
8999	9	83	184*	72*	145*	102
44	9	80	544*	177*	283*	153
9633	4.9	77*	253*	43*	205*	110
7794A	2.8	84	3650*	284*	215*	220*
7777	1.3	77*	897*	181*	300*	138
3924A	1.0	66*	1128*	72*	240*	94
3683F	0.5	67*	903*	203*	255*	277*
9618A2	0.4	64*	4366*	608*	338*	266*

* Significantly different from its control ($p < 0.05$).

Enzyme activities were calculated in nmol/hr/mg protein and the protein content as mg/g wet weight. Results are expressed as percentages of corresponding normal control liver values. Four or more rats were in each group. Growth rate is expressed as mean transplantation time, i.e., months between inoculation and growth to a size of 1.5 cm diameter.

TABLE 5. *Specific activities of pentose phosphate metabolic enzymes in tumors*

Enzymes	E.C. no.	Control tissue* (%)	Hepatoma 3683F (% of liver)	MK-3 kidney tumor (% of kidney)
Pentose phosphate synthesis				
Direct oxidation				
Glucose-6-phosphate DH	1.1.1.49	100	903	1,103
6-Phosphogluconate DH	1.1.1.44	100	203	867
Indirect oxidation				
Transaldolase	2.2.1.2.	100	255	454
Transketolase	2.2.1.1	100	277	198
Pentose phosphate utilization				
PRPP synthetase	2.7.6.1	100	278	259

* Activities were calculated in nmol/hr/mg protein and expressed as percentages of the values of the control tissues.
DH = dehydrogenase, PRPP = phosphoribosylpyrophosphate.

and 6-phosphogluconate dehydrogenases, transaldolase, and transketolase was made in hepatomas of different growth rates (Weber et al. 1974, Heinrich et al. 1976). The results in Table 4 show that the activities of glucose-6-phosphate dehydrogenase and transaldolase were increased in all hepatomas without showing a correlation with tumor growth rates. Since the activities were increased in all tumors, even in the slowest growing hepatomas, the increased activities of the enzymes were classified as transformation linked. In contrast, the activities of 6-phosphogluconate dehydrogenase and transketolase were increased in some tumors and were decreased or unchanged in others; therefore, these activities were not stringently linked with transformation or progression in the hepatoma spectrum. Measurement of these enzymic activities in the chemically induced, transplantable rat kidney tumor MK-3 showed increases in the activities of all four enzymes of pentose phosphate synthesis (Table 5).

Evidence for increased activity of the pentose-producing pathway

Isotope studies carried out in liver and hepatoma slices provided estimates indicating that the capacity for the direct oxidative pathway increased with increasing growth rate of the tumors (Sweeney et al. 1963).

Pentose Phosphate Utilization: Increased PRPP Synthetase Activity

There are two parallel metabolic pathways in which a sequence of steps is involved in the production of ribose-5-phosphate. However, the utilization of ribose-5-phosphate for production of PRPP is accomplished by one key enzyme, PRPP synthetase. The specific activity of this enzyme was increased in every hepatoma examined so far, and the rise correlated positively with the tumor growth rates (Balo and Weber, unpublished data).

An example of the linking of an enzymic activity to transformation and progression is noted in the behavior of PRPP synthetase. Since this enzymic activity is elevated in all the tumors, it is transformation linked; because it increased with the rise in growth rate, the activity is also linked with the progressive expression of neoplastic properties.

Evidence for Reprogramming of Gene Expression in Cancer Cells

The molecular correlation concept identified a pattern of ordered alterations in the biochemistry of tumor cells, and from the evidence we concluded that the metabolic imbalance in cancer cells is a manifestation of the reprogramming of gene expression (Weber 1977a, 1977b). This interpretation of the altered phenotype in cancer cells is based on the demonstration of changed concentrations in the end products of gene expression, the enzymes. In evaluating the alterations in enzymic activities, two assumptions were made: (1) that the activity of the enzyme, determined in the presence of optimum substrate and cofactor conditions yielding linear kinetics, was equivalent to the amount of the enzyme in the tissue; (2) that the amount of enzyme was an indicator of gene expression under the specified steady-state conditions. In the identification of changes in enzyme concentrations, two independent methods were used to measure enzyme amounts. Enzyme concentration was determined by (1) assay of enzymic activity, where proportionality between enzymic activity and added amount of enzyme was insured, and (2) immunotitration of the enzyme concentration by specific, antienzyme serum.

To gain an insight into the integrated pattern of the behavior of glycolysis, pentose phosphate production, and purine and pyrimidine metabolism, a key enzyme was selected from each metabolic pathway. This work demonstrated that the key enzymes of glycolysis (6-phosphofructokinase), of pentose phosphate production (glucose-6-phosphate dehydrogenase), of purine biosynthesis (amidophosphoribosyltransferase), and of pyrimidine biosynthesis (CTP synthetase) were increased in concentration, as shown by the two independent techniques of enzymic assay of activities and immunotitration of the concentrations of enzyme proteins (Figure 1). These results strengthen our interpretation that the biochemical pattern discovered in hepatomas with different growth rates indicates a reprogramming of gene expression because of the marked changes observed in the concentrations of the key enzymes in the liver neoplasms (Tzeng et al. 1981, Weber 1977a, 1977b, Weber et al. 1980b, 1981b).

Specificity to Neoplasia of Alterations in Carbohydrate and Pentose Phosphate Metabolism in Neoplasia

There is extensive evidence, reviewed elsewhere, that the enzymic imbalance pinpointed in neoplastic liver is characteristic of neoplasia (Weber 1977a, 1977b). Normal and regenerating liver in adult animals and fetal and developing livers

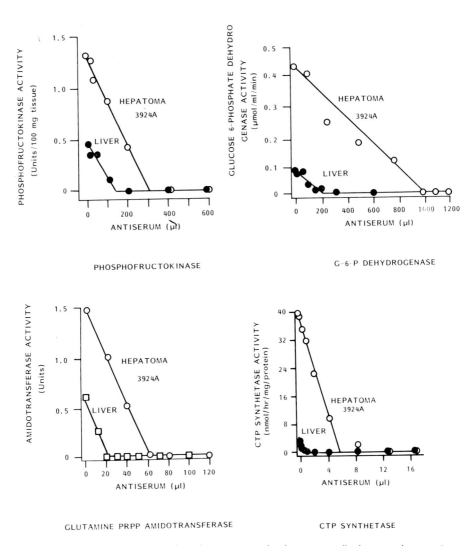

FIG. 1. Evidence for reprogramming of gene expression in cancer cells. Increased concentrations of key enzymes of carbohydrate (6-phosphofructokinase), pentose phosphate (glucose-6-phosphate dehydrogenase), purine (glutamine PRPP amidotransferase, amidophosphoribosyltransferase), and pyrimidine (CTP synthetase) metabolism.

in growing animals provided the appropriate controls. Although the rapidly growing hepatoma 3924A and the differentiating and regenerating livers had similar growth rates, each of these systems had a different enzymic pattern. It is important to bear in mind that although some alterations noted in the neoplastic liver also occurred in some of the control systems, the overall biochemical pattern of the neoplastic cells can be clearly distinguished from any one of the proliferating control systems and from adult liver.

Selective Advantages Conferred on Cancer Cells by Alterations in Carbohydrate and Pentose Phosphate Metabolism

In cancer cells, the increase in activities of key glycolytic enzymes and the decrease in those of gluconeogenic ones should lead to the glycolytic utilization of glucose, and the decrease or abolition of the recycling by gluconeogenesis should support the proliferative capabilities of cancer cells. Replacement of the high K_m, hormonally and nutritionally responsive isozyme population with that of low K_m enzymes that do not respond to regulation provides an escape from physiological control mechanisms for the cancer cells (Weber 1977a, 1977b). The increased activities of glucose-6-phosphate dehydrogenase and transaldolase should yield an increased capability of channeling glucose monophosphates to pentose phosphate production. These enzymic alterations are in line with the results of isotope studies that indicated a capacity for increased glycolysis and pentose phosphate formation. The transformation- and progression-linked increase in PRPP synthetase activity should increase the potential to produce PRPP, which may be utilized in the salvage and de novo synthetic pathways of purine and pyrimidine biosynthesis. The integrated enzymic and metabolic imbalance should confer selective growth advantages on the cancer cells (Figure 2).

Biochemistry of the Commitment to Proliferation in Cancer Cells

The elevated ability of the cancer cells to provide pentoses and PRPP appears to be critical in the biochemical program of liver cancer. In the presence of high concentrations of ribonucleotides in normal resting adult liver there are low pools of deoxynucleotides; the conversion to deoxyribonucleotides occurs at the level of ribonucleoside diphosphates. This conversion to deoxynucleotides occurs only in trace amounts because of the very low activity of the enzyme responsible for this conversion, the ribonucleotide reductase. Measurements in this laboratory in freeze clamp preparations demonstrated that in hepatomas the pools of dATP, dGTP, dCTP, and dTTP were elevated, and the rise paralleled the increase in growth rates of the tumors (Jackson et al. 1980, Weber et al. 1980b). These alterations in the hepatomas were clearly distinguishable from those occurring in differentiating and regenerating liver. The transformation- and progression-linked increase of the deoxynucleotide pools in the hepatomas emerged without significant changes in the amount of the immediate precursors, the ribonucleoside diphosphates (Figure 3).

The increased activity of ribonucleotide reductase (Elford et al. 1970), which was recognized as a transformation- and progression-linked alteration in the hepatoma spectrum (Takeda and Weber 1981), is responsible in large part for the increased conversion of the ribonucleotides to the deoxynucleoside triphosphate pool. It was emphasized that the transformation- and progression-linked increase in the activities of other strategic enzymes, carbamoyl-phosphate synthetase II (Aoki and Weber 1981), CTP synthetase (Kizaki et al. 1980), thymidine

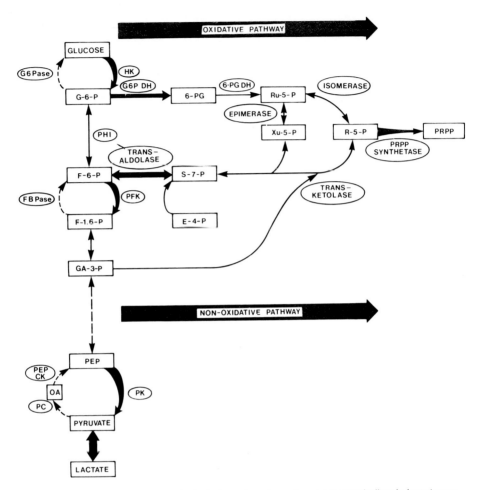

FIG. 2. Enzymic imbalance in carbohydrate and pentose phosphate metabolism in hepatomas. The thick, straight arrows indicate transformation-linked alterations, the tapered arrows indicate progression-linked alterations. The dotted arrows indicate decreased activities.

Abbreviations: E-4-P = erythrose-4-phosphate; F-1,6-P = fructose-1,6-phosphate; F-6-P = fructose-6-phosphate; FBPase, FDPase = fructose-bisphosphatase; GA-3-P = glyceraldehyde-3-phosphate; G-6-P = glucose-6-phosphate; G6Pase = glucose-6-phosphatase; G6P DH = glucose-6-phosphate dehydrogenase; HK = hexokinase; OA = oxaloacetate; PC = pyruvate carboxylase; PEP = phosphoenolpyruvate; PFK = 6-phosphofructokinase; 6-PG = 6-phosphogluconate; 6-PG DH = 6-phosphogluconate dehydrogenase; PHI = phosphohexose isomerase; PK = pyruvate kinase; PRPP = phosphoribosylpyrophosphate; R-5-P = ribose-5-phosphate; Ru-5-P = ribulose-5-phosphate; S-7-P = sedoheptulose-7-phosphate; Xu-5-P = xylulose-5-phosphate.

kinase (Weber et al. 1978b), IMP dehydrogenase (Weber et al. 1980b), and deoxycytidine kinase (Harkrader et al. 1980), was also critical in the integrated pattern of biosynthesis. The elevation in the activities of the key enzymes of carbohydrate catabolism and pentose phosphate, purine, and pyrimidine synthe-

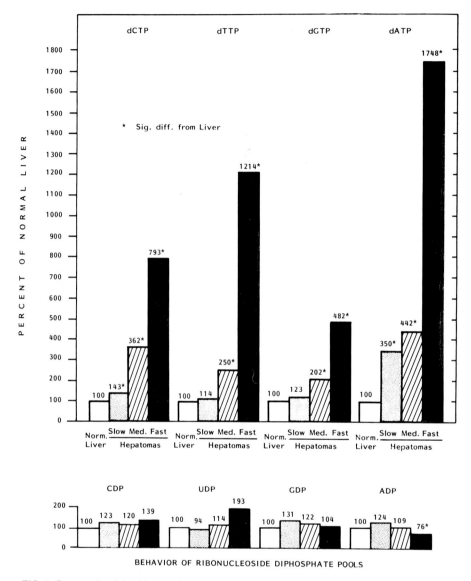

FIG. 3. Progression-linked increase in deoxynucleotide pools in hepatomas of different growth rates. There was no significant change in the concentration of the immediate precursors, ribonucleoside diphosphates.

sis concurrently with the decrease in the synthetic enzymes of carbohydrate metabolism and the catabolic enzymes of nucleic acid biosynthesis are essential elements in the biochemical commitment to replication of the hepatoma cells. A schematic figure summarizes some of the key features of the biochemical aspects of this commitment (Figure 4).

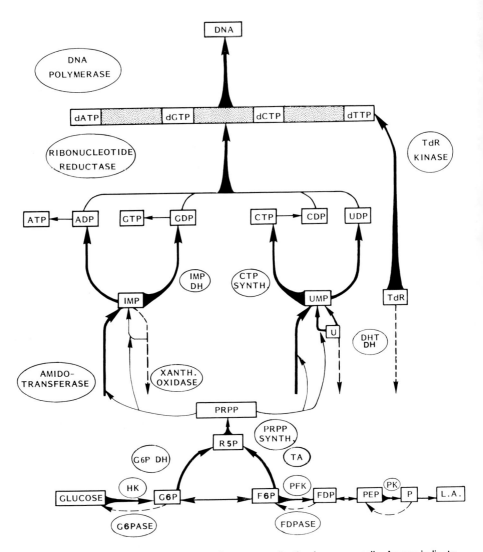

FIG. 4. Biochemical program of the commitment to replication in cancer cells. Arrows indicate changes as in Figure 2.

Abbreviations: DHT DH = dihydrothymine dehydrogenase; F-6-P = fructose-6-phosphate; FBPase, FDPase = fructose-bisphosphatase; FDP = fructose diphosphate (bisphosphate); G-6-P = glucose-6-phosphate; G6Pase = glucose-6-phosphatase; G6P DH = glucose-6-phosphate dehydrogenase; HK = hexokinase; IMP DH = IMP dehydrogenase; L.A. = lactic acid; P = pyruvate; PEP = phosphoenolpyruvate; PFK = 6-phosphofructokinase; PK = pyruvate kinase; PRPP = phosphoribosylpyrophosphate; PRPP Synth. = phosphoribosylpyrophosphate synthetase; R-5-P = ribose-5-phosphate; TA = transaldolase; TdR = thymidine; Xanth. oxidase = xanthine oxidase.

TABLE 6. *Lack of effect of starvation on hepatoma enzymic activity*

Enzymes	Specific activity (% of fed)	
	Normal liver	Hepatoma 3924A
Glycolysis		
Hexokinase	84	93
6-Phosphofructokinase	37*	94
Pyruvate kinase	39*	97
Pyrimidine synthesis		
TdR kinase	73*	88
CTP synthetase	58*	92
OMP decarboxylase	80*	96
Orotate phosphoribosyltransferase	62*	103
Uracil phosphoribosyltransferase	61*	117
Uridine kinase	69*	93
Uridine phosphorylase	118*	101
Pentose phosphate synthesis		
6-Phosphogluconate dehydrogenase	58*	101
Transaldolase	93	99

* Significantly different from values in fed rats ($p < 0.05$). Activities (nmol/hr/mg protein) were expressed as percentage of values in fed rats.
TdR = thymidine, OMP = orotidine 5′-phosphate.

Lack of Effect of Starvation on Enzymic Activities in Hepatoma

The stability of the activities of key enzymes in various metabolic pathways in the tumor was analyzed by a study of the effect of 3-day starvation in normal rats and in rats carrying hepatoma 3924A. The specific activities were compared in liver and tumors before and after starvation. The data summarized in Table 6 indicated that in the normal rat liver the activities of the key enzymes of glycolysis, pentose phosphate synthesis, and pyrimidine biosynthesis significantly decreased, but these enzymic activities did not change in hepatoma 3924A. These results emphasized the fact that the enzymic programs in the tumors failed to respond to nutritional regulation, which corresponds with examples of the decreased functional responsiveness of tumor cells to physiological regulatory stimuli (Weber et al. 1980b).

GENERALIZATION: APPLICABILITY OF THE ALTERED ENZYMOLOGY TO HUMAN NEOPLASMS

Extensive evidence has been obtained in studies in this laboratory that the enzymic imbalance observed in chemically induced, transplantable hepatomas and kidney tumors (Williamson et al. 1970) in the rat applies to other rodent tumors, including colon carcinomas in rats and mice, sarcoma in rats, and myeloma, lymphosarcoma, and lymphocytic leukemia in mice (Weber et al. 1977). The enzymic imbalance also applies to a virus-induced, transplantable hepatoma in chickens (Kovalszky et al. 1976, Prajda et al. 1979).

Our studies showed the applicability of the results to human hepatocellular carcinoma (Weber et al. 1976, 1978a) and kidney tumors (Weber 1980, Jackson et al. 1979, Weber et al. 1977). Further investigations showed the relevance of the altered enzyme pattern to human colon tumor xenografts of different degrees of differentiation and growth rates (Weber et al. 1981a). Recent studies revealed that the activities of hexokinase, pyruvate kinase, glucose 6-phosphate, and 6-phosphogluconate dehydrogenases and transaldolase were increased in human primary colon adenocarcinomas compared with the values in normal human colon mucosa (Weber et al. 1980a). Current results from 40 cases of human renal cell carcinomas demonstrated that the biochemical pattern originally discovered in the chemically induced, transplantable rat liver and kidney tumors also applied to human primary renal cell carcinomas (G. Weber and J. P. Donohue, unpublished data).

The integrated imbalance and the transformation- and progression-linked ordered enzymic program discovered in a model system of chemically induced, transplantable hepatomas of different growth rates in the rat (Weber 1971, 1977a, 1977b, 1980) applies to 14 animal and human tumors (Weber et al. 1980b) (Table 7). The broad applicability of these programs indicates that strategic segments of the altered gene program in neoplastic cells have been identified. It is important that the biochemical programs displayed are independent from the carcinogenic agent that produced the neoplasms, since the tumors analyzed

TABLE 7. *Shared enzymic programs identified in 14 tumor types*

Rat	Hepatomas of different growth rates*
	Renal cell carcinomas MK-1, MK-2, MK-3*
	Colon adenocarcinoma*
	Sarcoma*
Mouse	Colon adenocarcinoma*
	Plasma cell myeloma*
	Mecca lymphosarcoma*
	Lymphocytic leukemia*
Avian	MC-29 virus-induced hepatoma†
Human	Hepatocellular carcinoma‡
	Renal cell carcinoma‡
	Lung adenocarcinoma‡
	Colon carcinoma‡
	Colon xenografts§

* Chemically induced, transplantable.
† Virus-induced, transplantable.
‡ Spontaneous, primary.
§ Spontaneous, transplanted in nude mice.

include those produced by chemical and viral agents, as well as primary human neoplasms. These new insights should help in the selective targeting of chemotherapy against cancer cells in animals and man.

ACKNOWLEDGMENTS

The research work outlined in this paper was supported by grants from the United States Public Health Service, National Cancer Institute, Grant Nos. CA-05034 and CA-13526.

REFERENCES

Aisenberg, A. C., and H. P. Morris. 1961. Energy pathways of hepatoma No. 5123. Nature 191:1314–1315.

Aoki, T., and G. Weber. 1981. Carbamoyl-phosphate synthetase (glutamine-hydrolyzing): Increased activity in cancer cells. Science 212:463–465.

Ashmore, J., G. Weber, and B. R. Landau. 1958. Isotope studies on the pathways of glucose-6-phosphate metabolism in the Novikoff hepatoma. Cancer Res. 18:974–979.

Burt, M. E., and M. F. Brennan. 1981. Nutritional support of the cancer patient, in Contemporary Issues in Clinical Nutrition, vol. 3, Surgical Nutrition, M. Yarborough and W. P. Curreri, eds. Churchill-Livingston, London (in press).

Copeland, E. M., III, J. M. Daly, D. M. Ota, and S. J. Dudrick. 1979. Nutrition, cancer and intravenous hyperalimentation. Cancer 43:2108–2116.

Elford, H. L., M. Freese, E. Passamani, and H. P. Morris. 1970. Ribonucleotide reductase and cell proliferation. I. Variations of ribonucleotide reductase activity with tumor growth rate in a series of rat hepatomas. J. Biol. Chem. 245:5228–5233.

Harkrader, R. J., R. C. Jackson, D. A. Ross, and G. Weber. 1980. Increase in liver and kidney deoxycytidine kinase activity linked to neoplastic transformation. Biochem. Biophys. Res. Commun. 96:1633–1639.

Heinrich, P. C., H. P. Morris, and G. Weber. 1976. Behavior of transaldolase (EC 2.2.1.2) and transketolase (EC 2.2.1.1) activities in normal, neoplastic, differentiating and regenerating liver. Cancer Res. 36:3189–3197.

Jackson, R. C., F. J. Goulding, and G. Weber. 1979. Enzymes of purine metabolism in human and rat renal cortex and renal cell carcinoma. JNCI 62:749–754.

Jackson, R. C., M. S. Lui, T. J. Boritzki, H. P. Morris, and G. Weber. 1980. Purine and pyrimidine nucleotide patterns of normal, differentiating and regenerating liver and of hepatomas in rats. Cancer Res. 40:1286–1291.

Kizaki, H., J. C. Williams, H. P. Morris, and G. Weber. 1980. Increased cytidine 5'-triphosphate synthetase activity in rat and human tumors. Cancer Res. 40:3921–3927.

Kovalszky, I., A. Jeney, R. Asbot, and K. Lapis. 1976. Biochemistry and enzyme induction in MC-29 virus-induced transplantable avian hepatoma. Cancer Res. 36:2140–2145.

Lin, Y. C., J. C. Elwood, A. Rosado, H. P. Morris, and S. Weinhouse. 1962. Glucose metabolism in a low-glycolysing tumour, the Morris hepatoma 5123. Nature 195:153–155.

Lowry, O. H., N. J. Rosebrough, A. L. Farr, and R. J. Randall. 1951. Protein measurement with the Folin phenol reagent. J. Biol. Chem. 193:265–275.

Morris, H. P., and B. P. Wagner. 1968. Induction and transplantation of rat hepatomas with different growth rate (including "minimal deviation" hepatomas) in Methods in Cancer Research, vol. 4, H. Busch, ed. Academic Press, New York, pp. 125–152.

Ota, D. M., E. M. Copeland III, H. W. Strobel, Jr., J. Daly, E. T. Gum, E. Guinn, and S. J. Dudrick. 1977. The effect of protein nutrition on host and tumor metabolism. J. Surg. Res. 22:181–188.

Prajda, N., S. Eckhardt, Z. Suba, and K. Lapis. 1979. Biochemical behavior of MC-29 virus-induced transplantable chicken hepatoma. J. Toxicol. Environ. Health 5:503–508.

Reynolds, H. M., J. M. Daly, B. J. Rowlands, S. J. Dudrick, and E. M. Copeland III. 1980.

Effects of nutritional repletion on host and tumor response to chemotherapy. Cancer 45:3069–3074.

Sweeney, M. J., J. Ashmore, H. P. Morris, and G. Weber. 1963. Comparative biochemistry of hepatomas. IV. Isotope studies of glucose and fructose metabolism in liver tumors of different growth rates. Cancer Res. 23:995–1002.

Takeda, E., and G. Weber. 1981. Role of ribonucleotide reductase in expression of the neoplastic program. Life Sci. 28:1007–1014.

Tzeng, D. Y., S. Sakiyama, H. Kizaki, and G. Weber. 1981. Increased concentration of CTP synthetase in hepatoma 3924A: Immunological evidence. Life Sci. 28:2537–2543.

Warburg, O. 1956. On the origin of cancer cells. Science 123:309–314.

Weber, G. 1961. Behavior of liver enzymes during hepatocarcinogenesis. Adv. Cancer Res. 6:403–494.

Weber, G. 1968. Carbohydrate metabolism in cancer cells and the molecular correlation concept. Naturwissenschaften 55:418–429.

Weber, G. 1977a. Enzymology of cancer cells, Part 1. N. Engl. J. Med. 296:486–493.

Weber, G. 1977b. Enzymology of cancer cells, Part 2. N. Engl. J. Med. 296:541–551

Weber, G. 1980. Enzymic programs of human renal cell carcinoma, in Renal Adenocarcinoma, G. Sufrin and S. A. Beckley, eds. UICC Publications, Geneva, pp. 44–50.

Weber, G., F. J. Goulding, R. C. Jackson, and J. N. Eble. 1978a. Biochemistry of human renal cell carcinoma, in Characterization and Treatment of Human Tumors, W. Davis and K. R. Harrap, eds. Excerpta Medica, Amsterdam, pp. 227–234.

Weber, G., J. C. Hager, M. S. Lui, N. Prajda, D. Y. Tzeng, R. C. Jackson, E. Takeda, and J. N. Eble. 1981a. Biochemical programs of slowly and rapidly growing human colon carcinoma xenografts. Cancer Res. 41:854–859.

Weber, G., R. C. Jackson, J. C. Williams, F. J. Goulding, and T. J. Eberts. 1977. Enzymatic markers of neoplastic transformation and regulation of purine and pyrimidine metabolism. Adv. Enzyme Regul. 15:53–77.

Weber, G., H. Kizaki, T. Shiotani, D. Tzeng, and J. C. Williams. 1978b. The molecular correlation concept of neoplasia. Recent advances and new challenges, in Morris Hepatomas, H. P. Morris and W. E. Criss, eds. Plenum Publishing, New York, pp. 89–116.

Weber, G., H. Kizaki, D. Tzeng, T. Shiotani, and E. Olah. 1978c. Colon tumor: Enzymology of the neoplastic program. Life Sci. 23:729–736.

Weber, G., M. S. Lui, E. Takeda, and J. E. Denton. 1980a. Enzymology of human colon tumors. Life Sci. 27:793–799.

Weber, G., R. A. Malt, J. L. Glover, J. C. Williams, N. Prajda, and C. D. Waggoner. 1976. Biochemical basis of malignancy in man, in Biological Characterization of Human Tumours, W. Davis and C. Maltoni, eds. Excerpta Medica, Amsterdam, pp. 60–72.

Weber, G., H. P. Morris, W. C. Love, and J. Ashmore. 1961. Comparative biochemistry of hepatomas. II. Isotope studies of carbohydrate metabolism in Morris hepatoma 5123. Cancer Res. 21:1406–1411.

Weber, G., E. Olah, J. E. Denton, M. S. Lui, E. Takeda, D. Y. Tzeng, and J. Ban. 1981b. Dynamics of modulation of biochemical programs in cancer cells. Adv. Enzyme Regul. 19:87–102.

Weber, G., E. Olah, M. S. Lui, H. Kizaki, D. Y. Tzeng, and E. Takeda. 1980b. Biochemical commitment to replication in cancer cells. Adv. Enzyme Regul. 18:3–26.

Weber, G., M. Stubbs, and H. P. Morris. 1971. Metabolism of hepatomas of different growth rates in situ and during ischemia. Cancer Res. 31:2177–2183.

Weber, G., A. Trevisani, and P. C. Heinrich. 1974. Operation of pleiotropic control in hormonal regulation and in neoplasia. Adv. Enzyme Regul. 12:11–41.

Weinhouse, S. 1955. Oxidative metabolism of neoplastic tissues. Adv. Cancer Res. 3:269–325.

Weinhouse, S. 1982. Changing perceptions of carbohydrate metabolism in tumors, in Molecular Interrelations of Nutrition and Cancer (UT System Cancer Center 34th Annual Symposium on Fundamental Cancer Research), M. S. Arnott, J. van Eys, and Y.-M. Wang, eds. Raven Press, New York, pp. 167–181.

Williamson, D. H., H. A. Krebs, M. Stubbs, M. A. Page, H. P. Morris, and G. Weber. 1970. Metabolism of renal tumors in situ and during ischemia. Cancer Res. 30:2049–2054.

Molecular Interrelations of Nutrition and Cancer,
edited by M. S. Arnott, J. van Eys, and Y.-M. Wang.
Raven Press, New York © 1982.

Lipids and Cancer

David Kritchevsky

The Wistar Institute of Anatomy and Biology, Philadelphia, Pennsylvania 19104

Recently, the role played by dietary lipid in the neoplastic process has been the subject of discussion and review (Carroll and Khor 1975, Kritchevsky and Klurfeld 1981). Nutrients can modify carcinogens or procarcinogens or, by affecting enzymic function, cell permeability, hormone levels, or the action of the intestinal flora. The ensuing discussion will focus on selected aspects of lipids and cancer.

Epidemiological studies summarized by Carroll and Khor (1975) and Drasar and Irving (1973) suggest a high positive correlation between the intake of fat and incidence of breast and colon cancer in many populations. There are further suggestions that animal fat is the actual culprit. However, Berg (1975) has raised the possibility that total calories, not specific sources of calories, may explain the epidemiological observations.

Hill et al. (1979) reported on colon cancer mortality and diet in residents of Hong Kong who were divided into three socioeconomic groups. Their data are summarized in Table 1. Cancer mortality for males was $26.7/10^5$ in the highest income group and $11.7/10^5$ in the lowest; fecal bile acid excretion in the highest income group was double that in the lowest. However, the ingestion of all nutrients increased as a function of income. Calculation of caloric intake suggests that the low-, moderate-, and high-income groups ingested approximately 2,630, 3,000, and 3,900 calories/day, respectively. One can extract data from Table 1 to support almost any dietary hypothesis. Burke et al. (1980) compared the dietary intakes of men and women with benign and malignant gastrointestinal disease and found virtually no differences in either caloric level or dietary pattern. The daily caloric intake for subjects who showed no weight loss ranged from about 2,100 to 2,300. The intakes of protein, carbohydrate, and fat (as percentage of calories) were 13.5%, 47.3%, and 39.2%, respectively.

Animal studies show that both type and amount of dietary fat influence chemically induced carcinogenesis. Watson and Mellanby (1930) found that increased levels of dietary fat increased the incidence of coal tar-induced skin tumors in mice. Lavik and Baumann (1941, 1943) made a similar observation in mice

TABLE 1. *Colorectal mortality, diet, and income in Hong Kong**

	Family income		
	Low	Moderate	High
Mortality (per 100,000)			
Males	11.7	17.6	26.7
Females	11.2	16.2	—
Fecal bile acids			
(mg/g dry wt.)	2.2	3.1	4.7
Diet (g/day)			
Vegetable protein (V)	26	41	52
Animal protein (A)	98	111	144
A/V	2.72	2.71	2.77
Fat (% of calories)	79(27)	93(28)	127(29)
Carbohydrate	327	358	458
Sugars	9	12	16
Alcohol	6	7	10
Fiber-rich foods			
Rice, cereals	287	298	338
Vegetables	175	189	228
Fresh fruit	58	86	106
Total	520	573	672

* After Hill et al. 1979.

treated with methylcholanthrene (MCA). They also found, however, that tumor incidence in mice fed a low-fat, low-calorie diet was zero. Tumor incidence in MCA-treated mice fed a low-fat, high-calorie diet was 54%, and in mice fed a high-fat, high-calorie diet it was 66%. When they fed a high-fat, low-calorie diet, tumor incidence was only 28%. Their data thus implicate total calories rather than fat.

Carroll and Khor (1971) fed a variety of fats to rats treated with 7,12-dimethyl-benz(a)anthracene (DMBA) and found that tumor incidence was considerably higher in the animals fed unsaturated fat (Table 2). Reddy (1975) compared the effects of corn oil and lard on the induction of colon tumors using 1,2-dimethylhydrazine (DMH). When the two fats were used at a level of 5%, rats fed corn oil exhibited a much higher incidence of tumors; at 20% of the diet the two fats yielded identical tumor incidence. Broitman et al. (1977) have obtained similar results when comparing the effects of coconut and safflower oils on DMH-induced tumors. It has been suggested (Hillyard and Abraham 1974) that unsaturated fat affects the immune system, possibly via prostaglandin synthesis.

One line of reasoning that links dietary fat to tumor incidence is that dietary cholesterol plays a role because it is converted to bile acids, which may act as promotors of carcinogenesis. However, epidemiological studies (Enstrom 1975) show that between 1940 and 1970, when beef consumption in the United States doubled, the incidence of colon cancer mortality was virtually unchanged. In a specific case-controlled study, Graham et al. (1978) found no relationship

TABLE 2. *Influence of dietary fats on DMBA-induced mammary tumors in rats**

Fat (20%)	Iodine value†	Rats with tumors (%)	Tumors per tumor-bearing rat	Tumors per 30 rats
Sunflower seed oil	148	96.6	4.8	130
Soybean oil	139	100.0	3.4	103
Corn oil	130	90.0	4.0	110
Cottonseed oil	123	93.3	4.5	127
Olive oil	84	86.6	4.5	117
Lard	59	93.3	3.4	97
Tallow	39	80.0	3.0	72
Butter	34	86.6	3.3	88
Coconut oil	6	96.6	2.5	73

* After Carroll and Khor (1971).
† Calculated from published fatty acid spectra.

between frequency of meat consumption and colon cancer. Furthermore, the incidence of colon cancer is the same in Seventh Day Adventists, who eat meat sparingly (Phillips 1975), and Mormons, who consume a conventional diet (Lyon et al. 1976).

A metabolic clue to the effect of animal fats may be available from examination of the fecal steroids of populations exhibiting low or high incidence of colon cancer. In the intestine, cholesterol is normally hydrogenated to coprostanol. Coprostanol and its oxidation product, coprostanone, are, along with cholesterol, the principal neutral steroids found in the feces. One might adduce effects on cholesterol metabolism by examining the ratio of cholesterol to its neutral metabolites. The principal hepatic metabolites of cholesterol are the bile acids. The liver converts cholesterol to cholic (3,7,12-trihydroxycholanoic) and chenodeoxycholic (3,7-dihydroxycholanoic) acids. These are the primary bile acids. The intestinal flora possess a dehydroxylating enzyme that converts cholic acid to deoxycholic (3,12-dihydroxycholanoic) acid and chenodeoxycholic to lithocholic (3-hydroxycholanoic) acid. These are the secondary bile acids. Fecal bacteria convert the normal bile acids to a variety of other acidic products, but the ratio of primary to secondary bile acids might be another means to judge normal versus abnormal metabolism.

Reddy (1979) has summarized data on fecal steroids in normal subjects or subjects with colon cancer or adenomatous polyps. The findings are shown in Table 3. In the neutral sterol fraction the ratio of cholesterol to its metabolites is higher in the colon cancer cases. This may be an after-the-fact finding, indicating an inability to metabolize cholesterol. In the acidic fraction, the ratio of primary to secondary bile acids is somewhat higher in the control patients. The ratio of primary to total bile acids is similar in all groups. The absolute amount of excreted steroids (mg/g dry feces) is much lower in the control subjects, which could reflect the health status of the patients. Comparison of fecal steroid excretion in five populations of varying susceptibility to colon cancer

TABLE 3. *Fecal steroids (mg/g dry feces) in three groups of subjects**

Steroid	Colon cancer (35)†	Adenomatous polyps (15)	Control (40)
Neutral			
Cholesterol (CH)	12.6	6.4	3.2
Coprostanol (CO)	18.7	19.6	12.9
Coprostanone (CN)	3.9	4.0	1.9
CH/(CO + CN)	0.56	0.27	0.22
Acids			
Cholic	0.5	0.4	0.4
Chenodeoxycholic	0.5	0.3	0.2
Deoxycholic	7.0	0.3	3.7
Lithocholic	6.5	5.4	3.1
Other	5.1	4.2	3.5
Primary/secondary	0.074	0.061	0.088
Primary/all others	0.054	0.045	0.058

* After Reddy (1979).
† Number of subjects.

(Reddy 1979) also gives variable results (Table 4). The concentration of fecal steroids may play a decisive role, however. Residents of Kuopio, Finland, who have a low incidence of colon cancer, excrete the same daily amount of bile acids as do New Yorkers, but the steroid concentration is much higher in the New York group because of their smaller fecal bulk. Mower et al. (1974) compared bile acid excretion in Japanese in Hawaii and Japanese in Akita, Japan. The former exhibit a threefold to fourfold higher incidence of colon cancer. The ratio of primary to secondary bile acids is 0.61 in the residents of Hawaii and 0.65 in the residents of Akita.

TABLE 4. *Daily excretion of fecal steroids in five populations**

	Population				
	US (High fat)	US (Vegetarian)	US (SDA)†	Japanese	Chinese
Number	17	12	11	17	11
Total steroids (S) (mg/day)	818	318	266	266	195
Bile acids (B) (mg/day)	256	318	54	83	54
S/B	3.20	2.39	4.39	3.20	3.61
CH/CO + CN‡	0.038	0.270	0.385	0.130	0.625
P/S§	0.043	0.127	0.025	0.079	0.071

* After Reddy (1979).
† Seventh Day Adventists.
‡ Cholesterol/(Coprostanol + Coprostanone).
§ Primary/secondary bile acids.

TABLE 5. *Influence of cholestyramine on chemically induced large bowel tumors in rats**

Inducer	Diet	Number of tumors	
		Proximal	Distal
1,2 Dimethylhydrazine	Normal diet (ND)	15	1
	ND + 2% cholestyramine (NDC)	31	29
Azoxymethane	ND	19	8
	NDC	33	36
Methylazoxymethanol	ND	4	2
	NDC	18	15

* After Nigro et al. (1973).

If bile acids are a factor in the establishment of colon cancer, it would be logical to suppose that substances that enhance their excretion would inhibit experimental colon carcinogenesis. Bran (Barbolt and Abraham 1978) and cellulose (Freeman et al. 1980) will inhibit DMH-induced colon cancers in rats, but neither substance binds bile acids to any appreciable extent (Story and Kritchevsky 1976). However, Nigro et al. (1973) tested the effects of cholestyramine, a bile acid–binding resin, on large bowel tumors induced by three different agents. In every case, addition of cholestyramine to the diet significantly increased the incidence of tumors (Table 5).

We (Watanabe et al. 1979) studied the effects of dietary pectin, bran, and alfalfa on colon tumors induced by intramuscular injection of azoxymethane (AOM) or intrarectal instillation of methylnitrosourea (MNU). Table 6 shows that pectin and bran inhibited AOM-induced tumors but did not affect the action of MNU. Alfalfa, on the other hand, enhanced the incidence of MNU-induced tumors. These data show the interaction of type of fiber and mode of carcinogen administration. Our experiments (Kritchevsky and Story 1974, Story and Kritchevsky 1976, Vahouny et al. 1980) have shown that different types of fiber bind bile acids to varying extents. The extent correlates with the severity of mucosal damage (Cassidy et al. 1980,1981) (Table 7). The bile acid effect

TABLE 6. *Influence of dietary fiber (15%) on colon tumors induced by injected azoxymethane (AOM) or intrarectal methylnitrosourea (MNU)**

Regimen	Rats with tumors (%)		Tumors/tumor-bearing rat	
	AOM	MNU	AOM	MNU
Alfalfa	53.3	83.3	1.3	2.8
Pectin	10.0	58.6	1.0	1.7
Bran	33.0	60.0	1.2	1.3
Control	57.7	69.0	1.5	1.5

* After Watanabe et al. (1979).

TABLE 7. *Effect of dietary fiber (15%) on ultrastructural topography of rat colon and jejunum* *

Dietary additive	Average bile acid–binding capacity (%)	Intestinal villi or colonic ridges with structural deviations (%)	
		Colon	Jejunum
Alfalfa	15	58.6 ± 4.3	32.8 ± 7.2
Bran	5	15.0 ± 4.9	5.0 ± 1.1
Cellulose	0	22.1 ± 4.1	7.5 ± 2.1
Cholestyramine	80–100	39.5 ± 10.5	64.2 ± 4.7
Pectin	—	29.4 ± 8.0	30.7 ± 4.7

* After Cassidy et al. (1981).

may be mechanical rather than metabolic. More work remains to be done to secure this point.

Another aspect of lipids relating to cancer is emerging. Pearce and Dayton (1971) studied the effect of a hypocholesterolemic diet on coronary disease mortality in men. Over an 8-year period, the diet, which was high in polyunsaturated fat, resulted in fewer coronary deaths but had no effect on total mortality; many of the deaths in the test group were attributable to cancer. Miettinen et al. (1972) carried out a similar study in Finland and found the ratio of malignancies between test and control subjects in men and women was 1.27 and 1.10, respectively. A recent trial involving a hypocholesterolemic drug (clofibrate; ethyl p-chlorophenoxyisobutyrate) showed more malignancies among the subjects given the drug or in the low cholesterol control group than in the hypercholesterolemic controls. These findings raise a question concerning the possible connection between low serum cholesterol levels and cancer.

Feldman and Carter (1971) examined lipid levels in postmenopausal women with metastatic breast cancer and compared them with those of controls. Serum triglyceride and phospholipid levels were identical in the two groups, but cholesterol levels were significantly lower (236 ± 5.0 mg/100 ml vs 274 ± 6.8 mg/100 ml, p < 0.01) in the cancer patients, although lipoprotein distribution was not altered. Bjelke (1974) has reported a correlation between colon cancer and low serum cholesterol levels, as have Nydegger and Butler (1972). It can be argued that the low serum cholesterol levels observed in the cancer patients only reflect the nature of the disease. However, recent retrospective studies by Beaglehole et al. (1980) in New Zealand, Kark et al. (1980) in Evans County, Georgia, and Williams et al. (1981) in Framingham, Massachusetts, show that the subjects at the lower end of the serum cholesterol spectrum had the highest incidence of cancer. On the other hand, a survey in Norway (Bjelke 1974) showed no association between serum cholesterol and cancer in over 3,700 men examined 10 years after their enrollment in a heart disease study. How can these observations be explained? Did sera drawn from healthy subjects 10 to 20 years earlier already reflect a neoplasm? Do low levels of serum cholesterol reflect a more rapid flux of sterol through the intestine? Are rates of conversion of cholesterol to bile acids involved?

Low levels of circulating cholesterol mean low levels of β-lipoprotein, which, in turn, reflects reduced transport of other substances such as retinol, which may be protective. Another possibility is that reduced cholesterol levels or increased levels of unsaturated fatty acids, or both, may affect stability and fluidity of cell membranes (Inbar and Shinitzky 1974, Scandella et al. 1979). At present, we have conflicting epidemiological data concerning serum cholesterol levels and malignancy and some experimental data relating to the effects of unsaturated fat. Unsaturated fat affects cholesterolemia, which is the thread that relates these observations. More experimental and epidemiological data are needed to provide a reasonable understanding of the relationship, if any, between cancer and low cholesterol levels.

As one test of the falling cholesterol hypothesis, we studied DMH-treated Fischer 344 rats (Klurfeld, Aglow, Tepper, and Kritchevsky, manuscript submitted). One group of rats was maintained on a semipurified diet (SP) containing 47% dextrose, 21.7% casein, 10% coconut oil, and 5% corn oil. Another group was fed the same diet except that 2% of the dextrose was replaced with cholesterol (1.5%) and bile salts (0.5%) (Diet SPBC). After a 6-week acclimatization period, the rats were given weekly oral doses of DMH (30 mg/kg). After 3 weeks of treatment, one third of the rats in group SPBC were placed on diet SP, one third were placed on a diet containing 0.5% bile salt but no cholesterol (SPB), and the remaining third continued to eat diet SPBC. Three more doses of DMH were given and the rats maintained for 6 more months. Table 8 presents the data obtained. Presence of cholesterol and bile acid in the diet resulted in a higher tumor frequency, larger tumor size, and increased malignant transformation. Reversion to a hypocholesterolemic regimen decreased tumor frequency and size, while reversion to a bile acid–containing diet did not affect either of these parameters. These data suggest that the presence of bile acids in the diet affects tumor frequency and size, whereas cholesterol may play a role in malignant transformation.

This experiment was undertaken to examine the possibility that a hypocholesterolemic regimen in DMH-treated rats would give results similar to those re-

TABLE 8. *Influence of dietary change on DMH-induced colon tumors in Fischer 344 rats**

Regimen	Serum cholesterol (mg/dl)	Tumor incidence	Tumor/rat	Tumor size (mm)	Carcinoma (%)
SP	106 ± 13	21/30	1.4 ± 0.2	2.3 ± 0.2	25.9
SPBC	146 ± 15	23/30	2.3 ± 0.3	4.2 ± 0.4	42.0
SPBC → SP	92 ± 3	15/29	1.7 ± 0.2	3.2 ± 0.5	26.9
SPBC → SPB	109 ± 8	24/29	2.4 ± 0.2	3.9 ± 0.4	24.6

* After Klurfeld, Aglow, Tepper, and Kritchevsky (manuscript submitted).

ported in various clinical trials in man (Committee of Principal Investigators 1978, Miettinen et al. 1972, Pearce and Dayton 1971). Reversion to the semipurified diet actually reduced tumor incidence (from 70% to 52%) but gave a 21% increase in the number of tumors per rat and a 39% increase in tumor size. The reasons for this discrepancy may be due to differences in species (man vs rat), type of tumor (spontaneous vs induced) or diet. Experiments involving more rapid fluxes of serum lipid levels are in progress.

ACKNOWLEDGMENTS

This work was supported, in part, by a Research Career Award (HL-00734) from the National Institutes of Health and a grant-in-aid from the Commonwealth of Pennsylvania.

REFERENCES

Barbolt, T. A., and R. Abraham. 1978. The effect of bran on dimethylhydrazine-induced colon carcinogenesis in the rat. Proc. Soc. Exp. Biol. Med. 157:656–659.

Beaglehole, R., M. A. Foulkes, I. A. M. Prior, and E. Eyles. 1980. Cholesterol and mortality in New Zealand Maoris. Br. J. Med. 280:285–287.

Berg, J. W. 1975. Can nutrition explain the pattern of international epidemiology of hormone-dependent cancers? Cancer Res. 35:3345–3350.

Bjelke, E. 1974. Colon cancer and blood-cholesterol. Lancet 1:1116–1117.

Broitman, S. A., J. J. Vitale, E. Vavrousek-Jokuba, and L. S. Gottlieb. 1977. Polyunsaturated fat, cholesterol and large bowel tumorigenesis. Cancer 40:2453–2463.

Burke, M., E. I. Bryson, and A. E. Kark. 1980. Dietary intakes, resting metabolic rates and body composition in benign and malignant gastrointestinal disease. Br. Med. J. 280:211–215.

Carroll, K. K., and H. T. Khor. 1971. Effect of level and type of dietary fat on incidence of mammary tumors induced in female Sprague-Dawley rats by 7,12-dimethylbenz(a)anthracene. Lipids 6:415–420.

Carroll, K. K., and H. T. Khor. 1975. Dietary fat in relation to tumorigenesis. Prog. Biochem. Pharmacol. 10:308–353.

Cassidy, M. M., F. G. Lightfoot, L. E. Grau, T. R. Roy, J. A. Story, D. Kritchevsky, and G. V. Vahouny. 1980. Effect of bile salt-binding resins on the morphology of rat jejunum and colon— A scanning electron microscope study. Dig. Dis. Sci. 25:504–512.

Cassidy, M. M., F. G. Lightfoot, L. E. Grau, J. A. Story, D. Kritchevsky, and G. V. Vahouny. 1981. Effect of intake of dietary fibers on the ultrastructural topography of rat jejunun and colon—A scanning electron microscope study. Am. J. Clin. Nutr. 34:218–228.

Committee of Principal Investigators. 1978. A cooperative trail in the primary prevention of ischemic heart disease using clofibrate. Br. Heart J. 40:1069–1118.

Drasar, B. S., and D. Irving. 1973. Environmental factors and cancer of the colon and breast. Br. J. Cancer 27:167–172.

Enstrom, J. E. 1975. Colorectal cancer and consumption of beef and fat. Br. J. Cancer 32:432–439.

Feldman, E. B., and A. C. Carter. 1971. Circulating lipids and lipoproteins in women with metastatic breast cancer. J. Clin. Endocrinol. Metab. 33:8–13.

Freeman, H. J., G. A. Spiller, and Y. S. Kim. 1980. A double-blind study on the effects of differing purified cellulose and pectin fiber diets on 1,2-dimethylhydrazine-induced rat colonic neoplasia. Cancer Res. 40:2661–2665.

Graham, S., H. Dayal, M. Swanson, A. Mittelman, and G. Wilkinson. 1978. Diet in the epidemiology of cancer of the colon and rectum. JNCI 61:709–714.

Hill, M., R. Mac Lennan, and K. Newcombe. 1979. Diet and large-bowel cancer in three socioeconomic groups in Hong Kong. Lancet 1:436.

Hillyard, L. A., and S. Abraham. 1974. Effect of dietary polyunsaturated acids on growth of mammary adenocarcinomas in mice and rats. Cancer Res. 39:4430–4437.

Inbar, M., and M. Shinitzky. 1974. Cholesterol as a bioregulator in the development and inhibition of leukemia. Proc. Natl. Acad. Sci. USA 71:4229–4231.

Kark, J. D., A. H. Smith, and C. G. Hames. 1980. The relationship of serum cholesterol to the incidence of cancer in Evans County, Georgia. J. Chron. Dis. 33:311–322.

Kritchevsky, D., and D. M. Klurfeld. 1981. Fat and cancer, *in* Nutrition and Cancer: Etiology and Treatment, G. R. Newell and N. M. Ellison, eds. Raven Press, New York, pp. 173–188.

Kritchevsky, D., and J. A. Story. 1974. Binding of bile salts in vitro by non-nutritive fiber. J. Nutr. 104:458–462.

Lavik, P. S., and C. A. Baumann. 1941. Dietary fat and tumor formation. Cancer Res. 1:181–187.

Lavik, P. S., and C. A. Baumann. 1943. Further studies on the tumor-promoting action of fat. Cancer Res. 3:749–756.

Lyon, J. L., M. R. Klauber, J. W. Gardner, and C. R. Smart. 1976. Cancer incidence in Mormons and non-Mormons in Utah 1966–1970. N. Engl. J. Med. 294:129–133.

Miettinen, M., O. Turpeinin, M. J. Karvonen, R. Elosus, and E. Paavilainin. 1972. Effect of cholesterol-lowering diet on mortality from coronary heart-disease and other causes. Lancet 2:835–838.

Mower, H. F., R. M. Ray, R. Shoff, G. N. Stemmerman, A. Nomura, G. A. Glober, S. Kamiyama, A. Shimada, and H. Yamakawa. 1974. Fecal bile acids in two Japanese populations with different colon cancer risks. Cancer Res. 39:328–331.

Nigro, N. D., N. Bhadrachari, and C. Chomchai. 1973. A rat model for studying colonic cancer: Effect of cholestyramine on induced tumors. Dis. Colon Rectum 16:438–443.

Nydegger, U. E., and R. E. Butler. 1972. Serum lipoprotein levels in patients with cancer. Cancer Res. 32:1756–1760.

Pearce, M. L., and S. Dayton. 1971. Incidence of cancer in men on a diet high in polyunsaturated fat. Lancet 1:464–467.

Phillips, R. L. 1975. Role of life-style and dietary habits in risk of cancer among Seventh-Day Adventists. Cancer Res. 35:3513–3522.

Reddy, B. S. 1975. Role of bile metabolites in colon carcinogenesis. Cancer 36:2401–2406.

Reddy, B. S. 1979. Nutrition and colon cancer. Advances in Nutritional Research. 2:199–218.

Scandella, D. J., J. A. Hayward, and N. Lee. 1979. Cholesterol levels and plasma membrane fluidity in 3T3 and SV101–3T3 cells. J. Supramol. Struct. 11:477–483.

Story, J. A., and D. Kritchevsky. 1976. Comparison of the binding of various bile acids and bile salts in vitro by several types of fiber. J. Nutr. 106:1292–1294.

Vahouny, G. V., R. Tombes, M. M. Cassidy, D. Kritchevsky, and L. L. Gallo. 1980. Dietary fibers. V. Binding of bile salts, phospholipids and cholesterol from mixed micelles by bile acid sequestrants and dietary fibers. Lipids 15:1012–1018.

Watanabe, E., B. S. Reddy, J. H. Weisburger, and D. Kritchevsky. 1979. Effect of dietary alfalfa, pectin and wheat bran on azoxymethane or methylnitrosourea-induced colon carcinogenesis in F344 rats. JNCI 63:141–145.

Watson, A. F. and E. Mellanby. 1930. Tar cancer in mice. II. The condition of the skin when modified by external treatment or diet, as a factor in influencing the cancerous reaction. Br. J. Exp. Pathol. 11:311–322.

Williams, R. R., P. D. Sorlie, M. Feinleib, P. M. McNamara, W. B. Kannel, and T. R. Dawber. 1981. Cancer incidence by levels of cholesterol. JAMA 24:247–252.

Molecular Interrelations of Nutrition and Cancer,
edited by M. S. Arnott, J. van Eys, and Y.-M. Wang.
Raven Press, New York © 1982.

Effects of Unsaturated Fatty Acids on the Development and Proliferation of Normal and Neoplastic Breast Epithelium

William R. Kidwell, Richard A. Knazek, Barbara K. Vonderhaar,
and Ilona Losonczy

Laboratory of Pathophysiology, National Cancer Institute, Bethesda, Maryland 20205

Epidemiological studies have shown a strong positive correlation between per capita fat consumption and the incidence of human breast cancer in various countries (Lea 1966, Carroll et al. 1968, Wynder 1968, Dewaard 1969). Province-by-province analyses in Japan by Hirayama (1978) confirm this selective relationship between fat and mammary cancer development and show that, within the same population, breast cancer incidence has been increasing in proportion to increasing fat consumption.

These epidemiological findings were preceded by early investigations of Tannenbaum (1942), who found that elevated dietary fat facilitated the development of both spontaneous and carcinogen-induced mammary tumors in mice. This observation in an animal model system and numerous others that followed (Carroll 1975, Hopkins et al. 1976, Rao and Abraham 1976b, Chan and Dao 1981, Ip et al. 1980) indicate that dietary lipids are causally involved in the tumorigenic process.

Recent studies have suggested that high-fat consumption might be selective for enhancing mammary tumor formation because of enhanced production of pituitary hormones such as prolactin, which is thought to be a mitogen for mammary epithelium (Chan et al. 1975, Hill and Wynder 1976). This is a reasonable concept, since tumor promoters are generally mitogenic (Boutwell 1978) and since experiments of Carroll (1975) and Nishizuka (1978) have presented evidence for a promotional role of dietary fat.

While hormonal involvement is possible, even likely, it is probable that other factors are involved as well. For example, epidemiological and experimental animal studies indicate that skin tumor incidence is enhanced by high dietary fat, and it is unlikely that the same hormonal mitogens control growth of skin and mammary epithelium (Carroll 1975). Second, Ip et al. (1980) found that hypothalamic lesions in rats elevate serum prolactin levels and that a high-fat diet still dramatically increases 7,12-dimethylbenz(α)anthracene-induced mammary tumor incidence above that of low fat controls. Thus, while elevated serum prolactin levels may be necessary, they are insufficient for maximal tumor yield. Third, the earliest studies of dietary fat and mammary cancer incidence, those of Tannenbaum (1942), showed that spontaneous mouse mammary tumor incidence was elevated by high-fat diets. These spontaneous mouse mammary tumors are almost invariably hormone independent (ovarian independent), as are about two thirds of human mammary tumors (Desombre and Jensen 1980).

Concerning a more direct action of fats on the gland, several proposals have been made. One proposition is that lipophilic carcinogens may be concentrated in the adipose tissue of the mammary gland (Janss et al. 1972). This is not likely to be an important factor, since the efficiency of methylnitrosourea-induced rat mammary tumors is also potentiated by high-fat diets. Methylnitrosourea is a short-lived, nonlipophilic carcinogen (Chan and Dao 1981). Additionally, it has been shown that the capability of high-fat diets to enhance DMBA-induced mammary cancer still exists when the high-fat diet is not begun until 2 weeks after carcinogen administration (Carroll 1975). The lipophilic estrogens also do not appear to concentrate differentially in mammary glands of animals on high-fat diets (Carroll 1975).

A proposition that we favor is that elevated dietary lipids, in addition to peripheral actions, act directly on the mammary gland to affect the growth and development of the glandular epithelium. Experimental evidence leading to this conclusion and a model of how dietary fat excess [or as Wynder (1979) put it, ". . . unbalanced metabolism from dietary excesses . . ."] leads to increased tumor incidence will be presented.

THE ROLE OF UNSATURATED FATTY ACIDS IN THE GROWTH OF MAMMARY EPITHELIAL CELLS

Clues from a Mammary Tumor Cell Line

Our interest in the role of fatty acids in mammary tumorigenesis was aroused by our discovery that a rat mammary tumor cell line, WRK1, was dependent on linoleic acid for growth (Kidwell et al. 1978). This cell line was isolated from a DMBA-induced rat mammary adenocarcinoma and passaged continuously in culture in medium containing rat and fetal calf serum. Under these conditions, a large number of lipid droplets accumulated in these cells and growth was rapid. Upon removal of the rat serum or replacement of it with additional fetal calf serum, the lipid droplets rapidly disappeared and the cells died.

To identify the rat serum component necessary for cell growth, the serum was fractionated into total lipid and total protein fractions (Rothblatt et al. 1976), and these fractions were tested individually and in combination for their ability to promote WRK1 cell growth. As seen in Figure 1, almost all of the growth-promoting activity was present in the lipid component of rat serum. An analysis of rat serum and fetal calf serum lipids revealed one major difference,

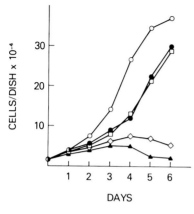

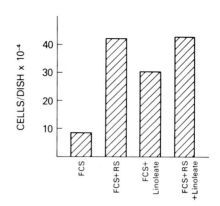

FIG. 1. Stimulation of cell growth by the lipid fraction of rat serum. WRK1 mammary tumor cells were plated in total serum lipid fraction, ●——●; the total serum protein fraction, ◇——◇; a combination of the two, □——□; or with no additions, ▲——▲. For comparisons, WRK1 cells were grown in medium supplemented with unfractionated rat serum, ○——○. (Reproduced from Kidwell et al. 1978, with permission of *Cancer Research*.)

FIG. 2. Growth promotion of WRK1 mammary tumor cells with linoleic acid. The stimulatory activity of rat serum is largely contained in its linoleic acid moiety. (Reproduced from Kidwell et al. 1978, with permission of *Cancer Research*.)

the amount of linoleic acid, which was almost 20-fold higher in rat than in fetal calf serum. Linoleic acid was almost surely the active principle in the rat serum, because the rat serum requirement for WRK1 cell growth was supplantable by pure linoleic acid (Figure 2).

Modulation of Normal and Neoplastic Mammary Cell Growth in Primary Culture by Fatty Acids

The stimulatory effect of linoleic acid on WRK1 cell growth was unexpected. Most cell lines that had been studied were not markedly affected by this or other unsaturated fatty acids (Bailey and Dunbar 1973). One possible explanation for this lack was that the selective pressure of growing cells in culture medium deficient in linoleic acid resulted in the selection of variant cells capable of growth in the absence of this fatty acid.

To see if the results obtained with WRK1 cells were indicative of an unsaturated fatty acid dependency of mammary epithelium, we developed techniques for the isolation and cultivation of pure mammary epithelium directly from normal rat mammary glands or from rat mammary tumors and analyzed the effects of various fatty acids on cell growth (Wicha et al. 1979). As seen in Figures 3 and 4, unsaturated fatty acids did indeed stimulate growth of both normal and neoplastic mammary cells. Since the plating efficiency was greater than 80%, there was no possibility that cell selection was a factor.

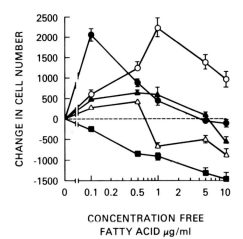

FIG. 3. Growth-response curve for the major fatty acids of the rat mammary gland. Isolated rat mammary ducts and alveoli were plated in 10% lipid-free serum containing hormones at the concentrations indicated in Table 2. ○——○, linoleic acid; ▲——▲, oleic acid; ●——●, linolenic acid; △——△, arachidonic acid; ■——■, stearic acid. (Reproduced from Wicha et al. 1979, with permission of *Cancer Research*.)

Experiments with normal human mammary epithelium from reduction mammoplasty (Figures 5 and 6) showed that rodent and human cells have similar requirements for unsaturated fatty acids and that both are inhibited by saturated fatty acids. The freshly isolated structures are depicted in Figure 5, and their appearance after culturing is illustrated in Figure 6. Upon culturing these cells, we found that the number of colonies that grew was increased threefold by linoleic acid supplementation of the growth medium. Addition of palmitic

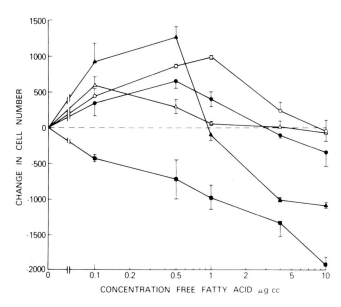

FIG. 4. Growth-response curve for fatty acids obtained with primary cultures of rat mammary tumor cells. Conditions and symbols are the same as for Figure 3.

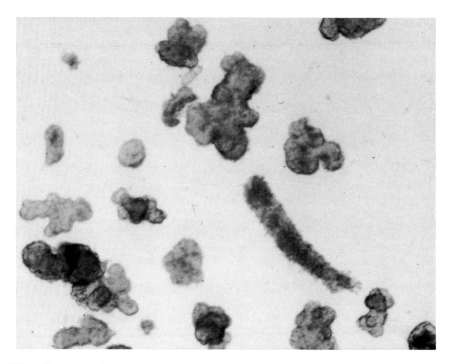

FIG. 5. Ducts and alveoli from human reduction mammoplasty tissue. The organoids, which have a high plating efficiency, were isolated and provided by R. C. Hallowes, Imperial Cancer Research Fund, London. Isolation methods were those of Stampfer et al. (1980).

acid, on the other hand, reduced the number of colonies per dish by one half (Table 1).

The unsaturated fatty acids do not initiate cell division, but rather enhance the growth rate of cells triggered to divide by the appropriate hormonal stimulus (Table 2).

Physiological Relevancy of In Vitro Studies

There is little question that the adipose tissue surrounding the mammary glandular epithelium plays an important role in the modulation of the growth of the epithelium. When pieces of the gland are transplanted to suitable hosts, the growing epithelium does not escape the confines of the fatty tissue component of the explant (Hoshino 1962). The role of the fatty matrix is also emphasized by the observations of DeOme and Faulkin (1959), who found that transplanted hyperplastic and normal mouse epithelium grow particularly well in mammary fat pads.

Although the mammary fat pads contain structural and cellular components other than adipocytes that might confer specificity for mammary epithelial cell

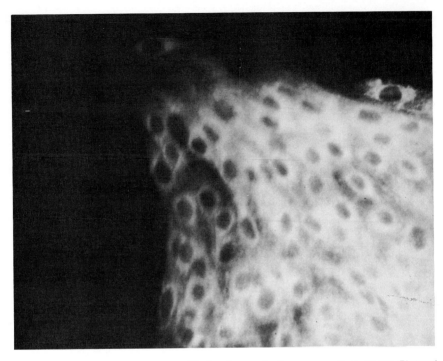

FIG. 6. Cultures of human mammary epithelium from reduction mammoplasty tissue. Photomicrographs taken 3 days after plating. The cells depicted were air dried and stained by indirect immunofluorescence for laminin, a component of basement membranes that is synthesized by mammary epithelium (Kidwell et al. 1980).

growth, our experiments suggest that it is the adipocytes that are important. The evidence is as follows. When rat mammary epithelium is acutely stimulated to proliferate by the administration of perphenazine, a drug that induces massive release of pituitary prolactin (Ben-David 1968, Wicha et al. 1979), the total fatty acid composition of the gland is altered, favoring the growth potential of the epithelium. As seen in Table 3, the amount of unsaturated fatty acids (growth promoting) relative to saturated (growth inhibiting) is increased by about 25% in the glands of perphenazine-treated animals. Since more than 98% of the fatty acids of the mammary gland are contained in the triglycerides of adipocytes, these changes in total glandular fatty acid composition must take place in the adipocytes, although other cells are possibly also involved.

A second relationship between the fatty acid composition of the mammary gland and the growth potential of unsaturated fatty acids detected in culture provides further confidence in the utility of the in vitro culture approach. The relative amounts of the unsaturated fatty acids in normal rat mammary glands are oleic acid $\cong$ linoleic acid $>>$ arachidonic acid $>$ linolenic acid (Wicha et al. 1979). The concentration optimum for these fatty acids determined in tissue culture has the same rank order. In other words, the concentration needed

TABLE 1. *Effect of various fatty acids on the growth of human mammary cells in culture*

Fatty acid added	Conc. (μl/ml)	Colonies per dish
Linoleic acid	0.1	4.8 ± 0.1
Linoleic acid	1.0	8.7 ± 1.0
Palmitic acid	0.1	2.3 ± 0.1
Palmitic acid	1.0	2.0 ± 0.2
None	—	3.3 ± 0.3

The organoids (alveoli and ductal fragments) as depicted in Figure 5 were plated in Eagle's medium containing 10% delipidized serum, 0.1 μg/ml insulin, 0.3 μg/ml prolactin, 0.5 μg/ml hydrocortisone and antibiotics. Colonies were counted 2 weeks after plating.

for optimal cell growth determined in vitro is proportional to the abundance of the unsaturated fatty acids in vivo.

Changes in the Mammary Epithelial Membrane Phospholipids during Proliferation

As demonstrated in Table 2, normal mammary epithelium does not proliferate in the culture system in the absence of the appropriate hormonal support. Thus, unsaturated fatty acids promote the rate at which cells divide after hormonal

TABLE 2. *Stimulation of the growth of normal and neoplastic rat mammary epithelium in primary culture*

Additions	Doubling time (hr)	[³H]Thymidine incorporation (10^3 × cpm/cell)
A. Normal epithelium		
No addition	0*	6.7 ± 1.2†
Hormones‡	58 ± 5	20.8 ± 0.5
Linoleic acid	0*	5.8 ± 0.5
Linoleic acid + hormones	34 ± 4	30.0 ± 1.6
Stearic acid + hormones	76 ± 8	15.5 ± 0.7
B. DMBA-induced tumor epithelium		
No addition	132 ± 12	33.9 ± 1.1
Hormones	89 ± 8	60.1 ± 1.5
Hormones + linoleic acid	35 ± 5	90.1 ± 1.8
Hormones + stearic acid	210 ± 40	ND§

Note that for the normal cells there is an absolute requirement for hormonal support for growth regardless of whether linoleic acid is present or not. Hormonal supplements are the same as in Table 1. Reprinted from Wicha et al. (1979) with permission of *Cancer Research*.
  * No detectable cell growth.
  † Mean ± S.E.
  ‡ Hormones, concentrations as in Table 1.
  § ND, not done.

TABLE 3. *Effects of perphenazine stimulation on the relative amounts of total saturated and unsaturated fatty acids in rat mammary glands*

	Linoleic:palmitic		Oleic:palmitic		Unsaturated: saturated*	
	Exp. 1*	Exp. 2	Exp. 1	Exp. 2	Exp. 1	Exp. 2
Normal (untreated)	1.39	1.47	1.57	1.60	2.77	2.81
Perphenazine	2.01	2.13	2.30	2.16	3.53	3.40

* Exp. 1 and 2 represent separate experiments.
Reprinted from Wicha et al. (1979) with permission of *Cancer Research.*

stimulation. How the unsaturated fatty acids bring this about is unknown, but it is thought to be via their insertion into membrane phospholipids. This apparently leads to changes in membrane fluidity and lateral mobility of receptors (Horwitz et al. 1974), increased membrane enzyme activation (Coleman 1973), enhanced amino acid transport (Kaduce et al. 1977), the differential exposure of cell membrane proteins (Shinitzky and Rivnay 1977), etc.

If changes in the degree of unsaturation of membrane phospholipids are a requisite part of the mitogenic process of the mammary epithelium, then analysis of membranes from proliferating vs. nonproliferating epithelium should reveal these changes. It has, as shown in Table 4. The phospholipids of epithelial cell membranes from the glands of unstimulated animals are only one half as

TABLE 4. *Changes in the membrane phospholipids of mammary epithelial cells in response to perphenazine-induced proliferation*

Experiment no.	% Linoleic acid in stimulated membrane phospholipid / % Linoleic acid in control membrane phospholipid
1	3.4
2	1.8
3	1.3
	(Average = 2.2)

Rat mammary ducts and alveoli were isolated according to Wicha et al. (1979) with or without prior stimulation of animals with perphenazine. Membranes were isolated according to Warren (1974). The lipids were subfractionated on silica gel plates in hexane:ether:acetic acid (4:1:0.05, by volume). Following saponification the fatty acids were methylated with Methyl–8 reagent (Pierce Chemical Co.), then separated and quantitated by gas chromatography on Silar 10 C capillary columns from Quadrex.

rich in linoleic acid as the membrane phospholipids of rapidly proliferating epithelium isolated from perphenazine-treated animals (Table 4). Cell membranes isolated from the ducts and alveoli of the glands of pregnant animals are also enriched in unsaturated fatty acids compared with those of membranes of virgin animals (not shown).

These results are consistent with the concept of a substitution of unsaturated fatty acids in the membranes of cells as a part of the response of the cells to mitogenic stimuli. The enrichment of unsaturated fatty acids in dividing cell membranes is at the expense of palmitic and stearic acids, suggesting that a saturated acyl moiety of membrane phospholipids is not conducive to optimum cell growth. When viewed in these terms, the growth-stimulating potential of unsaturated fatty acids and the growth-inhibitory properties of saturated fatty acids observed in culture are understandable.

The Source of Fatty Acids Utilized by Proliferating Mammary Epithelium

The two most likely sources of fatty acids required by the glandular epithelium are serum lipids and the lipid stores of the fat cells adjacent to the epithelium. Several observations from our laboratory suggest that the glandular adipocytes are an important source. First, as mentioned earlier, the magnitude of the change in total fatty acid composition of the mammary gland in response to perphenazine-induced proliferation indicates that fat cells are involved. Second, the average diameter of fat cells most proximal to proliferating epithelium is smaller than that of more distal adipocytes. Third, prolactin stimulates the release of fatty acids from explants of mammary glands. For example, in mammary explants in culture, prolactin (300 ng/ml) brings about the release of approximately four times as much free fatty acids in 24 hours as from explants with prolactin omitted (Figure 7).

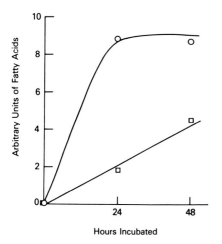

FIG. 7. Prolactin-stimulated release of free fatty acids by explants of intact mammary glands from C3H/HeN virgin mice. Approximately 100 mg tissue was cut into 50 pieces, and these were randomly distributed into four dishes. Ten milliliters growth medium (Eagle's minimal essential growth medium containing bovine serum albumin) was added to the dishes. After incubation for 24 hours (o——o, with prolactin; □——□, without prolactin) the tissue was removed. The free fatty acids liberated into the growth medium were extracted into an organic solvent and quantitated by titration with dilute NaOH.

These results do not indicate that the released fatty acids originate from the adipocyte component of the explants, but this origin is probable. When isolated epithelial cells were tested, they were found to *take up* unsaturated fatty acids selectively when prolactin was included in the growth medium, so that the total fatty acid concentration of the growth medium was lowered rather than increased (Table 5).

If the adipocytes are indeed the source of fatty acids released from mammary explants in response to prolactin stimulation, the prolactin effect is indirectly manifest. This is the case because mammary glands cleared of their epithelial component do not contain prolactin receptors (Bhattacharya and Vonderhaar 1979), i.e., the prolactin receptors are confined to the epithelial cells of the gland. It follows then that prolactin-stimulated epithelium signals fat cells to release fatty acids.

Comparisons of the release of fatty acids from glands cleared of epithelium vs. intact glands (see Figure 8) show that there is indeed a difference in lipid metabolism that depends on whether or not the glandular epithelium is present in mammary tissue. A most interesting difference between the two tissues is that relative to saturated fatty acids, there is more unsaturated fatty acid released in cleared glands (without epithelium) than in intact glands (with epithelium). In other words, the presence of the epithelium inhibits the release by the explants of the class of fatty acids required for maximizing epithelial cell growth (Table 6).

The foregoing observations can be integrated into a physiologically meaningful model as follows. When the epithelium receives a mitogenic stimulus, it transmits a signal to the adjacent fat cells, which causes them to release free fatty acids. There is then a differential resorption of unsaturated fatty acids, particularly oleic and linoleic acid, some of which replace the saturated fatty acid moieties

TABLE 5. *Prolactin stimulation of the uptake of fatty acids by nondividing rat mammary epithelial cells*

Fatty acid	Fatty acid remaining in the growth medium (μg)		Prolactin-stimulated fatty acid uptake (μg)
	Minus prolactin	Plus prolactin	
Palmitate	43.3	43.1	0.2
Stearate	17.6	16.0	1.6
Oleate	33.1	20.2	12.9
Linoleate	35.9	7.9	28.0

The ducts and alveoli from 10 animals were isolated and cultured in Eagle's minimal essential medium containing 1 g/100 ml bovine serum albumin with or without prolactin (NIH S12). After 24 hours incubation in bacterial plastic dishes to which the cells do not attach (and therefore do not divide), the medium was harvested and analyzed for free fatty acid content as described in Table 4.

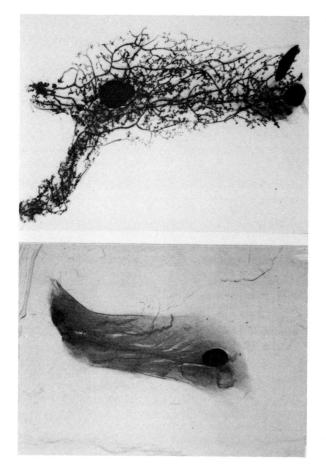

FIG. 8. Intact mammary glandular tissue (top) and the tissue from the same animal cleared of epithelium (bottom). In young animals, surgical removal of the nipple and surrounding tissue eliminates the epithelium. Surgery was generally performed at about 3 weeks. The tissue illustrated is from an animal that was 4 months old. (3×).

of membrane phospholipids. This condition speeds the rate at which the epithelial cells go through the division cycle.

What is the nature of the signal that the epithelium transmits to the fat cell? One possible candidate is a prostaglandin. We have found that 1 ng prostaglandin $f_{2\alpha}$ can effect the release of as much fatty acid from mammary explants as can 300 ng prolactin. A second candidate is the adipocyte lipase-activating factor that a number of tumors produce (Masuno et al. 1981). It will be interesting to see if this factor, a 75,000-dalton protein, is produced by normal mammary epithelium. This recruitment of unsaturated fatty acids from adjacent fat cells by lipase-activating factors may be especially important for mammary tumors as well as normal epithelium, because fatty acid desaturase of some mammary tumors does not increase to compensate for dietary deficiencies of unsaturated fatty acids (Rao and Abraham 1976a).

TABLE 6. *Effect of epithelial cells on the release of fatty acids by mammary tissue*

Animal no.	Intact (18:2/16:0)[*] Cleared (18:2/16:0)
1	0.80
2	0.57
3	0.79
4	0.90
5	0.68
	(Average = 0.75)

Mammary glands were cleared of epithelium on one side of the animal only, leaving the glands on the other side intact. Clearing was done by the method of DeOme and Faulkin (1959). Three months after clearing, the glands were removed from both sides of an animal and introduced into culture as described in Figure 7. Prolactin, 100 ng/ml, was included in the cultures. After incubation for 24 hours, the growth medium was harvested and the fatty acid species quantitated as described in Table 4.

[*] As an indication of the relative amount of unsaturated vs. saturated fatty acids released, the data are expressed as the ratio of linoleic acid to palmitic acid released from intact glands divided by the ratio of linoleic acid to palmitic acid released from cleared glands.

Fatty Acid Effects on the Development of Mammary Epithelium

In addition to the ability to facilitate the growth of adult mammary glandular epithelium, unsaturated fatty acids have a marked effect on the development of the gland. This is especially so for the essential fatty acids. A most pronounced failure of alveolar and ductal development is seen in adult animals deprived of essential fatty acids prenatally (Knazek et al. 1980). But even when the essential fatty acid deficiency is delayed to near weaning (wherein the essential fatty acid deficiency is less marked), there is a progressive inability to maintain alveolar and ductal structures of the mammary gland. A morphological example of this is presented in Figure 9 and a quantitation of the phenomenon is given in Figure 10. Animals on normal diets have an increase in the number of glandular alveoli present, which peaks around 16 weeks of age and then tends to level off. Animals on deficient diets also show an increased accumulation of

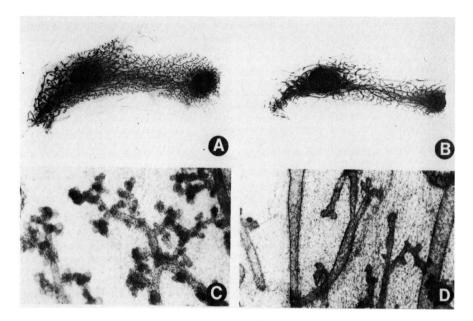

FIG. 9. Whole mounts of the fourth abdominal mammary glands of C3H/HeN mice on normal (A and C) or essential fatty acid-deficient diets (B and D). Animals were placed on the deficient diets at weaning and whole-mount preparations were made 18 weeks later. (Top, 4 ×; bottom, 55 ×.)

Note that the glands of animals on diets containing essential fatty acids had numerous, well-developed alveoli, while these structures were reduced in number and size in the glands of animals on essential fatty acid–free diets. In this latter group, the ducts were also distended and thinned.

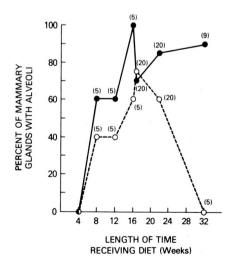

FIG. 10. Effect of essential fatty acid deficiency on the development of alveoli in mouse mammary glands. ●——●, normal diet; ○——○, deficient diets. Numbers in parentheses refer to the number of glands analyzed. (Reproduced from Knazek et al. 1980, with permission of *The Journal of the National Cancer Institute*.)

alveoli, peaking at about the same age, but the alveolar elements diminish rapidly thereafter until none are present in the glands at 32 weeks of age.

The major implication of this latter observation, so far as the role of lipids in breast cancer incidence is concerned, is that a dietary deficiency in essential fatty acids could reduce the number of mammary epithelial cells of the gland at risk for transformation. The nonarithmetic increase in carcinogen-induced mouse mammary tumors as a function of the amount of corn oil in the diet that Tannenbaum observed (1942) is indicative of a minimum requirement for essential fatty acids. This conclusion was also reached by Hopkins and Carroll (1979).

Obviously, the key question that needs to be answered is whether there is a further expansion of the mammary epithelial cell population with dietary essential fatty acid levels that exceed this minimum requirement. In experimental animals, such a quantitation is not an impossible task, especially with computerized scans of whole-mount mammary preparations. However, if mammary stem cells are especially affected by essential fatty acids and these are, as suspected, the prime targets of carcinogens, such a quantitation of total epithelium would be of limited value. At present we have no means of identifying, much less quantitating, mammary stem cells.

Dietary Fatty Acids Affect Prolactin Receptors

Most, if not all, hormones and growth factors are effectors of cell function only if the cells contain receptors for these factors. This is a unique way in which the specificity and control of tissue function are manifest in a multicellular organism. Since many of the cell's receptors are strategically located on cell membranes, it is not surprising that changes in membrane composition can alter the number, affinity, and functionality of such receptors. A classic example is adult-onset diabetes in which the functionality of the insulin receptor is impaired. This impairment is correlated with obesity, and the severity of the diabetic condition is lessened when the obese patient fasts.

Prolactin receptors are also sensitive to dietary factors. This hormone, by unknown mechanisms, induces its own receptors, but its ability to do so is dependent on sufficient levels of essential fatty acids in the diet (Knazek and Liu 1979). When animals on normal diets are treated with injections of prolactin, the number (but not the affinity) of prolactin-binding sites per unit of liver membrane protein is increased threefold to fourfold. In contrast, prolactin has little or no effect on the number of prolactin receptors in animals on essential fatty acid–deficient diets (Figure 11). These results indicate that the functionality of existing prolactin receptors is impaired in the essential fatty acid–deficient animal or that the ability of the cell to express new prolactin receptors is dependent on the availability (directly or indirectly) of essential fatty acids.

The fact that protein synthesis inhibitors do not block the ability of prolactin to induce its own receptor suggests that receptor expression results from changes

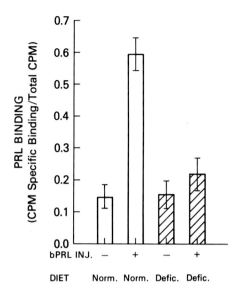

FIG. 11. Essential fatty acid dietary requirements for the maintenance and induction of prolactin receptors in mouse livers. The normal diets were the same composition as the deficient diets except for the substitution of corn oil for the medium chain triglyceride component of the deficient diets. The latter was free of essential fatty acids. Animals were begun on the diets 1–2 weeks after weaning. Prolactin (50 μg) or control vehicle was administered every 4 hours for 44 hours, after which liver membranes were prepared and assayed for prolactin receptor content. (Reproduced from Knazek et al. 1979, with permission of the Society for Experimental Biology and Medicine.)

in membrane composition, which lead to the exposure of cryptic receptors. Our studies have shown that prolactin (or drugs that stimulate prolactin release in animals) can change membrane phospholipid composition. Additionally, we have shown that a direct modification of membrane phospholipids, such as the methylation of phosphatidylethanolamine with endogenous membrane transmethylases and S-adenosylmethionine, increases the number of prolactin receptors (Bhattacharya and Vonderhaar 1980). Furthermore, prostaglandin I_2 has been found to increase the number of prolactin-binding sites on liver cell membranes in broken cell preparations. Changes in membrane composition were probably involved in this process, since membrane fluidity was increased in the prostaglandin-treated preparations (Dave and Knazek 1980). Further characterizations of membrane components in control vs. prolactin-treated cells will be needed to identify which membrane composition changes are physiologically important in the regulation of prolactin receptors and to what extent these changes are affected by dietary fat.

SUMMARY AND CONCLUSIONS

Excess fat in the diet is probably causally involved in the mammary tumorigenic process in humans. Since the process is fairly selective for tumors of the mammary gland, we have examined the role of fatty acids in the proliferation of mammary epithelium.

A combined in vivo–in vitro approach has led us to conclude that saturated fatty acids of membrane phospholipids are replaced by unsaturated fatty acids as a part of the proliferative response of the normal mammary epithelium to hormonal stimuli. The immediate source of the unsaturated fatty acid replacements appears to be the adjacent mammary adipocytes, which, upon a signal from the stimulated epithelium, release both saturated and unsaturated fatty acids. The epithelium then selectively takes up unsaturated fatty acids by some prolactin-dependent process.

The implication from these results is that an intimate relationship exists between lipid metabolism and prolactin action. This relationship is especially highlighted by the observation that essential fatty acids are required for the induction of prolactin receptors by prolactin. It is also suggested by the fact that the mammary glandular epithelium, a target tissue for prolactin, is exquisitely sensitive to essential fatty acid deficiencies. Further emphasis is provided by the ability of high-fat consumption to elevate serum prolactin levels (Chan et al. 1975, Wynder and Hill 1976, Ip et al. 1980).

We have emphasized the positive effect of unsaturated fatty acids on the rate of proliferation of normal and neoplastic mammary epithelium and the inhibitory effect of saturated fatty acids on this process. In view of this latter phenomenon, it is important to determine why high levels of saturated fatty acids in the diet can enhance mammary tumor formation in response to carcinogens (Hopkins and Carroll 1979) and why breast cancer mortality in humans correlates with total fat consumption but not with vegetable fat consumption (Carroll 1975).* Our results indicate that prolactin differentially stimulates the uptake of unsaturated fatty acids by the epithelium and that the inhibitory effect of saturated fatty acids on the growth of the epithelium is reversed by the addition of unsaturated fatty acids (Wicha et al. 1979). From the data of Hopkins and Carroll (1979), it appears that the ratio of saturated to unsaturated fatty acids in the diet can be as high as 6 to 1 and give the same tumor yield as diets in which this ratio is 1 to 10.

This seems to be a reflection of a threshold requirement for unsaturated fatty acids coupled with a high tolerance for these fatty acids above this threshold. This tolerance may be considered as a biological buffering system that effectively limits the availability of free fatty acids to the glandular epithelium. This buffering system also appears to be selective for unsaturated fatty acids, since the relative amounts of unsaturated vs. saturated fatty acids in mammary fat is increased in response to restricting food intake.

The shifting of the fatty acid buffering capacity of the mammary adipocyte to yield increased unsaturated fatty acid availability is apparently a physiological growth control mechanism. It follows then that dietary or environmental factors that shift this buffering equilibrium could affect the abundance of mammary epithelium at risk for transformation. They could also enhance the growth rate

---

* See, however, the report of Enig et al. (1978). These authors have reevaluated the dietary fat consumption trends in the U.S. and have concluded that the major change has been in the increased consumption of vegetable fat, which is higher in unsaturated than saturated fatty acids. Also indicated is the observation that animal fat consumption has dropped considerably during the last 60 years.

of already transformed mammary cells. It thus seems important to identify factors that affect this equilibrium.

ACKNOWLEDGMENT

We wish to thank Dr. Pietro Gullino for constant advice and encouragement during the course of these investigations and for critically reviewing the manuscript.

REFERENCES

Bailey, M. J., and L. M. Dunbar. 1973. Essential fatty acid requirements of cells in tissue culture. Exp. Mol. Pathol. 18:142–161.

Ben-David, M. 1968. Mechanism of induction of mammary differentiation in Sprague-Dawley female rats by perphenazine. Endocrinology 83:1217–1223.

Bhattacharya, A., and B. K. Vonderhaar. 1979. Thyroid hormone regulation of prolactin receptors of mouse mammary glands. Biochem. Biophys. Res. Commun. 88:1405–1411.

Bhattacharya, A., and B. K. Vonderhaar. 1980. Phospholipid methylation stimulates lactogenic hormone binding in mouse mammary gland membranes. Proc. Natl. Acad. Sci. USA 76:4489–4492.

Boutwell, R. K. 1978. Biochemical mechanisms of tumor promotion, *in* Mechanisms of Tumor Promotion and Carcinogenesis, T. J. Slaga, A. Sivak, and R. K. Boutwell, eds. Raven Press, New York, pp. 49–58.

Carroll, K. K. 1975. Experimental evidence of dietary factors and hormone dependent cancers. Cancer Res. 35:3374–3383.

Carroll, K. K., E. B. Gamal, and E. R. Plunkett. 1968. Dietary fat and mammary cancer. Can. Med. Assoc. J. 98:590–594.

Chan, P. C., and T. Dao. 1981. Enhancement of mammary carcinogenesis by a high fat diet in Fisher, Long-Evans and Sprague-Dawley rats. Cancer Res. 41:164–167.

Chan, P. C., F. Didato, and L. A. Cohen. 1975. High dietary fat, elevation of serum prolactin and mammary cancer. Proc. Soc. Exp. Biol. Med. 149:133–135.

Coleman, R. 1973. Membrane bound enzymes and membrane ultrastructure. Biochim. Biophys. Acta 300:1–30.

Dave, J. R., and R. A. Knazek. 1980. Prostaglandin I_2 modifies both prolactin binding capacity and fluidity of mouse liver membranes. Proc. Natl. Acad. Sci. USA 77:6597–6600.

DeOme, K. B., and L. Faulkin. 1959. Mammary tumor development from hyperplastic alveolar nodules and normal lobules transplanted into mammary gland-free fat pads and in the dorsal subcutis of female C3H mice. Proc. Am. Assoc. Cancer Res. 3:16–17.

Desombre, E., and E. Jensen. 1980. Estrophilin assays in breast cancer. Cancer 46:2783–2788.

Dewaard, F. 1969. The epidemiology of breast cancer: Review and prospects. Int. J. Cancer 4:577–586.

Enig, M. R., R. J. Munn, and M. Keeny. 1978. Dietary fat and cancer trends—a critique. Fed. Proc. 37:2215–2220.

Hill, P., and E. Wynder. 1976. Diet and prolactin release. Lancet 2:806–807.

Hirayama, T. 1978. Epidemiology of breast cancer with reference to the role of the diet. Prev. Med. 7:173–195.

Hopkins, G. J., and K. K. Carroll. 1979. Relationship between amount and type of dietary fat in promotion of mammary carcinomas induced by DMBA. JNCI 62:1009–1012.

Hopkins, G. J., C. E. West, and G. C. Hard. 1976. Effect of dietary fats on the incidence of 7,12-dimethylbenz(α)anthracene-induced tumors in rats. Lipids 4:328–333.

Horwitz, A. F., M. E. Hatten, and M. M. Burger. 1974. Membrane fatty acid replacements and their effect on growth and lectin-induced agglutinability. Proc. Natl. Acad. Sci. USA 71:3115–3119.

Hoshino, K. 1962. Morphogenesis and growth potentiality of mammary glands in mice. JNCI 29:835–851.

Ip, C., P. Yip, and L. Bernardis. 1980. Role of prolactin in the promotion of DMBA-induced mammary tumors by dietary fat. Cancer Res. 40:374–378.

Janss, D. H., R. C. Moon, and C. C. Irving. 1972. The binding of 7,12-DMBA to mammary parenchyma DNA and protein in vivo. Cancer Res. 32:254–262.

Kaduce, T. L., A. B. Awad, L. J. Fontenelle, and A. A. Spector. 1977. Effect of fatty acid saturation on the transport of α-aminobutyric acid in Ehrlich ascites cells. J. Biol. Chem. 252:6624–6630.

Kidwell, W. R., M. E. Monaco, W. S. Wicha, and G. S. Smith. 1978. Unsaturated fatty acid requirements for the growth and survival of a rat mammary tumor cell line. Cancer Res. 38:4091–4100.

Kidwell, W. R., W. S. Wicha, D. Salomon, and L. A. Liotta. 1980. Differential recognition of basement membrane collagen by normal and neoplastic mammary cells, in Cell Biology of Breast Cancer, M. Brennan, C. M. McGrath, and M. Rich, eds. Academic Press, New York, pp. 17–33.

Knazek, R. A., and S. C. Liu. 1979. Dietary essential fatty acids are required for the maintenance and induction of prolactin receptors. Proc. Soc. Biol. Med. 162:346–350.

Knazek, R. A., S. C. Liu, J. S. Bodwin, and B. K. Vonderhaar. 1980. Requirement of essential fatty acids in the diet for the development of the mouse mammary gland. JNCI 64:377–382.

Lea, A. J. 1966. Dietary factors associated with death-rates from certain neoplasms in man. Lancet 2:332–333.

Masuno, H., N. Yamasaki, and H. Okuda. 1981. Purification and characterization of the lipolytic factor (toxohormone-L) from cell free fluid from ascites sarcoma 180. Cancer Res. 41:284–288.

Nishizuka, Y. 1978. Biological influence of fat intake on mammary cancer and mammary tissue: Experimental correlates. Prev. Med. 7:218–224.

Rao, G. A., and S. Abraham. 1976a. Stearoyl-CoA desaturase activity in mammary adenocarcinomas carried by C3H mice. Lipids 10:835–839.

Rao, G. A., and S. Abraham. 1976b. Enhanced growth rate of transplantable mammary adenocarcinomas induced in C3H mice by dietary lineolate. JNCI 56:431–432.

Rothblatt, G. H., L. Y. Abrogast, L. Oulette, and B. V. Howard. 1976. Preparation of delipidized serum for use in cell culture systems. In Vitro 12:554–557.

Shinitzky, M., and B. Rivnay. 1977. Degree of exposure of membrane proteins determined by fluorescence quenching. Biochemistry 16:982–986.

Stampfer, M., R. C. Hallowes, and A. J. Hackett. 1980. Growth of normal human mammary cells in culture. In Vitro 16:415–425.

Tannenbaum, A. 1942. The genesis and growth of tumors. III. Effects of a high fat diet. Cancer Res. 2:49–53.

Warren, L. 1974. Isolation of plasma membranes from tissue culture L cells. Methods Enzymol. 31:156–162.

Wicha, M. S., L. A. Liotta, and W. R. Kidwell. 1979. Effects of free fatty acids on the growth of normal and neoplastic rat mammary epithelial cells. Cancer Res. 39:426–435.

Wynder, E. L. 1968. Current concepts of the aetiology of breast cancer, in Prognostic Factors in Breast Cancer, Proceedings of the First Tenovus Symposium. Livingston, Edinburgh, pp. 32–49.

Wynder, E. L. 1979. Dietary habits and cancer epidemiology. Cancer 43:1955–1961.

Wynder, E., and P. Hill. 1976. Diet and prolactin release. Lancet 2:806–807.

Molecular Interrelations of Nutrition and Cancer,
edited by M. S. Arnott, J. van Eys and Y.-M. Wang.
Raven Press, New York © 1982.

The Role of Lipids in Tumorigenesis

Kenneth K. Carroll and Martha B. Davidson

Department of Biochemistry, University of Western Ontario,
London, Ontario, Canada N6A 5C1

There is now abundant experimental evidence showing that animals fed high-fat diets develop mammary tumors and intestinal tumors more readily than those fed low-fat diets under comparable conditions (Carroll 1980, Reddy et al. 1980). Although evidence relating dietary fat to tumorigenesis has been accumulating since 1930 (Tannenbaum 1959), it has only recently stimulated widespread interest in the scientific community. This interest stems largely from the realization that in human populations mortality from cancer at sites such as breast and colon also shows a strong positive correlation with the amount of fat available for consumption (Carroll 1980, Reddy et al. 1980). Increasing numbers of scientists are therefore beginning to study this relationship with the hope that a better understanding of the effects of dietary fat on tumorigenesis can be applied to the prevention and treatment of cancer in humans.

This article will deal with some of the information that has been obtained in experiments with animals and will include a discussion of mechanisms by which dietary fat may influence tumorigenesis.

EFFECTS OF DIFFERENT TYPES OF DIETARY FAT

In the earlier studies on enhancement by high-fat diets of mammary tumorigenesis in animals, a number of different kinds of fat were used, but it was not possible from those studies to assess the relative effectiveness of different types of dietary fat (Carroll and Khor 1975). The first experiment carried out in our laboratory on dietary fat in relation to mammary tumors induced in rats by 7,12-dimethylbenz(α)anthracene (DMBA) showed that a diet containing 20% by weight of corn oil markedly increased the number of tumors compared to diets containing 20% coconut oil or 0.5% corn oil (Gammal et al. 1967). Subsequent studies with a variety of different dietary fats and oils showed that polyunsaturated fats were generally more effective than fats containing mainly saturated and monounsaturated fatty acids (Carroll and Khor 1971).

The ability of any particular fat or oil to increase the tumor yield did not, however, seem to be directly proportional to its content of polyunsaturated

fatty acids. Olive oil, for example, was as effective as some of the more polyunsaturated oils, while rapeseed oil had little or no effect, in spite of its relatively
high degree of unsaturation. The rapeseed oil used in this case had a high
content of erucic acid, and a subsequent experiment with rapeseed oil having
a high oleic and low erucic acid content showed that it was at least as effective
as other polyunsaturated oils (Carroll 1977). In another study, Dayton et al.
(1977) found no marked differences in the number of mammary tumors induced
by DMBA in rats fed a high-oleic safflower oil from a mutant variety, compared
to the normal high-linoleic safflower oil.

More recent studies in our laboratory appear to have provided at least a
partial explanation for these somewhat puzzling observations (Hopkins and Carroll 1979). These experiments confirmed our earlier findings that 20% saturated-
fat diets (coconut oil or beef tallow) produced no increase in the number of
mammary tumors that developed in rats treated with DMBA, compared to a
low-fat diet (3% sunflower-seed oil). However, when sunflower-seed oil was
used to replace 3% of the coconut oil or tallow in the diets containing 20%
saturated fat, the rats developed more than twice as many tumors following
treatment with DMBA, and the tumor yields were comparable to that obtained
by feeding a diet containing 20% sunflower-seed oil (Figure 1).

In another experiment (Hopkins et al. 1981), the tumor yield was also markedly
enhanced by using ethyl linoleate to replace 3% of the fat in a 20% coconut
oil diet, whereas it was not increased by using 3% ethyl oleate as replacement.
The effect did not seem to be specific for linoleate, however, since menhaden
oil, a fish oil containing polyunsaturated fatty acids belonging mainly to the
linolenate family, appeared to be about as effective as ethyl linoleate (Hopkins
et al. 1981).

These observations on mixtures of dietary fats appear to be compatible with
epidemiological data on breast cancer mortality in humans in relation to dietary
fat (Carroll 1980). In most countries, the fat available for consumption would
probably provide amounts of polyunsaturated fatty acids equivalent to at least
2% linoleate, and the results of our experiments suggest that, in the animal
model, larger amounts of linoleate have no additional effect on tumor yield.
As illustrated in Figure 1, rats fed 3% sunflower-seed oil (equivalent to about
2% linoleate), together with either 17% coconut oil or 17% beef tallow, developed at least as many tumors as those fed 20% sunflower-seed oil.

These experiments also indicated that a high-fat diet is required in addition
to a minimum amount of polyunsaturated fat to produce an increase in tumor
yield. This can be seen by comparing results with the low-fat diet containing
3% sunflower-seed oil to those with the high-fat diets containing 17% coconut
oil or tallow in addition to 3% sunflower-seed oil (Figure 1). It was not clear
from these experiments, however, whether the two requirements are separate
or interrelated. An attempt was therefore made to obtain more information
bearing on this question by a further experiment with diets containing 10%
fat. The results are illustrated in Figure 2.

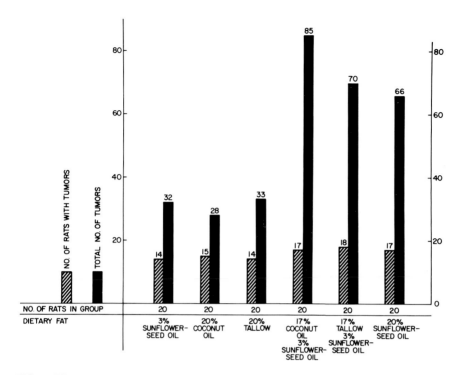

FIG. 1. Effects of type and level of dietary fat on development of mammary tumors in female Sprague-Dawley rats treated with DMBA. The rats were maintained on Purina Chow and were given 5 mg of DMBA in 0.5 ml of sesame oil by stomach tube at 50 days of age. One week later they were transferred to semipurified diets containing the fats indicated. The rats were killed and autopsied 4 months after receiving the DMBA. Both palpable and nonpalpable tumors are included in the results shown. (Reproduced from Carroll and Hopkins 1979 by permission of *Lipids*.)

Rats fed a diet containing 10% sunflower-seed oil developed nearly as many tumors after treatment with DMBA as rats fed a diet containing 20% sunflower-seed oil, whereas the animals fed a diet containing 7% coconut oil with 3% sunflower-seed oil showed no increase in tumor yield over those fed 3% sunflower-seed oil alone. A diet containing 10% coconut oil produced fewer tumors than the low-fat diet. These results contrast with those obtained with the mixture of 17% coconut oil and 3% sunflower-seed oil compared to 20% sunflower-seed oil (Figure 1). They suggest that as the level of fat in the diet decreases, the proportion of polyunsaturated fat must be increased in order to produce an increase in tumor yield. This is an indication that the two requirements are interrelated.

In our experiments, no attempt was made to determine the limiting amount of polyunsaturated fat required to produce the full effect on tumor yield by a diet containing 20% fat. However, 3% sunflower-seed oil may be close to the

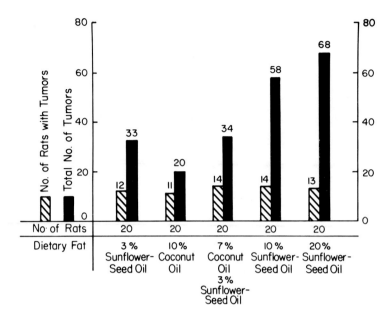

FIG. 2. Effects of type and level of dietary fat on development of mammary tumors in female Sprague-Dawley rats treated with DMBA. Experimental conditions were as described for Figure 1, except that the DMBA was given in olive oil.

limit, since King et al. (1979) reported that in rats treated with DMBA a diet containing 18% stripped, hydrogenated coconut oil and 2% linoleic acid gave a lower tumor yield than a diet containing 20% stripped corn oil.

Our studies with rapeseed oil are also of interest in relation to possible interactions between essential fatty acids and other dietary fat. The failure of high erucic rapeseed oil to increase the yield of mammary tumors, in spite of its relatively high content of linoleate, may be due to an effect of erucic acid on the distribution or metabolism of essential fatty acids. Earlier experiments in our laboratory provided evidence of reproductive disturbances reminiscent of essential fatty acid deficiency in rats fed erucic acid (Carroll and Noble 1957). These experiments also showed that postpartum development of the mammary gland and lactation were impaired by erucic acid.

There are some indications in the literature that effects of dietary fat on tumors at sites other than the mammary gland may likewise be influenced by the type as well as the level of dietary fat. Reddy et al. (1976, 1980) observed that intestinal tumors induced by 1,2-dimethylhydrazine developed more readily in rats fed 5% corn oil compared to those fed 5% lard, although both fats were equally effective at the 20% level. Roebuck et al. (1980) recently reported that a high level of unsaturated fat in the diet promoted pancreatic cancer induced in rats by azaserine, whereas saturated fat was ineffective.

MECHANISMS BY WHICH DIETARY FAT MAY INFLUENCE CARCINOGENESIS

The effect of dietary fat on tumorigenesis can be observed with spontaneous tumors, as well as with tumors induced by a variety of different agents. The latter include mammary tumors induced by chemical agents such as stilbestrol, acetylaminofluorene, DMBA, and N-nitrosomethylurea (Carroll 1980) or by exposure to X-irradiation (Silverman et al. 1980), and intestinal tumors induced by azoxymethane, 1,2-dimethylhydrazine, methylnitrosourea, or methylazoxymethanol acetate (Reddy et al. 1980). Furthermore, the effect can be demonstrated for chemically induced tumors by feeding the high-fat diet only after treatment with the carcinogen (Carroll and Khor 1975, Bull et al. 1979). These observations suggest that dietary fat acts as a promoter rather than affecting initiation of tumors.

Other studies also lend support to the idea that dietary fat affects the promotional stage of carcinogenesis. The work of Abraham and his associates (Rao and Abraham 1976, Hillyard and Abraham 1979) and that of Hopkins and West (1977) have shown that the growth and development of transplantable mammary tumors can be influenced by dietary fat. King et al. (1979) found that mammary tumors induced by DMBA also grew at a much faster rate in rats fed high-fat diets compared to those fed a low-fat diet.

Assuming that the effects of dietary fat are exerted at the promotional stage of carcinogenesis, there are still many ways in which the effect could be mediated (Reddy et al. 1980). In considering possible mechanisms, it should be kept in mind that dietary fat appears to affect only some types of tumors, whereas caloric restriction seems to have a general inhibitory effect on all types of tumors for which it has been investigated (Carroll and Khor 1975). It does not seem likely, therefore, that dietary fat influences tumorigenesis simply by serving as a nutritional source of calories.

Since the endocrine system plays an important role in mammary carcinogenesis, it is not surprising that attempts have been made to explain the effects of dietary fat on mammary tumors in terms of hormonal balance. Chan and Cohen (1975) suggested that high fat intake may enhance growth and development of normal and neoplastic mammary gland tissue by increasing the prolactin:estrogen ratio, but more recent studies have cast some doubt on this hypothesis (Cave et al. 1979, Ip et al. 1980, Hopkins et al. 1981). However, this does not preclude the possibility that the fat effect is mediated by endocrine effects. For example, high-fat diets may alter prolactin or estrogen receptors in the mammary gland and thus influence the availability of these hormones to the glandular cells.

It has been suggested that dietary fat enhances the development of intestinal tumors by increasing the concentration of bile acids in the intestinal contents. This idea is supported by animal studies showing that bile acids can act as tumor promoters when administered intrarectally (Reddy et al. 1980). Furthermore, it has been observed that feeding cholestyramine to rats treated with azoxymethane or surgically diverting bile to the middle of their small intestines increases the yield of intestinal tumors in them (Nigro et al. 1973, Chomchai et al. 1974).

Polyunsaturated fatty acids and prostaglandins are both capable of inhibiting certain immune functions (Meade and Mertin 1978, Vitale and Broitman 1981, Pelus and Strausser 1977), and it is possible that effects of dietary fat on tumorigenesis are mediated by the immune system (Hopkins and West 1976). Polyunsaturated fatty acids have also been found to stimulate the activity of guanylate cyclase, which catalyzes the synthesis of cyclic guanidine monophosphate (cGMP) (Goldberg and Haddox 1977, Murad et al. 1979). Since elevated concentrations of cGMP are consistent with this cyclic nucleotide's playing a role in cellular proliferation (Zeilig and Goldberg 1977), this stimulation represents another mechanism by which dietary fat may influence tumorigenesis.

Effects such as those on immune responses or on cGMP could very well be related to changes in the composition of cellular membranes brought about by dietary fat. Preliminary studies in our laboratory on the fatty acid composition of mammary tissue lipids in rats fed different types of dietary fat provided some evidence of a correlation between the degree of unsaturation of mammary tissue phospholipids and susceptibility to mammary tumorigenesis in rats treated with DMBA (Hopkins et al. 1981). This was of interest because phospholipids would be expected to be concentrated primarily in cellular membranes. Further studies along these lines were therefore carried out to obtain more information on the effects of dietary fat on the phospholipid fatty acid composition of rat mammary tissue.

For these experiments, rats were fed diets containing 3% sunflower-seed oil, 20% coconut oil, a mixture of 17% coconut oil and 3% sunflower-seed oil, or 20% sunflower-seed oil. In rats killed after 1, 2, or 3 months on diet, the degree of unsaturation of the phospholipid fatty acids was not consistently higher in animals fed the last two diets, as would be expected if there were a positive correlation between fatty acid unsaturation and susceptibility to mammary tumorigenesis (Figure 1). In another experiment, rats were killed after 4 months on the above diets, and the different phospholipid classes of the mammary gland were separated by thin-layer chromatography (Touchstone et al. 1980) prior to fatty acid analysis by gas-liquid chromatography. The fatty acids of the individual phospholipid classes again failed to show consistently higher unsaturation indices in rats fed the diets containing 20% sunflower-seed oil or the mixture of 17% coconut oil and 3% sunflower-seed oil.

Hillyard et al. (1980) studied the effect of dietary fat on the fatty acid composition of transplantable mouse and rat mammary adenocarcinomas. In their experiments, the rate of tumor growth could not be correlated with the levels of arachidonic acid in all murine mammary adenocarcinomas. Furthermore, linoleate added to the diet in amounts sufficient to enhance tumor growth in mice had little effect on the fatty acid composition of tumor lipids. In spite of these findings, it is still possible that dietary fat affects tumorigenesis by altering the fatty acid composition of specific membranes such as the plasma membrane. Another possibility is that the effects of dietary fat on tumorigenesis are mediated by prostaglandins or other biologically active compounds formed from polyunsaturated fatty acids (Hillyard and Abraham 1979, Hillyard et al. 1980).

LIMITING FACTORS IN TUMORIGENESIS

Until recently, most of the emphasis in cancer research has been placed on factors involved in tumor initiation. However, the concepts of tumor promotion (Berenblum 1979) and progression (Foulds 1969) have led to the view that cancer develops in stages, with initiation being only the first step of the process. Thus, the limiting factors in tumorigenesis are not necessarily those that control initiation. The course of events following initiation depends on the inherent characteristics of the initiated cell and on local environmental conditions, which determine whether the cell survives and how rapidly it proliferates.

It is clear from experiments with transplantable tumor cells that appreciable numbers of such cells can be injected into animals without any tumors appearing. As larger numbers of tumor cells are injected, the likelihood of a tumor developing increases, and beyond a certain point, this likelihood becomes almost a certainty. However, with exposure to intermediate numbers of cells, the result can be influenced by other factors, such as dietary fat (Hopkins and West 1977). Similar considerations evidently apply to tumor cells formed in situ by interaction with a carcinogenic agent. The tumor yield is clearly a function of the dose of carcinogen, but the results can also be influenced by dietary fat over a range of exposure to the carcinogenic stimulus (Carroll and Khor 1970).

If an initiated cell survives, it may remain dormant for a time, or it may proliferate for a limited period and then cell division may cease because of lack of nutrients or other adverse conditions. In some circumstances, the constant stimulus of a promoting agent may be required for continued growth. Thus, tumors do not always grow at a steady rate, and if tumor cells begin to die at a faster rate than new ones are formed by cell division, the tumor will inevitably regress.

Because of the multiplicity of factors that can initiate tumor cells, and the widespread occurrence of such factors, concentration on tumor initiation does not necessarily represent the best approach to prevention of tumorigenesis. Another possibility is to investigate factors, such as dietary fat, that appear to influence the promotional stage of tumorigenesis. A better understanding of the mechanisms by which such factors exert their effects may suggest new and better ways of preventing or inhibiting tumor development.

ACKNOWLEDGMENTS

This work was supported by the National Cancer Institute of Canada. Dr. Carroll is a Career Investigator of the Medical Research Council of Canada. Martha Davidson is the recipient of an Ontario Graduate Fellowship. Diana

Girard's technical assistance with original work reported in this article is gratefully acknowledged.

REFERENCES

Berenblum, I. 1979. Theoretical and practical aspects of the two-stage mechanism of carcinogenesis, *in* Carcinogens: Identification and Mechanisms of Action (Proceedings of The University of Texas System Cancer Center 31st Annual Symposium on Fundamental Cancer Research, 1978) A. C. Griffin and C. R. Shaw, eds. Raven Press, New York, pp. 25–36.

Bull, A. W., B. K. Soullier, P. S. Wilson, M. T. Hayden, and N. D. Nigro. 1979. Promotion of azoxymethane-induced intestinal cancer by high-fat diet in rats. Cancer Res. 39:4956–4959.

Carroll, K. K. 1977. Dietary factors in hormone-dependent cancers. Curr. Concepts Nutr. 6:25–40.

Carroll, K. K. 1980. Lipids and carcinogenesis. J. Environ. Pathol. Toxicol. 3(4):253–271.

Carroll, K. K., and G. J. Hopkins. 1979. Dietary polyunsaturated fat versus saturated fat in relation to mammary carcinogenesis. Lipids 14:155–158.

Carroll, K. K., and H. T. Khor. 1970. Effects of dietary fat and dose level of 7,12-dimethylbenz(α)anthracene on mammary tumor incidence in rats. Cancer Res. 30:2260–2264.

Carroll, K. K., and H. T. Khor. 1971. Effects of level and type of dietary fat on incidence of mammary tumors induced in female Sprague-Dawley rats by 7,12-dimethylbenz(α)anthracene. Lipids 6:415–420.

Carroll, K. K., and H. T. Khor. 1975. Dietary fat in relation to tumorigenesis. Progr. Biochem. Pharmacol. 10:308–353.

Carroll, K. K., and R. L. Noble. 1957. Influence of a dietary supplement of erucic acid and other fatty acids on fertility in the rat. Sterility caused by erucic acid. Can. J. Biochem. Physiol. 35:1093–1105.

Cave, W. T., Jr., J. T. Dunn, and R. M. MacLeod. 1979. Effects of iodine deficiency and high-fat diet on N-nitrosomethylurea-induced mammary cancers in rats. Cancer Res. 39:729–734.

Chan, P.-C., and L. A. Cohen. 1975. Dietary fat and growth promotion of rat mammary tumors. Cancer Res. 35:3384–3386.

Chomchai, C., N. Bhadrachari, and N. D. Nigro. 1974. The effect of bile on the induction of experimental intestinal tumors in rats. Dis. Colon Rectum 17:310–312.

Dayton, S., S. Hashimoto, and J. Wollman. 1977. Effects of high-oleic and high-linoleic safflower oils on mammary tumors induced in rats by 7,12-dimethylbenz(α)anthracene. J. Nutr. 107:1353–1360.

Foulds, L. 1969. Neoplastic Development, Vol. 1. Academic Press, New York.

Gammal, E. B., K. K. Carroll, and E. R. Plunkett. 1967. Effects of dietary fat on mammary carcinogenesis by 7,12-dimethylbenz(α)anthracene in rats. Cancer Res. 27:1737–1742.

Goldberg, N. D., and M. K. Haddox. 1977. Cyclic GMP metabolism and involvement in biological regulation. Annu. Rev. Biochem. 46:823–896.

Hillyard, L. A., and S. Abraham. 1979. Effect of dietary polyunsaturated fatty acids on growth of mammary adenocarcinomas in mice and rats. Cancer Res. 39:4430–4437.

Hillyard, L., G. A. Rao, and S. Abraham. 1980. Effect of dietary fat on fatty acid composition of mouse and rat mammary adenocarcinomas. Proc. Soc. Exp. Biol. Med. 163:376–383.

Hopkins, G. J., and K. K. Carroll. 1979. Relationship between amount and type of dietary fat in promotion of mammary carcinogenesis induced by 7,12-dimethylbenz(a)anthracene. JNCI 62:1009–1012.

Hopkins, G. J., and C. E. West. 1976. Possible roles of dietary fats in carcinogenesis. Life Sci. 19:1103–1116.

Hopkins, G. J., and C. E. West. 1977. Effect of dietary polyunsaturated fat on the growth of a transplantable adenocarcinoma in C3HA^vyfB mice. JNCI 58:753–756.

Hopkins, G. J., T. G. Kennedy, and K. K. Carroll. 1981. Polyunsaturated fatty acids as promoters of mammary carcinogenesis induced in rats by 7,12-dimethylbenz(a)anthracene. JNCI 66:517–522.

Ip, C., P. Yip, and L. L. Bernardis. 1980. Role of prolactin in the promotion of dimethylbenz(a)anthracene-induced mammary tumors by dietary fat. Cancer Res. 40:374–378.

King, M. M., D. M. Bailey, D. D. Gibson, J. V. Pitha, and P. B. McCay. 1979. Incidence and growth of mammary tumors induced by 7,12-dimethylbenz(a)anthracene as related to the dietary content of fat and antioxidant. JNCI 63:657–663.

Meade, C. J., and J. Mertin. 1978. Fatty acids and immunity. Adv. Lipid Res. 16:127–165.

Murad, F., W. P. Arnold, C. K. Mittal, and J. M. Braughler. 1979. Properties and regulation of guanylate cyclase and some proposed functions for cyclic GMP. Adv. Cyclic Nucleotide Res. 11:175–204.

Nigro, N. D., N. Bhadrachari, and C. Chomchai. 1973. A rat model for studying colonic cancer: Effect of cholestyramine on induced tumors. Dis. Colon Rectum 16:438–443.

Pelus, L. M., and H. R. Strausser. 1977. Prostaglandins and the immune response. Life Sci. 20:903–914.

Rao, G. A., and S. Abraham. 1976. Enhanced growth rate of transplanted mammary adenocarcinoma induced in C3H mice by dietary linoleate. JNCI 56:431–432.

Reddy, B. S., L. A. Cohen, G. D. McCoy, P. Hill, J. H. Weisburger, and E. L. Wynder. 1980. Nutrition and its relationship to cancer. Adv. Cancer Res. 32:237–345.

Reddy, B. S., T. Narisawa, D. Vukusich, J. H. Weisburger, and E. L. Wynder. 1976. Effect of quality and quantity of dietary fat and dimethylhydrazine in colon carcinogenesis in rats. Proc. Soc. Exp. Biol. Med. 151:237–239.

Roebuck, B. D., J. D. Yager, Jr., and D. S. Longnecker. 1980. Dietary promotion of azaserine induced pancreatic carcinogenesis. Proc. Am. Assoc. Cancer Res. 21:109.

Silverman, J., C. J. Shellabarger, S. Holtzman, J. P. Stone, and J. H. Weisburger. 1980. Effect of dietary fat on X-ray-induced mammary cancer in Sprague-Dawley rats. JNCI 64:631–634.

Tannenbaum, A. 1959. Nutrition and cancer, *in* The Physiopathology of Cancer, F. Homburger, ed., 2nd Ed. Hoeber-Harper, New York, pp. 517–562.

Touchstone, J. C., J. C. Chen, and K. M. Beaver. 1980. Improved separation of phospholipids in thin layer chromatography. Lipids 15:61–62.

Vitale, J. J. and S. A. Broitman. 1981. Lipids and immune function. Cancer Res. 41:3706–3710.

Zeilig, C. E., and N. D. Goldberg. 1977. Cell-cycle-related changes of 3'5'-cyclic GMP levels in Novikoff hepatoma cells. Proc. Natl. Acad. Sci. USA 74:1052–1056.

Nutritional Modulation of Cell Proliferation

Molecular Interrelations of Nutrition and Cancer,
edited by M. S. Arnott, J. van Eys and Y.-M. Wang.
Raven Press, New York © 1982.

The Role of Nutrients in Control of Normal and Malignant Cell Growth

Wallace L. McKeehan

W. Alton Jones Cell Science Center, Lake Placid, New York 12946

Malignancy seems . . . to consist in a change in the mode of alimentation of the cells . . . conception of the malignant cell . . . should be . . . based on the nutritional properties of each cell type. Carrel (1929).

The proliferation of unicellular organisms such as bacteria and yeast is controlled by the availability of nutrients in the external environment. Survival of unicellular organisms is dependent on the ability of cells to adapt and proliferate within their available and often unpredictable nutritive environment. When the nutrient supply is adequate, cells proliferate until the nutrient supply or the available space becomes limiting to further proliferation. The specialization of individual cells and the evolution of multicellular organisms require that the proliferation of different cell types occur only on demand in the interest of the organism.

HYPOTHESIS: NUTRIENT REQUIREMENTS AS CONTROLLING FACTORS OF CELL PROLIFERATION

To alleviate the vagaries of the nutritional environment, multicellular organisms have evolved a system for distribution of nutrients that maintains a relatively similar and constant supply of nutrients to the cells of the organism. Despite this favorable condition for proliferation, the growth of many individual cell types within an organism is restrained and only occurs on the demand of distal signals such as hormones or spatial disruptions in the tissue (i.e., wounding). One hypothesis to account for this restraint is that specialized nutrient requirements evolved concurrently with cellular specialization and the external nutrient supply such that the normal extracellular concentration of nutrients is suboptimal and limiting for cell proliferation. Unique plasma membrane permeability properties, intracellular compartmentalization of the access of nutrients to key metabolic processes, and specialized metabolic requirements for nutrients determine cell nutrient requirements. These barriers to cell proliferation are altered on demand by external messengers such that the external nutrient supply is transiently optimal for cell proliferation until the external signal is removed. An abnormal and potentially malignant situation arises when the external nutrient supply is constitutively optimal for proliferation. This can occur due to the abnormal, continued presence of the external growth signal, or a constitutive alteration in permeability barriers, or metabolic patterns that determine the cell nutrient requirements for proliferation.

NUTRIENT AND SERUM GROWTH FACTOR REQUIREMENTS FOR PROLIFERATION OF NORMAL AND TRANSFORMED FIBROBLASTS IN CULTURE

Kinetic Analysis

The proliferation of isolated cells in culture, released from restrictions imposed by tissue and the organism, can be controlled by manipulation of both nutrients and macromolecular growth regulatory factors in the environment (McKeehan and McKeehan 1981). We have borrowed the principles of enzyme kinetic analysis to quantitate the relationship between the level of nutrients and growth factors in the medium to the multiplication rate of normal human diploid fibroblasts. An experimental system was designed in which (1) all defined nutrient concentrations and other environmental conditions were optimal for cell survival and multiplication (Ham and McKeehan 1979; McKeehan et al. 1978), and (2) an exponential increase in the cell population could be determined in near steady-state conditions when multiplication was stimulated by nonnutritive macromolecular growth factors from fetal bovine serum (McKeehan and McKeehan 1981). The multiplication rate responded to an increase in the concentration of individual nutrient or macromolecular serum factors in a manner characteristic of a dissociable, saturable interaction between cells and the nutrient. A plot of multiplication rate versus nutrient concentration or serum factors yielded the rectangular hyperbola that is described by the Henri-Michaelis-Menten equa-

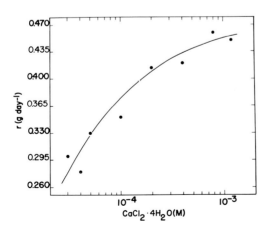

FIG. 1. Multiplication rate of normal human lung fibroblasts as a function of increasing $CaCl_2 \cdot 4H_2O$ concentration. Clonal multiplication of 100 cells was analyzed in $CaCl_2 \cdot 4H_2O$-deficient medium MCDB 105 (McKeehan et al. 1978) containing 500 μg per ml FBSP with the indicated levels of $CaCl_2 \cdot 4H_2O$ added to the medium. The data were fitted to a single rectangular hyperbola. Multiplication rate is expressed in cell generations (g) per day. (Reproduced from McKeehan and McKeehan 1980b.)

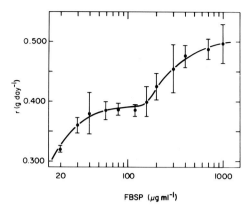

FIG. 2. Effect of serum growth factors on rate of multiplication of normal cells. The indicated concentrations of FBSP (see Figure 1) were added to the medium containing 100 cells. A right rectangular hyperbola was fitted to data from 20 to 120 μg per ml and another to the data for 175 to 1,000 μg FBSP per ml. (Reproduced from McKeehan and McKeehan 1981, with permission of Alan R. Liss, Inc.)

tion, as the response changed from first-order, to mixed-order, to zero-order kinetics (Figures 1,2). Linearization and regression analysis of the data yielded the kinetic parameters $S_{0.50}$ and R_{max} that relate the external nutrient or serum factor concentration to the multiplication rate of the cell population (Figures 3,4). The $S_{0.50}$ value is the concentration of nutrient or growth factor that promotes a half-maximal rate of cell multiplication. R_{max} is the maximal rate of proliferation of the cell population under the condition.

Normal Human Lung Fibroblasts

Table 1 summarizes the $S_{0.50}$ values for serum factors and nutrients for normal human lung fibroblasts (N-HLF). The multiplication response of N-HLF to fetal bovine serum factors (FBSP) was so clearly biphasic that the response was dissected into hyperbolic regions and two $S_{0.50}$ values were assigned (Figures 2,4). In contrast, the multiplication response of N-HLF to most nutrients was fitted to a single hyperbola, and a single $S_{0.50}$ value was assigned (Figures 1,3).

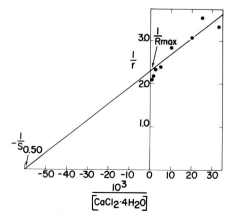

FIG. 3. Double-reciprocal plot of multiplication rate versus $CaCl_2 \cdot 4H_2O$ concentration. The best linear plot was fitted to the data from Figure 1 by least squares estimate. Regression to the intercepts yielded an $S_{0.50}$ value of 1.7×10^{-5} M and a R_{max} value of 0.444 g day^{-1}. (Reproduced from McKeehan and McKeehan 1980b.)

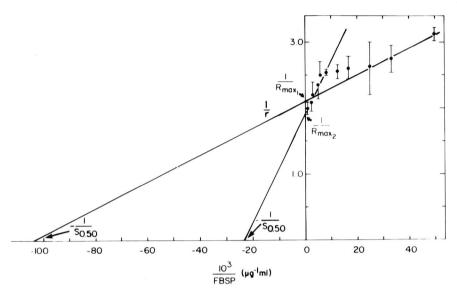

FIG. 4. Double-reciprocal (Lineweaver-Burk) transformation of multiplication rate of normal cells versus serum factor concentration. The data from Figure 2 were transformed to $1/r$ and 10^3 ml μg^{-1}/FBSP. Since the data in Figure 2 are clearly biphasic, two linear plots were fitted to the data by least squares estimate. Regression of both plots yielded two sets of kinetic parameters. The ordinate intercepts yielded the maximal growth rate ($1/R_{max}$) possible under the condition. The abscissa intercepts yielded the FBSP concentration ($S_{0.50}$) where multiplication rate was half-maximal ($R_{max}/2$). The kinetic parameters for the data were $S_{0.50}$ = 9.7 μg ml^{-1}, R_{max} = 0.475 g day^{-1} for the first phase response, and $S_{0.50}$ = 43.1 μg ml^{-1} = 0.520 g day^{-1} for the second phase of the response. (From McKeehan and McKeehan 1981, with permission of Alan R. Liss, Inc.)

$S_{0.50}$ values for amino acids ranged from 5.6 nM for tryptophan to 16 μM for glycine. The average $S_{0.50}$ value for essential amino acids was 4 μM. Cellular synthesis of alanine, aspartic acid, asparagine, glutamic acid, and proline was sufficient to support a maximal rate of multiplication, and no external requirement could be demonstrated. The multiplication response to water-soluble vitamins, trace elements (other than Fe and Se ions), H^+, Na^+, Cl^-, SO_4^{2-}, HCO_3^-, CO_2, and O_2 was insufficient for kinetic analysis, or the data did not fit the Michaelis-Menten equation.

Differences Between Requirements for Growth of Normal and Virally Transformed Human Lung Fibroblasts

Following infection of cultured normal human fibroblasts with SV40 virus, continuous cell lines evolve that exhibit multiple phenotypic properties that are associated with malignant cells in vivo (Girardi et al. 1966, Kahn and Shin 1979). Using SV40-transformed cells (SV-HLF) as a malignant cell prototype,

TABLE 1. $S_{0.50}$ values for multiplication of normal and transformed human lung fibroblasts*

Nutrient	N-HLF	SV-HLF
Arg	1.5($\pm$ 0.56)E-6	1.3($\pm$ 0.28)E-6
Cys†	2.4($\pm$ 1.9)E-6	9.3($\pm$ 1.8)E-7
Gln†	1.1($\pm$ 0.38)E-5	1.1($\pm$ 0.28)E-6
Gly‡	1.6($\pm$ 2.7)E-5	6.8($\pm$ 4.4)E-6
His†	1.5($\pm$ 0.68)E-6	5.0($\pm$ 2.5)E-7
Ile‡	4.0($\pm$ 3.9)E-7	1.8($\pm$ 1.4)E-7
Leu	5.2($\pm$ 6.8)E-7	3.8($\pm$ 0.56)E-7
Lys	1.5($\pm$ 0.83)E-5	1.6($\pm$ 1.9)E-5
Met‡	9.6($\pm$ 6.1)E-8	4.9($\pm$ 5.6)E-8
Phe†	3.0($\pm$ 2.6)E-6	9.5($\pm$ 0.54)E-8
Ser	8.0($\pm$ 0.28)E-7	7.0($\pm$ 1.0)E-8
Thr§	1.8($\pm$ 0.65)E-6	1.1($\pm$ 1.4)E-6
Trp†	5.6($\pm$ 3.7)E-9	zero order
Tyr‡	1.4($\pm$ 0.79)E-7	2.0($\pm$ 1.2)E-7
Val†	1.5($\pm$ 1.7)E-6	4.1($\pm$ 0.83)E-6
Ade†	1.4($\pm$ 0.20)E-8	zero order
Choline†	9.5($\pm$ 4.2)E-7	2.0($\pm$ 1.9)E-8
dThd†	1.3($\pm$ 1.7)E-8	zero order
Glc	2.7($\pm$ 2.3)E-5	3.5($\pm$ 3.1)E-5
Inositol†	3.3($\pm$ 1.5)E-7	1.1($\pm$ 0.36)E-7
Pyruvic acid	3.4($\pm$ 1.5)E-6	2.9($\pm$ 0.85)E-6
Ca^{2+}†	1.3($\pm$ 1.1)E-5	2.4($\pm$ 1.3)E-5
Mg^{2+}†	3.5($\pm$ 3.4)E-5	2.5($\pm$ 2.0)E-6
K$^+$	5.1($\pm$ 4.6)E-4	3.2($\pm$ 4.3)E-4
Pi	1.0($\pm$ 0.72)E-6	8.1($\pm$ 2.5)E-7
Fe†	3.3($\pm$ 2.5)E-8	zero order
Se†	2.7($\pm$ 1.4)E-10	zero order

* The $S_{0.50}$ values for each nutrient are indicated for normal (N-HLF) and transformed (SV-HLF) human lung fibroblasts. Kinetic analysis was carried out in medium MCDB 104 to 107 minus the nutrient under consideration and containing 250 μg FBSP per ml. The indicated $S_{0.50}$ values were assigned from pooled results of multiple experiments obtained over a 4-year period. $S_{0.50}$ values are in units of moles per liter. An abbreviated exponential notation is used. For example, 1.5($\pm$0.56)E-6 denotes an $S_{0.50}$ value of 1.5 $\times$ 10^{-6} M. $\pm$0.56 $\times$ 10^{-6} M is a 95% confidence limit for the $S_{0.50}$ value. "Zero order" indicates that no stimulatory effect on multiplication rate due to increasing the concentration of the component in the medium could be detected. The probability (P) that the difference between $S_{0.50}$ values for N-HLF and SV-HLF were due to chance was determined by Students t test.
† $P \leq 0.001$.
‡ $P \leq 0.10$.
§ $P \leq 0.01$.
No footnote symbol, $P \geq 0.10$
(Reproduced from McKeehan et al. 1981.)

we compared their nutrient and serum factor requirements for multiplication to those of normal parent cells (Table 1).

Serum Factors

When all nutrient concentrations were optimal and in steady-state, the response of SV-HLF to growth regulatory signals in serum was similar to that of the normal cells (N-HLF) (Figure 5). The multiplication response was bimodal. In the combined results of multiple experiments, there was no significant difference in the quantitative serum factor requirements for multiplication of the normal and transformed cells (Table 2).

Nutrients

When serum growth factor concentration was held constant, SV-HLF required only reduced levels of many nutrients in order to multiply (Table 1). The requirement for five (cysteine, glutamine, histidine, phenylalanine, tryptophan) of the 13 normally essential amino acids was reduced. Although the multiplication rate of N-HLF was stimulated by external adenine (or other purines) and thymidine (or other pyrimidines), multiplication of SV-HLF was independent of external purines or pyrimidines. Of the two major energy sources most utilized by cultured fibroblasts, glutamine and glucose (Zielke et al. 1978), the requirement for one, glutamine, for multiplication was reduced by transformation. The requirement of N-HLF and SV-HLF for glucose was similar (Table 1). Viral transformation reduced the inositol and choline requirement for multiplication.

Although the multiplication response of normal cells to Ca ions could be fitted to a single hyperbola, the response of SV-HLF was complex and different from that of N-HLF (McKeehan and McKeehan 1980a). SV-HLF multiply at a suboptimal rate without additional Ca^{2+}. SV-HLF responded to additional

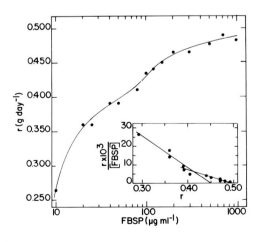

FIG. 5. Multiplication response of transformed cells to FBSP. Multiplication of 100 cells was assessed at the indicated concentrations of FBSP as described for normal cells in Figures 2 and 4. The inset is an Eadie-Scatchard plot of the data. (Reproduced from McKeehan and McKeehan 1981, with permission of Alan R. Liss, Inc.)

TABLE 2. *Quantitative requirement for FBSP for multiplication of normal and transformed human lung fibroblasts* *

N-HLF $S_{0.50} \pm$ S.E.		SV-HLF $S_{0.50} \pm$ S.E.	
1.2 ± 0.86	17.9 ± 2.7	7.0 ± 0.85	15.3 ± 1.3
6.8 ± 2.2	48.9 ± 2.1	28.3 ± 2.4	81.3 ± 8.9
11.3 ± 3.0	59.6 ± 12.1	4.2 ± 3.0	13.9 ± 5.0
4.3 ± 0.10	38.8 ± 5.2	5.7 ± 1.3	34.4 ± 10.4
3.1 ± 1.4	58.5 ± 11.6	—	13.7 ± 5.0
1.5 ± 0.40	45.6 ± 10.6	6.9 ± 0.80	10.2 ± 4.5
3.7 ± 0.80	103 ± 23	Mean $\pm$ S.D.	
1.2 ± 0.10	17.1 ± 3.7	10.4 ± 10.1	28.1 ± 27.4
1.2 ± 0.20	27.3 ± 7.7		
8.2 ± 1.8	17.1 ± 4.0		
7.1 ± 1.3	44.9 ± 2.3		
Mean $\pm$ S.D.			
4.5 ± 3.4	43.5 ± 25.3		

* The multiplication response of normal (N-HLF) and transformed (SV-HLF) cells to FBSP was analyzed in medium MCDB 104 to 107 as described in Figures 2, 4, and 5. The $S_{0.50}$ for FBSP is in units of micrograms per milliliter. Paired values represent the $S_{0.50}$ values calculated from each hyperbolic phase of the biphasic response to FBSP from single experiments. (Reproduced from McKeehan et al. 1981.)

Ca^{2+} in a hyperbolic fashion, and an $S_{0.50}$ value for Ca^{2+} could thus be assigned (Table 1). At 250 $\mu g/ml$ FBSP in the medium, the Ca^{2+} requirement for a maximal multiplication rate of SV-HLF was actually higher than that of N-HLF (Table 1). This difference was dependent on the level of serum growth factors in the medium (discussed later). SV-HLF required significantly less Mg^{2+} than N-HLF at all levels of FBSP in the medium (Table 1) (McKeehan and McKeehan 1980a). At 250 $\mu g/ml$ FBSP in the medium, the K^+ requirement of N-HLF and SV-HLF was similar (Table 1). However, as shown later in the text, a reduced K^+ requirement of SV-HLF for multiplication became apparent at lower levels of FBSP. SV-HLF also exhibited a reduced requirement for the ions of Fe and Se. Although N-HLF multiplied within a narrow pH range, the rate of multiplication of SV-HLF was unaffected by variations in pH of the medium from 6.8 to 7.8 (Figure 6). Less significant reductions in the requirement of SV-HLF for threonine, glycine, isoleucine, methionine, and tyrosine were apparent. No differences in the requirement for arginine, leucine, serine, lysine, pyruvic acid, and phosphate ions were detected (Table 1).

In summary, when the nutrient supply was optimal and constant, SV-HLF had no selective growth advantage over N-HLF, regardless of the level of nonnutritive regulatory factors from serum that were present in the medium. In contrast, SV-HLF had a growth advantage under conditions in which at least 12 of 26 different individual nutrients limited the multiplication rate of N-HLF.

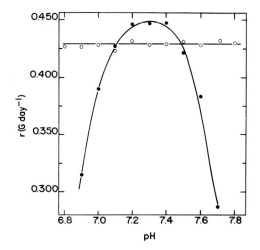

FIG. 6. Effect of pH on multiplication rate of normal and transformed cells. The indicated pH occurs under incubation conditions of 37°C in a humidified atmosphere of 2% CO_2 and 98% air. ●—●, Normal cells; ○—○, Transformed cells. (Reproduced from McKeehan et al. 1981.)

CONTROL OF CELL NUTRIENT REQUIREMENTS BY GROWTH REGULATORY FACTORS

Specific Growth Factors Transiently Modify Nutrient Requirements of Normal Cells

The majority of serum-derived, nonnutritive cell growth regulatory factors that have been elucidated thus far are hormone-like polypeptides or steroids (Gospodarowicz and Moran 1976, Barnes and Sato 1980). Much is known about the interaction of growth factors with cell-associated receptors and subsequent events in factor-receptor metabolism (Hopkins 1980). However, less is understood about how the growth factor-receptor interactions cause the biochemical and morphological changes that culminate in cell division.

We have proposed that some serum growth factors control the multiplication rate of normal cells in a manner similar to the way that "allosteric effectors" control the velocity of enzyme reactions (McKeehan and McKeehan 1980b). Serum growth factors may affect the rate of cell proliferation by modification of the cellular "K_m" ($S_{0.50}$) value for specific nutrients required for proliferation. Of over 30 individual nutrients examined, serum factors modified the cellular environment ($S_{0.50}$ value) for only Ca^{2+}, K^+, Mg^{2+}, phosphate ions, and 2-oxocarboxylic acids, such as pyruvate and 2-oxoglutarate. Cellular requirements for the 20 amino acids, glucose, adenine (and other purines), thymidine (and other pyrimidines), choline, inositol, and polyamines were independent of serum factors.

Individual chemically defined growth factors also modify the cellular requirement for specific nutrients (McKeehan and McKeehan 1979). Purified epidermal growth factor (EGF) controls the external Ca^{2+} requirement for proliferation of human skin fibroblasts (McKeehan and McKeehan 1979) and normal human prostatic epithelial cells (Lechner and Kaighn 1979). Fibroblast growth factor (FGF) reduces the Ca^{2+} requirement for multiplication of bovine endothelial cells (personal communication, Dr. J. Smith, W. Alton Jones Cell Science Center). In addition to Ca^{2+}, EGF controls the Mg^{2+} and pyruvic acid requirement for multiplication of human skin fibroblasts but not the K^+ requirement (our unpublished results). Thus, different growth factors within serum may control the cellular requirement for different nutrients. These results strongly support the hypothesis that nonnutritive, hormone-like growth signals in serum control the nutrient requirements for cell multiplication. Such growth regulatory factors most effectively govern the cell multiplication rate when the specific nutrients involved are at multiplication-limiting concentrations in the environment.

Oncogenic Transformation Overrides Control of Nutrient Requirements by Serum Growth Factors

Balk et al. (1973) established a relationship between a reduced cellular Ca^{2+} requirement for multiplication and a reduced requirement for a growth factor unique in serum (as opposed to cell-free plasma) for multiplication of Rous sarcoma virus-infected chicken fibroblasts (RSV-CEF). In medium containing plasma, the Ca^{2+} requirement for multiplication of normal chicken embryo fibroblasts (N-CEF) was much larger than for RSV-CEF. The serum factor reduced the Ca^{2+} requirement of N-CEF to that of RSV-CEF. The multiplication rate of RSV-CEF was independent of the serum factor and proceeded to an equal extent in either serum or plasma. Thus, in plasma-containing medium, RSV-CEF had a striking growth advantage over N-CEF, especially at a low Ca^{2+} concentration. These results enabled the isolation and purification of the serum factor as a polypeptide growth factor, released from platelets (Ross and Vogel 1978) during the preparation of normal serum but absent from cell-free plasma. The original observations of Balk et al. (1973) for normal and RSV-transformed chicken fibroblasts have been confirmed in normal and SV40 virus-transformed human skin fibroblasts (Sher et al. 1979). Lechner and Kaighn (1979) demonstrated similar relationships among purified EGF, external Ca^{2+}, and the multiplication rate of normal and tumorigenic human prostate epithelial cells. These studies, using different experimental models and different modes of oncogenic transformation, show that a constitutive alteration in cell Ca^{2+} requirement for proliferation overrides the transient control of the requirement by specific growth factors. Under conditions in which external Ca^{2+} and serum growth factors limit normal cell proliferation, the transformed cells have a distinct growth advantage because of their reduced demand for Ca^{2+}.

In addition to Ca^{2+}, external K^+ and Mg^{2+} requirements for multiplication of human lung fibroblasts are reduced constitutively by transformation by SV40 virus (Table 3). Although the Ca^{2+} requirement of SV-HLF was influenced by serum factors, at low levels of serum factors the Ca^{2+} requirement for multiplication of N-HLF was much greater than that of SV-HLF. Increasing levels of

TABLE 3. Effect of FBSP concentration on $S_{0.50}$ values for Ca^{2+}, K^+, Mg^{2+}, pyruvic acid, and Pi for multiplication of normal and transformed human fibroblasts*

	100 μg ml⁻¹ FBSP		250 μg ml⁻¹ FBSP		500 μg ml⁻¹ FBSP	
	N	T	N	T	N	T
Ca^{2+}	5.4(± 2.9)E-4	2.7(± 0.50)E-5	2.7(± 0.50)E-5	†2.5(± 0.60)E-5	1.9(± 0.30)E-5	1.3(± 0.30)E-5
K^+	4.8(± 3.0)E-3	2.3(± 0.80)E-4	6.0(± 3.9)E-4	†1.8(± 0.60)E-4	5.2(± 3.4)E-4	1.9(± 0.30)E-4
Mg^{2+}	8.0(± 2.0)E-5	9.4(± 6.4)E-6	6.0(± 1.3)E-5	4.6(± 1.8)E-6	3.1(± 0.90)E-5	6.9(± 2.3)E-6
Pyruvic acid	2.3(± 0.20)E-5	3.0(± 2.0)E-5	2.4(± 1.2)E-6	2.9(± 0.33)E-6	zero order	zero order
Phosphate ions	8.2(± 1.8)E-7	8.8(± 0.20)E-7	7.8(± 2.2)E-7	†1.1(± 0.10)E-6	3.7(± 1.2)E-7	5.4(± 0.40)E-7

* $S_{0.50}$ (± SE) in units of moles per liter were determined for each nutrient at the indicated concentration of FBSP in the medium. N = normal cells; T = transformed cells.

† Indicated $S_{0.50}$ values were determined at 200 μg FBSP per ml instead of 250 μg per ml.

(Reproduced from McKeehan et al. 1981.)

serum factors reduced the Ca^{2+} requirement of N-HLF compared with that of SV-HLF. Although the K^+ and Mg^{2+} requirement for multiplication of normal cells was stringently dependent on the level of serum factors in the medium, the multiplication requirement for K^+ and Mg^{2+} was a constitutive property of SV-HLF and unaffected by serum factors. At low levels of serum factors in the medium, the K^+ and Mg^{2+} requirement for multiplication of N-HLF was much greater than that of SV-HLF. Serum factors reduced the K^+ requirement of N-HLF to that of SV-HLF. Serum factors also reduced, but not to zero, the difference in the Mg^{2+} requirements of N-HLF and SV-HLF. Thus, in human lung fibroblasts, Ca^{2+}, K^+, and Mg^{2+} ions emerge as key nutrients whose requirement for normal cells to multiply is stringently controlled by serum factors. Viral transformation overrides the influence of serum factors on the requirement for all three ions. When the external concentration of Ca^{2+}, K^+, or Mg^{2+} is limiting, serum factors effectively control the multiplication rate of normal cells. Under this condition, alterations in the Ca^{2+}, K^+, and Mg^{2+} requirement for transformed cells to multiply are expressed as a selective growth advantage and override the control of the normal cell multiplication rate by serum-derived growth factors.

CONCLUSION

Alterations in Nutrient Requirements as Clues to Cellular Processes That Are Altered by Oncogenic Agents

By cell culture methodology, we have been able to pinpoint specific differences in nutritive requirements of a virally transformed malignant cell prototype from its normal parent. Viral infection and evolution of the phenotypically transformed cell line causes a general relaxation of the quantitative requirements of cells for nutrients they need to multiply. Although multiple alterations in cell nutrient requirements were apparent, changes occurred in the requirement for specific nutrients of the total set generally required by most cell types. Thus, it is unlikely that a general, nonspecific defect such as an increased membrane permeability for all nutrients accounts for all the differences. The differences probably reflect specific alterations in multiple metabolic processes, including those that control permeability, that normally set the overall quantitative requirement for specific nutrients of cells to multiply. The specific differences in growth requirements for the normal and transformed cell prototypes studied here provide valuable clues to metabolic processes that may be targets of alteration during malignant transformation (McKeehan et al. 1981). Transformation altered the requirement for nutrients involved in multiple domains of metabolism whose rates may regulate cell proliferation. These nutrients included five different amino acids whose end products may be important in metabolic processes other than protein synthesis (Meister 1965). The reduced requirement for glutamine is especially noteworthy, since it is a key component in multiple pathways whose products may limit cell proliferation (Prusiner and Stadtman 1973). These pathways include purine, pyrimidine, asparagine, amino sugars, and pyridine nucleotide bio-syntheses as well as basic energy metabolism (Zielke et al. 1978). The reduced requirement for an external purine and pyrimidine further suggests the impor-tance of purine and pyrimidine metabolism. The reductions in inositol and cho-line suggest that phospholipid metabolism may be important in control of normal and transformed cell growth. Ca^{2+}, K^+, and Mg^{2+} are potential regulators of multiple domains of metabolism whose end products may control proliferation. Although these three ions have long been implicated in the stimulation of diverse cell functions by external regulatory signals, much new information concerning their role in cell proliferation has recently emerged (Leffert 1980). As we have emphasized earlier, Ca^{2+}, K^+, and Mg^{2+} ions may be especially important in the escape of malignant cells from the control of some external growth regulatory signals.

Physiological Significance of Differences in Nutritional Requirements

The significance of alterations that occur in the nutritional requirements of transformed cells depends on whether the changes confer a growth advantage over their normal cell counterparts under physiological conditions. The reduced requirements of malignant cells for a nutrient will be of most serious consequence when the normal external concentration of the nutrient limits the proliferation of normal cells. Unfortunately, the normal levels of nutrients in the microenviron-ment of tissue cells in vivo, such as the fibroblasts used in this study, cannot be precisely determined with current technology. The levels of nutrients in human plasma or serum are usually employed as a best estimate, although these values are probably overestimates, since concentration gradients exist from blood plasma to the cellular microenvironment. This is especially true if concentrations of only the free, unbound ions are important.

Table 4 indicates that plasma levels for most nutrients are 7 to 9,000 times the cell $S_{0.50}$ values for multiplication. Although transformed cells have a reduced requirement for the nutrients shown in Table 4, there is little growth advantage conferred if the plasma levels represent the effective external nutrient concentra-tions in tissue. However, the reduced requirements could confer an advantage to the transformed cells if physiological conditions are ever such that the microen-vironmental concentration of the indicated nutrients are at or below the $S_{0.50}$ value for normal cell proliferation.

In contrast to the levels of most nutrients (Table 4), plasma levels of free Ca^{2+} and K^+ (Table 5) would limit normal fibroblast proliferation, especially when regulatory growth signals from serum are low or absent from the environ-ment. However, plasma levels of Ca^{2+} and K^+ are six to seven times the $S_{0.50}$ for proliferation of transformed cells, and therefore adequate to support their proliferation. Clearly, the reduced Ca^{2+} and K^+ requirements for proliferation of the transformed cells would confer a growth advantage on them under

TABLE 4. *Comparison of plasma nutrient levels and $S_{0.50}$ values for nutrients for multiplication of normal and transformed fibroblasts**

Nutrient	Concentration in plasma (μM)	$\dfrac{\text{Plasma}}{S_{0.50}}$ for N-HLF	$\dfrac{\text{Plasma}}{S_{0.50}}$ for SV-HLF
Cys	33	14	35
Gln	568	52	368
His	74	49	148
Phe	51	17	537
Trp	54	9,000	∞
Ade	0.7–1	7–100	∞
Choline	440	440	22,000
dThd	2	200	∞
Inositol	26	87	236

* Plasma concentrations and $S_{0.50}$ values are in units of μmoles per liter. Plasma levels of nutrients except adenine (ade) and thymidine (dThd) were obtained from Dittmer (1961). Ade values were from Hamet (1975) and de Verdier et al. (1977). dThd was from Mitchell et al. (1975).

these conditions. The plasma level of free Mg^{2+} exceeds the $S_{0.50}$ value of both normal and transformed cells (Table 5). Thus, the reduced Mg^{2+} requirement for proliferation of transformed cells would not confer a growth advantage. However, if plasma Mg^{2+} levels are greater than the external microenvironmental levels of free Mg^{2+} in tissue by a factor of seven or greater, then the reduced Mg^{2+} requirement would become selectively advantageous to transformed cell growth (Table 5).

Malignant cells are heterogenous in phenotypic properties and the degree to which they have escaped the growth-controlling elements of the organism. Tumor cells that arise from different tissues have different properties, and tumors

TABLE 5. *Comparison of plasma levels of free Ca^{2+}, K^+, and Mg^{2+} and the $S_{0.50}$ value for proliferation of normal and transformed fibroblasts*

Nutrient	Concentration in plasma (μM)	Plasma $S_{0.50}$					
		FBSP 10 μg/ml		FBSP 100 μg/ml		FBSP 1000 μg/ml	
		N	T	N	T	N	T
Ca^{2+}	1180	$\ll 1$	6	2	44	118	60
K^+	1400	$\ll 1$	7	0.3	6	5	7
Mg^{2+}	530	7	66	7	56	18	65

* The indicated concentrations in plasma are the free ion levels estimated by Walser (1961) for Ca^{2+} and Mg^{2+}. Levels of free K^+ were from Dittmer (1961). $S_{0.50}$ and plasma levels are in units of μmoles per liter. FBSP = fetal bovine serum proteins (see Figure 1). N = normal cells; T = transformed cells.

that arise from the same type of tissue often differ from each other. Moreover, cells within the same tumor have heterogenous properties. When transformation is studied in vitro, the properties of the resultant malignant cells are equally heterogenous and vary with the oncogenic agent employed to induce transformation. Thus, it is difficult to extrapolate the specific differences in nutritional requirements that we have uncovered from a single in vitro model, normal and SV40-transformed human lung fibroblasts, to malignant cells in general. Fibroblasts and their in vitro transformants have been criticized as being invalid models for real cancers (Shields 1976). Yet the general pattern of reduced nutritional requirements of transformed fibroblasts that we have revealed here cannot be ignored. It is a clue to the nature of the growth advantage possessed by malignant cells in general. Different gradations and combinations of alterations in the cellular requirements for different nutrients may actually account for the extreme diversity of observed malignant cell phenotypes. Clearly needed are rigorous, systematic comparative studies of the quantitative differences in nutritional requirements between a variety of normal and malignant cell types under the defined and controlled conditions offered by cell culture methodologies.

ACKNOWLEDGMENTS

This investigation was supported by Grant No. 26110 from the National Cancer Institute, Grant No. 27194 from the National Institute of General Medical Sciences, and the W. Alton Jones Foundation.

REFERENCES

Balk, S. D., J. F. Whitfield, T. Youdale, and A. Braun. 1973. Roles of calcium, serum, plasma, and folic acid in the control of proliferation of normal and Rous sarcoma virus-infected chicken fibroblasts. Proc. Natl. Acad. Sci. USA 70:675–679.

Barnes, D., and G. Sato. 1980. Serum-free cell culture: A unifying approach. Cell 22:649–655.

Carrell, A. 1929. The nutritional properties of malignant cells. Proceedings of the American Philosophical Society 58:129–139.

de Verdier, C. H., A. Ericson, F. Niklasson, and M. Westman. 1977. Adenine metabolism in man. I. After intravenous and peritoneal administration. Scan. J. Clin. Invest. 37:567–575.

Dittmer, D. S., ed. 1961. Blood and Other Body Fluids. Biological Handbooks, Federation of American Society for Experimental Biology, Washington.

Girardi, A. J., D. Weinstein, and P. S. Moorhead. 1966. SV40 transformation of human diploid cells. Annales Medicinae Experimentalis et Biologiae Fenniae 44:242–254.

Gospodarowicz, D., and J. S. Moran. 1976. Growth factors in mammalian cell culture. Annu. Rev. Biochem. 45:531–558.

Ham, R. G., and W. L. McKeehan. 1979. Media and growth requirements. Methods Enzymol. 58:44–93.

Hamet, M. 1975. Micro-estimation of adenine by a method of enzymatic kinetic and isotopic dilution. Ann. Biol. Clin. (Paris) 33:131–138.

Hopkins, C. R. 1980. Epidermal growth factor and mitogenesis (Editorial). Nature 286:205–206.

Kahn, P., and S.-L. Shin. 1979. Cellular tumorigenicity in nude mice. J. Cell. Biol. 82:1–16.

Lechner, J. F., and M. E. Kaighn. 1979. Reduction of the calcium requirement of normal human epithelial cells by EGF. Exp. Cell Res. 121:432–435.

Leffert, H. L., ed. 1980. Growth Regulation by Ion Fluxes. Ann. N.Y. Acad. Sci. vol. 339.

McKeehan, W. L., D. P. Genereaux, and R. G. Ham. 1978. Assay and partial purification of factors from serum that control multiplication of human diploid fibroblasts. Biochem. Biophys. Res. Commun. 80:1013–1021.

McKeehan, W. L., and K. A. McKeehan. 1979. Epidermal growth factor modulates extracellular Ca^{2+} requirement for multiplication of normal human skin fibroblasts. Exp. Cell Res. 123:397–400.

McKeehan, W. L., and K. A. McKeehan. 1980a. Calcium, magnesium, and serum factors in multiplication of normal and transformed human lung fibroblasts. In Vitro 16:475–485.

McKeehan, W. L., and K. A. McKeehan. 1980b. Serum factors modify the cellular requirement for Ca^{2+}, K^+, Mg^{2+}, phosphate ions, and 2-oxocarboxylic acids. Proc. Natl. Acad. Sci. USA 77:3417–3421.

McKeehan, W. L., and K. A. McKeehan. 1981. Extracellular regulation of fibroblast multiplication: A direct kinetic approach to analysis of role of low molecular weight nutrients and serum growth factors. J. Supramol. Struc. 115:83–110.

McKeehan, W. L., K. A. McKeehan, and D. Calkins. 1981. Extracellular regulation of fibroblast multiplication. Quantitative differences in nutrient and serum factor requirements for multiplication of normal and SV40 virus transformed human lung cells. J. Biol. Chem. 256:2973–2981.

Meister, A. 1965. The Biochemistry of the Amino Acids. Academic Press, New York.

Mitchell, R. S., S. D. Balk, O. Frank, H. Baker, and M. J. Cristine. 1975. The failure of methotrexate to inhibit chicken fibroblast proliferation in a serum-containing culture medium. Cancer Res. 35:2613–2615.

Prusiner, S., and E. R. Stadtman, eds. 1973. The Enzymes of Glutamine Metabolism. Academic Press, New York.

Ross, R., and A. Vogel. 1978. The platelet-derived growth factor. Cell 14:203–210.

Sher, C. D., R. C. Shepard, H. N. Antoniades, and C. D. Stiles. 1979. Platelet-derived growth factor and the regulation of mammalian fibroblast cell cycle. Biochim. Biophys. Acta 560:217–241.

Shields, R. 1976. Transformation and tumorigenicity (Editorial). Nature 262:348.

Walser, M. 1961. Ion association. VI. Interactions between calcium, magnesium, inorganic phosphate, citrate and protein in normal human plasma. J. Clin. Invest. 40:723–730.

Zielke, H. R., P. T. Ozand, T. T. Tildon, D. A. Sevdalian, and M. Cornblath. 1978. Reciprocal regulation of glucose and glutamine utilization by cultured human diploid fibroblasts. J. Cell Physiol. 95:41–48.

Molecular Interrelations of Nutrition and Cancer,
edited by M. S. Arnott, J. van Eys and Y.-M. Wang.
Raven Press, New York © 1982.

Nuclear Events in Normal and Malignant Cells and the Control of Cell Proliferation

Norbel Galanti,* Yoshihiro Tsutsui,† Gerald Jonak, Shoji
Kawasaki, Kenneth Soprano, and Renato Baserga

*Department of Pathology and Fels Research Institute, Temple University School of
Medicine, Philadelphia, Pennsylvania 19140*

While nutrients and growth factors in the environment regulate the extent
of cell proliferation, their mechanism of action must ultimately result in certain
cellular responses that cause the cell to grow. For cell division to occur, at
least three fundamental things must take place: (1) the cell must grow in mass,
i.e., a cell must double all its cellular components; (2) the cell must replicate
DNA; and (3) the cell must undergo mitosis. It has been often taken for granted
that these three processes are strictly interrelated to the point that, for instance,
cell DNA synthesis is equated with cell proliferation. It may not necessarily
be so, and in this presentation, we wish to show that the increase in cell mass
and cell DNA replication are under separate and independent controls, and
that the information for these two fundamental aspects of cell proliferation is
encoded in separate and distinct gene sequences.

In addition, we will show that transforming viruses can induce cell DNA
synthesis in the absence of certain intracellular functions that are required by
serum-stimulated cells. The implication is that transforming genes can overrule
not only nutritional but even intracellular requirements for growth.

Before we look at the actual experiments, let us introduce two simplifications
we have used in order to reduce the problem of cell proliferation to manageable
proportions. The first is the use of viruses, specifically SV40 and adenoviruses,
which are known to induce cell DNA synthesis and mitosis in quiescent cells
(for a review, see Weil 1978). The advantage of using viruses is that their genomes
are of limited size. For instance, the genome of SV40 consists of 5,243 base
pairs, fully sequenced (Tooze 1980), obviously much more amenable to analysis
than the approximately 3×10^9 base pairs of the mammalian genome. By genetic
experiments and by the microinjection experiments of Graessmann and collaborators (see below), the product of the A gene, called the T antigen, has been

---

* Present Address: Departamento de Biologia Celular, Universidad de Chile, Santiago

† Present Address: Nagoya University School of Medicine, The 2nd Department of Pathology,
65, Tsuruma-cho, Showa-ku, Nagoya 466, Japan

shown to contain all the necessary information to induce growth in size, cell DNA replication, and mitosis in resting cells. Thus, one protein can induce in resting cells all the necessary changes leading to mitosis. The adenovirus genome is somewhat more complicated than the SV40 genome, since it consists of 35,000 base pairs instead of 5,243, but still considerably less complex than the mammalian genome.

The second simplification we have made is that growth in size can be measured by measuring the synthesis or the accumulation of ribosomal RNA (rRNA). This is reasonable: nucleic acids and proteins constitute 50% of the dry weight of a cell, and rRNA constitutes about 70% of all nucleic acids and is an essential part of ribosomes, where proteins are synthesized. Thus, rRNA genes constitute a reasonable target for a stimulus to grow in size.

METHODS AND MATERIALS

Cell Lines

NIH 3T3 cells and ts13 cells were used. The growth and maintenance of these cell lines have been described in a previous paper (Galanti et al. 1981).

Cloned Genes

pSV2G is a recombinant plasmid containing a fragment of SV40 genome, extending from map units 1.0/0 counterclockwise to map units 0.144, cloned in pBR322. The construction and characterization of this plasmid has been described in detail (Galanti et al 1981). For restriction endonuclease assays, the reaction conditions were as recommended by New England Biolabs. The separation and isolation of DNA restriction fragments from agarose gel electrophoresis have been described in detail by Galanti et al. (1981).

Microinjection of Fragments

DNA and DNA fragments were delivered directly into nuclei of cells by the glass capillary microinjection technique described by Graessmann and coworkers (1976, 1979). Samples were dissolved in 10 mM Tris·HCl, pH 7.5, at 25°C and routinely centrifuged for 15 min in an Eppendorf centrifuge before microinjection. At least 100 cells were microinjected for each experiment.

Detection of T Antigen by Immunofluorescence

The cells were fixed in cold methanol for 15 min at 4°C. SV40 T antigen was visualized by the indirect immunofluorescence technique of Pope and Rowe (1964) with hamster anti-T antisera and, as a second antibody, fluorescein-conjugated goat anti-hamster IgG. The antibody used was an anti-T antibody prepared in our laboratory by immunization of hamsters with an SV40-transformed hamster cell line.

Autoradiography

The cells were continuously labeled with ^{3}H-thymidine (New England Nuclear Corp., 6.7 Ci/mmol 0.7 μCi/ml) added immediately after microinjection, and autoradiographs were made and analyzed as described by Baserga and Malamud (1969).

Cell Transformation

For cell transformation experiments, NIH 3T3 cells were microinjected with pSV2G (0.25 mg/ml), SV40 DNA (0.25 mg/ml), or restriction fragments obtained from pSV2G. Cells were kept 2 days at 37°C in fresh 10% fetal calf serum and Dulbecco's medium, then transferred to Dulbecco's medium supplemented with 1% fetal calf serum. This last medium was changed every 3 days. Between 10 and 15 days after microinjection, clones were growing in the microinjected area. The clones were trypsinized and replated in Dulbecco's medium supplemented with 10% fetal calf serum. The clones were tested for T positivity by indirect immunofluorescence and were then expanded in 10% fetal calf serum.

Growth of Transformed Cell Lines in 10% and in 1% Serum

Growing populations of transformed cells were trypsinized and replated in either 10% or 1% serum in 35-mm Petri dishes at a concentration of 5 × 10^4 cells per dish and incubated at 37°C. Each day for 10 days, cells were trypsinized and suspended in 3 ml of Dulbecco's medium and counted. The same procedure was used for NIH 3T3 cells.

Growth of Cells in Soft Agar

This was carried out as described by MacPherson and Montagnier (1964).

Tumorigenesis

NIH 3T3 cells transformed by microinjection of cloned SV40 DNA or by microinjection of fragments prepared from cloned SV40 DNA treated with restriction endonucleases were washed in calcium- and magnesium-free Hanks' balanced salt solution, detached by trypsinization, and resuspended in Dulbecco's medium supplemented with 10% calf serum. The cells were counted and adjusted to a concentration of 10^7 cells/ml. An aliquot of 0.2 ml was injected subcutaneously in each side of the back of nude mice. Control experiments were carried out with untransformed NIH 3T3 cells.

Immunoprecipitation of T Antigen

The technique of Schwyzer (1977) was used as described.

RESULTS

Microinjection Technique

The manual microinjection technique offers unique possibilities for introducing new information into viable mammalian cells. Among the macromolecules that have been microinjected are DNA (Mueller et al. 1978, Floros et al. 1981), cRNA (Graessmann and Graessmann 1976), mRNA (Richardson et al. 1980, Bravo and Celis 1980, Floros et al. 1981) and proteins (Tjian et al. 1978, Kreis et al. 1979). These macromolecules can induce in the microinjected cells both phenotypic (Stacey 1980, Feramisco 1979, Mueller et al. 1978, Tjian et al. 1978, Soprano et al. 1981) and genotypic changes (Graessmann et al. 1979, Anderson et al. 1980). The advantages of manual microinjection, in the case of viral genes, are that the genes can be introduced even into cells that lack receptors for a given virus and that nonviable mutants, or defined segments of viral genes, cloned in an appropriate vector, can also be efficiently introduced.

We will first deal, briefly, with the fate of the microinjected genes and with the production of transformants. For these studies, we used pSV2G, a recombinant plasmid derived from pBR322, that contains the entire SV40 A region coding for the T antigens (Galanti et al. 1981).

Fate of Microinjected SV40 DNA Fragments

In a typical experiment, pSV2G DNA was microinjected into groups of ts13 cells, each group consisting of 100 cells each. The number of T-positive cells in the circle of microinjected cells was determined at different times after microinjection. The results are shown in Table 1. The number of T-positive cells increased progressively after microinjection, doubling every day, until day 3. Then, the number of T-positive cells decreased suddenly and precipitously, so that on days 6 and 7, only one or two weakly T-positive cells could be detected. If the cultures were kept for longer periods, clones of transformants could be detected (see below).

It should be noted that these results were obtained only when ts13 cells were incubated, after microinjection, in 10% serum. If the microinjected cells were kept in 1% serum, about 80% were T-positive after 24 hours, but the

TABLE 1. *Number of T-positive cells at different times after microinjection of a cloned SV40 DNA fragment**

Hours	No. T+ cells/ microinjected circle
24	73
48	380
72	452
96	405
120	—
144	—

* 100 ts13 cells were microinjected in each circle, and the number of T-positive (T+) cells was determined as described in Methods and Materials.
—, none consistently detectable.

number did not increase in subsequent days and, in fact, after 72 hours, no T-positive cells could be detected in the microinjected circle.

Transformation of Cells Microinjected with Fragments of SV40 DNA

Although a number of cell lines were microinjected with SV40 DNA, thus far we have obtained positive results only with 3T3 cells. Three different sources of SV40 DNA were used: (1) DNA prepared from SV40-infected cells by the Hirt procedure (Hirt 1967); (2) pSV2G DNA (see above); and (3) an HpaII-Pst I restriction fragment obtained from pSV2G. This fragment includes that part of the SV40 early region that extends from the origin of replication to 0.27 map units. It therefore lacks approximately the last 300 base pairs of the A gene. Transformants were obtained with all three sources of DNA. These cells were judged to be SV40 transformed by the following criteria: (1) after cloning, 100% of the cells were strongly T-positive, with the typical fluorescent nuclei and dark nucleoli; (2) the transformed cells grew more vigorously in 1% serum than the parent 3T3 cell line (Figure 1); (3) the transformed cell lines grew in soft agar, whereas 3T3 cells did not (Table 2); (4) transformed cells induced tumors in nude mice, while 3T3 cells did not (Table 2); and (5) the transformed cells produced T antigens recognizable by slab gel electrophoresis of immunoprecipitates (Figure 2). The last requires some further comments. Note that cells transformed by microinjection of SV40 DNA fragments produce several recognizable forms of large T antigen. Note also that cells transformed with an HpaII-Pst I fragment from pSV2G produce a large T antigen that

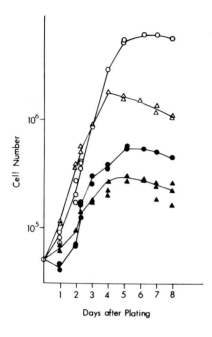

FIG. 1. Growth curves of 3T3 and NC-1 cells in medium supplemented with either 1% or 10% serum. Initially, 5 × 10⁵ cells were plated and the number of cells at different times after plating was determined by counting in a hemocytometer. NC-1 cells are 3T3 cells that were microinjected with pSV2G DNA (see text). ○ NC-1 cells in 10% serum; △ NC-1 cells in 1% serum; ● 3T3 cells in 10% serum; ▲ 3T3 cells in 1% serum.

has the same (apparent) molecular weight of the large T antigen in NG-1 and NG-2 cells.

Induction of Cell DNA Synthesis in G_1-Specific Temperature-Sensitive Mutants

G_1-specific ts mutants are operationally defined as mutants that arrest at the nonpermissive temperature in the G_1 phase of the cell cycle, but grow normally at the permissive temperature. The definition of G_1 ts mutants implies, also, that (1) when collected by mitotic detachment and plated at the nonpermissive temperature, the cells do not enter S phase; (2) when made quiescent by serum restriction and subsequently stimulated at the nonpermissive temperature, the cells do not enter S phase; (3) the cells enter S phase at the permissive temperature whether plated after mitotic detachment or stimulated after nutritional deprivation; (4) the parental cell line must be capable of entering S phase at both temperatures; and finally (5) the cells arrest in G_1 only, even when shifted up to the nonpermissive temperature in other phases of the cell cycle. The mutant cell line we used for these studies are ts13 cells, which are derived from BHK cells. BHK cells are capable of entering S phase even at temperatures of 41°C, whereas ts13 cells shifted up to the nonpermissive temperature of 39.6°C arrest in G_1 (Talavera and Basilico 1977, Floros et al. 1978).

pSV2G or SV40 DNA was microinjected into the nuclei of ts13 cells and caused these cells to become T positive according to indirect immunofluorescence. The microinjection of these fragments of viral genes induced cell DNA

TABLE 2. *Growth of 3T3 cells transformed by microinjection of SV40 DNA*

Cell line	Growth in soft agar	Growth in nude mice
3T3	no	no
NC-1*	yes	yes
NC-2†	yes	not done
Bear-1‡	yes	not done

* NC-1 cell line was derived as described in Fig. 1.

† NC-2 cells were derived from 3T3 cells microinjected with SV40 DNA.

‡ Bear 1 cells were derived from 3T3 cells microinjected with an HpaII-Pst I fragment obtained by digestion of pSV2G DNA. Growth in soft agar and in nude mice was determined as described in Methods and Materials.

replication in ts13 cells at both the permissive temperature of 34°C and the nonpermissive temperature of 39.6°C (Floros et al. 1981). The stimulation of cell DNA replication by microinjected SV40 DNA was inhibited when antibody anti-T antigen was simultaneously microinjected with the SV40 DNA. This indicates that the effect of the microinjected genes on cell DNA replication is mediated through the product of the SV40 genome, the T antigen (Floros et al. 1981).

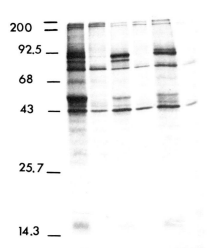

FIG. 2. Slab gel electrophoresis of ³⁵S-labeled proteins immunoprecipitated by anti-T antiserum. Labeling, immunoprecipitation, and electrophoresis are described in the text. Lanes 1, 3, and 5: cell extracts immunoprecipitated with antiserum anti-SV40-T antigen. Lanes 2, 4, and 6: cell extracts treated with pre-immune serum. Lanes 1, 2: NC-1 cells (see Fig. 1). Lanes 3, 4: G2N2 cells (3T3 cells transformed by microinjection with SV40 DNA). Lanes 5, 6: cells transformed by microinjection of an HpaII-Pst I fragment of SV40 DNA.

Induction of Cellular DNA Replication in G_1-Specific ts Mutants by Adenovirus 2

We used another temperature-sensitive mutant, tsAF8 cells, which also were derived from BHK cells (Meiss and Basilico 1972). This mutant is also a bona fide G_1 ts mutant, since it arrests only in G_1 when shifted up to the nonpermissive temperature of 40.6°C. Adenovirus 2 infection causes stimulation of cell DNA synthesis in serum-deprived tsAF8 cells at 34°C. Furthermore, infection with adenovirus 2 also stimulates cell DNA replication in tsAF8 cells at the nonpermissive temperature of 40.6°C (Rossini et al. 1979). The most interesting result of these experiments, however, is that adenovirus 2, although capable of stimulating cell DNA replication in tsAF8 cells as well as in other cell lines, stimulated neither the synthesis (Soprano et al. 1980) nor the accumulation (Pochron et al. 1980) of rRNA. This means that the adenovirus 2 genome contains information for the stimulation of cell DNA replication but not for the stimulation of rRNA synthesis, that is, not for the growth in size of the cells. We shall return to this finding a little later.

The combined experiments with adenovirus 2 and with microinjected SV40 DNA show that at least two G_1 cellular functions necessary for the G_0 to S transition in serum-stimulated cells can be dispensed with at least for one round of DNA synthesis. Regardless of one's views of the cell cycle, one must say that these G_1 ts mutants have a ts defect in a cellular function that is required for the progression of cells from mitosis or G_0 to S under standard nutritional conditions. These functions are no longer needed for entry into S when quiescent cells are provided with information from the early region of the SV40 genome or from adenovirus 2.

The Role of RNA Polymerase II in Cellular DNA Synthesis

tsAF8 cells have been identified as having a mutation in RNA polymerase II (Rossini and Baserga 1978, Rossini et al. 1980). At the nonpermissive temperature of 40.6°C, the RNA polymerase II molecules disappear from tsAF8 cells with a half-life of 10 to 12 hours. At 34°C in tsAF8 or in BHK cells at either temperature, RNA polymerase II remains at constant levels. RNA polymerase I activity is not affected by the shift to the nonpermissive temperature, and the cells remain viable for at least 60 hours, although RNA polymerase II activity is virtually gone by 24 hours after shift up. A rapid survey of protein synthesis indicated that protein synthesis is not affected for at least 30 hours at the nonpermissive temperature (Rossini et al. 1980). Furthermore, studies by flow cytophotometry demonstrated that in tsAF8 cells RNA accumulates just as effectively at the nonpermissive temperature as at the permissive temperature (Ashihara et al. 1978). These studies indicate, therefore, that (1) a functional RNA polymerase II is necessary for the entry of cells into S phase, and (2) a functional RNA polymerase II is not required for the growth in size of cells, since the synthesis of rRNA and proteins remains unaffected for at least 30 hours after the RNA polymerase II molecules have disappeared. These findings clearly separate the requirements for cell DNA replication from those for growth in size. It should also be made clear that cell size, in itself, is not sufficient for entry into S. Indeed, in human diploid fibroblasts, an inverse relationship appears to exist between growth rate and cell volume (Mitsui and Schneider 1976).

The Information for Growth in Size and for Cell DNA Replication Is Encoded In Different DNA Sequences

We have mentioned above that adenovirus 2 contains information for the stimulation of cell DNA synthesis in quiescent mammalian cells but not the information for growth in size (Rossini et al. 1979, Pochron et al. 1980). It is therefore conceivable that the information for cell DNA replication is encoded in DNA sequences that do not contain the information for growth in size. This hypothesis has been confirmed in a series of experiments with SV40.

SV40 infection can stimulate cell DNA replication and mitosis in quiescent mammalian cells (for a review, see Weil 1978). We investigated whether the capacity to stimulate growth in size can be dissociated from the capacity to stimulate cell DNA replication by using adeno-SV40 hybrid viruses and mutants of SV40 that were cloned in plasmids and can be microinjected directly into the nuclei of quiescent cells. A number of mutants and hybrid viruses (Lewis 1977) were used for this purpose. Their map coordinates in terms of the SV40 genome are given in Table 3, which summarizes our results in a number of studies. To determine whether a given virus or fragment of virus can stimulate cell DNA synthesis, we microinjected DNA into quiescent cells, usually ts13 cells. Stimulation of cell DNA synthesis was determined by autoradiography after exposure of the cells to [³H]thymidine as previously described (Baserga and Malamud 1969).

Stimulation of rRNA synthesis was instead studied by determining the ability of the virus or the viral fragment to reactivate silent rRNA genes in human-mouse hybrid cells. Hybrids between human and rodent cells express only the rRNA of the dominant species (usually the rodent), the dominant species being the one whose chromosomes are not segregated. The rRNA genes of the recessive species, when present, are not expressed. The two species of RNA can be distinguished because human 28S rRNA migrates in gels at a slightly slower speed than 28S rRNA of rodents (Eliceiri and Green 1969). For our studies, we selected 55-54 cells, a hybrid cell line between human fibrosarcoma HT1080 cells and BALB/c macrophage in which the human species is dominant. The hybrid cells have retained all human chromosomes and 18 mouse chromosomes, including chromosomes 12, 15, and 18, where the mouse genes for rRNA are located (Croce 1976). These hybrid cells express human 28S rRNA but not mouse 28S rRNA, although mouse rRNA genes are present (Croce et al. 1977). Infection of 55-54 cells with SV40 reactivates the silent mouse rRNA genes (Soprano

TABLE 3. *Sequences of SV40 genome required for induction of cell DNA synthesis or reactivation of ribosomal RNA genes*

SV40 information (map units)	Induction of cell DNA replication	Reactivation of ribosomal RNA genes
1.00/0	+	+
1.00/0.144	+	+
0.73/0.27	+	+
0.70/0.33	+	+
0.76/0.375	+	−
0.71/0.42	+	−
△ 0.59/0.54	+	+
△ 0.65/0.51	+	+
0.28/0.11	ND	−
0.39/0.11	ND	+
0.44/0.11	ND	+
0.59/0.11	ND	+

The map units are given counterclockwise on the conventional SV40 map. The first eight fragments of SV40 were tested by manual microinjection, the last four by infection with adeno-SV40 hybrid viruses.

△, deletion; ND, not done.

Data summarized from Soprano et al. (1981) and Galanti et al. (1981).

et al. 1979), but infection with adenovirus 2 does not (Soprano et al. 1980).

In Table 3 we have summarized our studies on the map coordinates of SV40 that contain the information necessary and sufficient for either the stimulation of cell DNA replication or the reactivation of silent rRNA genes. These studies are the summary of two separate papers by Soprano et al. (1981) and by Galanti et al. (submitted for publication). From Table 3 it is evident that the information for these two fundamental processes of cell proliferation, growth in size and cell DNA replication, is encoded in different DNA sequences on the same SV40 genome. The information for cell DNA replication maps between map units 0.51 and 0.42 of the SV40 genome, while the information for rRNA synthesis stimulation maps between 0.39 and 0.33 map units of the genome. In other words, we can get viruses and mutant viruses that can stimulate cell DNA replication only or can stimulate synthesis of rRNA only. These processes, therefore, have different molecular bases.

DISCUSSION AND CONCLUSIONS

The conclusions that one can draw from these experiments are: (1) There are genes that can stimulate cell DNA replication and there are genes that can stimulate rRNA synthesis, i.e., growth in size. (2) Cell DNA replication is dependent on a functional RNA polymerase II, which means it is dependent on the transcription of unique copy genes. In contrast, growth in size is independent from a functional RNA polymerase II, although it requires an active RNA polymerase I. (3) Viral genes, like those of SV40 and adenovirus, can induce cell DNA replication in the absence of certain G_1 cellular functions that are required by serum-stimulated cells.

In terms of nutrition, these studies clearly indicate that transforming genes can lower the requirements not only for nutrients and growth factors but also for certain intracellular functions that are necessary for orderly progression in the cell cycle.

The implication of these findings and conclusions are manifold, but we would like to point out a few corollaries that may be of immediate interest to the problem of nutrition and cancer. It is apparently possible to stimulate cell DNA replication while avoiding increase in cell size. A condition like this usually results in unbalanced growth, which leads to the death of the cell. It is conceivable that in the foreseeable future one could actually kill tumor cells by inducing them into DNA synthesis while restraining them from growing in size. This is a rather unorthodox approach in the sense that in such a procedure we would do the opposite of what one usually does, i.e., try to kill cancer cells by inhibiting cell DNA synthesis.

A second implication is that the growth factors and nutrients that control cell proliferation in the environment may be different, i.e., there may be growth factors that stimulate cell growth while others stimulate cell DNA replication. Indeed, there are some cases, for instance estrogens (Hamilton 1968) or ACTH (Alvarez and Lavender 1974), in which the effect on cells is largely due to a growth in size rather than to cell DNA synthesis, but up to now no one has been able to separate clearly growth factors that stimulate growth in size from growth factors that stimulate cell DNA replication. Since these two processes can be separated at the gene level, it is possible that they will also be separable at the level of nutrients and growth factors.

Finally, one can advance the hypothesis that similar gene sequences are present in normal cells and that a fundamental difference between normal and cancer cells is that these genes are under tighter control in normal cells than they are in transformed cells. In other words, it may be possible that the same gene sequences are expressed in normal cells only under optimal conditions of nutrition and growth factors, whereas they are expressed in cancer cells even when the nutritional and growth factor environment is considerably below optimal. This approach is the first demonstration that cell proliferation can now be studied at a molecular level inside the cell and that this molecular basis may eventually be related to the nutritional conditions of the environment.

ACKNOWLEDGMENTS

This work was supported by U.S. Public Health Service Research Grants CA 14907 and CA 12923.

REFERENCES

Alvarez, M. R., and K. Lavender. 1974. Nuclear cytochemical changes in rat adrenal glands stimulated by adrenocorticotrophic hormone. Exp. Cell Res. 83:1–8.

Anderson, W. F., L. Killos, L. Sanders-Haigh, P. J. Kretschmer, and E. G. Diacumakos. 1980. Replication and expression of thymidine kinase and human globin genes microinjected into mouse fibroblasts. Proc. Natl. Acad. Sci. USA 77:5399–5403.

Ashihara, T., F. Traganos, R. Baserga, and Z. Darzynkiewicz. 1978. A comparison of cell cycle-related changes in postmitotic and quiescent AF8 cells as measured by cytofluorometry after acridine orange staining. Cancer Res. 38:2514–2518.

Baserga, R., and D. Malamud. 1969. Autoradiography: Techniques and applications. Hoeber, New York, 281 pp.

Bravo, R., and J. E. Celis. 1980. Direct microinjection of rabbit globin mRNA into mouse 3T3 cells. Exp. Cell Res. 126:481–485.

Croce, C. 1976. Loss of mouse chromosomes in somatic cell hybrids between HT-1080 human fibrosarcoma cells and mouse peritoneal macrophages. Proc. Natl. Acad. Sci. USA 73:3248–3252.

Croce, C. M., A. Talavera, C. Basilico, and O. J. Miller. 1977. Suppression of production of mouse 28S ribosomal RNA in mouse-human hybrids segregating mouse chromosomes. Proc. Natl. Acad. Sci. USA 74:694–697.

Eliceiri, G. L., and H. Green. 1969. Ribosomal RNA synthesis in human-mouse hybrid cells. J. Mol. Biol. 41:253–260.

Feramisco, J. R. 1979. Microinjection of fluorescently labeled α-actinin into living fibroblasts. Proc. Natl. Acad. Sci. USA 76:3967–3971.

Floros, J., T. Ashihara, and R. Baserga. 1978. Characterization of ts13 cells. A temperature-sensitive mutant of the G_1 phase of the cell cycle. Cell Biol. Int. Rep. 2:259–269.

Floros, J., G. Jonak, N. Galanti, and R. Baserga. 1981. Induction of cell DNA replication in G_1 specific ts mutants by microinjection of SV40 DNA. Exp. Cell Res. (in press).

Galanti, N., G. J. Jonak, K. J. Soprano, J. Floros, L. Kaczmarek, S. Weissman, V. B. Reddy, S. M. Tilghman, and R. Baserga. 1981. Characterization and biological activity of cloned SV40 DNA fragments. J. Biol. Chem. (in press).

Graessmann, A., and M. Graessmann. 1976. "Early" simian virus-40-specific RNA contains information for tumor antigen formation and chromatin replication. Proc. Natl. Acad. Sci. USA 73:366–370.

Graessmann, A., M. Graessmann, W. C. Topp, and M. Botchan. 1979. Retransformation of a simian virus 40 revertant cell line, which is resistant to viral and DNA infections, by microinjection of viral DNA. J. Virol. 32:989–994.

Hamilton, T. H. 1968. Control by estrogen of genetic transcription and translation. Science 161:649–661.

Hirt, B. 1967. Selective extraction of polyoma DNA from infected mouse cell cultures. J. Mol. Biol. 26:365–369.

Kreis, T. E., K. H. Winterhalter, and W. Birchmeier. 1979. In vivo distribution and turnover of fluorescently labeled actin microinjected into human fibroblasts. Proc. Natl. Acad. Sci. USA 76:3814–3818.

Lewis, A. M. 1977. Defective and nondefective Ad2-SV40 hybrids. Prog. Med. Virol. 23:96–139.

MacPherson, I., and L. M. Montagnier. 1964. Agar suspension culture for the selective assay of cells transformed by polyoma virus. Virology 23:291–294.

Meiss, H. K., and C. Basilico. 1972. Temperature-sensitive mutants of BHK 21 cells. Nature New Biol. 239:66–68.

Mitsui, Y., and E. L. Schneider. 1976. Relationship between cell replication and volume in senescent human diploid fibroblasts. Mech. Ageing Dev. 5:45–56.

Mueller, G., A. Graessmann, and M. Graessmann. 1978. Mapping of early SV40 specific functions by microinjection of different early viral DNA fragments. Cell 15:579–585.

Pochron, S., M. Rossini, Z. Darzynkiewicz, F. Traganos, and R. Baserga. 1980. Failure of accumulation of cellular RNA in hamster cells stimulated to synthesize DNA by infection with adenovirus 2. J. Biol. Chem. 255:4411–4413.

Pope, J. H., and W. P. Rowe. 1964. Detection of specific antigen in SV40 transformed cells by immunofluorescence. J. Exp. Med. 120:121–130.

Richardson, W. D., B. J. Carter, and H. Westphal. 1980. Vero cells injected with adenovirus type 2 mRNA produce authentic viral polypeptide patterns: Early mRNA promotes growth of adenovirus-associated virus. Proc. Natl. Acad. Sci. USA 77:931–935.

Rossini, M., and R. Baserga. 1978. RNA synthesis in a cell cycle-specific temperature sensitive mutant from a hamster cell line. Biochemistry 17:858–863.

Rossini, M., S. Baserga, C. H. Huang, C. J. Ingles, and R. Baserga. 1980. Changes in RNA polymerase II in cell cycle-specific temperature-sensitive mutant of hamster cells. J. Cell. Physiol. 103:97–103.

Rossini, M., R. Weinmann, and R. Baserga. 1979. DNA synthesis in temperature-sensitive mutants of the cell cycle infected by polyoma virus and adenovirus. Proc. Natl. Acad. Sci. USA 76:4441–4445.

Schwyzer, N. 1977. Purification of SV40 T antigen by immunoaffinity chromatography on staphylococcal protein A sepharose. INSERM. Early Proteins of Oncogenic DNA Viruses 69:63–68.

Soprano, K. J., V. G. Dev, C. M. Croce, and R. Baserga. 1979. Reactivation of silent rRNA genes by simian virus 40 in human-mouse hybrid cells. Proc. Natl. Acad. Sci. USA 76:3885–3889.

Soprano, K. J., G. J. Jonak, N. Galanti, J. Floros, and R. Baserga. 1981. Identification of an SV40 DNA sequence related to the reactivation of silent rRNA genes in human>mouse hybrid cells. Virology 109:127–136.

Soprano, K. J., M. Rossini, C. Croce, and R. Baserga. 1980. The role of large T antigen in simian virus 40-induced reactivation of silent rRNA genes in human-mouse hybrid cells. Virology 102:317–326.

Stacey, D. 1980. Behavior of microinjected molecules and recipient cells, *in* Introduction of Macromolecules into Viable Mammalian Cells, R. Baserga, C. Croce, and G. Rovera, eds. Alan Liss, New York, pp. 125–134.

Talavera, A., and C. Basilico, 1977. Temperature-sensitive mutants of BHK cells affected in cell cycle progression. J. Cell Physiol. 92:425–436.

Tjian, R., G. Fey, and A. Graessmann. 1978. Biological activity of purified simian virus 40 T antigen proteins. Proc. Natl. Acad. Sci. USA 75:1279–1283.

Tooze, J. 1980. DNA Tumor Viruses. Cold Spring Harbor Laboratory, Cold Spring Harbor.

Weil, R. 1978. Viral 'tumor antigens:' A novel type of mammalian regulator protein. Biochim. Biophys. Acta 516:301–388.

Molecular Interrelations of Nutrition and Cancer,
edited by M. S. Arnott, J. van Eys and Y.-M. Wang.
Raven Press, New York © 1982.

Nutritional Manipulations of the Growth Kinetics of Normal and Malignant Cells in vivo

James J. Stragand

Department of Laboratory Medicine, The University of Texas M. D. Anderson Hospital and Tumor Institute at Houston, Houston, Texas 77030

Malignant disease has often been characterized as a disorder of cell proliferation, and this concept has formed the basis for many treatment strategies, specifically the use of agents cytotoxic to actively dividing cells. This strategy suffers from the disadvantage that the patient represents an integrated system of proliferative compartments, both tumor and normal. Typically, the human tumor proliferates much slower than the normal tissue counterpart (Baserga and Kisieleski 1962, Bottomley and Cooper 1973, Hill 1978) and as such is less sensitive to therapy. As a consequence, for each treatment directed against the tumor, one may expect to produce at least an equal amount of normal tissue toxicity. The success of the treatment protocol then depends on the extent of damage and the timing of recovery of normal tissue versus that of the tumor.

One approach to the problem of differential cell killing involves the use of agents or procedures designed to minimize the proliferative difference between the tumor and normal tissues. These agents would ideally increase tumor cell proliferation, thereby increasing the susceptibility to therapy, or reduce normal tissue proliferation, minimizing normal tissue toxicity. Historically, tumor cell proliferation has been enhanced by applying an initial bolus of drug or radiation designed to "recruit" the large nonproliferative tumor cell population into the proliferative cycle (Van Putten et al. 1976). This initial dose is then followed, at an appropriate interval, by a second agent designed to exploit the increased tumor proliferation. The obvious disadvantage of this approach lies in its inherent toxicity. Other approaches have employed pretreatment with protein synthesis inhibitors such as cycloheximide to reduce the subsequent damage from cytotoxic challenge (Ben-Ishay and Farber 1976).

What I would like to address in this chapter is the possible use of the host's nutritional status to modify selectively normal and tumor cell proliferation and the resultant damage from cycle-active chemotherapy. It has been known for many years that nutrition can markedly influence the growth kinetics of both normal and malignant tissues (Rous 1914). In vivo animal studies indicate that caloric "underfeeding" or the elimination of specific dietary components such

TABLE 1. *Effect of diets on experimental tumors*

Dietary component or nutritional manipulation	System	Effect	Reference
Fats			
Low-fat or saturated fat (p.o.)	Mouse C3H/BA adenocarcinoma	Reduced tumor growth	Rao and Abraham 1976
High-linoleate (p.o.)	Mouse C3H/BA adenocarcinoma	Enhanced tumor growth	Rao and Abraham 1976
Corn oil (saturated) (i.p.)	Rat hepatoma 7777 and 7800	Reduced tumor growth	Gilbertson et al. 1977
High-lipid (IVH)	Rat mammary adenocarcinoma	Host growth without tumor stimulation	Buzby et al. 1978
Proteins—amino acids			
Low phenylalanine (p.o.)	Mouse L1210 leukemia	Reduced tumor growth	Pine 1978
High-protein (IVH)	Rat mammary adenocarcinoma	Enhanced tumor growth	Buzby et al. 1978
Low-protein (p.o.)	Rat intestine	Reduced proliferation	Hooper et al. 1968
Low valine, threonine, isoleucine, or methionine (p.o.)	Mouse BW 10232 adenocarcinoma	Reduced tumor mass	Theuer 1971
Minerals			
Low Mg^{++} or K$^+$ (p.o.)	Rat Yoshida or Walker 256 carcinoma	Reduced tumor mass	Young and Parsons 1977
Zinc (i.p.)	Mouse L1210 leukemia	Reduced tumor mass	Phillips and Sheridan 1977
Fasting and refeeding with elemental diet + FeCl$_3$ (p.o.)	Mouse intestine	Colonic hyperplasia	Stragand and Hagemann 1978a
Fasting and refeeding with elemental diet + NaCl (p.o.)	Mouse intestine	No colonic hyperplasia	Stragand and Hagemann 1978a
Low-zinc (p.o.)	Rat Walker 256 carcinoma	Reduced tumor growth	McQuitty et al. 1970
Vitamins			
Increased vitamin A (p.o.)	Mouse C3HBA adenocarcinoma	Reduced tumor growth	Rettura et al. 1975
Hypervitaminosis A	Rabbit Shope papilloma	Reduced tumor growth	McMichael 1965
High-dose ascorbic acid	Human rectal polyps	Reduced mass	Decosse et al. 1975
High-dose ascorbic acid	Mouse sarcoma 180	Reduced tumor growth	Yamafuji et al. 1971

General			
Starvation	Mouse Ehrlich ascites, T1699 mammary	Reduced tumor mass	Sandor 1976
Starving and refeeding	C3H/HeJ spontaneous mammary tumor	G_1 block and synchronization and recruitment	Stragand et al. 1979
Starving and refeeding	SW 620 human colonic adenocarcinoma xenografts	G_2 block and synchronization	Stragand et al. 1980b
Hyperalimentation (IVH)	Rat hepatoma 7777	Increased mitotic index	Cameron and Paviat 1976
Elemental diet	Mouse intestine	Reduced proliferation	Lehnert 1979

as proteins tend to reduce the incidence of spontaneous neoplasm and retard the establishment and growth of transplantable tumors. Hyperalimentation or an alteration of the dietary composition can increase the incidence and growth of malignant tissues (Table 1). In vitro nutritional studies have also established a disparity in the kinetic responses of normal cells and their virus-transformed counterparts. When deprived of serum or essential amino acids, normal cells became blocked at a point in mid G_1 termed the "restriction point" (Pardee 1974). The cells remained blocked until adequate nutritional conditions were reestablished. In contrast, transformed cells were delayed randomly throughout the cell cycle, indicating a loss of the restriction point function.

The use of nutrition in the treatment of malignant disease may offer a significant advantage over recruitment procedures employing cytotoxic agents only. The nutritional status of cancer patients is often dramatically compromised by the anorexia and oligophagia attendant on the disease and its therapy (Costa 1977). This poor nutritional status is often corrected through intravenous hyperalimentation (IVH) techniques (Copeland and Dudrick 1975, Copeland et al. 1975). In essence, the cancer patient may routinely experience hypercaloric and hypocaloric states as a consequence of the disease or therapy. If these various nutritional states are reflected by specific cytokinetic responses within the tumor or normal tissues, it is conceivable that these changes could be exploited through the proper selection and scheduling of systemic chemotherapy.

In this chapter, I will describe how altered nutritional states can selectively affect the cytokinetic profiles of normal and malignant murine tissues and human tumors in a tissue-specific manner. It is also my hope to show how these altered nutritional states may be used to enhance the subsequent tumor response to cycle-active chemotherapy. Previous studies have established that kinetically directed therapy may be used to enhance the tumor response (Braunschweiger and Schiffer 1978, Schenken 1976, Skipper et al. 1967).

MATERIALS AND METHODS

Animals

All animals employed in these studies were maintained in temperature-controlled rooms with a 12-hour photoperiod and had access to water *ad libitum* throughout. Studies of intestinal cell renewal employed HA/ICR female mice (20–25 g). Murine mammary tumor studies employed the spontaneous mammary tumor (SMT) of the C_3H/HeJ retired female breeders (9–12 months old) and T-1699 transplantable mammary tumor (TMT) in DBA/2J mice (20–22 g). Human colonic tumor xenografts were established by subcutaneous inoculation of 5×10^7 SW 620 human colonic adenocarcinoma cells into female BALB/c athymic mice (18–20 g) housed under laminar flow hoods in isolation rooms maintained at 27.6°C.

Nutritional Manipulations: Fasting-Refeeding

Animals were fasted for periods of 48 to 72 hours, beginning at 1200 hours, in metabolism cages to eliminate the ingestion of bedding or fecal materials. A fast of this duration produces a 15–20% loss in body weight with no apparent harm to the animal. After fasting, animals were refed *ad libitum* with laboratory chow (Purina) or with defined pellet diets based on the Purina formula. These diets were either complete or lacking in one or more dietary components. All food supply was weighed before and after the animals ate to determine diet palatability and consumption.

Cell Kinetic Analysis

Normal Tissues

Cell Kinetic analysis of intestinal tissue was based on the technique of Hagemann et al. (1970). Briefly, animals received a single intraperitoneal injection of 2 μCi tritiated thymidine ([³H]Thd) per gram body weight 30 min prior to sacrifice. Samples of the terminal ileum and ascending colon were removed, weighed, fixed in Clark's solution to remove unincorporated [³H]Thd, and solubilized, and disintegrations were counted by standard liquid scintillation counting techniques. The data were expressed as disintegrations per minute per milligram of tissue (dpm/mg). This technique is based on the observation that over 95% of the cells that incorporate [³H]Thd are the proliferative S-phase cells of the adult intestinal mucosa. If macroscopic germinal lymphatic centers are avoided during sampling, the dpm/mg parameter provides a reliable estimate of intestinal S-phase cellularity (Stragand and Hagemann 1978b). When necessary, we did more detailed studies by the crypt dissection technique of Wimber et al. (1960), which allows for the direct quantitation of the number of crypt cells that incorporate [³H]Thd, expressed as labeled nuclei (LN) per crypt. In studies employing BALB/c athymic mice, samples of the esophagus, stomach (fundus), duodenum, jejunum, ileum, ascending and descending colon, and femurs were analyzed. The femurs were removed, cleaned of adherent muscle, and solubilized in 2.0 ml Soluene-100 (Packard) at 37°C for 48 hours. Disintegrations were counted and the data expressed as disintegrations per minute per milligram of intestinal tissue or per total femur.

Tumor Tissue

Tumor tissue kinetics were analyzed by in vitro techniques based on the primer available DNA polymerase (PDP) assay to estimate the tumor growth fraction (GF), by single [³H]Thd labeling studies to determine the thymidine-labeling index ([³H]Thd L.I.), and by double thymidine labeling to determine the S-phase duration. These procedures are described in great detail elsewhere (Schiffer et al. 1976, Braunschweiger et al. 1976, Stragand et al. 1979).

Briefly, approximately 0.5 to 1.0 cm³ of tumor was minced in Ham's F-10 medium, filtered through a stainless steel screen, washed twice, and resuspended in fresh medium. Aliquots of this sample were taken and cytocentrifuge preparations were made for use in the PDP assay. In this assay, the sample nuclei are provided with the necessary materials for DNA synthesis, including tritiated thymidine triphosphate. When both αDNA polymerase and DNA template are present in the nuclei, DNA synthesis occurs and can be quantitated by autoradiography. The percentage of labeled nuclei is termed the PDP index and has been shown to provide a good estimate of the GF in murine solid tumors, as determined from mathematical calculations of percentage of labeled mitoses (PLM) data (Schiffer et al. 1976). One thousand cells were examined for each PDP index.

The remaining tumor sample was incubated with [³H]Thd (2.5 μCi/ml, 20 Ci/mmol) at 37°C for 30 min in [³H]Thd L.I. studies or for 60 min in double-labeling T_s determinations. In the latter case [¹⁴C]Thd (0.25 μCi/ml, 51 Ci/mmol) was added after 60 min for an additional 30 min. Labeling was terminated on ice, and viable cells were isolated on a Ficoll-Hypaque gradient. The cells were then washed and cytocentrifuge preparations were made. One thousand cells were examined for each [³H]Thd L.I. determination, while 200 labeled cells were evaluated for the T_s estimate.

RESULTS

Nutritional Effects on Intestinal Cell Renewal

The effects of a 72-hour period of fasting followed by refeeding with standard laboratory chow on the proliferative activity of the intestinal epithelium in HA/ICR female mice is shown in Figure 1. As indicated, both the large and small bowel showed a decline in proliferation during the fasting period, as measured by both dpm/mg and LN/crypt. During this period, the ileum also exhibited a significant cell loss, which reached 60% of the control value after 72 hours. The colon, in contrast, maintained its cellularity throughout the fast. Following refeeding, ileal proliferative indices exhibited a gradual return to control values, with a moderate overshoot observed in LN/crypt value at 24 hours. During this same period, the colonic epithelium showed a dramatic increase in proliferation, reaching four times the fasting level by 8 hours of refeeding, plateauing at 16–24 hours and regaining the control values by 36 hours.

The mechanism underlying this differential tissue-specific response of the small and large bowel, separated by only 2 cm, is suggested by PLM experiments and temporal appearance of LN and mitotic figures (MF) following refeeding. PLM data (Table 2) for the ileum indicated a lengthening of all cell cycle phases during fasting. With refeeding, a simultaneous increase in both LN and

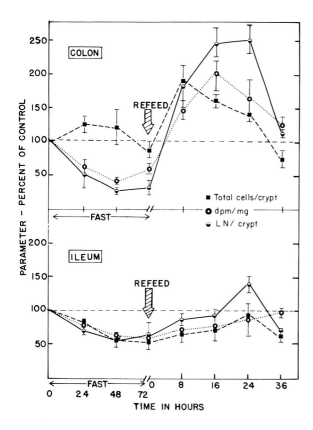

FIG. 1. Effects of fasting and refeeding on the proliferative activity and cellularity of the ileum and colon in HA/ICR mice. Mean ± one standard error, 5–10 mice per point. (Reproduced from Hagemann and Stragand 1977, with permission of *Cell and Tissue Kinetics*.)

MF/crypt was observed. These data suggest an overall lengthening of the cell cycle during fasting and subsequent shortening of the cell cycle following refeeding. In contrast, colonic PLM data indicate a lengthening of only the G_1 phase during fasting, with all other cycle phases remaining constant. Within 4 hours

TABLE 2. *Cell cycle times for the ileum and colon in control, fasting, and refed animals**

	T_c (hr)	G_1 (hr)	S (hr)	$G_2 + 0.7$ M (hr)
Ileum				
Control	12.6	5.3	5.9	1.4
Fasting	20.1	9.3	9.3	1.5
Refed	10.8	3.8	5.6	1.4
Colon				
Control	18.2	9.9	7.1	1.2
Fasting	35.3	26.1	7.6	1.6
Refed	14.8	5.8	7.0	2.0

* Cycle times were mathematically determined from graphic data by the asymmetry technique of Mendelsohn and Takahashi (1971).

of refeeding, the colon exhibited a twofold to threefold increase in the LN/ crypt value, followed at 12 hours by a similar increase in MF/crypt (see Figure 4, panel A). This sequential appearance of LN followed by MF suggests the induction of a cell cycle block in the G_1 period during fasting, which is released upon refeeding, causing a parasynchronous progression of cells into DNA synthesis and mitosis. This parasynchronized progression will be discussed in more detail later.

Other factors contributing to the disparity in the responses of the small and large bowel concern changes in crypt cellularity. As indicated in Figure 1, the colonic crypt maintained control cellularity levels during fasting. This maintenance of the normal crypt compartment size may place the colonic crypt in a configuration whereby it was able to respond significantly to the refeeding stimulus. In contrast, the ileal crypt showed a marked reduction in crypt cellularity during fasting. As a result, the refeeding signal elicited its effects on a depleted ileal crypt compartment, reducing the overall magnitude of the ileal refeeding response. These differential changes in crypt cellularity are believed to be based on differences in intestinal transit times during the fasting and refeeding periods.

The causal mechanism underlying the response to fasting and refeeding in the colonic epithelium obviously lies in the physiological/nutritional aspects of food ingestion. The physiological component includes the abrasive and distending nature of food entering the colonic lumen; the nutritional aspect deals with the food composition and the resultant blood-borne elements.

In order to determine whether the physical presence of food in the gut lumen was required to initiate the refeeding response, the following experiment was performed. Mice were fasted for 24 hours to remove any material from the gut lumen. The colon was then surgically ligated approximately 2 cm from the ileocecal junction with gastrointestinal suture. The ligations were performed in such a manner that the superior mesenteric artery was not disturbed. It was assumed that all mice therefore had an intact blood supply to all colonic regions. Following ligation, the fast was continued for an additional 48 hours, for a total fasting interval of 72 hours. The mice was then refed for 8 hours and the colonic proliferative activity determined as described previously. The rationale for this procedure is as follows: The side of the colon proximal to the ligation will receive both physical and nutritional stimulation from the refed diet, whereas the distal side will receive only nutritional stimulation. If the proliferative signal is based on nutritional factors, both proximal and distal colonic regions should respond equally. Alternatively, if the signal is based on the physical aspects of refeeding, only the proximal region will respond. The results of these ligation studies are presented in Table 3. As indicated by line 7, the side of the colon proximal to the ligation and in contact with the food showed a dramatic proliferative response to refeeding, whereas the side distal to the ligation remained at the hypoproliferative fasting level. This indicated that the physical presence of food in the lumen was required in part to initiate the colonic refeeding response and perhaps to maintain the steady-state renewal

TABLE 3. *Effect of food restriction on the colonic refeeding response*

Treatment	dpm/mg, % Control
1. Sham ligation	100 ± 10*
2. Sham ligation + 48-hr fast	63 ± 5
3. Sham ligation + 72-hr fast	42 ± 10
4. Sham ligation + 72-hr fast + 8-hr refeed	208 ± 20
5. Ligation + 48-hr fast	
Proximal to ligation	81 ± 25
Distal to ligation	40 ± 10
6. Ligation + 72-hr fast	
Proximal to ligation	241 ± 28
Distal to ligation	59 ± 8
7. Ligation + 72-hr fast + 8-hr refeed	
Proximal to ligation	425 ± 75
Distal to ligation	82 ± 2

* Mean value of 5–10 mice ± one standard error.

rate as suggested previously in IVH studies. (Bounous et al. 1971a, 1971b).

A possible role for physical stimulation is evidenced in Table 3, line 6. In ligated animals, 72 hours of *fasting without refeeding* produced a hyperplasia ($241 \pm 28\%$ control) similar to that of a control animal after 72-hour fast and refeeding (line 4). An explanation for this is that the ligation procedure resulted in a significant accumulation of fluids on the proximal side of the ligation, producing a colonic distention. The diameter of the proximal colonic region of a ligated animal after 48 hours of fasting (0.45 ± 0.3 cm) was 1.5 times that of control animals and 2.6 times that of the distal region (0.17 ± 0.1 cm). However, this fluid-induced distention was similar to that seen in non-ligated animals after 2–8 hours of refeeding (0.48 ± 0.06 cm). It is assumed, therefore, that at least part of the colonic refeeding signal was associated with the physical presence of food in the large bowel, perhaps in the form of distention. In studies to ascertain the mitogenic activity of the distending fluid itself, no proliferative stimulation was seen in control animals or when the fluid was transferred to the distal colonic regions.

In order to examine the effects of nutrition on the colonic refeeding response, the following experiments were performed. Animals were fasted for 72 hours and refed *ad libitum* with Purina lab chow or one of several defined diets, based on the composition of the lab chow. These various diets were prepared utilizing the following materials in the percentages listed.

Carbohydrate: sucrose, reagent grade (Fisher), 67%.
Protein: casein hydrolysate (ICN Pharmaceuticals), 22%.
Fat: polyethylated vegetable oil, EL-620 (GAF Corp.), 5%.
Minerals: balanced salt mixture (ICN Pharmaceuticals).
Vitamins: vitamin diet fortification mixture (ICN Pharmaceuticals), 2%.
Fiber: nonnutritive cellulose fiber (Teklad Mills Labs). Fiber added at 10% (w/w) of the above components.

The synthetic diets were mixed in various combinations (Figure 2) and made into pellets with a mechanical pelleter (Parr Inst., Moline, Ill.), with water and fat as binding agents. A low-bulk calcium-free diet (GIBCO) was also employed. After 16 hours of refeeding, proliferative activity in the colon was determined, as described previously, by [³H]Thd incorporation. The results of these studies are presented in Figure 2. As indicated, the majority of diets possessed the capacity to restore colonic proliferation from the hypoproliferative fasting level to those of control during the 16-hour refeeding period. However, only three diets were able to induce the colonic hyperplasia seen after refeeding with chow. The factors common to the three diets were: sugar, casein (amino acids), and a dietary salt mixture (excluding calcium). These three components appear to represent the minimum essential dietary requirements for the refeeding hyperplasia, since elimination of any one of the three reduced the response dramatically. It was hypothesized that one or all of these agents were involved in the removal of the fasting-induced G_1 block and subsequently provided the factors required for the entry of cells into DNA synthesis. Both sugar and protein may represent basic nutritional requirements for the fasted animal to return to the normal physiological state. The mineral requirement could represent

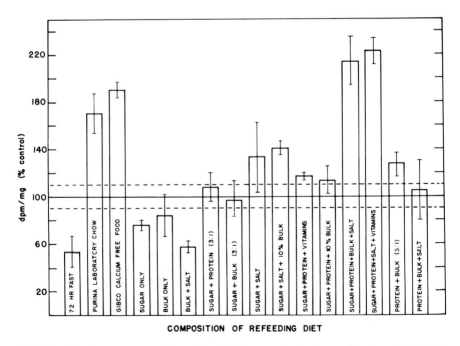

FIG. 2. Proliferative response of the colon at 16 hours of refeeding with various diets. Mean of 5–10 mice per point ± one standard error. Horizontal lines delimit range of control mice. (Reprinted from Stragand and Hagemann 1977, with permission of *American Journal of Clinical Nutrition.*)

the need for specific ions similar to the calcium requirement in the hepatic response to partial hepatectomy (McManus et al. 1975).

In order to investigate further this mineral requirement in the refeeding response, the following experiment was performed. Animals were fasted for 72 hours and refed with one of the following diets: (1) lab chow; (2) a complete diet prepared in the laboratory as described previously; (3) a diet based on diet 2 but without salt; (4) specific salt diets composed of diet 3 plus 3% of the monovalent and divalent salt groups described by Kenny and Munson (1959); or (5) diet 3 plus 3% of specific salts. The proliferative response of the colon to refeeding with these various diets is presented in Figure 3. Animals refed with a diet containing a complete salt mixture duplicated the response observed with standard laboratory chow. If, however, the salt component was deleted

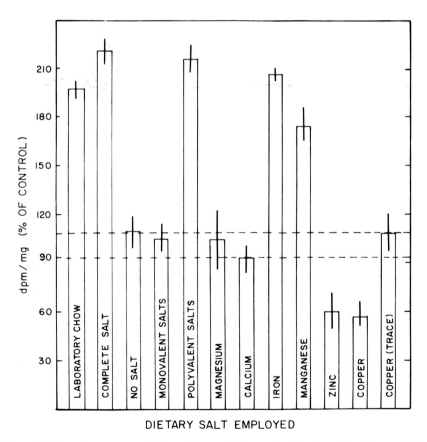

FIG. 3. Proliferative response of the colon at 16 hours of refeeding with diets containing varying mineral components. Mean of five mice per point ± one standard error. All salts at 3% (w/w) except "trace" = 0.3%. (Reproduced from Stragand and Hagemann 1978a, with permission of *Cell and Tissue Kinetics.*)

or replaced with monovalent salts, no stimulated entry into S-phase by refeeding was observed. Substitution of specific polyvalent salts for the dietary mineral requirement showed iron and, to a lesser extent, manganese to be effective inducers of the colonic hyperplasia. Magnesium, calcium, zinc, and copper failed to increase the proliferative activity over control levels.

The detailed cytodynamic response of the colon to refeeding with: (1) standard laboratory chow, (2) a salt-free diet, or (3) a diet containing 3% ferric chloride as the sole mineral component is presented in Figure 4. Refeeding with standard lab chow (panel A) resulted in the rapid accumulation of labeled nuclei, followed some 12 hours later by a similar increase in the mitotic figures/crypt. If mice were refed with a salt-free diet (panel B), there was no hyperplasia or evidence of a parasynchronous progression through the cell cycle. However, when iron was substituted as the sole mineral component (panel C), colonic S-phase cellular-

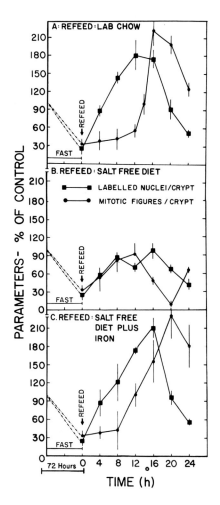

FIG. 4. Temporal response of the colon to fasting and refeeding with diets with and without iron salts. Mean of five mice per point ± one standard error. (Reproduced from Stragand and Hagemann 1978a, with permission of *Cell and Tissue Kinetics.*)

ity was markedly increased, and the colonic cell progression through the subsequent cell cycle was again parasynchronized.

The results further show a distinct synchronization of the colonic crypt cells following fasting and refeeding with standard laboratory chow. The duration of the colonic S phase in untreated animals is approximately 8 hours, with a G_1 of approximately 10 hours (Hagemann and Stragand 1977). The timing and sequential appearance of labeled nuclei and mitotic figures would suggest that this synchronization is the result of a prompt removal of a fasting-induced cycle block in G_1. The presence of this G_1 block following fasting would agree with the "restriction point" block following serum deprivation in vitro as proposed by Pardee (1974). In the present study the exact position of this cycle block cannot be ascertained with certainty. The rapid increase in labeled nuclei upon refeeding would suggest the block to be operant near the G_1/S border. However, it is not possible to distinguish this possibility from a cycle blockage at an earlier G_1 period, with an accelerated transit through late G_1 following refeeding. That the synchronous movement of cells is not observed following refeeding with a salt-free diet suggests an incomplete removal of the block. Substituting iron as the sole dietary mineral component again produces the synchronous hyperplasia with refeeding. These results suggest that iron is a major cofactor required in the removal of the G_1 block or that the lack of iron in the refeeding diet is itself producing a cycle block at some point between the nutritional block and the G_1-S boundary.

A dietary mineral requirement in normal steady-state colonic cell renewal has been established (Stragand and Hagemann 1977). The present results would suggest a potential role for iron in the continued maintenance of the colonic epithelium in nutritionally complete animals. At the cellular level these findings may not be unique to the colon. An iron requirement for DNA synthesis has been shown in HeLa cells (Robbins et al. 1972) and human lymphocytes (Hoffbrand et al. 1976).

Nutritional Effects on Murine Tumor Cell Renewal

The effect of fasting-refeeding on tumor cell proliferation was examined in two very different experimental mammary adenocarcinomas, the T-1699 transplantable mammary tumor (TMT) and the C_3H/HeJ spontaneous mammary tumor (SMT). These tumors were selected for nutritional studies on the basis of their divergent cell kinetic and morphological characteristics. The C_3H SMT is a slow growing, well-differentiated mammary adenocarcinoma, while the T-1699 TMT is fast growing and poorly differentiated.

Tumor-bearing mice were fasted for periods of 48 and 72 hours. Tumor growth was monitored by caliper measurements in two dimensions, tumor volumes were calculated ($V = LW^2 [\pi/6]$), growth curves constructed, and the tumor volume doubling times (T_D) estimated. Tumor cell kinetics were determined, as before, using the PDP assay and single- and double-thymidine labeling studies.

Calculations based on these measurements provide estimates of tumor cell cycle times (Steel 1977).

The effect of fasting and refeeding on the growth kinetics of the TMT and SMT are given in Table 4. Untreated control TMTs had a T_D of approximately 72 hours, while during fasting, animals showed a tumor regression of 5–20% and negative T_D values. Refeeding after 48 hours resulted in a sharp increase in tumor growth, attaining age-matched control tumor volumes by day 6. Refeeding at 72 hours resulted in a slower recovery. The T_Ds during refeeding were similar to the prefasting values, while in the age-matched controls the T_D had increased to 168 hours.

The T_D for untreated SMTs was approximately 13 days. During a 72-hour fast, the reduction in SMT volume ranged from 20% to 60%, with a mean reduction of 40% ± 7%. Refeeding resulted in a prompt resumption of growth; however, tumor volumes remained below age-matched control values for the remainder of the observation period.

In the TMT, 48 hours of fasting resulted in a 13% reduction in the tumor growth fraction (significant at $p \leq 0.05$) with a concomitant 45% reduction in the [³H]Thd L.I. The T_S value increased by a factor of 2, while the calculated cell cycle time increased by a factor of 3. The cytokinetic changes observed after 72 hours of fasting were of similar magnitude to those observed after 48 hours. In the SMT, fasting resulted in no significant change in the tumor growth fraction, but an 80% reduction in [³H]Thd L.I. was observed. The T_S increased slightly from 10.9 to 12 hours, while the calculated cell cycle time lengthened by a factor of 5 to over 110 hours.

The temporal cytokinetic response to fasting and refeeding in the T-1699 TMT is presented in Figure 5. Refeeding after a 48-hour fast resulted in a recovery to the age-matched control growth fraction by 24 hours. Refeeding after 72 hours of fasting resulted in a much slower recovery in the growth fraction. [³H]Thd L.I. following refeeding at 48 hours exhibited an initial sharp fluctuation and then a slow recovery to control levels during the next 72 hours. Refeeding after 72 hours of fasting produced no changes in the [³H]Thd L.I. until 72 hours after refeeding. Both the PDP and [³H]Thd indices increased

TABLE 4. *Cell kinetic parameters for control and fasting T-1699 TMT and C3H/HeJ SMT*

	T-1699 TMT			C3H/HeJ SMT	
	Control	48-hr fast	72-hr fast	Control	60-hr fast
T_D (hr)	72	−264†	−216†	312	−96
PDP-I (%)	70.6 ± 3.0	61.4 ± 4.1	49.9 ± 4.0	16.6 ± 0.4*	18.5 ± 3.5
[³H]Thd L.I. (%)	25.4 ± 1.2	13.4 ± 2.1	15.2 ± 1.9	6.9 ± 0.6*	1.5 ± 0.7
T_s (hr)	6.9 ± 0.2	15.2 ± 0.7	12.4 ± 0.1	10.9 ± 0.2*	12.0 ± 0.5
T_c (hr)	17.6	58.9	35.9	20.5	111.3

* From Braunschweiger et al. 1976.
† Negative value indicates time to 50% regression.

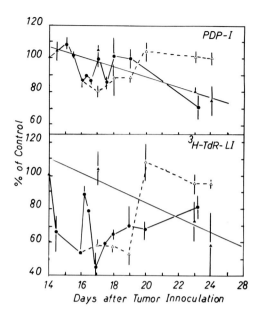

FIG. 5. Temporal response of the T-1699 TMT to a 48-hour (●) or 72-hour (△) fast versus control (▲—▲). Animals were fasted on day 14 and refed on day 16 or 17. Mean of five mice per point ± one standard error. (Reproduced from Stragand et al. 1979, with permission of *European Journal of Cancer.*)

over age-matched controls between days 3 and 7 after refeeding. However, in terms of kinetically directed therapy, in no instance were the refeeding-induced changes more advantageous than the cell kinetic profiles observed prior to fasting.

The temporal cytokinetic response to refeeding in the C_3H SMT is presented in Figure 6. A 2.7-fold increase in the tumor growth fraction was observed after 24 hours of refeeding, with control values being regained by 72 hours. The [^{3}H]Thd L.I. increased within 6 hours of refeeding, reaching a maximum value at 24 hours. The T_S value exhibited a fourfold increase over the control values at 6 hours and a twofold increase between 12 and 36 hours. Control T_S durations were reestablished by 48 hours and remained constant for the rest of the observation period.

As stated earlier, these tumors were selected for nutritional studies because of their divergent cytokinetic and morphological characteristics. In both tumors, nutritional deprivation produced a significant reduction in tumor volume. Upon refeeding of the animals, both tumors recovered rapidly, regaining their prefasting control growth rates within 1 to 2 days. Volume changes in both systems can be attributed to a pronounced depression in cell production, coupled with a continuing rate of cell loss. The cytodynamic basis for this diminished cell production, however, was unique to each system. In the TMT, fasting produced a generalized lengthening of the cell cycle, as evidenced by a twofold to threefold increase in both the T_S and cell cycle times. Upon refeeding, increases in the [^{3}H]Thd and PDP indices were observed within 24 hours after a 48-hour fast, while a *delayed* response was observed after a 72-hour fast. This suggests a dose-response type of relationship for the fasting stress in this poorly differenti-

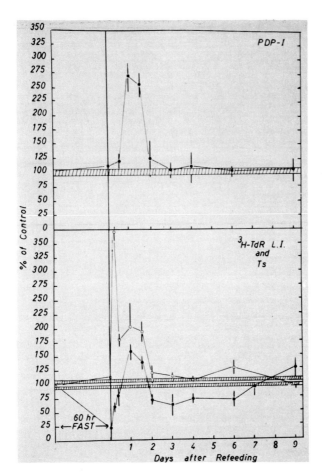

FIG. 6. Effect of a 60-hour fast plus refeeding on the PDP index, [³H]Thd L.I. (●—●), and Ts (○—○) of the C₃H SMT. Mean of three to five mice per point ± one standard error. Horizontal lines delimit control values ± one standard error. (Reproduced from Stragand et al. 1979, with permission of *European Journal of Cancer*.)

ated mammary adenocarcinoma. In contrast, the C₃H SMT showed a marked lengthening of the cell cycle during fasting, with only a slight increase in the duration of S-phase, together with an 80% reduction in the [³H]Thd L.I. The refeeding response of the [³H]Thd L.I. was initiated promptly, but increases in the PDP index were not observed until 24 hours after the refeeding signal. These observations are consistent with the presence of the cell cycle block near the G₁/S border, its prompt release upon refeeding, and a resulting parasynchronous movement of tumor cells into S phase. The division of these cells then produces the observed increase in the PDP index. Synchronization is further evidenced by the marked lengthening of T_S immediately after refeeding, reflective of a large cohort of cells entering S without a concomitant movement of cells into G₂. These events would tend to elevate the T_S measurement. The sustained increase in T₂ observed between 12 and 36 hours could be accounted for by the movement of cells into S, which exceeded the movement of cells into G₂ as would be expected during a recruitment period. Further evidence for the recruitment of noncycling tumor cells is given by the increase in the PDP index during refeeding. The magnitude of this increase (270% of control) was greater than that which could be expected from the division of the synchronous cohort of cells in mitosis, i.e., 200%.

In an effort to evaluate the therapeutic relevance of the cytokinetic events induced during nutritional manipulations in the C_3H SMT, the following experiments were performed. C_3H, tumor-bearing animals (0.5–0.8 cm^3) were fasted for 60 hours and then refed with standard lab chow. At 24 hours after refeeding, the animals were treated with methotrexate (MTX, 6 mg/kg) and 5-fluorouracil (5-FU, 42 mg/kg) to coincide with the increase in the tumor [^{3}H]Thd L.I. and PDP indices. Additional animals received chemotherapy without the fasting-refeeding pretreatment. The results of these studies are presented in Figure 7.

As indicated, MTX plus 5-FU alone produced a 20% reduction in tumor volume after 48 hours, with a subsequent rapid tumor recovery. Nutritional manipulations alone produced a 25% reduction in tumor volume, again with a rapid recovery upon refeeding. No tumor water loss was observed during fasting, indicating cellular material was lost. However, the administration of MTX + 5-FU at 24 hours of refeeding to coincide with the increased [^{3}H]Thd and PDP indices produced a significantly greater reduction in tumor volume and slowed the subsequent tumor recovery. A second course of fasting, refeeding, and chemotherapy initiated on day 15 produced a further reduction in tumor

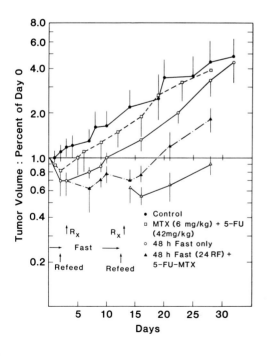

FIG. 7. Effects of fasting and feeding (○); MTX and 5-FU only (□); fasting and refeeding and MTX and 5-FU once (▲) or twice (△) versus control (●) C_3H SMT tumor growth. Mean of two to five mice per point ± one standard error.

volume and delayed tumor recovery. Between days 30 and 35, tumor volumes of these twice-treated animals exhibited a 10-fold difference from the age-matched untreated animals.

Nutritional Studies in Human Colonic Adenocarcinoma Xenografts

In an effort to validate these nutritional cell kinetic concepts in a human tumor model, stock cultures of SW 620 human colonic adenocarcinoma cells were harvested and aliquots of 5×10^7 cells were inoculated subcutaneously into the right flank of BALB/c athymic female mice. SW 620 cells were originally established from metastases in lymph nodes of a patient with histologically confirmed colonic adenocarcinoma.

Previous studies have shown these colonic xenograft models to exhibit an undifferentiated morphology, as in the parent cell line, and the cell kinetic properties expected for human colonic tumors in situ. Athymic mice bearing 0.3 to 0.5 cm³ SW 620 xenografts were fasted for 48 hours and refed wtih chow *ad libitum*. Tumor cell kinetics were measured as described previously,

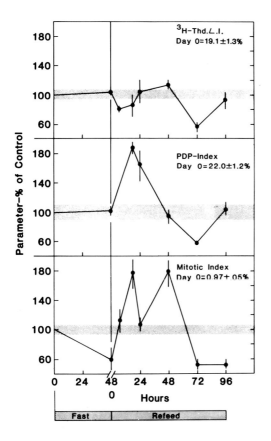

FIG. 8. Cell kinetic response of the SW 620 xenograft to fasting and refeeding. Points represent the mean of three mice ± one standard error. Horizontal stippling delimits range of control values.

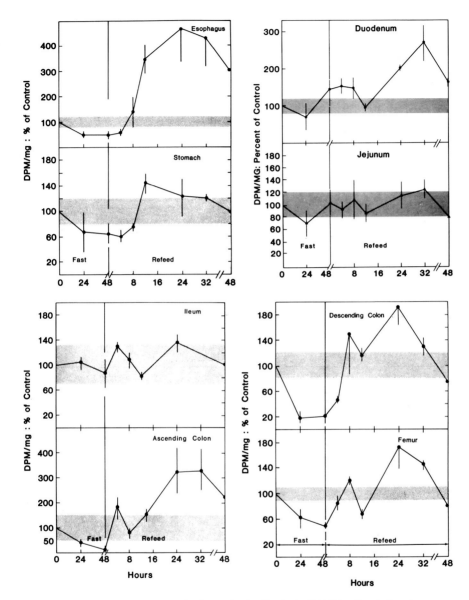

FIG. 9. Normal tissue responses to fasting and refeeding in the BALB/c athymic female mouse. Mean of three mice per point ± one standard error. Horizontal stippling delimits the range of control values.

employing the PDP assay to estimate the tumor growth fraction and single- and double-thymidine labeling. In parallel studies, [³H]Thd incorporation into the esophagus, stomach, duodenum, jejunum, ileum, ascending and descending colon, and femur was analyzed as an estimate of normal tissue proliferation.

The fasting-refeeding procedure produced only a transient delay in the SW 620 growth, which resumed promptly upon refeeding. The cell kinetic events in the xenograft accompanying these nutritional manipulations are presented in Figure 8. As indicated, no changes in the tumor growth fraction or [³H]Thd L.I. were noted during the 48-hour fast, although a 40% reduction in the mitotic index was observed. Following refeeding, a twofold increase in the PDP and mitotic indices at 16–24 hours was noted, followed by a 20% increase in [³H]Thd L.I. at 48 hours. This recovery sequence may suggest the presence of a G_2 cycle block induced during fasting with apparent parasynchronous progression of cells following refeeding. The lack of an increase in the [³H]Thd L.I. of a similar magnitude to the PDP and mitotic indices may reflect the failure of these G_2-blocked cells to remain in the cycle and reenter the S period.

Results of the normal tissue response are given in Figure 9. As indicated, the normal tissue responses to nutritional manipulations in the BALB/c athymic mice appeared to be tissue specific. In general, the esophagus, duodenum, ascending and descending colon, and femur respond to refeeding with a twofold to fourfold increase in proliferation, whereas the stomach, jejunum, and ileum response is greatly reduced. These tissue responses agree with previously reported findings on the small and large bowel in normal mice (Hagemann and Stragand 1977).

SUMMARY

The present studies have indicated that nutrition can affect the cell kinetic characteristics of normal and tumor tissues in a pronounced and tissue-specific manner. The significance of these studies lies in the potential to exploit the nutritional consequences of malignant disease in terms of cycle-active chemotherapy. For example, a patient receiving complete intravenous nutritional support, i.e., complete bowel rest, should exhibit a reduced intestinal proliferation concomitant with the expected tumor cell renewal rate. In this instance, we could expect reduced gut toxicity during chemotherapy without compromising the tumor response. These observations have been confirmed by Bounous et al. (1971a, 1971b). Additional studies are needed to elucidate specific nutritional control points for tumor tissues similar to the iron requirement in intestinal cell renewal. In addition, if the cell kinetic events associated with the transposition between hypocolonic and hypercolonic conditions during IVH therapy could be established, it would be possible to exploit these in protocols employing cycle-active agents.

REFERENCES

Baserga, R., and W. E. Kisieleski. 1962. A comparative study of the kinetics of cellular proliferation in normal and tumorous tissues using tritiated thymidine. JNCI 28:331–339.

Ben-Ishay, F., and E. Farber. 1976. Protective effects of an inhibitor of protein synthesis, cyclohexamide, on bone marrow damage induced by ara-C or nitrogen mustard. Lab. Invest. 33:478–487.

Bottomley, J. P., and E. H. Cooper. 1973. Cell proliferation in colonic mucosa and carcinoma of the colon. Proc. R. Soc. Med. 66:1183–1184.

Bounous, G., J. S. Hugon, and J. M. Gentile. 1971a. Elemental diet in management of intestinal lesions produced by 5-fluorouracil in the rat. Can. J. Surg. 14:298–311.

Bounous G., J. M. Gentile, and J. S. Hugon. 1971b. Elemental diet in management of intestinal lesions produced by 5-fluorouracil in man. Can. J. Surg. 14:312–324.

Braunschweiger, P. G., L. Poulakos, and L. M. Schiffer. 1976. In vitro determination in gold activation and autoradiography for determination of labeling index and DNA synthesis times in solid tumors. Cancer Res. 36:1748–1753.

Braunschweiger, P. G., and L. M. Schiffer. 1978. Therapeutic implications of cell kinetic changes after cyclophosphamide treatment in spontaneous and transplantable mammary tumors. Cancer Treat. Rep. 62:727–735.

Buzby, G. P., J. L. Mallen, T. P. Stein, E. E. Miller, C. L. Hobbs, and E. F. Rosata. 1978. Host-tumor interaction and nutrient supply. Cancer. 45:2940–2948.

Cameron, I. L., and W. A. Paviat. 1976. Stimulation of growth of a transplantable hepatoma in rats by parenteral nutrition. JNCI 56:597–599.

Copeland, E. M., and F. J. Dudrick. 1975. Cancer nutritional concepts. Semin. Oncol. 2:329–335.

Copeland, E. M., D. V. MacFadyen, M. A. Rapp, and S. J. Dudrick. 1975. Hyperalimentation and immune competence in cancer. Surg. Forum 26:138–140.

Costa, G. 1977. Cachexia, the metabolic component of malignant disease. Cancer Res. 37:2327–2335.

DeCosse, J. J., M. B. Adams, J. F. Kuzma, P. LoGerfo, and R. E. Condon. 1975. Effect of ascorbic acid on rectal polyps of patients with familial polyposis. Surgery 78:605–612.

Gilbertson, J. R., R. A. Gelman, P. Ove, and M. L. Coetzee. 1977. Inhibition of growth of Morris hepatomas 7777 and 7800 by corn oil. Oncology 34:62–64.

Hagemann, R. F., C. P. Sigdestad, and S. Lesher. 1970. A method for the quantitation of proliferative cells of the intestinal mucosa on a weight basis: Some values for C57B1/6 mice. Cell Tissue Kinet. 3:21–27.

Hagemann, R. F., and J. J. Stragand. 1977. Fasting and refeeding: Cell kinetic response of jejunum, ileum and colon. Cell Tissue Kinet. 10:3–14.

Hill, B. T. 1978. The management of human solid tumors: Some observations of the irrelevance of traditional cell cycle kinetics and the value of certain recent concepts. Cell Biol. Int. Rep. 2:215–230.

Hoffbrand, A. V., K. Ganeshaguru, W. C. Hooter, and M. H. N. Tattersall. 1976. Effect of iron deficiency and desferrioxamine on DNA synthesis in human cells. Br. J. Haematol. 33:517–526.

Hooper, A. F., P. M. Rose, and R. W. Wannemacher. 1968. Cell population changes in the intestinal epithelium of the rat following starvation and protein depletion. Proc. Soc. Exp. Biol. Med. 128:695–703.

Kenny, A. D., and P. L. Munson. 1959. A method for the biological assay of phosphaturic activity in parathyroid extracts. Endocrinology 64:513–518.

Lehnert, S. 1979. Changes in growth kinetics of jejunal epithelium in mice maintained on an elemental diet. Cell Tissue Kinet. 2:239–248.

McManus, J. P., J. F. Whitfield, R. H. Rixon, A. L. Boynton, T. Youdale, and S. Swirenga. 1975. The positive control of cell proliferation by the interplay of calcium ions and cyclic nucleotides: A review. Adv. Cyclic Nucleotide Res. 5:719–739.

McMichael, H. 1965. Inhibition of growth of Shope rabbit papilloma by hypervitaminosis A. Cancer Res. 25:947–955.

McQuitty, J. T., W. D. DeWys, L. Monaco, W. H. Strain, C. G. Rob, J. Apgar, and W. J. Pories. 1970. Inhibition of tumor growth by dietary zinc deficiency. Cancer Res. 30:1387–1390.

Mendelsohn, M. L., and M. Takahashi. 1971. A critical evaluation of the fraction of labelled mitoses method as applied to the analysis of tumor and other cell cycles, in The Cell Cycle and Cancer, R. Baserga, ed. Marcel Dekker, New York, pp. 55–96.

Pardee, A. B. 1974. A restriction point for control of normal animal cell proliferation. Proc. Natl. Acad. Sci. USA 71:1286–1290.

Phillips, J. L., and P. J. Sheridan. 1977. Effect of zinc administration on the growth of L1210 and BW5147 tumors in mice. JNCI 57:361–363.

Pine, M. 1978. Effects of low phenylalanine diet on murine leukemia L1210. JNCI 60:633–641.

Rao, G. A., and S. Abraham. 1976. Enhanced growth rate of transplanted adenocarcinoma induced in C₃H mice by dietary linoleate. JNCI 56:431–432.

Rettura, G., A. Schitter, M. Hardy, S. M. Levenson, A. Demetriou, E. Seifter. 1975. Antitumor action of vitamin A in mice inoculated with adenocarcinoma cells. JNCI 54:1489–1491.

Robbins, E., J. Fant, and W. Nanton. 1972. Intracellular iron binding macromolecules in HeLa cells. Proc. Natl. Acad. Sci. USA 69:3708–3713.

Rous, P. 1914. The influence of diet on transplantable and spontaneous mouse tumors. J. Exp. Med. 20:433–451.

Sandor, R. S. 1976. Effect of fasting on growth and glycolysis of the Erlich ascites tumor. JNCI 56:247–248.

Schenken, L. 1976. Proliferative character and growth modes of neoplastic disease as determinants of chemotherapeutic efficacy. Cancer Treat. Rep. 60:1761–1776.

Schiffer, L. M., A. M. Marcoe, and J. S. Nelson. 1976. Evaluation of the tumor growth fraction in murine tumors by the PDP assay. Cancer Res. 36:2415–2418.

Skipper, H. E., F. M. Schabel, and W. S. Wilcox. 1967. Experimental evaluation of potential anticancer agents. XXI. Scheduling of arabinosylcytosine to take advantage of its S-phase specificity against leukemia cells. Cancer Chemother. Rep. 51:125–165.

Steel, C. G. 1977. Basic theory of growing cell populations, *in* Growth Kinetics of Tumors, Chapter 2. Clarendon Press, Oxford, England, pp. 56–85.

Stragand, J. J., J-P. Bergerat, R. A. White, J. Hokanson, and B. Drewinko. 1980a. Biologic and cell kinetic properties of a human colonic adenocarcinoma (LoVo) grown in athymic mice. Cancer Res. 40:2846–2852.

Stragand, J. J., P. G. Braunschweiger, A. A. Pollice, and L. M. Schiffer. 1979. Cell kinetic alterations in murine mammary tumors following fasting and refeeding. Eur. J. Cancer 15:281–286.

Stragand, J. J., and R. F. Hagemann. 1977. Dietary influence of colonic cell renewal. Am. J. Clin. Nutr. 3:918–923.

Stragand, J. J., and R. F. Hagemann. 1978a. An iron requirement for the synchronous progression of colonic cells following fasting and refeeding. Cell Tissue Kinet. 11:513–518.

Stragand, J. J., and R. F. Hagemann. 1978b. Effect of lumenal contents on colonic cell renewal. Am. J. Physiol. 233(3):E208–211.

Stragand, J. J., R. A. White, and B. Drewinko. 1980b. Cytodynamic properties of a human colonic xenograft (SW 620) growth in athymic mice. Cancer Res. (in press).

Theuer, R. C. 1971. Effect of essential amino acid restriction on the growth of female C₅₇B1 mice and their implanted B210232 adenocarcinomas. J. Nutr. 101:223–232.

Van Putten, L. M., H. J. Keizer, and J. H. Mulder. 1976. Synchronization in tumor chemotherapy. Eur. J. Cancer 12:79–85.

Wimber, D. E., H. Quastler, O. L. Stein, and D. R. Wimber. 1960. Analysis of tritium incorporation into individual cells by radioautography of squash preparations. J. Biophys. Biochem. Cytol. 8:327–347.

Yamafuji, J., Y. Makamura, H. Omura, T. Soeda, and J. Cyotoku. 1971. Patency of ascorbic, dehydroascorbic or 2,3-diketogularic acid and their action of deoxyribonucleic acid. Clin. Oncol. 76:1–7.

Young, C. A., and F. M. Parsons. 1977. The effects of dietary deficiencies of magnesium and potassium on the growth and chemistry of transplanted tumors and host tissues in the rat. Eur. J. Cancer 13:103–113.

Molecular Interrelations of Nutrition and Cancer,
edited by M. S. Arnott, J. van Eys and Y.-M. Wang.
Raven Press, New York © 1982.

Nutrient Control of Proliferation in Normal and Tumor Cell Populations

George M. Padilla and Ivan L. Cameron

*Department of Physiology, Duke University Medical Center, Durham, North Carolina
27710 and Department of Anatomy, The University of Texas Health Science Center at
San Antonio, San Antonio, Texas 78284*

Nutrition may be viewed as the availability and uptake of substrates, ions, and other essential compounds that provide the energy and precursors for growth and cellular proliferation. Heitman and Cameron (1981) have recently summarized extensively the variables encountered in studies on the effect of general and limited undernourishment on cell proliferation. In order to assess the relation between nutrition and proliferation, one must accurately monitor and control the diet provided to an experimental animal. This is best accomplished by total parenteral nutrition techniques involving the continuous infusion of nutrients in liquid form via an indwelling catheter (Steiger et al. 1972). The following questions may then be asked: Can a tumor-bearing animal be protected from the onset of an inordinate weight loss (cachexia) by hyperalimentation? Do cancer and host cells differ in their response to varying nutritional levels in terms of their proliferative behavior? What is the cellular and metabolic basis that imparts a proliferative advantage to cancer cells? We will outline below experiments that provide some answers to these questions and point to future goals in this area of cancer research.

NUTRITIONAL INFLUENCES ON TUMOR AND HOST CELL POPULATIONS

The Measurement and Classification of Proliferative Cell Populations

To assess the impact of nutrition on cellular proliferation, we must have at hand precise indices of proliferative activities in the host tissues and the tumor cell population. The mitotic index, which is the percentage of cells in mitosis at a given time, can be used to establish the turnover time of a population of proliferating cells, provided a reliable estimate of the duration of mitosis is obtained. Since not all cells have the same duration of mitosis, a direct estimate must be made (Leblond 1959). This can be accomplished by using mitotic spindle poisons such as Colcemid to determine the kinetics of accumulation of metaphase-arrested cells (Heitman and Cameron 1981). For example, a quadrupling of the mitotic index in 2 hours would indicate a mitotic time of 0.5 hours.

A more sensitive index of proliferative activity is the DNA synthetic or labeling index obtained by the combined use of tritiated thymidine and tissue autoradiography. Most mammalian cells spend 5 to 8 hours in the S phase of the cell cycle, an interval approximately 10 times longer than mitosis. In spite of the heightened sensitivity of this index, the mammalian body contains tissues whose cells are renewed very slowly, making chronic or repeated administration of tritiated thymidine necessary to obtain reliable values for the rate of entry into the S phase (Cameron 1968, 1971).

This experimental approach permits us to classify cell populations of adult nongrowing mice as static, rapidly or slowly renewing, marginally proliferative, and neoplastic (Table 1) (Cameron 1970). Static populations include neurons of the central and peripheral nervous system and cardiac muscle cells of the heart ventricles as their major types. Rapidly renewing cells, with turnover

TABLE 1. *Proliferative behavior of cell populations of nongrowing mice*

Type	Examples	Renewal time (days)
Static	Neurons of central and peripheral nervous system, muscle cells in heart and ventricle	
Renewing		
Rapid (renewal time < 30 days)	Epidermis	14–21
	Cornea	6
	Oral epithelium	7
	Gastric epithelium	4
	Intestinal epithelium	2–3
	Hemopoietic cells (maturation)	1–3
	Lymphopoietic cells	26–34
	Megakaryocytes (maturation)	2–3
Slow (renewal time > 30 days but < lifetime of animal)	Pulmonary epithelium	100
	Kidney cortex	170
	Hepatocytes and littoral cells	550, 160
	Pancreatic acinar and islet cells	520
	Salivary gland cells	250
	Adrenal cortex	90–600
	Dermal fibroblasts	60
Partially renewed (cells proliferate at such a slow rate that not all cells in the population are renewed during life span of animal)	Smooth muscle cells, harderian gland cells, glial cells in most areas of the brain, brown fat cells, osteocytes, kidney medullary tubule cells, zymogenic (chief) cells of stomach, transitional epithelium, adrenal medulla	
Neoplastic	Solid tumor cells, metastic cancer cells	

Adapted from Cameron (1970).

times of less than 30 days, include most alimentary tract epithelia, the epidermis, and cells from the hemopoietic and lymphatic system, as well as cells from the reproductive system. Cells with renewal times in excess of 30 days are quite varied: they include cells of the respiratory tract, kidney cortex, hepatocytes, parenchymal cells of several glands, and dermal fibroblasts. Lastly, populations with minimal proliferative activity (i.e., those in which only a portion of the cells are renewed during the lifetime of the animal) include smooth muscle cells, osteocytes, glial cells, transitional epithelial cells, and medullary cells in the kidneys and adrenals.

The experimental approach used by Cameron and co-workers (Heitman and Cameron 1981, Cameron et al. 1977, Cameron and Pavlat 1976, Cameron 1981, Grubbs et al. 1981) to study nutritional influences on cellular proliferation is based on total parenteral (intravenous) liquid feeding (Steiger et al. 1972). This technique avoids several of the variables encountered with *ad libitum* solid food feeding. For example, the frequency of feeding and quality of nutrients ingested can be carefully controlled at desired levels. The mechanical effects of solid food ingestion on the alimentary tract epithelia, which are thought to stimulate proliferation, are also eliminated. More importantly, this technique permits investigators to monitor total caloric intake (Cameron and Pavlat 1976), determine the role of nitrogen balance and growth of a transplantable tumor (Cameron et al. 1979, Grubbs et al. 1981), and investigate the relation between gluconeogenesis and cancer cachexia in tumor-bearing animals (Grubbs et al. 1979). The results of these studies in terms of the nutritional influences on cellular proliferation are summarized below.

Role of Parenteral Nutrition on Tumor-Host Responses

Large, rapidly growing hepatomas are accompanied by higher mortality, fluid retention, weight loss (cachexia), leukocytosis, and anemia in animals. As shown in the data summarized in Table 2, there was also a marked drop in serum transferrin and IgG. The metabolizable caloric intake of animals with large tumors was considerably lower than the control animals, except for those fed parenterally (i.e., liquid i.v. feeding). Likewise, the nitrogen balance of tumorous animals under parenteral nutrition was not significantly lower than their tumor-free control counterparts. Lastly, the tumor-bearing animals on a liquid diet had a fluid intake-to-output ratio and a caloric intake that exceeded that of the control rats. Taken together, these data indicate that even though hyperalimented rats take in sufficient quantities of nutrients to maintain them in a seemingly positive nitrogen balance, the nutritional demands of the tumor cannot be fully met. The question then arises, are the metabolic and nutritional imbalances imposed upon the host animal by a rapidly growing tumor as evidenced by cachexia and anemia reflected in the proliferative activity of host tissues?

To answer this question, the proliferative activity of two distinct populations of cells, the ear epidermis and epithelium of the small intestines, was monitored.

TABLE 2. *Effect of parenteral nutrition on tumor-host responses**

	Without tumor			With tumor		
	Solid food p.o.	Liquid food i.v.	p.o.	Solid food p.o.	Liquid food i.v.	p.o.
% Mortality during experiment	0	13	0	25	33	0
% Terminal carcass weight as % of body weight	81	84	86	73	71	75
Terminal water content of carcass (%)	63	62	62	65	65	64
Terminal leukocyte count ($\times 10^3 \cdot cm^{-3}$)	11	13	12	22	25	19
Terminal hematocrit (%)	49	48	49	29	27	34
Terminal serum transferrin (% of total protein)	10.4	8.5	10.3	5.9	5.1	4.9
Terminal serum IgG (% of standard IgG)	74	64	69	26	27	42
Metabolizable caloric intake in first 5 days (100^{-1}g b.w.)	97	120	102	30	123	75
Nitrogen balance, last 2 days [(mg N in − mg N out)/100 g b.w.]	—	103	104	—	100	56
Fluid balance (fluid in/urine out/100 g b.w.)	1.29	2.65	2.82	1.46	3.31	3.14

* No animals died during the first 5 days; thus nonterminal data include all rats and terminal data include those rats killed at 7 days.
From Cameron et al. 1979.

Sixty-one young male rats (Buffalo strain) were divided into two groups. Experimental animals were inoculated s.c. in the flank with a suspension of Morris hepatoma cells (no. 7777; Cameron and Pavlat 1976). Control animals were injected with saline. All rats were kept in metabolic cages. At regular intervals the rats were weighed, and 3 weeks after inoculation, the control and experimental animals were randomly placed into separate feeding regimens as follows. Two sets of rats were fed solid food and water *ad libitum.* One set containing control and experimental animals was sacrificed at the beginning of the feeding regimen to serve as the 0-time controls (shown at the top of Table 3). The other set of rats was fed solid food for 7 days along with three other sets of rats fed a liquid formula either p.o. or i.v. At the end of 7 days, the animals were sacrificed. One hour before this, they were injected with tritiated thymidine, and after sacrifice labeling indices were determined on cells from the tumors, ear epidermis, and epithelium of the small intestine (Cameron 1981).

As shown in Table 3, animals with small tumors (3.5% of body weight) did not differ from controls. Note that the tumor had a labeling index in excess of 50%. This alone indicates a very high proliferative activity even when compared to the ear epidermis, which is typical of a tissue with a rapidly renewing cell population (Table 1). One week later, rats on solid food showed a significant drop in the labeling index of the ear epidermis and a slight but statistically

TABLE 3. *Effect of tumor size and method of feeding on proliferative activity of tumor and host tissues*

Feeding method and tumor size (% b.w.)	(n)	Labeling index*		
		Tumor (% within 37 μm of blood vessel)	Ear epidermis (% in basal layer)	Ileum (no. labeled cells per crypt)
Solid food (p.o.)†				
−tumor	7	–	4.2 ± 0.4	23.4 ± 1.5
+tumor (3.5%)	8	54.7 ± 1.8	3.5 ± 0.1	26.5 ± 1.5
−tumor	5	–	3.4 ± 0.1	26.1 ± 1.8
+tumor (13.1%)	5	45.3 ± 2.9	1.2 ± 0.6	21.8 ± 0.8
Liquid (i.v.)				
−tumor	8	–	2.9 ± 0.5	15.6 ± 3.8
+tumor (14.1%)	8	54.5 ± 3.2	1.9 ± 0.2	15.7 ± 0.9
Liquid (p.o.)				
−tumor	7	–	3.3 ± 0.5	17.5 ± 0.9
+tumor (10.6%)	7	43.5 ± 1.9	2.3 ± 0.5	18.4 ± 0.9
CDBM‡				
$p < 0.05$		7.4	1.4	3.3
$p < 0.01$		10.0	1.8	4.4

* Rats were injected with ^{3}H-thymidine 1 hr before sacrifice.
† The first 2 groups of animals represent "0 time" controls, other groups were all harnessed and started on their feeding procedures at this time.
‡ Critical differences between means were obtained by analysis of variance and multiple range test. Values given show when the differences between pairs of means in each column become significant for the values given.
Adapted from I. L. Cameron 1981.

significant decrease in the number of labeled intestinal cells per crypt. The labeling of the tumor was also decreased to a significant level ($p < 0.05$) (Cameron 1981). Rats parenterally fed showed a labeling index in the tumor that was increased to the level of the 0-time rats with smaller tumors, but the ear epidermis labeling index remained significantly lower than the 0-time control rats. Control rats on a liquid i.v. diet also had a somewhat depressed labeling index in the ear epidermal cells. Note that in control and tumorous rats the number of cells labeled per crypt was markedly reduced when a liquid diet was used. Presumably, this reduction reflects the lack of stimulation on the small intestine by solid food.

In summary, the data presented in Table 3 indicate that the host cannot manage maintenance of normal cell proliferation activity in the ear epidermis with a tumor in excess of 10% of its body weight, and therefore the proliferative activity of at least some of its cell populations is inhibited in spite of the caloric relief offered by parenteral hyperalimentation. Was such inhibition of cell proliferation and carcass weight loss a result of subtle nutritional imbalances that would have become manifest in time regardless of the size of the tumor, or was the size of the tumor critical?

To answer this question, an experiment was performed in which the duration of the experiment was extended to 13 days in animals harboring tumors of about 3% of body weight or less. Growth, carcass mass, and the nitrogen balance were carefully monitored at 3-day intervals. Sixteen days after inoculation, the rats were sacrificed, and analyses of terminal body weights and carcass and tumor weights were performed (Grubbs et al. 1981). The results of this study showed that a rat is able to maintain a small tumor without any loss of weight or differences in weight gain, caloric intake, and positive nitrogen balance from control rats. In fact, in both tumorous and control rats there was a significant rise in the positive nitrogen balance at the end of the parenteral feeding period. This study indicates that the size of the tumor is critical to maintenance of carcass weight loss.

Since parenteral hyperalimentation alone did not prevent cancer cachexia in rats bearing tumors in excess of a few percent of their body weight, the hypothesis that gluconeogenesis is a vital link in the process of a host's weight loss was tested. The blood levels of glucose and amino acids were kept high by parenteral nutrition, and hydrazine sulfate was used to block the enzyme phosphoenolpyruvate carboxykinase (PEP-CK), which is a key enzyme involved in the process of gluconeogenesis (Gold 1974). Three groups of rats were used in this study: one group was fed a liquid formula i.v., and hydrazine sulfate (15 mg-kg^{-1}) was injected twice daily i.p. for 5 days. A second group of rats was fed the same liquid formula p.o. *ad libitum*. Thus, all animals were fed the same liquid formula (Grubbs et al. 1979). A portion of the results from this study are summarized in Table 4. Rats fed parenterally and treated with hydrazine sulfate (H.S.) for 5 days showed carcass weight of 84% of initial body weight, a value similar to rats without tumors (i.e., a carcass weight of 85% is similar to that of the nontumorous rats listed in Table 2). Animals fed orally *ad libitum* showed a terminal carcass weight drop to 64% of initial body weight. Animals without any H.S. treatment and *ad libitum* feeding showed a carcass weight loss to 76% of initial body weight. Hydrazine sulfate only

TABLE 4. *Effect of hydrazine sulfate on body and carcass weight and tumor growth*

Feeding method	Drug*	Terminal body weight† (g)	Body weight (% of initial)	Carcass weight (% of initial)	Tumor growth rate‡ Before therapy	Tumor growth rate‡ After therapy
i.v.	+HS	410 ± 7.9	107 ± 0.8	84 ± 1.2	0.44 ± 0.01	0.81 ± 0.3
p.o. *ad lib.*	+HS	298 ± 8.3	88 ± 0.5	64 ± 0.7	0.62 ± 0.06	−0.20 ± 0.14
p.o. *ad lib.*	none	342 ± 5.7	97 ± 0.6	76 ± 0.7	0.79 ± 0.07	0.81 ± 0.06

* Hydrazine sulfate, 15 mg/kg, twice daily, i.p.
† Initial body weight was not significantly different in the three groups of rats.
‡ Computed from slope of curve describing change in cross-sectional area per day.
Modified from Grubbs et al. (1979).

inhibited the growth of tumors in rats being fed *ad libitum*. Grubbs et al. (1979) also found that, with the exception of animals under parenteral feeding, the net loss in body weight resulted from a reduced food intake in the rats fed *ad libitum*. Grubbs et al. (1979) also noted a significant and marked drop in the net positive nitrogen balance for rats being treated with H.S. and fed *ad libitum* from 40.7 mg $N_2/100$ g/24 hr on the second day to 7.3 mg $N_2/100$ g/24 hr on the fifth day. The rats being fed parenterally and treated with H.S. had a net positive nitrogen balance of 83.6 mg $N_2/100$ g/24 hr on the second and 74.7 mg $N_2/100$ g/24 hr on the fifth day. Rats on solid food without H.S. had an intermediate nitrogen balance that did not change in the course of the experiment (27 mg $N_2/100$ g/24 hr).

It is thus clear that H.S. induced a reduction in the nitrogen balance that was largely overcome by parenteral feeding, and more importantly it was this combination that prevented the onset of cancer cachexia, as noted by changes in carcass weight. These results suggest that further experiments need to be done to find a combination of parenteral nutrition and selected metabolic inhibitors in the management of the cancer patient that will prevent cancer cachexia and allow aggressive cancer therapy.

IMPACT OF GLUCOSE METABOLISM AND CELLULAR TRANSPORT PROCESS ON CELL PROLIFERATION IN TUMOR AND HOST

We have shown that total parenteral hyperalimentation in combination with inhibition of gluconeogenesis can temporarily prevent the onset of cancer cachexia, but it seems apparent that a large and rapidly growing tumor will eventually overcome the caloric relief and inhibit the cell proliferation rate in host tissues. What lesion endows cancer cells with an ability to continue cell proliferation even when the host is nutritionally deprived? Is it a change in the transport or ion flux properties of the tumor cell membrane or are there fundamental changes in the energy-yielding metabolic pathways, as suggested by the experiments on the inhibition of gluconeogenesis in tumorous rats? We would like, at this point, to consider the relations that may exist between cell membrane functions in proliferating and nonproliferating cells that may impinge on some key metabolic processes. We would especially like to consider those alterations in the internal milieu of the cell (e.g., internal pH, ionic balances). Although it is too early to place the demonstrable differences between normal and cancer cells in a fixed hierarchy of relevance, it does seem useful to see if they are interrelated.

Figure 1 illustrates the possible loci at which differences between cancerous and normal cells become manifest. This figure is offered to guide this discussion, for it incorporates in a simplified way some of the concepts recently presented by Gillies (1981), Wenner and Tomei (1981), Koren (1980), and Eigenbrodt and Glossmann (1980).

It is clear that proliferating cells show an increased transport of nutrients

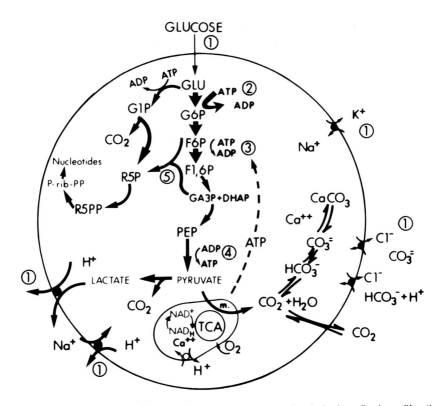

FIG. 1. Possible relationships between transport processes and carbohydrate flux in proliferating and tumor cells.

and ions through an alteration of the membrane, as first proposed by Holley (1972, 1975) and by Pardee (1975). For the present discussion, we include in the "proliferating" category tumor cells as well as any other cell type stimulated to divide. Figure 1 shows the various types of transport processes that appear to be modified (enhanced) in proliferating cells (see #1 on the figure). The figure also shows some ion/ion and ion/proton exchanges that maintain electro-neutrality and cause alkaline internal pH as discussed by Gillies (1981). Such a pH shift may influence, for example, the catalytic activity of some key enzymes as noted below.

In reference to Figure 1, let us examine a proposed sequence of events that takes place as growth-arrested cells are stimulated to proliferate.

Recent reports suggest that most, if not all, stimulated cells possess a common sequence of events leading to cell reproduction (Cameron and Pool 1981). Knowing and understanding the sequential events leading to cell reproduction is important for at least two reasons. First, the sequence of events will help us understand the normal growth duplication cycle and give us valuable clues on how we might intervene to regulate cell reproduction. Second, as we learn more about the normal sequence of events upon stimulation of cell reproduction, we will eventually come to understand the loss of growth control (lesion) that characterizes tumor cells. It seems reasonable to believe that once such a tumor cell lesion is established, the lesion itself will provide a point of therapeutic attack.

Upon stimulation, the earliest event involves an influx of Na^+ that may be associated with the antitransport of H^+ out of the cell, causing alkalinization of the cytoplasm. The Na^+ influx may be associated with the cotransport of glucose and other cellular nutrients.

How can the early ionic and pH change bring about alterations in the cell's metabolic pathway? For example, one of the characteristics of rapidly dividing normal and tumor cells is their increased glycolytic capacity and their high rate of lactic acid production under aerobic conditions.

Upon transformation of a normal cell to a tumor cell or the stimulation of proliferation of normal cells, the activity of several key enzymes [Figure 1: cytoplasmic hexokinase (2), phosphofructokinase (3), pyruvate kinase (4), transketolase-transaldolase (5)] is modified so that the carbon flux favors the formation of lactate, which is released to the outside, and the formation of ribose-5-phosphate and subsequently 5-phosphoribose-1-pyrophosphate (P-rib-PP), which is a precursor of purine and pyrimidine biosynthesis. Enzymes catalyzing the breakdown of this high-energy compound are increased by 200–300% in proliferating cells (Weber 1977). Eigenbrodt and Glossmann (1980) called *nucleigenic* those tumor and proliferating cells that direct their glucose metabolism toward the synthesis of nucleic acids as described above.

Eigenbrodt and Glossmann (1980) also noted that proliferating cells and rapidly growing cancer cells contain a pyruvate kinase isoenzyme (PK-M_2) whose activity is inactivated through phosphorylation by a cAMP-independent protein kinase. Such a phosphorylation is inhibited by fructose 1,6-diphosphate, P-rib-PP, and P_1-P_5, di(adenosine-5'-pentaphosphate). The net result of the interaction of these various glycolytic metabolites on pyruvate kinase is to channel the carbohydrate flow selectively in the direction of P-rib-PP at low glucose concentrations. At high glucose concentrations, elevated levels of fructose 1,6-diphosphate and P-rib-PP most likely overcome the protein kinase–mediated inactivation of PK-M_2 (Eigenbrodt and Glossmann 1980). In this way, tumor and proliferating cells are able to synthesize nucleic acids and proteins without as great a dependence on the external level of glucose.

Note that several of these enzymes, phosphofructokinase in particular, and some of the protein kinases are thought to be controlled by the internal pH of the cells (Gillies 1981). This hypothesis rests on the observation that glycolysis itself is inhibited by internal acid pH. The mechanism of inhibition is not known, although Gillies (1981) suggests that the affinity of several glycolytic enzymes for specific membrane proteins is dependent on the internal pH. Another control mechanism might include the effect of pH on various phosphorylation reactions that are known to regulate the activity of such enzymes as phosphofructokinase

(Furuya and Uyeda 1980). Several aspects of this question are discussed elsewhere in this symposium monograph.

One can explain the loss of growth control in tumor cells by postulating that a lesion exists in the cell membrane that does not allow the cancer cell to return to a nonproliferating state. For example, the cancer cell membrane may be permanently leaky to Na^+ or the Na^+-K^+-ATPase pump may be inefficient (Spector et al. 1980). In either case, the transformed malignant cell would not be able to return to a nonproliferative state.

The tumor cell in the host may have a lesion that allows it to proliferate even when proliferation of normal host cells is depressed. According to Gold (1974), the proliferating tumor cell avidly uses glucose for glycolysis and produces lactate in large quantities. The energy needs of the tumor are adequately met by this inefficient process. The lactate produced by the tumor cells is transported to the host's liver, where the lactate is converted back to glucose by gluconeogenesis. The energy required for gluconeogenesis is greater than that derived by glycolysis in the tumor cells. Thus, this tumor glycolysis and host gluconeogenesis system constitutes a net energy-losing cycle in the host. We propose that this energy-losing cycle in the host is associated with cancer cachexia and with the observed depression of cell proliferation in the host tissue. A lesion in the membrane of the tumor cell, as discussed above, can be used: (1) to explain the failure of cancer cells to respond to normal growth and nutrient control and (2) to explain cancer cachexia of the host. Thus, to meet adequately the nutritional requirements of the cancer patient, we must understand the nature of the lesion in the cancer cell.

REFERENCES

Cameron, I. L. 1968. A method for the study of cell proliferation and renewal in the tissue of mammals, *in* Methods in Cell Physiology, Vol. 3, D. M. Prescott, ed. Academic Press, New York, pp. 261–276.

Cameron, I. L. 1970. Cell renewal in the organs and tissues of the non-growing adult mouse. Texas Rep. Biol. Med. 28:203–248.

Cameron, I. L. 1971. Cell proliferation and renewal in the mammalian body, *in* Cellular and Molecular Renewal in the Mammalian Body, I. L. Cameron and J. D. Thrasher, eds. Academic Press, New York, pp. 45–85.

Cameron, I. L. 1981. Total parenteral nutrition on tumor-host responses in rats. Cancer Treat. Rep. (in press).

Cameron, I. L., W. J. Ackley, and W. Rogers. 1977. Responses of hepatoma-bearing rats to total parenteral hyperalimentation and to *ad libitum* feeding. J. Surg. Res. 23:189–195.

Cameron, I. L., and W. A. Pavlat. 1976. Stimulation of a transplanted hepatoma in rats by parenteral nutrition. JNCI 56:597–602.

Cameron, I. L., W. A. Pavlat, M. D. Stevens, and W. Rogers. 1979. Tumor-host responses to various nutritional feeding procedures in rats. J. Nutr. 109:671–684.

Cameron, I. L., and T. B. Pool, eds. 1981. The Transformed Cell. Academic Press, New York, 435 pp.

Eigenbrodt, E., and H. Glossmann. 1980. Glycolysis—one of the keys to cancer? Trends in Pharmacological Science 1:240–245.

Furuya, E., and K. Uyeda. 1980. Regulation of phosphofructokinase by a new mechanism. J. Biol. Chem. 255:11656–11659.

Gillies, R. J. 1981. Intracellular pH and growth control in eukaryotic cells, *in* The Transformed Cell, I. L. Cameron and T. B. Pool, eds. Academic Press, New York, pp. 347–395.

Gold, J. 1974. Inhibition of gluconeogenesis at the phosphoenolpyruvate carboxykinase and pyruvate carboxylase reactions, as a means of cancer chemotherapy. Oncology 29:74–89.

Grubbs, B., W. Rogers, and I. L. Cameron. 1979. Combining total parenteral nutrition and inhibition of gluconeogenesis to overcome cancer cachexia. Oncology 36:216–223.

Grubbs, B. S., W. Rogers, and I. L. Cameron. 1981. Total parenteral nutrition for maintenance of growth, carcass mass, and positive nitrogen balance in rats with a small transplantable tumor. Oncology (in press).

Heitman, D. W., and I. L. Cameron. 1981. Nutritional influences on cell proliferation, *in* Comparative Animal Nutrition, M. Rechcigl, ed. S. Karger, Basel (in press).

Holley, R. W. 1972. A unifying hypothesis concerning the nature of malignant growth. Proc. Natl. Acad. Sci. USA 69:2840–2841.

Holley, R. W. 1975. Control of growth of mammalian cells in cell culture. Nature (London) 258:487–490.

Koren, R. 1980. The relevance of the state of growth and transformation of cells to their patterns of metabolic uptake. Int. Rev. Cytol. 68:127–172.

Leblond, C. P. 1959. Classical techniques for the study of the kinetics of cellular proliferation, *in* The Kinetics of Cellular Proliferation, F. Stohlman, Jr., ed. Grune and Stratton, New York, pp. 31–47.

Pardee, A. B. 1975. The cell surface and fibroblast proliferation. Some current research trends. Biochim. Biophys. Acta 417:153–172.

Spector, M., S. O'Neal, and E. Racker. 1980. Reconstitution of the Na^+-K^+ pump of Ehrlich ascites tumor and enhancement of efficiency by quercetin. J. Biol. Chem. 255:5504–5507.

Steiger, E., H. M. Vaks, and S. J. Dudrick. 1972. A technique for long-term intravenous feeding in unrestrained rats. Arch. Surg. 104:330–332.

Weber, G. 1977. Enzymology of cancer cells. N. Engl. J. Med. 296:486–493.

Wenner, C. E., and L. D. Tomei. 1981. Phenotypic expression of malignant transformation and its relationship to energy metabolism, *in* The Transformed Cell, I. L. Cameron and T. B. Pool, eds. Academic Press, New York (in press).

Nutritional Modulation of Cell Transformation

Molecular Interrelations of Nutrition and Cancer,
edited by M. S. Arnott, J. van Eys, and Y.-M. Wang.
Raven Press, New York © 1982.

Inhibition of In Vitro Neoplastic Transformation by Retinoids

John S. Bertram, Lawrence J. Mordan, Krystyna Domanska-Janik, and Ralph J. Bernacki

Cancer Drug Center, Roswell Park Memorial Institute, Buffalo, New York 14263

Clinical symptoms of vitamin A deficiency were described in the last century and consisted of xerophthalmia and night blindness. Studies in experimental animals have added keratinizing metaplasia of skin and mucous membranes, sterility, and bone defects (Moore 1967, McLaren 1967). Following the discovery that the pigment content of plants correlated well with their biological activity as sources of vitamin A, the plant pigment carotene was isolated and shown to prevent clinical symptoms of deficiency (Moore 1929). β-Carotene, the most potent plant pigment, is broken down in the intestine to yield retinaldehyde, which, after conversion to retinol in the gut epithelium, is esterified and absorbed into the body in the chylomicron fraction of lymph (Goodman et al. 1966). These esters are removed by the liver and stored as long-chain fatty esters, principally of palmitic acid. Large quantities of vitamin A can be stored in the liver and are released in response to tissue needs. In response to demand, deesterification takes place, and retinol is released bound to a specific binding protein (RBP), which in the circulation complexes with serum prealbumin to form a tertiary complex. The binding chemically stabilizes retinol and prevents its excretion by the kidney (for a review, see Goodman 1980).

VITAMIN A AND CANCER PREVENTION IN EXPERIMENTAL ANIMALS

Current interest in vitamin A and its synthetic analogs (retinoids) stems from early observations that symptoms of vitamin A deficiency in epithelial tissues, characterized as hyperkeratosis of skin and metaplastic changes in internal epithelia (Wolbach and Howe 1925), were similar to epithelial lesions (e.g., leukoplakia) known to be premalignant. Animal experiments then demonstrated that the chemical induction of cancer could be prevented or delayed by systemic retinol or retinyl palmitate (Chu and Malmgren 1965, Saffioti et al. 1967). Subsequent work has shown that natural or certain synthetic compounds having vitamin A–like activity (Mayer et al. 1978) are capable of inhibiting the chemical induction of cancer in a variety of organs, including the mammary gland (Moon et al. 1979, Maiorana and Gullino 1980), skin (Bollag 1972, Brown et al. 1977), bladder (Grubbs et al. 1977, Becci et al. 1978), lung (Smith et al. 1975, Nettesheim et al. 1979), colon (Newberne and Suphakarn 1977), and oral cavity (Shklar et al. 1980) of experimental animals. In converse experiments, animals made deficient in vitamin A by dietary means were shown to be more susceptible to chemically induced tumors of the respiratory tract (Nettesheim and Williams 1976), bladder (Cohen et al. 1976), and colon (Newberne and Rogers 1973). (For reviews, see Sporn et al. 1976, Sporn and Newton 1979.)

VITAMIN A AND CANCER PREVENTION IN MAN

In man, interventional therapy of this kind is being actively considered by the National Cancer Institute. Limited clinical studies have been performed by Bollag's group in Switzerland and success has been reported in the treatment of precancerous lesions of the skin. Regressions have been reported in the treatment of squamous cell carcinomas (Bollag 1975). Highly suggestive evidence for the potential role of vitamin A in the prevention of human cancer comes from epidemiological studies of natural "experiments" that have been progressing in vitamin A–deficient individuals. Significantly increased risk factors for cancer of the lungs (Mettlin et al. 1979), bladder (Mettlin and Graham 1979), and esophagus (Mettlin et al. 1981) have been found in individuals with low intake of vitamin A and its precursor β-carotene. Furthermore, a recent prospective study has shown significantly lower blood retinol levels to be associated with males who subsequently demonstrated an increased incidence of lung cancer. Increased cancer frequencies at other sites were also detected in the low-retinol group, but the small number of subjects involved did not allow conclusions to be drawn (Wald et al. 1980).

EXPERIMENTAL STUDIES IN CELL CULTURES

In Vitro Neoplastic Transformation: The 10T½ System

Our group has been interested for a number of years in developing protocols to modify the carcinogenic process and thereby to develop tools to study mechanisms of carcinogenesis using an in vitro transformation system. We have employed the C3H/10T½ C18 (10T½) cell line in which quantitative neoplastic transformation can be induced by a variety of chemical and physical carcinogens (Reznikoff et al. 1973a). Transformed foci are readily distinguishable from the background of nontransformed cells and appear as dense, piled-up regions of randomly oriented polar cells (Figure 1). About 90% of foci of this morphological type (Type III) will produce sarcomas at the site of injection into immunosuppressed syngeneic mice (Reznikoff et al. 1973a, Bertram 1977). In these cells, morphological transformation occurs approximately 28 days after exposure of logarithmic growth phase cells to the carcinogenic stimulus, and microscopically

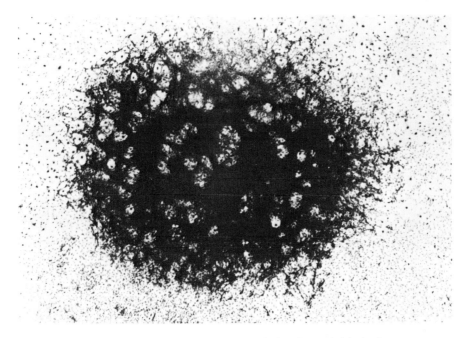

FIG. 1. Morphology of a type III transformed focus derived by methylcholanthrene treatment of 10T½ cells.

transformed foci occur by day 35 after treatment (Merriman and Bertram 1979). Cultures are generally exposed to the carcinogen 24 hours after plating of cells in a 60-mm Petri dish at a cell density that gives rise to about 250 clonogenic cells per dish. Cultures become confluent and cease dividing about 10 days after seeding; thus, transformed foci arise from a confluent background of quiescent cells. Parallel cultures seeded at a lower density of about 50 clonogenic cells per dish are usually employed to determine the effects of treatment on survival. These cultures are fixed and stained after 7 days and colonies counted (Reznikoff et al. 1973a).

Effects of Retinyl Acetate on de novo Transformation

When nontoxic concentrations of retinyl acetate were applied to replicate cultures that had been treated 7 days previously with a transforming concentration of 3-methylcholanthrene (MCA) (2.5 μg/ml for 24 hours), it was found that the expression of transformation was suppressed in a dose-responsive manner (Figure 2). A concentration of 0.02 μg/ml of retinyl acetate caused a 50% reduction in the MCA-induced transformation frequency, while 0.1 μg/ml virtually abolished transformation. The effects of retinol and retinal were comparable to retinyl acetate. However, all-trans-retinoic acid, which in many systems is

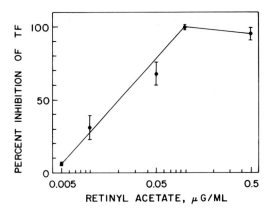

FIG. 2. Retinyl acetate inhibition of methylcholanthrene-induced neoplastic transformation. (Reproduced from Merriman and Bertram 1979, with permission of *Cancer Research.*)

the most potent of the retinoids in maintaining epithelial cell differentiation (Newton et al. 1980) and is highly active in vivo in inhibiting transformation in many other systems (Sporn et al. 1977), failed to inhibit transformation in this system. Indeed, at concentrations that caused some cytotoxicity, the induction of transformation was actually increased (Figure 3) (Bertram 1980). It is of interest that all-trans-retinoic acid has also been shown to increase the induction of skin tumors in mice exposed to UV irradiation (Forbes et al. 1979) and to repeated applications of dimethylbenz[a]anthracene (Verma et al. 1980a). This enhancing effect of retinoic acid on tumorigenesis in several systems must be viewed with concern (Food and Drug Administration 1978, Schroeder and Black 1980). All our subsequent studies have been performed with retinyl acetate, which is readily converted to retinol, an unequivocally natural form of vitamin A.

Reversibility of the Inhibition of Transformation

In order to determine if the inhibition of transformation caused by retinyl acetate was permanent or depended upon the continuous presence of the drug, replicate cultures were exposed to MCA, treated with 0.5 μg/ml retinyl acetate 7 days later, and maintained in retinyl acetate as previously described for an additional 4 weeks. At this point when no transformation was expressed in carcinogen-exposed cultures, the dishes were randomized: half were maintained on weekly retinyl acetate treatment, and half received only acetone (0.5%) as solvent control. The incidence of transformation was then monitored over the succeeding 5 weeks. As seen in Figure 4, inhibition of transformation was maintained at a high level until between 3–5 weeks after withdrawal of retinyl acetate. However, in dishes fixed and stained 5 weeks after drug removal, the frequency of transformation was the same as in control cultures treated only with MCA. In cultures kept on retinyl acetate, inhibition of transformation was maintained at the 70% level throughout this period. Thus the effects of retinyl acetate

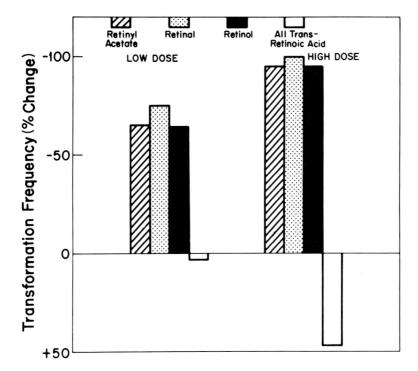

FIG. 3. Comparative activities of retinyl acetate, retinal, retinol (0.5 and 0.05 μg/ml), and retinoic acid (0.01 and 0.001 μg/ml) on inhibition of methylcholanthrene-induced neoplastic transformation. (Redrawn from Merriman and Bertram 1979 and Bertram 1980, with permission of *Cancer Research*.)

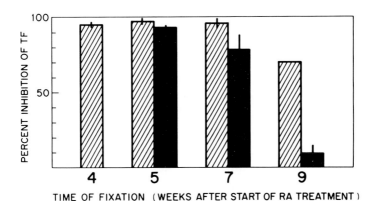

FIG. 4. Reversibility of the inhibition by retinyl acetate of methylcholanthrene-induced neoplastic transformation. Cultures were exposed to retinyl acetate for 4 weeks, then randomized into two groups. One group continued to receive drug (hatched bars) while a second group received solvent alone (solid bars). (Reproduced from Merriman and Bertram 1979, with permission of *Cancer Research*.)

depend upon the continued presence of the drug and upon drug withdrawal. Transformed cells do not immediately express themselves, but require a latent period of 3–5 weeks. This is precisely the period required for expression of transformation in carcinogen-only treated control cultures, and we suggested that retinyl acetate was acting by inhibiting the progression of an initiated cell to a phenotypically transformed cell (Merriman and Bertram 1979). This process takes about 28 days in 10T½ cells, many months in mice, and 10–20 years in humans. The reversibility of retinoid inhibition of transformation has since been confirmed in vivo (Thompson et al. 1979).

Effects on Transformed Cells

Having described the activity of retinyl acetate in this system, we next determined its mechanism of action. One question was whether transformation could be suppressed in established transformed cells in addition to cells transformed de novo by MCA. Although retinyl acetate has no effect on the growth rate of transformed cells obtained by cloning carcinogen-induced transformed foci, these were not the conditions under which the transformation assay was run. We set up reconstruction experiments of confluent monolayers of 10T½ cells and seeded about 100 transformed cells onto these monolayers. The capacity of these transformed cells to produce foci in the presence or absence of retinyl acetate or retinol was then assessed. As seen in Table 1, an increased number of colonies developed in treated dishes in comparison with acetone-treated controls, and these colonies tended to be larger than controls. Thus, it is clear that at concentrations up to 10-fold higher than concentrations causing inhibition of de novo transformation, retinyl acetate does not influence the expression of established transformed cells. We have also found that once transformation is expressed in carcinogen-treated cultures (i.e., 4 weeks after treatment) retinyl acetate is ineffective in reducing subsequent colony growth. Because of this lack of effect on transformed cells, we have concentrated our studies on the effects of retinyl acetate on the nontransformed 10T½ cells.

Pleiotropic Effects of Retinyl Acetate on 10T½ Cells

Saturation Density

The 10T½ cell line was originally selected to exhibit a high degree of postconfluence inhibition of cell division (Reznikoff et al. 1973b), which is seen operationally as a low cell density at confluence and the development of a stable cell monolayer. Neoplastically transformed cells, on the other hand, do not exhibit postconfluence inhibition of cell division, but continue to grow to produce multi-layered cell sheets (Reznikoff et al. 1973a, Bertram 1977). Autoradiographic studies after tritiated thymidine labeling for 1 hour have demonstrated that, whereas at confluence 10T½ cells have a labeling index of about 2%,

TABLE 1. *Effect of retinoids on the plating efficiency and growth of transformed cells plated on confluent monolayers of 10T½ cells* *

Retinyl acetate concentration (μg/ml)	Line A		Line B		Line C	
	No.	Size (% control)	No.	Size (% control)	No.	Size (% control)
0.1	137 ± 12†	103 ± 1	116 ± 15	123 ± 10	134 ± 5	126 ± 13
1.0	115 ± 3	114 ± 2	109 ± 8	131 ± 1	115 ± 13	120 ± 5

* Reconstruction experiments were performed using confluent monolayers of 10T½ cells grown in BME plus 5% serum. About 100 transformed cells were seeded onto the 10T½ monolayer, and after 24 hours replicate cultures received the appropriate concentration of retinyl acetate. Dishes were fixed and stained after 7 days of treatment without further medium change. Cultures were scored for the number and size of the transformed foci.

† Mean ± S.E. of two separate experiments using three dishes/data point (expressed as a percentage of the solvent only-treated controls). (From Merriman and Bertram 1979, with permission of *Cancer Research*.)

transformed cells at saturation density maintain a 45% labeling index (Bertram et al. 1977). This property of nontransformed fibroblasts is probably the single most important expression of their normal phenotype. When 10T½ cells are grown under conditions of increasing concentrations of fetal calf serum (FCS) in their growth medium, the saturation density rises (i.e., cells become more crowded), but conditions of postconfluence inhibition of cell division are always reached. In contrast, transformed cells respond little to serum concentrations between 2.5% and 20%, which cause such major alterations of saturation density in nontransformed cells (Figure 5). The addition of retinyl acetate to the growth medium of 10T½ cells growing under various conditions of serum concentration has the effect of reducing the saturation densities of confluent monolayers without affecting the logarithmic portion of the growth curve. As seen in Figure 6, retinyl acetate reduced the saturation density of cells in a dose-dependent manner, with the major effect being seen in those cultures growing under conditions of high serum concentration (10%). Regardless of serum concentration, a concentration of 0.1 μg/ml retinyl acetate produced the minimum saturation density of about 4.5×10^5 cells/dish, which may be the maximum degree to which cells can spread to occupy the active surface of the dish. Thus, retinyl acetate

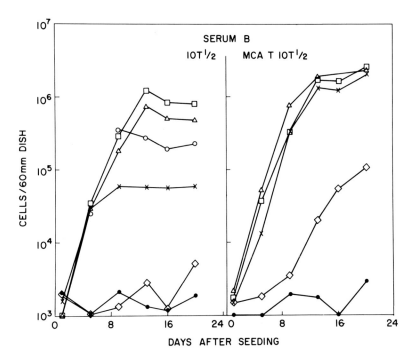

FIG. 5. Effects of serum concentration on the saturation density of nontransformed and transformed 10T½ cells. Left panel, 10T½ cells growing in BME + 20%, □; 10%, △; 5%, ○; 2.5%, x; 1%, ◇; and 0.1%, ●, serum. Right panel, methylcholanthrene-transformed cells, same symbols. (Reproduced from Bertram 1977, with permission of *Cancer Research.*)

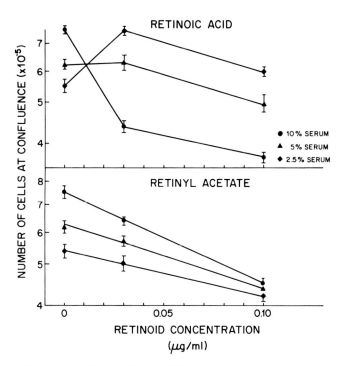

FIG. 6. Reduction of saturation density of 10T½ cells growing in 60-mm dishes by retinoic acid (upper panel) and retinyl acetate (lower panel). Cultures were seeded into the stated concentrations of serum and retinoids and grown to confluence.

enhances one aspect of the nontransformed phenotype in 10T½ cells. All-trans-retinoic acid produced very variable effects on saturation density in these cells (Figure 6, upper panel), and is thus again seen to behave very differently from retinyl acetate or retinol itself.

Cell Spreading

The decrease in saturation densities seen in retinyl acetate–treated cultures must be accompanied with an increase in cell spreading at confluence, since both control and treated cultures were confluent (i.e., formed a continuous cell sheet). To determine if similar effects were produced in logarithmic phase cultures in which cells are normally much less spread, we treated logarithmic phase cultures with 0.05 or 0.5 µg/ml retinyl acetate, or with acetone as control, for 3 days, then assessed the degree of cell spreading of a representative cell population. This was performed by preparing scanning electron micrographs of glutaraldehyde-fixed cell preparations. Morphological types were placed in one of six categories depending upon the degree of flatness. As seen in Table 2 the majority of confluent cells (92%) can be classified as flat, whereas only

TABLE 2. *Effect of retinyl acetate on the morphological types of 10T½ cells*

| | | | Logarithmic 10T½ | |
| | Confluent 10T½ (%) | Acetone control (%) | Retinyl acetate (μg/ml) 0.05 (%) | 0.50 (%) |
Morphological type*				
Flat	92.0	56.9	59.4	87.3†
Semi-flat	4.0	24.8	27.5	7.7†
Raised polygonal	2.0	13.4	10.1	3.0†
Rounded	0	1.3	0	1.0
Spindle	2.0	2.9	2.9	1.0†
No. cells analyzed	50	306	207	300
Cell density‡	302	69.2 ± 1.8	70.0 ± 6.3	67.3 ± 7.4

* Determined by scanning electron microscopy.
† Significant difference ($P < 0.05$) from control value.
‡ Number of cells/mm² ± standard deviation.

57% of logarithmic cells fall into this category. When cells in logarithmic growth phase were treated for 3 days with 0.5 μg/ml retinyl acetate, 87% of cells were classified as flat, and the profile of cell flatness within the population was similar to untreated confluent cells. However, this concentration did not reduce the growth rate of these cells; thus, flattening at confluence is clearly separable from growth inhibition at confluence. Treatment of transformed cells with retinyl acetate caused some degree of cell flattening, but much less than that seen in nontransformed cells. In control cultures, only about 20% of cells had a flattened morphology and this increased to 44% in retinyl acetate–treated cultures (0.5 μg/ml) (data not shown). Thus, by enhancing the degree of cell flattening, retinyl acetate enhances one of the morphological markers of a nontransformed phenotype in these fibroblasts.

Cell Substrate Adhesion

To determine if the increased cell spreading was associated with increased cell-substrate adhesion, we measured the rate at which confluent 10T½ cells could be detached from the plastic substrate by exposure to a 0.5% trypsin: EDTA, 2×10^{-4} M solution in phosphate-buffered saline. It was found that 0.3 or 0.03 μg/ml retinyl acetate decreased the number of cells that could be detached by a standard exposure to trypsin:EDTA and that about 3 days were required to produce maximal effect (Figure 7). In parallel studies, the time course of this release was studied over the first 4 min after addition of trypsin:EDTA to cells previously cultured for 3 days in the presence of retinyl acetate or certain synthetic retinoids shown to be active in inhibiting transformation (Figure 8). While retinyl acetate (panel A) clearly showed a dose-dependent increase in adhesion, retinylidene dimedone, which was approximately equipotent

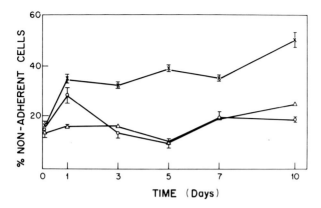

FIG. 7. Time course of production of increased adhesion of 10T½ cells to the plastic substrate. Confluent cultures in growth medium supplemented with 5% serum were treated with acetone (x---x), or retinyl acetate at 0.3 μg/ml (△---△) or 0.03 μg/ml (○---○). The rate of release of cells by a trypsin: EDTA solution was then determined at increasing times after treatment. (Reproduced from Bertram 1980, with permission of *Cancer Research*).

in the transformation assay, showed increased adhesion only at the highest dose tested (panel B), and 4-hydroxphenyl retinamide, which in the transformation assay was more potent than retinyl acetate (Bertram 1980), actually caused a decrease in adhesion (panel C). Transformed 10T½ cells are all released from the plastic substrate by a 4-min exposure to trypsin:EDTA, and retinyl

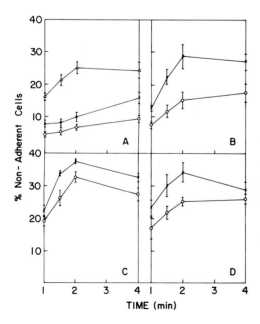

FIG. 8. Time course of release of 10T½ cells by trypsin: EDTA from a plastic substrate. Four days prior to assay, confluent cultures were treated with either high dose (○---○) or low dose (×---×) of the respective retinoid or with acetone as control (△---△). **Panel A,** retinyl acetate, 0.3 and 0.03 μg/ml; **B,** retinylidene dimedone, 0.3 and 0.1 μg/ml; **C,** N-4-hydroxyphenylretinamide, 0.3 and 0.1 μg/ml; **D,** N-ethylretinamide, 3.0 and 1.0 μg/ml.

acetate marginally slows this rate (data not shown). Thus, retinyl acetate again accentuates the differences between nontransformed and transformed cells. The effects of the synthetic analogs are difficult to interpret at this time. Clearly, however, increased adhesion per se is not related to inhibition of neoplastic transformation.

Microfilament Bundles

The possession by cultured fibroblasts of an organized system of microfilaments is seen only in nontransformed cells, in which microfilament bundles (MFB) are arrayed parallel to the long axis of the cell. The majority of these arrays are microfilaments associated with the lower (attached) surface of the cell as observed in transmission electron microscopy (Goldman et al. 1975). By a variety of labeling procedures, using antibodies to actin (Lazarides and Weber 1974) or antibodies to DNase (Wang and Goldberg 1978) and by binding of heavy meromyosin (Ishikawa et al. 1969), microfilaments have been shown to be composed of actin cables. Other studies have shown MFBs to be associated with attachment zones of cells to substrates ("feet"), and it now seems clear that these attachment zones serve as organizing centers for new MFBs as a cell migrates over a solid substrate (Goldman et al. 1976). This association between attachment sites and MFB is believed to allow cell flattening and spreading against the surface tension forces that would otherwise make a cell spherical. Exposure of cells to cytochalasin B, a disorganizer of MFBs (Goldman 1972), results in the rounding up of spread cells.

Many transformed cells examined fail to exhibit the organized architecture of MFBs, which are randomly distributed throughout the cytoplasm (Pollack et al. 1975). As discussed above, transformed cells are not attached as tightly to nor do they spread as much on a solid substrate as do nontransformed fibroblasts. Nontransformed fibroblasts must spread to replicate, while many nontransformed cells need not (Folkman and Moscona 1978), which presumably explains why transformed cells can grow in suspension in soft agar. Thus, the MFB system appears to be involved directly or indirectly in cellular growth control. It has been proposed by Puck (1977) that cytoskeletal defects can explain the pleiotropic changes that occur during neoplastic transformation.

An analysis of retinyl acetate–treated logarithmic phase 10T½ cells, which as shown above are more spread and firmly attached than otherwise untreated 10T½ cells or transformed 10T½ cells under any conditions, revealed an increasing frequency of MFBs as detected by light microscopic observation after Coomassie blue staining (Pena 1980). These stained organelles could also be labeled with anti-DNase, a highly specific actin label (Wang and Goldberg 1978). Retinyl acetate at 0.03 μg/ml, which in previous studies inhibited transformation by about 60% (Figure 2), caused an increased in MFBs from about 21/100 μm in controls to 54/100 μm in treated cells (Figure 9). We have not yet successfully analyzed transformed cells for similar effects, as the lack of cell spreading in

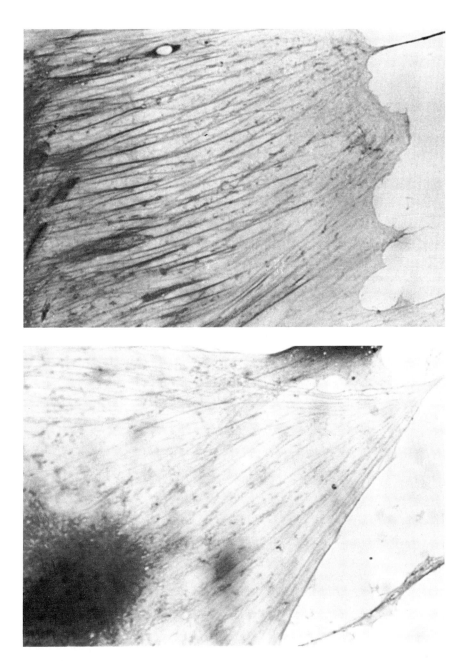

FIG. 9. Photomicrographs of microfilament bundles in control (top) or retinyl acetate–treated (0.1 μg/ml) (bottom) cells. Bundles were visualized by Coomassie blue staining (× 11,500).

control populations makes analysis difficult. Cell spreading induced by culturing cells in a low concentration of fetal calf serum did not induce the increased frequency of MFBs seen as a consequence of exposure to retinyl acetate; thus, this response is not simply a consequence of spreading (data not shown).

Membrane Biochemistry

Profound changes in membrane biochemistry have been reported to occur upon neoplastic transformation, involving both the lipid and protein constituents (for a review, see Warren et al. 1978). In an elegant series of papers, Hakomori's group has shown that the ganglioside components of the plasma membrane of neoplastic cells suffer from incomplete glycosylation, apparently as a result of decreases in specific glycosyltransferases (for a review, see Hakomori 1975). Although the relevance of these changes to aberrant growth control mechanisms of neoplastic cells is not known, because of the relative ease of analysis of these membrane components in comparison with the glycoproteins, and because similar patterns of incomplete glycosylation have been reported in chemically transformed cells derived from the 10T½ cell line (Langenbach and Kennedy 1978), we decided to study the effects of retinyl acetate on this aspect of membrane biochemistry.

Nontransformed 10T½ cells were treated for 3 days in logarithmic growth phase with either retinyl acetate (0.1 μg/ml, a concentration that virtually eliminates transformation, Figure 2) or with acetone as control. Cells were then harvested by scraping and the ganglioside fraction extracted by partition into organic solvents according to the methods of Yu and Ledeen (1972). This fraction was then chromatographed on thin-layer chromatography with a solvent system of chloroform/methanol/water/NH_3 (60:25:7:1) and carbohydrate-containing bands visualized by resorcinol staining. Identities of bands so visualized were confirmed by comparison with chromatography behavior of known reference standards of GM_2, GM_1, GDl_a, and GT_1. The identity of GDl_b and GM_3 was inferred from their chromatographic behavior. Quantitation of stained bands was performed by densitometric scanning, and tracing ganglioside patterns in treated and control populations is shown in Figure 10. Gangliosides containing a single sialic acid residue (i.e., GM_3, GM_2, GM_1) or GDl_a, which contains two nonlinked residues, are essentially unchanged quantitatively in treated and control cells, whereas proportions of those gangliosides containing linked sialic acid residues (i.e., GD_3, GDl_b, and GT_1) are increased in treated cells. This is depicted diagrammatically in Figure 11. The data suggest that retinyl acetate stimulates an alternate pathway of ganglioside biosynthesis, which results in the induction in normal cells of gangliosides with a more complex glycosylation pattern. This trend, as discussed above, counters the trend observed upon neoplastic transformation of many cell lines (Hakomori 1975), including 10T½ cells (Langenbach and Kennedy 1978), one of incomplete glycosylation of membrane components, resulting in a simplification of glycosylation patterns. Thus,

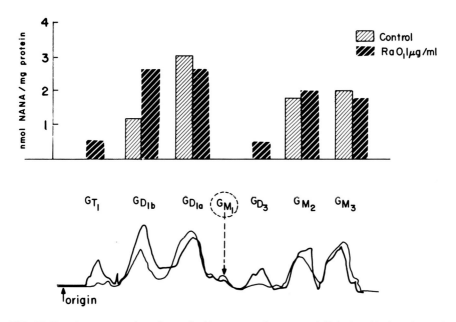

FIG. 10. Densitometer tracing of ganglioside patterns from control (light hatching) and retinyl acetate–treated (0.1 μg/ml) cells. Ganglioside notation is according to Svennerholm (1964).

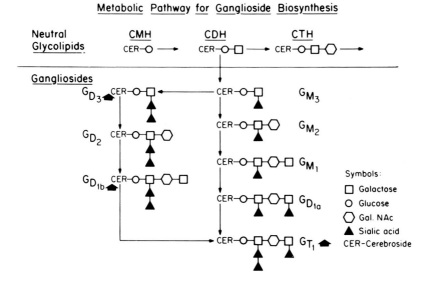

FIG. 11. Schematic synthetic routes for gangliosides. Gangliosides elevated by retinyl acetate (see Figure 10) indicated by ↑. Ganglioside notation according to Svennerholm (1964).

retinyl acetate again accentuates the normal phenotype in nontransformed cells.

Whether these alterations represent a primary effect of retinyl acetate or are a consequence of other alterations is unclear at this time. Also unclear is the relevance of these changes to the pleiotropic effects on cellular behavior observed in retinyl acetate–treated cells. In this context, it should be noted that several cell membrane receptors, including those for cholera toxin, are gangliosides (Gill 1977). Furthermore, Hakamori's group has shown that culturing cells in the presence of monovalent anti-GM_3 ganglioside antibody can prevent the phenotypic expression of transformation in a temperature-sensitive NRK cell line transformed by ovarian sarcoma virus, in which transformation results in a decrease in GM_3. Similar results have been obtained using anti-GM_1 in mouse sarcoma virus–transformed 3T3 cells, in which GM_1 is depleted upon transformation (Hakamori 1978). In several cell lines subject to postconfluence inhibition of cell division, but not in transformed cells, cell-cell contact stimulates intercellular glycosylation of gangliosides, suggesting that this glycosylation is somehow connected to the phenomenon of growth control (Hakomori 1970, Robbins and MacPherson 1971). This intercellular glycosylation was found to be stimulated by retinol (Yogeeswaran et al. 1974). Thus, evidence exists to suggest a role for gangliosides in cell growth control phenomena, and the interaction of retinol in the synthesis of these macromolecules offers an intriguing explanation for the complex effects of this drug.

CONCLUSIONS

Accentuation of the Normal Phenotype

As summarized in Table 3, we have shown that, for all parameters so far examined that differentiate a nontransformed cell from a neoplastic cell, retinyl acetate accentuates the nontransformed phenotype. This fact, together with the

TABLE 3. *Pleiotrophic effects of retinyl acetate on cultured cells*

Cellular property	Nontransformed cell		Transformed cell	
	Control	Retinyl acetate	Control	Retinyl acetate
Saturation density	Low	Lower	High	No change
Spreading	Medium	High	Low	Medium
Underlapping	Medium	Low	High	ND
Adhesion	High	Higher	Low	Increased
Microfilaments	Organized	More organized	Disorganized	?
Gangliosides	Complex	More complex	Less complex	ND

ND, not determined.

reversibility of retinoid effects seen both in vitro (Figure 4) and in vivo (Thompson et al. 1979), leads us to conclude that retinyl acetate acts by stabilizing the normal phenotype against neoplastic change. These conclusions do not apply to retinoic acid, which in our system behaves quite differently. From the evidence presented above indicating that retinyl acetate alters plasma membrane function (adhesion, spreading) and biochemistry (gangliosides) and from its implication in the biosynthesis of membrane glycolipids and glycoproteins, we have adopted a working hypothesis that the primary effect of this compound (or compounds leading to formation of retinol) is on the plasma membrane of 10T½ cells. Since established transformed cells are only minimally altered by retinyl acetate treatment (Table 1), it appears that this stabilizing effect can only influence preneoplastic initiated cells, which have not yet expressed the transformed phenotype. The "quantum leap" of change that accompanies phenotypic expression may be too extensive for correction by membrane alterations alone.

Relationship to Tumor Promoters

It is of great interest that the tumor-promoting phorbol esters, which act in the opposite manner to the retinoids in accelerating the neoplastic transformation of initiated cells, have been reported to mimic transformation in nontransformed cells (Weinstein et al. 1979). Thus, the actions of these compounds on many facets of cell behavior appear diametrically opposed, and in some situations retinoids will prevent phorbol ester–induced promotion (Verma et al. 1980b). Since phorbol esters have also been postulated to have a primary action on the plasma membrane (Weinstein et al. 1979), it appears likely that both compounds influence common regulatory mechanisms.

Possible Mechanisms for the Effects of Retinyl Acetate on Cellular Functions

Via epigenetic modifications of membrane biosynthesis

Retinol, which is readily formed from retinyl acetate in cells, has been implicated in the synthesis of glycoproteins and glycolipids via the intermediate retinol phosphate, which is further converted into mannosyl retinyl phosphate. This intermediate can function as a mannose donor to a growing polysaccharide chain of glycoprotein (Wolf et al. 1979, DeLuca et al. 1979). The involvement of retinol in glycosylation of lipids has been suggested from observation of the stimulation of membrane glycosylation by retinol and by retinol phosphate galactose (Yogeeswaran et al. 1974, Hakomori 1975).

Via alterations in gene expression by specific binding proteins

Specific cellular binding proteins for retinol (CRBP) and retinoic acid (CRABP) have been described in a number of tissues and malignancies, and the suggestion was made that these binding proteins could translocate to the nucleus and alter gene expression in a manner analogous to steroid hormones (Chytil and Ong 1979, Takase et al. 1979). We have been unable to detect either CRBP or CRABP in cultures of 10T½ cells (Libby and Bertram, unpublished results), and DeLuca (personal communication) has also been unable to detect these proteins in a number of cell lines in which retinol has biological effects. With the knowledge that negatives are hard to prove, we nevertheless feel that an association with specific binding proteins of this type is unlikely to be involved in the activity of retinol in the 10T½ system.

It is hoped that a deeper understanding of the mechanisms of the biological action of retinyl acetate and retinol on a model system such as that described above will lead to greater understanding of fundamental mechanisms of carcinogenesis and to the rational design of experimental and clinical chemoprevention studies.

ACKNOWLEDGMENTS

This work reported in this chapter was supported by USPHS Grants CA-25484 to JSB and Program Grant CA-13038.

REFERENCES

Becci, P. J., H. J. Thompson, C. J. Grubbs, R. A. Squire, C. C. Brown, M. B. Sporn, and R. C. Moon. 1978. Inhibitory effect of 13-cis-retinoid acid on urinary bladder carcinogenesis induced in C57B1/6 mice by N-butyl-N-(4-hydroxy-butyl)-nitrosamine. Cancer Res. 38:4463–4466.

Bertram, J. S. 1977. Effects of serum concentration on the expression of carcinogen-induced transformation in the C3H/10T½ C18 cell line. Cancer Res. 37:514–523.

Bertram, J. S. 1980. Structure activity relationships among various retinoids and their ability to inhibit neoplastic transformation and to increase cell adhesion in the C3H/10T½ C18 cell line. Cancer Res. 40:3141–3146.

Bertram, J. S., P. R. Libby, and W. M. LeStourgeon. 1977. Changes in nuclear actin levels with change in growth state of C3H/10T½ cells and the lack of response in malignantly transformed cells. Cancer Res. 37:4104–4111.

Bollag, W. 1972. Prophylaxis of chemically induced benign and malignant epithelial tumors by vitamin A acid (retinoic acid). Eur. J. Cancer 8:689–693.

Bollag, W. 1975. Therapy of epithelial tumors with an aromatic retinoic acid analog. Chemotherapy 21:236–247.

Brown, I. V., B. P. Lane, and J. Pearson. 1977. Effects of depot injections of retinal palmitate on 7,12-dimethylbenz(a)anthracene-induced preneoplastic changes in rat skin. JNCI 58:1347–1355.

Chu, E. W., and R. A. Malmgren. 1965. An inhibitory effect of vitamin A on the induction of tumors of forestomach and cervix in the Syrian hamster by carcinogenic polycyclic hydrocarbons. Cancer Res. 25:884–897.

Chytil, F., and D. E. Ong. 1979. Cellular retinol- and retinoic acid-binding proteins in vitamin A action. Fed. Proc. 38:2510–2514.

Cohen, S. M., J. F. Wittenberg, and G. T. Bryan. 1976. Effect of avitaminosis A and hypervitaminosis A on urinary bladder carcinogenicity of N-(4-5-nitro-2-furyl-2-thiazolyl)-formamide. Cancer Res. 36:2334–2339.

DeLuca, L. M., P. V. Blat, W. Sasak, and S. Adamo. 1979. Biosynthesis of phosphoryl and glucosyl phosphoryl derivatives of vitamin A in biological membranes. Fed. Proc. 38:2535–2539.

Food and Drug Administration. 1978. Retinoic acid and sun-caused skin cancer. FDA Drug Bull. Aug/Sept. 8, 20.

Folkman, J., and A. Moscona. 1978. Role of cell shape in growth control. Nature 273:345–349.

Forbes, P. D., F. Urbach, and R. E. Davies. 1979. Enhancement of experimental photocarcinogenesis by topical retinoic acid. Cancer Lett. 7:85–90.

Gill, D. M. 1977. Mechanism of action of cholera toxin, *in* Advances in Cyclic Nucleotide Research, P. Greengard and G. A. Robison, eds, Vol. 8. Raven Press, New York, pp. 85–118.

Goldman, R. 1972. The effects of cytochalasin B on the microfilaments of baby hamster kidney (BHK-21) cells. J. Cell Biol. 52:246–254.

Goldman, R., E. Lazarides, R. Pollack, and K. Weber. 1975. The distribution of actin in non-muscle cells. Exp. Cell Res. 90:333–344.

Goldman, R., J. Schloss, and J. Starger. 1976. Organizational changes in actin-like microfilaments during animal cell movement, *in* Cell Motility, R. Goldman, T. Pollard, and J. Rosenbaum, eds. Cold Spring Harbor Laboratory, Cold Spring Harbor, New York, pp. 217–245.

Goodman, D. S. 1980. Vitamin A metabolism. Fed. Proc. 39:2716–2722.

Goodman, D. S., R. Blomstrand, B. Werner, H. S. Huang, and T. Shiratori. 1966. The intestinal absorption and metabolism of vitamin A and β-carotene in man. J. Clin. Invest. 45:1615–1623.

Grubbs, C. J., R. C. Moon, R. A. Squire, G. M. Farrow, S. F. Stinson, D. G. Goodman, C. C. Brown, and M. B. Sporn. 1977. 13-Cis-retinoic acid: Inhibition of bladder carcinogenesis induced in rats by N-butyl-N-(4-hydroxybutyl)nitrosamine. Science 198:743–744.

Hakomori, S. 1970. Cell density-dependent changes of glycolipid concentrations in fibroblasts, and loss of this response in virus-transformed cells. Proc. Natl. Acad. Sci. USA 67:1741–1747.

Hakomori, S. 1975. Structures and organization of cell surface glycolipids: Dependency on cell growth and malignant transformation. Biochim. Biophys. Acta 417:55–89.

Hakomori, S. 1978. Glycolipid changes associated with oncogenesis and ontogenesis, and the inhibition of the process of transformation by monovalent anti-glycolipid antibodies. Adv. Pathobiol. 7:270–281.

Ishikawa, H., R. Bischoff, and H. Holtzer. 1969. Formation of arrowhead complexes with heavy meromyosin in a variety of cell types. J. Cell Biol. 43:312–328.

Langenbach, R., and S. Kennedy. 1978. Gangliosides and their cell density-dependent changes in control and chemically transformed C3H/10T½ cells. Exp. Cell Res. 112:361–372.

Lazarides, E., and K. Weber. 1974. Actin filaments: The specific visualization of actin filaments in non-muscle cells. Proc. Natl. Acad. Sci. USA 71:2268–2272.

Maiorana, A., and P. M. Gullino. 1980. Effect of retinyl acetate on the incidence of mammary carcinomas and hepatomas in mice. JNCI 64:655–663.

Mayer, H., W. Bollag, R. Hanni, and R. Ruegy. 1978. Retinoids, a new class of compounds with prophylactic and therapeutic activities: In oncology and dermatology. Experientia 34:1105–1119.

McLaren, D. 1967. Effects of vitamin A deficiency in man, *in* The Vitamins, W. H. Sebrell and R. S. Harris, eds., Vol. 1, 2nd Ed. Academic Press, New York, pp. 267–280.

Merriman, R. L., and J. S. Bertram. 1979. Reversible inhibition by retinoids of 3-methylcholanthrene-induced neoplastic transformation in C3H-10T½ clone 8 cells. Cancer Res. 39:1661–1666.

Mettlin, C., and S. Graham. 1979. Dietary risk factors in human bladder cancer. Am. J. Epidemiol. 110:255–263.

Mettlin, C., S. Graham, R. Priore, J. Marshall, and M. Swanson. 1981. Diet and cancer of the esophagus. Nutrition and Cancer 2:143–147.

Mettlin, C., S. Graham, and M. Swanson. 1979. Vitamin A and lung cancer. JNCI 62:1435–1438.

Moon, R. C., H. J. Thompson, P. J. Becci, C. J. Grubbs, R. J. Gander, D. L. Newton, J. M. Smith, S. L. Phillips, W. R. Henderson, L. T. Mullen, C. C. Brown, and M. B. Sporn. 1979. N-(4-hydroxyphenyl) retinamide, a new retinoid for prevention of breast cancer in the rat. Cancer Res. 39:1339–1346.

Moore, T. 1929. Relation of carotin to vitamin A. Lancet 2:380–381.

Moore, T. 1967. Effects of vitamin A deficiency in animals: Pharmacology and toxicology of vitamin A, *in* The Vitamins, W. H. Sebrell and R. S. Harris, eds., vol. 1, 2nd Ed. Academic Press, New York, pp. 246–266.

Nettesheim, P., C. Snyder, and J. C. Kim. 1979. Vitamin A and the susceptibility of respiratory tract tissues to carcinogenic insult. Environ. Health Perspect. 29:89–93.

Nettesheim, P., and M. L. Williams. 1976. The influence of vitamin A on the susceptibility of the rat lung to 3-methylcholanthrene. Int. J. Cancer 17:351–357.

Newberne, P. M., and A. E. Rogers. 1973. Rat colon carcinomas associated with aflatoxin and marginal vitamin A. JNCI 50:439–448.

Newberne, P. M., and V. Suphakarn. 1977. Preventive role of vitamin A in colon carcinogenesis in rats. Cancer 40(suppl.):2253–2556.

Newton, D. L., W. R. Henderson, and M. B. Sporn. 1980. Structure activity relationship of retinoids in hamster tracheal organ culture. Cancer Res. 40:3413–3425.

Pena, S. D. J. 1980. A new technique for the visualization of the cytoskeleton in cultured fibroblasts with Coomassie blue R250. Cell Biol. Int. Rep. 4:149–153.

Pollack, R., M. Osborn, and K. Weber. 1975. Patterns of organization of actin and myosin in normal and transformed cultured cells. Proc. Natl. Acad. Sci. USA 72:994–999.

Puck, T. T. 1977. Cyclic AMP, the microtubule-microfilament system, and cancer. Proc. Natl. Acad. Sci. USA 74:4491–4495.

Reznikoff, C. A., J. S. Bertram, D. W. Brankow, and C. Heidelberger. 1973a. Quantitative and qualitative studies of chemical transformation of cloned C3H mouse embryo cells sensitive to postconfluence inhibition of cell division. Cancer Res. 33:3239–3249.

Reznikoff, C. A., D. W. Brankow, and C. Heidelberger. 1973b. Establishment and characterization of a cloned line of C3H mouse embryo cells sensitive to postconfluence inhibition of cell division. Cancer Res. 33:2331–2338.

Robbins, P. W., and I. MacPherson. 1971. Control of glycolipid synthesis in a cultured hamster cell line. Nature 229:569–570.

Saffioti, U., R. Montesano, A. R. Sellakumar, and S. A. Borg. 1967. Experimental cancer of lung. Inhibition by vitamin A of the induction of tracheobronchial squamous metaplasia and squamous cell tumors. Cancer 20:857–864.

Shklar, G., P. Marefat, A. Kornhauser, D. P. Trickler, and K. D. Wallace. 1980. Retinoid inhibition of lingual carcinogenesis. Oral Surg. 49:323–332.

Schroeder, E. W., and P. H. Black. 1980. Retinoids: Tumor preventors or tumor enhancers? JNCI 65:671–674.

Smith, D. M., A. E. Rogers, and P. M. Newberne. 1975. Vitamin A and benzo(a)pyrene carcinogenesis in the respiratory tract of hamsters fed a semi-synthetic diet. Cancer Res. 35:1485–1488.

Sporn, M. B., and D. L. Newton. 1979. Chemoprevention of cancer with retinoids. (Abstract) Fed. Proc. 38:2528–2534.

Sporn, M. B., N. M. Dunlop, D. L. Newton, and J. M. Smith. 1976. Prevention of chemical carcinogenesis by vitamin A and its synthetic analogs (retinoids). Fed. Proc. 35:1332–1338.

Sporn, M. B., R. A. Squire, C. C. Brown, J. M. Smith, M. L. Wenk, and S. Springer. 1977. 13-Cis-retinoic acid: Inhibition of bladder carcinogenesis in the rat. Science 195:487–489.

Svennerholm, L. 1964. The gangliosides. J. Lipid Res. 5:145–155.

Takase, S., D. E. Ong, and F. Chytil. 1979. Cellular retinol-binding protein allows specific interaction of retinol with the nucleus in vitro. Proc. Natl. Acad. Sci. USA 76:2204–2208.

Thompson, H. J., P. J. Becci, C. C. Brown, and R. C. Moon. 1979. Effect of the duration of retinal acetate feeding on inhibition of 1-methyl-1-nitrosourea-induced mammary carcinogenesis in the rat. Cancer Res. 39:3977–3980.

Verma, A. K., E. A. Conrad, and R. K. Boutwell. 1980a. Induction of mouse epidermal ornithine decarboxylase activity and skin tumors by 7,12-dimethyl[a]anthracene: Modulation by retinoic acid and 7,8-benzoflavone. Carcinogenesis 1:607–611.

Verma, A. K., T. J. Slaga, P. W. Wertz, G. C. Mueller, and R. K. Boutwell. 1980b. Inhibition of skin tumor promotion by retinoic acid and its metabolite 5,6-epoxy retinoic acid. Cancer Res. 40:2367–2371.

Wald, N., M. Idle, and J. Boreham. 1980. Low serum-vitamin A and subsequent risk of cancer. Lancet 2:813–815.

Wang, E., and A. Goldberg. 1978. Binding of deoxyribonuclease I to actin: A new way to visualize microfilament bundles in nonmuscle cells. J. Histochem. Cytochem. 26:745–749.

Warren, L., C. A. Buck, and G. P. Turzynski. 1978. Glycopeptide changes and malignant transformation. A possible role for carbohydrate in malignant behavior. Biochim. Biophys. Acta 516:97–127.

Weinstein, I. B., L. Lee, P. B. Fisher, A. Mufron, and H. Yamashaki. 1979. Action of phorbol esters in cell culture: Mimicry of transformation, altered differentiation, and effects on cell membranes. J. Supramol. Struct. 12:195–208.

Wolbach, S. D., and P. R. Howe. 1925. Tissue changes following deprivation of fat soluble A vitamin. J. Exp. Med. 42:753–777.

Wolf, G., T. C. Kiorges, S. Masushige, J. B. Schneiber, M. J. Smith, and R. S. Anderson. 1979.

Recent evidence for the participation of vitamin A in glycoprotein synthesis. (Abstract) Fed. Proc. 38:2540–2543.

Yogeeswaran, G., R. A. Laine, and S. Hakomori. 1974. Mechanism of cell contact-dependent glycolipid synthesis: Further studies with glycolipid glass complex. Biochem. Biophys. Res. Commun. 59:591–599.

Yu, R. K., and R. W. Leedeen. 1972. Gangliosides of human, bovine and rabbit plasma. J. Lipid Res. 13:680–686.

Molecular Interrelations of Nutrition and Cancer,
edited by M. S. Arnott, J. van Eys, and Y.-M. Wang.
Raven Press, New York © 1982.

Vitamins and Micronutrients Modify Carcinogenesis and Tumor Promotion in Vitro

Carmia Borek

Radiological Research Laboratory, Departments of Radiology and Pathology, Cancer Center/Institute of Cancer Research, Columbia University, College of Physicians & Surgeons, New York, New York 10032

In recent years compelling evidence from epidemiological and animal data has implicated dietary factors in the pathogenesis of cancer (Nutrition in the causation of cancer, 1975), a disease whose progression is characterized by specific sequential events (Berenblum 1975).

The complex role of nutritional factors in modifying cancer incidence may be attributed in part to several modes of action. Dietary agents can act as: (a) an auxiliary to other environmental factors implicated in the induction of cancer, namely as potentiators or promotors (Borek and Ong 1981); (b) as causes of cancer (Miller and Miller 1979); or (c) as cancer-preventive factors (Sporn et al. 1976, Griffin 1979). In this latter role, nutritional elements would inhibit neoplasia induced and promoted by environmental agents such as radiation and chemicals and counteract the effect of dietary hazards.

While we are slowly becoming aware of (a) and (b), we are consistently in search for nutritional elements that would act as chemopreventive agents and fulfill the requirements of (c). Since a cancer-inducing agent can be its own promotor when delivered at the appropriately high dose to the right target tissue, the effectiveness of chemopreventive agents in suppressing carcinogenesis may also be related to dose and target tissue.

Cancer is an old disease. It already afflicted prehistoric animals as evidenced in the skeleton of Tyrannosaurus rex standing in the London Natural History museum. Yet awareness of oncogenic agents is recent. Recognition of the carcinogenic potential of chemicals is traced back only to the 18th century (Pott 1775) and that of radiation to the 19th century shortly after x-rays were discovered by Roentgen in 1895 (Brown 1936). More recently, interest in occupational carcinogenesis were developed with the realization that many potential physical and chemical carcinogens exist and are increasing in our environment (Occupational carcinogenesis 1976).

While epidemiological and animal data have contributed much to our knowledge of carcinogenesis, they have their limitation in studies on the hazardous effects of low doses and in evaluating cellular mechanisms regulating carcinogenesis.

In recent years it has become possible to grow animal cells in culture under defined nutritional conditions (for reviews, see Borek 1979, Borek 1981a, 1982). These in vitro systems have served as powerful tools in cancer research for comparing the carcinogenic potential of various agents found in the environment as well as those used in medical diagnosis and therapy. In addition they have served to evaluate agents and conditions that can modulate the induction or expression of neoplastic development.

In our earlier work using radiation as an oncogenic agent we showed that transformation in vitro consists of the following steps: (1) initiation, i.e., exposure of the cultured cells to the carcinogen (Borek and Sachs 1966); (2) fixation of the transformed state as a hereditary property requiring replication within hours after initiation (Borek and Sachs 1967, 1968); and (3) expression of the transformed state requiring several cell replications and resulting in a focus or colony that is morphologically distinct from the control (Borek and Sachs 1967, Reznikoff et al. 1973).

Similar to neoplastic development in vivo, transformation of cells in vitro into malignant cells is a multistage process. It is associated with the loss and acquisition of a large number of cellular structural and functional properties, some of which are illustrated in Table 1. The most obvious phenotypic change that enables the quantitative assessment of transformation in vitro is the loss of growth control resulting in a formation of dense multilayered colonies or foci, with irregular cell-cell orientation (Figures 1 and 2).

While initiation of carcinogenesis is irreversible, the effect of secondary events, which may serve as promotors, can be reversed. Thus, in modulating the neoplastic event we aim to prevent the induction and inhibit the expression and onset of neoplasia. We seek to associate primary events of induction with events at a genetic level, such as DNA damage. However, we cannot yet unequivocally associate initiation with particular biochemical or structural end points. Thus, we must evaluate preventive and protective measures by their ability to modify expression of the malignant state and neoplastic development and try, whenever possible, to correlate these end points with cellular and molecular changes. This has been our approach in recent work on prevention of carcinogenesis in which protease inhibitors (Borek et al. 1979, Borek and Cleaver 1981), retinoids (Borek et al. 1981a, 1981b, Miller et al. 1981) and hormonal factors (Guernsey et al. 1980) have been evaluated as preventive agents.

This chapter will deal with the inhibitory action of retinoids on radiogenic transformation and tumor promotion and the underlying molecular mechanisms involved. It will address the synergism we have found between radiation and food pyrolysates (Borek and Ong 1981) and the ability of retinoids to counteract this action. We will briefly discuss recent work that indicates that selenium, a micronutrient, is an effective inhibitor of carcinogenesis in vitro.

CELL CULTURES

While human cells are transformable by radiation (Borek 1981b) and by chemical carcinogens (Kakunaga 1978, Milo and DiPaolo 1978), rodent cells offer

TABLE 1. *Properties of fibroblasts and epithelial cells malignantly transformed in vitro distinguishing them from normal parental cells*

Characteristic	Fibroblasts	Epithelial
Morphology (light microscopy)	Pleomorphic, refractile criss-cross orientation, irregular growth pattern	Often not dramatically different from normal, somewhat more pleomorphic in some cases (e.g., liver)
Topography (scanning electron microscope)	Increase in surface features	Inconsistent changes, sometimes an increase in microvilli
Cell density	Increased saturation density, multilayering, and piling up of cells, loss of density-dependent inhibition of growth	Inconsistent, depends on cell line and tissue of origin, in some cell lines piling up of cells, in others maintenance of monolayer growth pattern
Serum requirement for growth	Decreased in rodent cells, less pronounced characteristic in transformed human cells, since normal human cells can grow in lower serum levels	Low as normal (in liver cells); not sufficiently studied in a variety of systems
Calcium dependence for growth	Reduced	Reduced
Altered cell surface glycoproteins	Yes	Yes
Agglutinability by low concentrations of lectins	Yes	Yes
Increased protease production	Yes	Inconsistent
Changes in cytoskeleton	Pronounced	Inconsistent
Growth in agar	Yes	Yes
Tumorigenicity	Yes	Yes

Modified from Borek 1979.

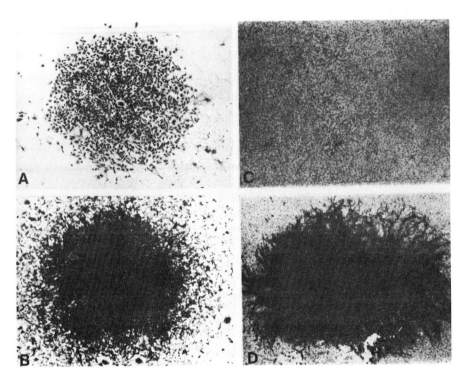

FIG. 1. Morphological criteria for transformation. (A,B) Clonal assay in hamster embryo cell cultures; (C,D) focus assay in mouse embryo 10T½ cells. (A) Normal hamster embryo cell clone, 14 days old. (B) A 14-day-old clone of hamster cells transformed in vitro by 300 rad x-rays. (C) A monolayer of untransformed 10T½ cells 6 weeks in culture. (D) A type III focus of 10T½ cells transformed by 300 rad of x-rays, 6 weeks in culture. (Reproduced from Borek et al. 1979.)

more defined systems for quantitative analysis. The investigations discussed here utilized two rodent cell systems: freshly cultured diploid hamster embryo (HE) cells (Borek and Sachs 1966, Borek 1979) and a heteroploid mouse cell line, 10T½, developed from C3H mouse embryos (Reznikoff et al. 1973).

Transformation as well as survival in the hamster cell system was assayed as described (Borek and Sachs 1966, Borek et al. 1978, Borek 1979). Briefly, the transformed hamster embryo cells grow as colonies that differ markedly from the surviving normal one (Figure 1A) by their piled up morphology and irregular cell-cell contact (Figure 1B). These morphological criteria have been associated with an ability of the cells to produce tumors in animals (Borek and Sachs 1966, Borek and Hall 1974). Transformation in the 10T½ cells was assayed in a focus formation assay as described (Reznikoff et al. 1973). The normal cells grow as contact-inhibited flat sheets (Figure 1C), whereas the transformed cells form multilayered foci with irregular boundaries (Figure 1D).

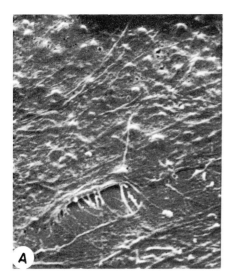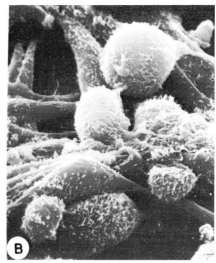

FIG. 2. A scanning electron micrograph of (A) normal cells derived from hamster embryo and (B) the same cell types transformed in vitro into malignant cells by 300 rad of X irradiation. Note the flat, smooth normal cells with tight intercellular junctional complexes. In contrast, the transformed cells are pleomorphic, grow in irregular fashion, and are rich in surface features. (A) SEM × 6000; (B) SEM × 2000.

RETINOIDS, RADIOGENIC TRANSFORMATION, AND TUMOR PROMOTORS

Retinoids

Within the last decade a variety of vitamin A analogs (retinoids) have been shown to inhibit the expression of malignancy both in experimental systems and in the clinic (for review, see Lotan 1980). At the same time interest has been revived and awareness increased about the effectiveness of compounds, mostly of plant origin and called tumor promotors, in enhancing carcinogenesis. One of these compounds, TPA (12–0 tetradecanoyl-phorbol 13-acetate) (Hecker 1971) has been used extensively in studies with cell culture systems.

While an antagonism between TPA and retinoids has been recognized in some in vitro carcinogenesis studies, in growth-related enzymatic systems in vivo and in vitro, and in differentiation in vitro (for review, see Lotan 1980), no studies have evaluated the effects of retinoids and TPA, alone or in combination, on oncogenic transformation in vitro.

Our early studies have shown that a vitamin A analog inhibits radiation-induced transformation in vitro (Harisiadis et al. 1978) and that retinoids and TPA exert antagonistic effects on vitamin A–binding protein production (Borek and Smith 1978). Our current studies are aimed at elucidating whether the antagonism between vitamin A and TPA on cell differentiation in vitro prevails in radiation-induced transformation in vitro. If it does, is the antagonism mediated via DNA damage as reflected in chromosomal sister chromatid exchanges (Perry and Evans 1975) or via other cellular and molecular events, for example at the level of the cell membrane?

Our protocol, which is detailed elsewhere (Borek et al. 1981a, Miller et al. 1981), consisted of the following: Cells were plated in the presence of the retinoid and irradiated 24 hours later with 300 rad (hamster cells), a dose that yields maximum transformation in this system (Borek and Hall 1974), or 400 rad for the 10T½ (Terzaghi and Little 1976). The retinoid used in the hamster cell system was β-all-trans retinoic acid, and that for the C3H 10T½ cells was a trimethylmethoxyphenyl analog of N-ethyl retinamide (TMMP). TPA was added immediately after irradiation for the duration of the experiment (2 weeks for HE and 6 weeks for 10T½). The retinoids were removed from the culture dishes 4 days after irradiation. Thus, if retinoids could inhibit cell transformation and interfere with the promotional effect of TPA, they had to do so within 4 days. As seen in Table 2, this was indeed the case. While TPA increased radiation-induced oncogenesis, retinoids inhibited radiogenic transformation irreversibly and eliminated any promotional effect of TPA.

DNA damage has been implicated in the process of transformation (Shilo and Weinberg 1981), and sister chromatid exchanges (SCE) reflect alterations in chromosomal DNA (Perry and Evans 1975). Thus, we set out to establish whether the striking inhibition of transformation and promotion by the retinoids is reflected in the patterns of SCE in the treated cells.

We found, as seen in Figure 3 and detailed elsewhere (Borek et al. 1981a), that whereas the inducing agent, x-rays, enhanced SCE twofold, the agents that modulated transformation did not express their modifying activity at the

TABLE 2. *TPA and retinoid modification of x-ray induced transformation in hamster embryo and C3H-10T½ cells*

	Hamster embryo		C3H-10T½	
Treatment	Surviving fraction	Mean rate of transformation $(10^{-3}) \pm$ standard error	Surviving fraction	Mean rate of transformation $(10^{-4}) \pm$ standard error
Control	1.00	0	1.00	0
TPA (0.16 μm)	0.70	0	0.93	0
Retinoid (7.1 μm)*	0.62	0	0.75	0
Retinoid, TPA	0.89	0	0.67	0
X-rays	0.42	6.99 ± 1.65	0.32	8.78 ± 1.29
X-rays, TPA	0.53	12.52 ± 1.81	0.52	16.15 ± 1.59
X-rays, retinoid	0.38	2.94 ± 0.79	0.30	4.37 ± 0.93
X-rays, retinoid, TPA	0.41	2.41 ± 0.85	0.36	2.46 ± 0.54

* C3H 10T½ cells were exposed to a trimethyl methoxyphenyl analog of N ethyl retinamide. The hamster embryo cells were exposed to β-all-trans retinoic acid.

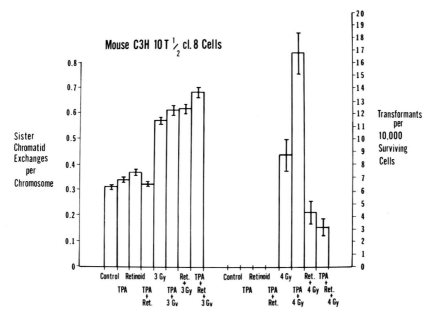

FIG. 3. Comparison of the effects of x-rays, retinoid TMMP-ERA, and TPA on transformation induction (right side) and sister chromatid exchanges (left side) in C3H/10T½ cells. Standard errors of the mean are indicated. For the SCE studies, cells were scored up to 20 hours after irradiation, while transformation incidence was assessed at 5 weeks after irradiation with TPA in continuous cell contact and retinoid present for 4 days only. (Reproduced from Miller et al. 1981, with permission of Academic Press.)

chromosomal level. The promoting TPA and the inhibitory retinoids both gave rise to increased SCE.

If retinoids were not acting at the chromosomal level, might they be affecting transformation at the membrane level? Membrane structural changes have been reported following cell treatment with retinoids (DeLuca et al. 1972). Our studies concentrated on membrane-associated ion transport enzymes, which are altered in the transformed state (Borek et al. 1981b). We evaluated the effects of the retinoids and TPA on $Na^+/K^+ATPase$, $Mg^+/ATPase$, and 5' nucleotidase (Borek et al. 1981b).

We found that regulation of cell transformation by the retinoids and TPA are reflected specifically in the level of $Na^+/K^+ATPase$. As seen in Table 3, TPA enhances the enzyme level; retinoids inhibit the Na^+/K^+ ATPase. When cells are plated with both agents, Na^+/K^+ ATPase returns to the control level. Retinoids modify transformation and inhibit promotion, therefore, at the level of gene expression and via the cell membrane. We are evaluating the molecular mechanism underlying these events. It is of interest to note in Table 3 that once cells are transformed, a condition against which preventive measures can no longer be effective, the retinoids do not modify the Na^+/K^+ ATPase.

TABLE 3. *The effect of all-trans retinoic acid (RA) and TPA on membrane enzyme activities in hamster embryo and C3H/10T½ cells**

Treatment	Na^+/K^+-ATPase	Mg^+-ATPase	5'-Nucleotidase
Hamster embryo			
Control	1.21 ± .21	1.35 ± .17	1.73 ± .28
TPA (0.16 μM)	1.53 ± .43	1.44 ± .45	1.89 ± .31
Retinoid (7.1 μM)	.78 ± .19	1.32 ± .36	1.75 ± .21
Retinoid, TPA	1.13 ± .27	1.19 ± .41	1.91 ± .32
C3H/10T½			
Control	1.79 ± .32	1.26 ± .31	.56 ± .08
TPA (0.16 μM)	2.18 ± .31	1.26 ± .26	.60 ± .12
Retinoid (7.1 μM)	1.13 ± .20	1.32 ± .26	.68 ± .05
Retinoid, TPA	1.73 ± .23	1.23 ± .28	.64 ± .10
Transformed hamster embryo			
Control	2.46 ± .27	1.54 ± .31	5.75 ± 1.21
TPA (0.16 μM)	2.31 ± .21	1.38 ± .21	5.90 ± 1.38
Retinoid (7.1 μM)	2.50 ± .29	1.42 ± .21	5.83 ± 1.10
Retinoid, TPA	2.34 ± .31	1.50 ± .32	5.92 ± 1.23
Transformed C3H/10T½			
Control	.97 ± .09	.87 ± .08	.40 ± .07
TPA (0.16 μM)	1.21 ± .12	1.38 ± .22	.46 ± .06
Retinoid (7.1 μM)	.82 ± .21	8.99 ± .06	.59 ± .02
Retinoid, TPA	1.04 ± .18	1.05 ± .10	.47 ± .16

All values are mean ± standard error in moles Pi/hr/mg protein.
* Modified from Borek et al. 1981b.

Further evidence indicating the inhibitory effect of retinoids on carcinogenesis is shown by their effects on the interaction between ionizing radiation and carcinogenic food pyrolysis products as described below.

RADIATION, TRYPTOPHAN, PYROLYSATE, AND RETINOIDS

While there is a growing awareness that potential carcinogens present in increasing amounts in our environment may interact in a way that is additive or synergistic, little is known about the selectivity and extent of these relationships. Such potentially harmful compounds may be found as chemical principals in our diet in naturally occurring substances (Miller and Miller 1979) or resulting from the processing of food. Several agents of this nature have been identified in Japan as pyrolysis products from charred surfaces of broiled protein foods such as meat and fish (Sugimura et al. 1977). Among them, a tryptophan pyrolysate has been shown to be mutagenic and induce DNA damage and to be carcinogenic both in vivo and in vitro (Sugimura et al. 1977, Takayama et al. 1977, Nagao and Sugimura 1978, Tohada et al. 1980).

Because of our interest in radiation carcinogenesis and the fact that radiation had been a potent cancer-inducing agent in Japan (Rossi and Kellerer 1974), we investigated the interaction between radiation and pyrolysis products on transformation. If they did interact, would retinoids modify this interaction?

We used the HE system described above. The pyrolysate product was D.L. tryptophan pyrolysate, a 3-amino-1-methyl-5H-pyrido (4,3-b) indol (Trp-P-2) (Sugimura et al. 1977) kindly donated by Drs. Sugimura and Sato.

For transformation experiments, cells were treated with 50 or 150 rad of x-rays as described (Borek and Ong 1981), and Trp-P-2 was added 24 hours after irradiation. Cultures that were neither irradiated nor treated with Trp-P-2 served as controls. Cultures that were irradiated but not treated with Trp-P-2 as well as others unirradiated but treated with Trp-P-2 served to evaluate the oncogenic potential of the single agents.

The results presented in Table 4 indicate that Trp-P-2 is a more effective carcinogen than x-rays. The transformation rate following radiation alone was related to the dose absorbed by the cells as previously reported (Borek and Hall 1973).

In the combined treatment experiments in which Trp-P-2 was added to the cells 24 hours after their exposure to x-rays, the transformation frequency was higher than in cultures treated with either radiation or Trp-P-2. The enhancement was related to the radiation absorbed. At 50 rad an additive effect cannot be excluded, but the combined treatment at 150 rad distinctly implies that synergism between the radiation and Trp-P-2 occurred in their oncogenic effects.

We next evaluated whether the retinoid all-trans retinyl acetate (RA) has any effect on the radiation- and pyrolysate-induced transformation. In experiments that will be detailed elsewhere, RA (gift of Dr. Sporn) was added to the cell cultures at 0.2 μg/ml, a concentration that produced little toxicity. The compound was added to the cells at plating time and removed 4 days later. As seen in Table 5 the retinoid suppressed both radiation- and pyrolysate-induced transformation and markedly inhibited the interaction between the two agents.

The inhibitory effect of the retinoids on Trp-P-2–induced transformation was similar when retinyl acetate was added 48 hours after the addition of the chemical, indicating that the inhibitory activity was not mediated by interference with cellular processing of the carcinogens.

TABLE 4. *In vitro cell transformation by x-rays and Trp-P-2*

Treatment	Surviving fraction	Transformation frequency ($\times 10^{-3}$)
Control	1.00	0
50 rad	0.98	0.8 ± 0.28
150 rad	0.88	2.2 ± 0.45
Trp-P-2	0.89	12.4 ± 0.63
50 rad + Trp-P-2	0.92	15.3 ± 0.47
150 rad + Trp-P-2	0.78	42.7 ± 0.67

TABLE 5. *Retinoid (RA) modification of cell transformation by x-rays and Trp-P-2 in hamster embryo cells*

Treatment	Surviving fraction	Transformation frequency ($\times10^{-3}$)
Control	1.00	0
150 rad	0.85	2.8
150 rad, RA	0.79	0.2
Trp-P-2	0.83	12.6
Trp-P-2, RA	0.76	2.6
150 rad, Trp-P-2	0.76	49.8
150 rad, Trp-P-2, RA	0.69	5.3

The problem of cocarcinogenesis is an important one, since daily life subjects us to a complex environment composed of a wide variety of agents. The difficulty lies in identifying the carcinogens that act in an additive or synergistic manner. Once recognized, measures may be sought to alter exposure to these agents or to find ways to modify their effects and interactions.

The potential role in carcinogenesis of food products presents a complex dilemma in terms of assessing the risk to the general public, since epidemiological data have shown that altered patterns of diet modify risks to certain malignancies (Oiso 1975, Weisburger et al. 1977).

The data presented indicate that in vitro a combined treatment of x-rays (50 or 150 rad) and Trp-P-2 (0.5 μg/ml) results in a higher frequency of transformation than that observed following treatment by the single agent, and that the enhancement is linked to the dose of radiation absorbed by the cells. The pyrolysis product seems to act as a potentiation rather than an adjunctive agent in producing oncogenic transformation, since the combined effects of radiation and the chemical are greater than the sum of the individual effects of either. At present we are ignorant of the mechanisms underlying this interaction. Each of these agents can interact with DNA and induce chromosomal changes. Since Trp-P-2 was added to the cells during the "fixation" period of the radiation-induced transformed state (Borek and Sachs 1967), a variety of complex events may be involved.

The fact that broiled meat and fish, which are commonly consumed in Japan (Nagao and Sugimura 1978, Oiso 1975, Sugimura et al. 1977), contain the ingredients that interact with radiation to enhance carcinogenesis further compounds the interpretation of cancer incidence in the Hiroshima and Nagasaki data, the most frequently quoted data base for carcinogenesis in humans. Our findings that retinoids can inhibit this interaction and inhibit radiation- and pyrolysate-induced transformation, alone or in combined treatment, is positive information. Similar to the retinoid action in suppressing radiation transformation and its promotion by TPA, RA exerted its effect within a short period and in an irreversible manner. We do not know whether RA modulates pyrolysate- and radiation-transforming action via genetic mechanisms or via the membrane as found for the other retinoids studied above, but studies are in progress.

We can conclude, however, on the basis of the above experiments that although in vitro systems do not fully represent the in vivo situation they are defined systems. They lend support to the notion that retinoids are effective suppressors of carcinogen-induced neoplastic development and could be used to antagonize both initiators and promotors present in our environment or encountered in the course of therapy.

While the effectiveness of retinoids has been demonstrated, one constantly seeks additional preventive agents that may perform similar functions, perhaps at lower and less toxic doses, or complement the activity of retinoids, perhaps by acting on a different stage in the carcinogenic process.

SELENIUM AS AN INHIBITOR OF ONCOGENESIS IN VITRO

Selenium, a ubiquitous element in nature and one used in industry, can be toxic and carcinogenic. It is, however, a micronutrient required in our diet (for a comprehensive review, see Griffin 1979). Selenium has been shown to exert an anticarcinogenic effect in vivo by inhibiting carcinogen-induced tumors. Yet it is not clear at which stage of neoplastic development Se is effective. To study these aspects and the cellular and molecular mechanisms involved, it is of great advantage to utilize defined systems such as cell cultures.

Recently, we began investigating the effects of selenium on chemical- and radiation-induced transformation. Our preliminary data, shown in Table 6, indicate that when mouse 10T½ cells are preincubated for 24 hours with selenium (0.1 μM, a nontoxic level) and then treated with benzo-(a)-pyrene at 1.2 μg/ml for 48 hours, pyrolysate Trp-P-2, or radiation, a marked inhibition of cell transformation by all agents is observed. Se, which was present throughout

TABLE 6. *The effect of selenium on radiation and chemically induced transformation in vitro*

Treatment	Transformed foci/ surviving cells	Transformation frequency
Control	0/14750	0
Selenium pretreatment*	0/7050	0
Pyrolysate†	19/27500	6.91×10^{-4}
Pyrolysate + selenium	4/11000	3.63×10^{-4}
Benzo-a-pyrene‡	25/23200	1.08×10^{-3}
Benzo-a-pyrene + selenium	6/27000	2.22×10^{-4}
400 rad	14/12000	1.16×10^{-3}
400 rad + selenium	7/11400	6.14×10^{-4}

* Na_2SeO_3 conc. = 0.25 mM.
† Trp-P-2 conc. = 0.5 μg/ml.
‡ Benzo-a-pyrene conc. = 1.2 μg/ml.

the experiment, may interfere with metabolic activation of the chemical carcinogens and thus elicit its inhibitory action. Yet the data on radiation indicates that there may be other mechanisms involved in the inhibitory process, for no activation process is involved in radiation-induced carcinogenesis. Thus, though extensive additional experimentation is required, the results shown here are promising. Perhaps Se, when added at particular concentrations and at specific times, might serve as a useful chemopreventive agent. Its effectiveness may complement the activity of retinoids, both acting to inhibit neoplastic development at the expression phase, but at different stages. We may still find out that Se activity is also effective at the initiating stage, which would make it a powerful chemopreventive agent. Studies are now in progress.

ACKNOWLEDGMENTS

This investigation was supported by Contract DE-AC02–78EV04733 from the Department of Energy and by Grant No. CA 12536–10 to the Radiological Research Laboratory/Department of Radiology, and by Grant No. CA 13696 to the Cancer Center/Institute of Cancer Research, awarded by the National Cancer Institute, Department of Health and Human Services.

REFERENCES

Berenblum, I. 1975. Sequential aspects of chemical carcinogenesis: Skin, *in* Cancer, A Comprehensive Treatise, Vol. 1, Etiology: Chemical and Physical Carcinogenesis, F. F. Becker, ed. Plenum Press, New York, pp. 323–344.

Borek, C. 1979. Malignant transformation in vitro: Criteria, biological markers, and application in environmental screening of carcinogen. Radiat. Res. 79:209–232.

Borek, C. 1981a. Differentiation, metabolic activation and malignant transformation in cultured liver cells exposed to chemical carcinogens, *in* Advances in Modern Environmental Toxicology, Vol. 1, Mammalian Cell Transformation by Chemical Carcinogens, N. Mishra, V. Dunkle, and M. Mehlman, eds. Senate Press, Inc., Princeton, New Jersey, pp. 297–318.

Borek, C. 1981b. X-ray induced in vitro neoplastic transformation of human diploid cells. Nature 283:776–778.

Borek, C. 1982. Radiation oncogenesis in culture. Adv. Cancer Res. (in press).

Borek, C., and C. Cleaver. 1981. Protease inhibitors neither damage nor interfere with DNA repair in human cells. Mutat. Res. 82:373–380.

Borek, C., and E. J. Hall, 1973. Transformation of mammalian cells in vitro by low doses of x-rays. Nature 243:450–453.

Borek, C., and E. J. Hall. 1974. Effect of split doses of x-rays on neoplastic transformation of single cells. Nature 252:499–501.

Borek, C., E. J. Hall, and H. H. Rossi. 1978. Malignant transformation in cultured hamster embryo cells produced by x-rays, 430-keV mono-energetic neutrons, and heavy ions. Cancer Res. 38:2997–3005.

Borek, C., R. C. Miller, C. R. Geard, D. L. Guernsey, R. S. Osmak, M. Rutledge-Freeman, A. Ong, and H. Mason. 1981a. The modulating effect of retinoids and a tumor promotor on malignant transformation, sister chromatid exchanges and Na/K ATPase. Ann. N.Y. Acad. Sci. 359:237–250.

Borek, C., R. C. Miller, C. R. Geard, D. L. Guernsey, and J. M. Smith. 1981b. In vitro modulation of oncogenesis and differentiation by retinoids and tumor promoters, *in* Carcinogenesis and Biological Effects of Tumor Promoters, E. Hecker, W. Kunz, F. Marks, N. E. Fusenig, and H. W. Thielmann, eds. Raven Press, New York (in press).

Borek, C., R. C. Miller, C. Pain, and W. Troll. 1979. Conditions for inhibiting and enhancing effects of the protease inhibitor antipain on x-ray induced neoplastic transformation in hamster and mouse cells. Proc. Natl. Acad. Sci. USA 76:1800–1803.

Borek, C., and A. Ong. 1981. The interaction of ionizing radiation and food pyrolysis products in producing oncogenic transformation in vitro. Cancer Lett. (in press).

Borek, C., and L. Sachs. 1966. In vitro cell transformation by x-irradiation. Nature 210:276–278.

Borek, C., and L. Sachs. 1967. Cell susceptibility to transformation by x-irradiation and fixation of the transformed state. Proc. Natl. Acad. Sci. USA 57:1522–1527.

Borek, C., and L. Sachs. 1968. The number of cell generations required to fix the transformed state in x-ray induced transformation. Proc. Natl. Acad. Sci. USA 59:83–85.

Borek, C., and J. E. Smith. 1978. Tumor promotor inhibits production of liver retinol binding protein. J. Cell. Biol. 79:78a.

Brown, P. 1936. American Martyrs to Science Through the Roentgen Ray. Charles C Thomas, Springfield, Illinois.

DeLuca, L., N. Maestri, F. Bonanni, and D. Nelson. 1972. Maintenance of epithelial cell differentiation: The mode of action of vitamin A. Cancer 30:1326–1331.

Griffin, A. C. 1979. Role of selenium in chemoprevention of cancer. Adv. Cancer Res. 34:419–442.

Guernsey, D. L., A. Ong, and C. Borek. 1980. Thyroid hormone modulation of x-ray-induced in vitro neoplastic transformation. Nature 288:591–592.

Harisiadis, L., R. C. Miller, E. J. Hall, and C. Borek. 1978. A vitamin A analog inhibits radiation induced oncogenic transformation. Nature (London) 274:486–487.

Hecker, E. 1971. Isolation and characterization of cocarcinogenic principles from croton oil. Methods in Cancer Research 6:439–489.

Kakunaga, T. 1978. Neoplastic transformation of human diploid fibroblast cells by chemical carcinogens. Proc. Natl. Acad. Sci. USA 75:1334–1338.

Lotan, R. 1980. Effects of vitamin A and its analogs (retinoids) on normal and neoplastic cells. Biochim. Biophys. Acta 605:33–91.

Miller, E. C., and J. A. Miller. 1979. Naturally occurring chemical carcinogens that may be present in foods. International Review of Biochemistry, Biochemistry of Nutrition 27:123–165.

Miller, R. C., C. R. Geard, R. S. Osmak, M. Rutledge-Freeman, A. Ong, H. Mason, A. Napholtz, N. Perez, L. Harisiadis, and C. Borek. 1981. Modification of sister chromatid exchanges and radiation-induced transformation in rodent cells by the tumor promoter 12-0-tetradecanoylphorbol-13-acetate and two retinoids. Cancer Res. 41:655–659.

Milo, G. E., Jr., and J. A. DiPaolo. 1978. Neoplastic transformation of human diploid cells in vitro after chemical carcinogen treatment. Nature 275:130–132.

Nagao, M., and T. Sugimura. 1978. Environmental mutagens and carcinogens. Ann. Rev. Genet. 12:117–159.

Nutrition in the causation of cancer: Proceedings of a symposium. 1975. Cancer Res. 35:3231–3550.

Occupational carcinogenesis. 1976. Ann. N.Y. Acad. Sci. 271:1–516.

Oiso, T. 1975. Incidence of stomach cancer and its relation to dietary habits and nutrition in Japan between 1900 and 1975. Cancer Res. 35:3254–3258.

Perry, P., and H. J. Evans. 1975. Cytological detection of mutagen-carcinogen exposure by sister chromatid exchanges. Nature (London) 258:121–125.

Pott, P. 1775. Cancer Scroti, *in* Chirurgical Observations. Howes, Clark, and Collins, London, pp. 65–68.

Reznikoff, C. A., J. S. Bertram, D. W. Brankow, and C. Heidelberger. 1973. Quantitative and qualitative studies of chemical transformation of cloned C3H mouse embryo cells sensitive to postconfluence inhibition of cell division. Cancer Res. 33:3239–3249.

Rossi, H. H., and A. M. Kellerer. 1974. The validity of risk estimates of leukemia incidence based on Japanese data. Radiat. Res. 58:131–140.

Shilo, B., and R. A. Weinberg. 1981. Unique transforming gene in carcinogen transformed mouse cells. Nature 289:607–609.

Sporn, M. B., N. M. Dunlop, D. L. Newton, and J. M. Smith. 1976. Prevention of chemical carcinogenesis by vitamin A and its synthetic analogs (retinoids). Fed. Proc. 35:1332–1338.

Sugimura, T., M. Nagao, T. Kawachi, M. Honda, T. Yahagi, Y. Seino, S. Sato, and N. Matsukura. 1977. Mutagen-carcinogens in food, with special reference to highly mutagenic pyrolytic products in broiled foods, *in* Origins of Human Cancer, H. H. Hiatt, J. D. Watson, and J. Winsten, eds. Cold Spring Harbor Laboratory, Cold Spring Harbor, New York.

Takayama, S., Y. Katoh, M. Tanaka, M. Nagao, K. Wakabayashi, and T. Sugimura. 1977. In vitro transformation of hamster embryo cells with tryptophan pyrolysis products. Proceedings of the Japan Academy 53:126–129.

Terzaghi, M., and J. B. Little. 1976. X-radiation-induced transformation in a C3H mouse embryo-derived cell line. Cancer Res. 36:1367–1374.

Tohada, H., A. Oikawa, T. Kawachi, and T. Sugimura. 1980. Induction of sister chromatid exchanges by mutagens from amino acids and protein pyrolysates. Mutat. Res. 71:65–69.

Weisburger, J. H., L. A. Cohen, and E. L. Wynder. 1977. On the etiology and metabolic epidemiology of the main human cancers, *in* Origins of Human Cancer, H. H. Hiatt, J. D. Watson, and J. Winsten, eds. Cold Spring Harbor Laboratory, Cold Spring Harbor, New York, pp. 567–602.

Molecular Interrelations of Nutrition and Cancer,
edited by M. S. Arnott, J. van Eys, and Y.-M. Wang.
Raven Press, New York © 1982.

Inhibition of Transformation and Oncogenic Progression by Ascorbic Acid: A Possible Role in Chemoprevention

William F. Benedict and Peter A. Jones

Division of Hematology-Oncology, Department of Medicine, Childrens Hospital of Los Angeles [*W.F.B., P.A.J.*], *and Departments of Pediatrics* [*W.F.B., P.A.J.*] *and Biochemistry* [*P.A.J.*], *University of Southern California School of Medicine, Los Angeles, California 90054*

Chemoprevention, the use of nontoxic agents to block, arrest, or reverse the development of neoplasia, is becoming a major new field of cancer research. Substances are being sought that can block the initiation of a cell by a carcinogen, prevent the formation of a tumor subsequent to cell initiation, or help elucidate those events that are important in the progression of an initiated cell to a tumorigenic stage. Such agents have included retinoids, antioxidants, phosphodiesterase inhibitors, and protease inhibitors.

It is our belief that ascorbic acid may be able to play an important role in chemoprevention as well as in isolating events necessary for oncogenic progression. Until the report from our laboratory (Benedict et al. 1980b), ascorbic acid had been considered to be of possible chemopreventive use mainly as a chemical to block cell initiation (See Cameron et al. 1979 for review). This later role included its antiviral activity and its ability to block the formation of nitrosamines from nitrite or nitrous acid, which are in turn carcinogenic.

Our observation that ascorbic acid at the noncytotoxic concentration of 1 μg/ml could completely inhibit transformation of mouse C3H/10T½ cells induced by 3-methylcholanthrene (MCA) when added daily as late as 3 weeks after a 24-hour exposure to MCA (Benedict et al. 1980b) was the first indication that ascorbate could also function at a level beyond the initiation step (Figure 1). In addition, transformation was completely inhibited if ascorbate was added the day after exposure to MCA and continued for only the first 23 days, the cultures being maintained and stained on day 42 (Figure 1). This latter finding suggested that the inhibition might be quite stable, unlike that of retinoids (Merriman and Bertram 1979), phosphodiesterase inhibitors (Bertram 1979), and protease inhibitors (Kuroki and Drevon 1979), which also inhibit chemically induced transformation in C3H/10T½ cells. These other agents inhibit only in a reversible manner, since the transformed cells appear or reappear once these agents are removed.

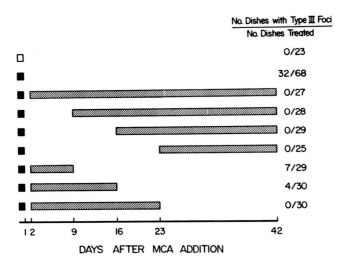

FIG. 1. Inhibition of MCA-initiated cells by ascorbic acid. Following a 24-hr exposure to 5 μg/ml of MCA (■) or acetone (□), ascorbic acid (1 μg/ml) was added daily for different periods of time (▨). The dish contents were then stained 6 weeks after the experiment was begun and scored for the presence of type III morphologically transformed foci. (Reproduced from Benedict et al. 1980b, with permission of *Cancer Research.*)

To extend our initial observations, we passaged cells from several dishes that contained a single MCA-induced morphologically transformed focus (Figure 2). Ascorbic acid (1 μg/ml) was then added daily to half the cultures. The transformed cells returned to a normal morphological pattern in approximately 75% of the first-passage cultures (Benedict et al. 1980b). Thus, ascorbic acid was able not only to completely inhibit MCA-induced transformation but also to revert certain morphologically transformed cells back to a normal morphological phenotype.

This reversion back to a normal morphology was often irreversible, since the ascorbic acid could be removed from these cells after exposure for four passages without any transformed foci reappearing (Figure 3). We have subsequently observed that the ascorbic acid needs to be present for only one or two passages to prevent the reappearance of transformed foci (see Figure 4).

In contrast, if the mass cultures containing the same transformed cells were passaged in the absence of ascorbate for four subcultures and then were treated daily with ascorbic acid, they no longer reverted to a normal morphological pattern (Figure 3). Thus, after a certain number of cell divisions, morphologically transformed cells cannot be reverted to a normal growth pattern by ascorbic acid.

Although the morphology of cells from most of the transformed foci returned to normal when subcultured at passage 1 in the presence of ascorbic acid, the transformed cells from some foci were totally unaffected by the ascorbate (Figure 2). Thus, it was possible that there were important phenotypic differences between

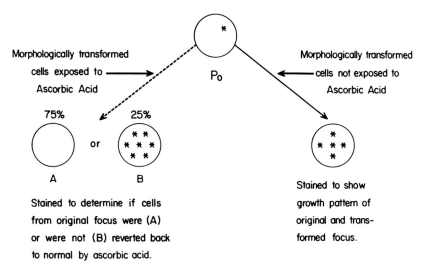

Morphologically transformed cells exposed to Ascorbic Acid

P_0

Morphologically transformed cells not exposed to Ascorbic Acid

75%   25%

or

A   B

Stained to determine if cells from original focus were (A) or were not (B) reverted back to normal by ascorbic acid.

Stained to show growth pattern of original and transformed focus.

FIG. 2. General scheme for determining if ascorbic acid reverts cells from a given morphologically transformed focus back to a normal growth pattern. Various cultures, each containing an independently derived type III focus, were subcultured into four dishes. One-half of the dishes received ascorbate daily at the noncytotoxic concentration of 1 μg/ml; the other half did not. One dish each was then fixed and stained at approximately 1 month after subculture. Numerous transformed foci were observed in cultures not treated with ascorbate. However, in approximately 75% of the dishes that received ascorbate, the morphologically transformed cells observed in P_0 returned to a normal pattern in the first subculture (A). A reversion back to a normal morphology was not seen in the remaining dishes treated with ascorbate (B). The complete protocol and results have been published elsewhere (Benedict et al. 1980b). Additional cultures that never received ascorbic acid were maintained. Cells from these cultures were later tested for their ability to form colonies in agarose and tumors in nude mice (Benedict et al., in press).

cells from type III morphologically transformed foci that initially responded to ascorbate and those that did not. We have recently found, in fact, that significant differences do exist between such transformed cells.

Our approach was first to isolate several transformed cell lines that either reverted back to a normal morphological pattern in the presence of ascorbic acid or did not. These cell lines then were tested at various passages for their ability to form colonies in agarose or to produce tumors in athymic (nude) mice. No cells tested for these properties had ever been exposed to ascorbic acid, since additional cells that never had received ascorbate were maintained at each passage.

All of the transformed cell lines initially unresponsive to ascorbic acid formed colonies in agarose (a measurement of the loss of anchorage-dependent growth) and produced tumors in nude mice during early passages. In contrast, the cell lines that initially responded to ascorbic acid did not form colonies in agarose nor were they tumorigenic at early passages (Benedict et al., in press). Subsequently, these latter cell lines developed the ability to form colonies in agarose,

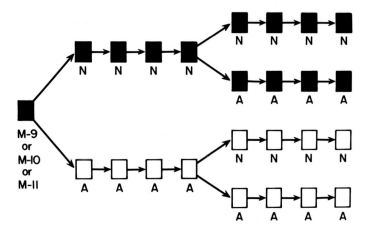

FIG. 3. Irreversible suppression of the transformed phenotype by ascorbic acid. Three separate cultures containing type III foci (M-9 through M-11) were subcultured as shown in Fig. 2. One-half of the dishes received ascorbate (A) and one-half did not (N). Contents of representative dishes were then stained and scored for the presence (■) or absence (□) of type III foci. All cultures treated with ascorbate contained no transformed foci (M-9-A through M-11-A), whereas all parallel cultures not exposed to ascorbic acid contained numerous foci (M-9-N through M-11-N). The cells from the remaining dishes that did not initially receive ascorbate were passaged an additional three times without ascorbate, and cells from the ascorbate-treated dishes were subcultured three more times in the presence of ascorbate. Subsequently, at passage 5, one-half of the cultures not previously exposed to ascorbate were treated with ascorbic acid, whereas ascorbate was removed from one-half of the cultures that had received ascorbic acid continuously from the first subculture. At each passage, dishes were stained and scored for the presence or absence of type III foci. (Reproduced from Benedict et al. 1980b, with permission of *Cancer Research*).

but only two of the eight cell lines initially tested became tumorigenic at any passage examined (Benedict et al., in press).

The above findings are important for two reasons. First, they imply that ascorbate may be able to revert the morphology of transformed cells only during an early stage in their progression to cells capable of producing tumors. Secondly, ascorbic acid can be utilized to isolate morphologically transformed cell variants at different stages during this progression. This will allow us to study in depth factors involved in the loss of anchorage dependency and the development of a tumorigenic phenotype.

It will be important also to determine whether ascorbic acid can prevent tumor formation following exposure to a carcinogen. In a recent preliminary report (Kallistratos and Fasske 1980), ascorbic acid was shown to suppress tumor formation in Wistar rats when it was added to their drinking water at the same time they were given a subcutaneous injection of the carcinogen benzo[a]pyrene (BP). We are presently repeating these studies using a larger number of animals and extending such experiments to include conditions in which ascorbate treatment is delayed for several days following the injection of BP. These studies will determine if the neoplastic process can be influenced in vivo by

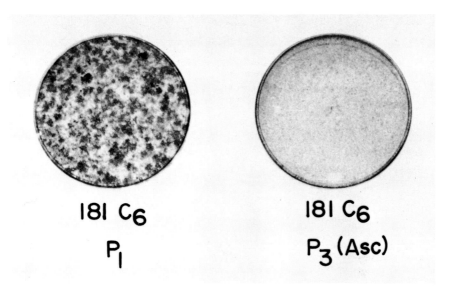

$181 \ C_6$
P_1

$181 \ C_6$
P_3 (Asc)

FIG. 4. Reversion of the transformed morphology to a normal growth pattern by ascorbic acid. A representative culture containing a type III focus was passaged in the absence of ascorbic acid (181 C_6P_1). Numerous transformed foci were distributed throughout each dish; they represented an expansion of the transformed cells present in the original focus. In contrast, when transformed cells from the same original focus were subcultured and ascorbic acid (1 $\mu g/ml$) was added daily thereafter, the transformed cells reverted to a normal morphology. The dish shown on the right (181 $C_6 \ P_3$) is a culture treated for two passages with ascorbic acid and from which ascorbate was removed in passage 3. No reappearance of the transformed foci was observed.

ascorbic acid subsequent to the initiation of cells by a carcinogen. They parallel our experiments in vitro.

Our initial findings need to be extended to other chemical carcinogens that are either direct acting or, like MCA, require further activation to their ultimate carcinogenic form. In addition, physical agents such as X-irradiation should be examined to determine if ascorbic acid can inhibit morphological transformation. Moreover, other transformation assays including the hamster embryo (Pienta et al. 1977, Benedict et al. 1980a) and mouse 3T3 models (Kakunaga 1973, Benedict et al. 1980a), as well as epithelial cell systems, need to be studied. The results from the above experiments will enable us to determine if our observation in 10T½ cells (Benedict et al. 1980b) can be generalized.

Finally, it has recently been suggested that combination chemoprevention might be as useful an approach to prevent cancer as combination chemotherapy is now to treat cancer (Sporn 1980). Since ascorbic acid already appears to inhibit transformation and revert transformed cells to a normal morphology by a different mechanism than retinoids, protease inhibitors, or phosphodiesterase inhibitors, it is logical to hypothesize that ascorbic acid could act additively or even synergistically as a chemopreventive agent with these other agents. We hope that the testing of this hypothesis together with the extension of our initial observations as described above will lead to new approaches for optimizing the use of ascorbic acid as a chemopreventive agent in man.

REFERENCES

Benedict, W. F., I. Chouroulinkov, P. B. Fisher, T. Kakunaga, H. Marquardt, R. J. Pienta, and H. Yamasaki. 1980a. Transformation in cell culture, *in* Long-Term and Short-Term Screening Assays for Carcinogens: A Critical Appraisal, IARC Monograph (Supplement 2). IARC, Lyons, France, pp. 185–199.

Benedict, W. F., W. L. Wheatley, and P. A. Jones. 1980b. Inhibition of chemically induced morphological transformation and reversion of the transformed phenotype by ascorbic acid in C3H/10T½ cells. Cancer Res. 40:2796–2801.

Benedict, W. F., W. L. Wheatley, and P. A. Jones. 1981. Differences in anchorage dependent growth and tumorigenicities between transformed C3H/10T½ cells whose morphologies are or are not reverted to a normal phenotype by ascorbic acid. Cancer Res. (in press).

Bertram, J. S. 1979. Modulation of cellular interaction between C3H/10T½ cells and their transformed counterparts by phosphodiesterase inhibitors. Cancer Res. 39:3502–3508.

Cameron, E., L. Pauling, and B. Leibowitz. 1979. Ascorbic acid and cancer: A review. Cancer Res. 39:663–681.

Kakunaga, T. 1973. A quantitative system for assay of malignant transformation by chemical carcinogens using a clone derived from BALB/3T3. Int. J. Cancer 12:463–473.

Kallistratos, G., and E. Fasske. 1980. Inhibition of benzo(a)pyrene carcinogenesis in rats with vitamin C. J. Cancer Res. Clin. Oncol. 97:91–96.

Kuroki, T., and C. Drevon. 1979. Inhibition of chemical transformation in C3H/10T½ cells by protease inhibitors. Cancer Res. 39:2755–2761.

Merriman, R. L., and J. S. Bertram. 1979. Reversible inhibition by retinoids of 3-methylcholanthrene-induced neoplastic transformation in C3H/10T½ clone 8 cells. Cancer Res. 39:1661–1666.

Pienta, R. J., J. A. Poiley, and W. B. Lebherz. 1977. Morphological transformation of early passage golden Syrian hamster embryo cells derived from cryopreserved primary cultures as reliable in vitro bioassay for identifying diverse carcinogens. Int. J. Cancer 19:642–655.

Sporn, M. 1980. Combination chemoprevention of cancer. Nature 287:197–208.

Nutrient Requirements and Modulation of Carcinogenesis

Molecular Interrelations of Nutrition and Cancer,
edited by M. S. Arnott, J. van Eys, and Y.-M. Wang.
Raven Press, New York © 1982.

Nutritional Modulation of Carcinogenesis

T. Colin Campbell

Nutrition and Cancer Program Project, Division of Nutritional Sciences, Cornell University, Ithaca, New York 14853

In recent years, an extremely impressive array of nutritional effects on the carcinogenic process have been reported. A rather casual scanning of the literature suggests that most nutrients have been examined in one or more experimental models; this symposium monograph itself has considered the effects of carbohydrates, lipids, vitamin A, vitamin C, vitamin E, zinc, and selenium. These results, coupled with the proliferation of epidemiological findings, have given rise to claims that upwards of 70% of all human cancer might be controlled through the appropriate use of diet (Doll and Peto 1981).

If all of these findings were significant for human health, the consumer would be totally perplexed and overwhelmed. Very likely he would accept nothing more from the scientific community and turn instead to the faith healer. As a matter of fact, I think that is precisely what accounts for the 1000% growth in the multibillion dollar health food business in the last 6 years (LeBovit 1977). Bits of scientific information on nutrient effects are balooned into sizable commercial ventures that owe their success to the careful nurturing of the public's fear of a disease such as cancer.

I make these rather off-handed comments because of my belief that the researchers of the diet-nutrition-cancer interrelations walk a very narrow path in the development of new information. On the one hand, our research community rather unfortunately demands rapid publication of new information; on the other, the public thirsts for new information on cancer because it dreads this disease and perceives that nutrition supposedly can do much for one's well being. Given the enormous complexities and apparent conflict of these new data, are any common themes emerging? If a few such themes could be constructed, not only might we gain some insight into the kind of research most needed but also we might find a few generalities to pass on to the public. The remainder of this chapter, then, will be a presentation of a few selected sets of data on the dietary protein effect on chemical carcinogenesis as these data illustrate, first, the difficulties of interpretation of experimental nutritional effects and, second, the generalities that might be drawn about nutrition effects.

Several years ago, we were impressed by the reports of Madhavan and Gopalan (1968) showing that when rats were fed less protein, the yield of liver tumors induced by aflatoxin B_1 (AFB$_1$) was greatly depressed. Although at that time AFB$_1$ was known to be metabolized to less-toxic metabolites (DeIongh et al. 1964, Butler and Clifford 1965), it was not clear how a lower protein intake could affect tumorigenicity through modification of metabolism. Previous work (Rouiller 1964) had indicated, for example, that the clearance of drugs was decreased with low protein diets. After AFB$_1$ was shown to be metabolized by the hepatic microsomal mixed-function oxidase (MFO) system (Portman et al. 1968) and after it was confirmed that the feeding of low-protein diets was associated with lower MFO enzyme activities (Mgbodile and Campbell 1972), a lower rate of AFB$_1$ clearance was indicated. However, it was not clear how a lower rate of AFB$_1$ clearance could be related to fewer tumors.

Subsequent work in the laboratory of the Millers (Garner et al. 1972, Swenson et al. 1973), however, suggested that AFB$_1$ underwent metabolic activation to a highly reactive, presumably electrophilic product that was capable of forming covalent adducts with macromolecules such as DNA, RNA, and protein. The putative reactive metabolite was suggested to be the 2,3-epoxide. That finding supported the Millers' electrophilic theory of chemical carcinogenesis (Miller 1970) and suggested that the amount of metabolic activation of AFB$_1$ by the MFO system should be a reasonably good indicator of its tumorigenicity. Thus, we then hypothesized that the lower protein diet might lower the in vivo formation of macromolecular adducts (Preston et al. 1976), that with DNA being the more important insofar as the somatic mutation theory of cancer is concerned. These results are shown in Table 1. This effect appeared quite impressive, considering the fact that the animals were fed the 5% casein diet for only 1–2 weeks, suggesting the possibility that a reduction in AF-DNA adduct formation could be responsible for the lower AFB$_1$ tumorigenicity.

We also examined varying levels of dietary casein, ranging from 5% to 40% casein, as well as varying periods of time following the initiation of feeding. The titration of DNA adduct formation with dietary protein intake (Figure 1)

TABLE 1. *Effect of protein deficiency on the binding of aflatoxin to nuclear macromolecules*

	Group 1	Group 2	Group 3
Dietary casein (%)	5	20	20
pmoles AF bound to chromatin per mg DNA	81.7 ± 16.0^a	187 ± 8^a	259 ± 36^b
pmoles AF bound to DNA per mg DNA	56.4 ± 9.6^a	141 ± 14^b	202 ± 21^c
pmoles AF bound to protein per mg protein	11.9 ± 3.2^a	$21.8 \pm 8.3^{a,b}$	35.2 ± 21^b

Data represent 3–5 rats per group, with standard errors. Statistical significance between dietary treatments indicated by lettered superscripts; data that are not significantly different at the 5% level of probability show the same letter (Preston et al. 1976).

Group 2 animals were pair-fed, to group 1, whereas group 3 animals were fed *ad libitum*.

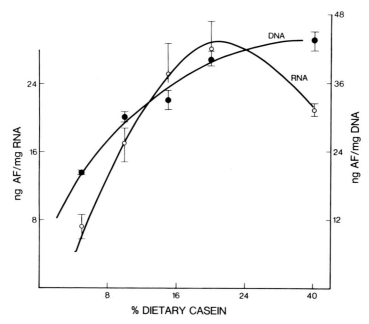

FIG. 1. Weanling rats fed semipurified diets containing various levels of casein for 15 days and then injected i.p. with [³H] AFB₁ (1 mg/kg). Ten hours after injection, animals were sacrificed and DNA and RNA were isolated and counted to determine the covalently bound AFB₁ metabolite. Animals were fed *ad libitum;* total food intakes of protein between 10% and 40% of diet (by weight) were not significantly different (Smolin and Campbell, unpublished observation).

showed that more modest changes in dietary protein level could also elicit a response (L. Smolin and T. C. Campbell, unpublished observation). The time required for an alteration in the level of AF-DNA adducts following the feeding of a low-protein diet (Figure 2) appeared somewhat delayed compared with the time required for the alteration of MFO activity (M. Maso, M. P. Goetchius, and T. C. Campbell, unpublished observation) (Figure 3). Thus, we were led to the notion that adduct formation was not necessarily dependent on the rate of activation by the MFO system and began to question the role of MFO activity as a primary rate limitation in the formation of AF-DNA adducts.

Evidence with phenobarbitone treatment also did not support a consistently close relationship between MFO activity and adduct formation, since in vitro MFO activity was increased but in vivo AF-DNA adduct formation was decreased (Garner 1975). One consideration was that there were other associative reactions possibly playing a significant role. For example, uridine diphosphoglucuronic acid transferase, which presumably catalyzes the formation of AF-glucuronide conjugates (Mabee and Chipley 1973) was increased by low-protein diets (Woodcock and Wood 1971). Also, kinetic evidence for epoxide hydrase, if its involvement in the degradation of the aflatoxin epoxide can be assumed, sug-

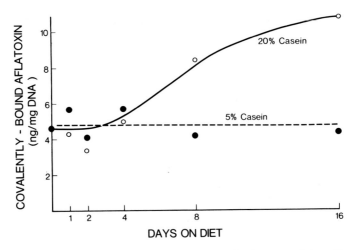

FIG. 2. Weanling Spraque-Dawley rats were fed isocaloric diets containing either 20% or 5% casein. Animals were injected i.p. with [³H]AFB₁ (1.0 mg/kg) in 0.06 ml dimethyl formamide and sacrificed 10 hours later (M. Maso, M. Goetchius, and T. C. Campbell, unpublished observation).

gested that this enzyme could influence the availability of the epoxide *but only at certain concentrations* of AFB₁ (Adekunle et al. 1977). That is, the relative activities of the MFO and epoxide hydrase enzymes could be theoretically reversed with different substrate concentrations as a result of a Km effect. These

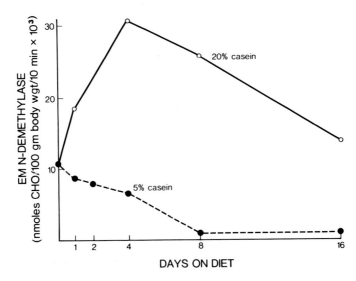

FIG. 3. Weanling Spraque-Dawley rats were fed isocaloric diets containing either 20% or 5% casein. Hepatic microsomal ethylmorphine N-demethylase activities were measured (M. Maso, M. Goetchius, and T. C. Campbell, unpublished observation).

data also suggested that in vitro enzyme activities have little or no meaning relative to physiological substrate concentrations.

Another factor confounding interpretation of in vitro enzyme activities, as they may relate to adduct formation, is the knowledge that the MFO "activity" is composed of multiple hemoproteins, each of which appears to have differing levels of activity for AFB_1 metabolism (Guengerich 1977). Moreover, unpublished data in our laboratory shows that the mixture of hemoproteins may be influenced by dietary protein level (J. Rapp, M. Root, and T. C. Campbell, unpublished observation). At this point we must conclude that estimation of AFB_1 activation and detoxification reaction rates with in vitro microsomal preparations cannot reliably predict in vivo formation of macromolecular adducts. Therefore, the more appropriate procedure to be used for AFB_1 activation appears to be the measurement of in vivo adducts (Figures 1 and 2).

One of the presumed major routes of detoxification for AFB_1 was suggested to be the formation of sulfur conjugates, particularly the mercapturic acids (Degan and Neumann 1978). Moreover, Mgbodile et al. (1975) had shown that the administration of diethyl maleate, which sequesters glutathione, could influence AFB_1-induced hepatotoxicity. Thus, we examined the effect of low-protein diets on hepatic glutathione levels and, quite surprisingly, found higher levels with the lower protein diet (Allen-Hoffmann and Campbell 1977). Thus, it was reasoned that the animal fed the low-protein diet had an additional advantage of being able to decrease the likelihood of adduct formation through the alternate formation of more glutathione conjugates. This presumably reasonable thought quickly vanished when we then found that the increased level of hepatic glutathione in the animals fed the low-protein diets was due to the supplementation of our casein-containing diets with an excess of the limiting amino acid, methionine (Mainigi and Campbell 1981). When methionine/casein ratios remained the same (with methionine being no higher than 1.5% of the casein), the total glutathione was lower on the low-protein diet, as expected.

Recently, however, we obtained data that question the relative importance of hepatic glutathione levels in the formation of in vivo covalent AF-macromolecular adducts (M. P. Goetchius, B. S. Appleton and T. C. Campbell, unpublished observation). AFB_1 was administered at doses ranging over five orders of magnitude (10 ng/kg body weight to 5.0 mg/kg body weight) and hepatic AF-DNA adducts were measured. Interestingly, the dose-response relationship was linear down to these very low doses of AFB_1. When diethyl maleate was administered, it was found to influence the amount of adduct formation only slightly and then primarily at the higher doses, which are those conventionally reported in the literature. We are currently left with the impression, therefore, that mercapturic acid formation with AFB_1 is neither significant at low AFB_1 doses nor significantly involved in the dietary protein effect on adduct formation.

During the time we concentrated much of our effort on AFB_1 metabolism and tumorigenicity as related to in vivo adduct formation, many other laboratories pursued similar studies with other carcinogens in order to evaluate similar relationships of in vivo adduct formation with carcinogenic potential. These studies have, in general, exhibited an impressive positive correlation (recently reviewed by Lutz 1979). We, too, have been encouraged to continue to dissect the metabolic mechanisms responsible for adduct formation with AFB$_1$. However, after having raised more questions than answers concerning the identity of the intracellular mechanism responsible for adduct formation, we are presently considering the possibility that the mechanism most responsible for distinguishing the difference between the high- and low-protein diets may not be as dependent on enzymatic reactions as it is on the initial capability of the cell to accumulate AFB$_1$.

Several years ago, for example, we found that a striking difference between the relatively resistant mouse and the more susceptible rat appeared to be primarily due to the transport of AFB$_1$ into the liver cell (Portman and Campbell 1970). Moreover, in numerous other studies employing risk factors such as dietary protein level, administration of phenobarbital, differing sex, and differing rat strain, the amount of AF-DNA adducts appears to exhibit a first-order relationship with the amount of aflatoxin present in the tissue. That is, after the administration of a radiolabeled dose of AFB$_1$, the amount of radioactivity present in the tissue homogenate closely correlates with the amount of macromolecular adducts. Not all of the homogenate radioactivity is the AFB$_1$ substrate, of course, although at a constant time after dosing the proportion of radioactivity represented by AFB$_1$ is approximately the same.

To investigate this in somewhat greater detail, the in vitro kinetics of AF-DNA adduct formation was examined (unpublished data from this laboratory). In the presence of constant enzyme activity and a constant amount of DNA, increasing the AFB$_1$ concentration to 250 μM resulted in a linear increase in the formation of AF-DNA adducts, indicating that neither the enzyme activity nor the availability of DNA receptor sites was limiting. Moreover, a concentration of 250 μM AFB$_1$ in vitro is far in excess of the amount expected to be present within the liver cell after a dose below 5 mg/kg. Thus, we currently believe that the differing capabilities for AF-DNA adduct formation with a variety of risk factors may be largely the result of the capacity of the cell to transport the AFB$_1$ across its membrane in the first place. This is somewhat of an oversimplification in that competing events for AFB$_1$ disposition may differ between risk factors, but these appear to be of considerably less quantitative importance.

Like many other investigators working with other carcinogens and other experimental models, we have emphasized the measurement of in vivo adducts because of the apparent correlation with carcinogenic potency, although we have been aware that there appear to be important exceptions. Moreover, total DNA adducts obviously include varying amounts of different base adducts, and certain base adducts will undoubtedly prove to be more relevant for the initiation event. Wogan and his group, for example, have identified several base adducts and have shown that their retention over time differs for individual adducts (Croy and Wogan 1981). Investigations on N-methyl-N-nitrosourea adducts have suggested, for example, that the O^6 adduct of guanine may be more indicative of carcinogenicity than is the N^7 adduct of guanine (Margison and Kleihues 1975). Both adducts are observed with AFB_1 (Croy and Wogan 1981).

Even though information should be continually sought on the mechanisms responsible for the formation and identification of the most relevant adducts, we must pause and ask ourselves what the relative importance is for such an adduct in distinguishing the manner in which risk factors are expressed. Measurement of the specific adduct may prove to be a good estimate of risk or carcinogenic potency of carcinogenic initiators that act through this mechanism. However, modification of the amounts of adducts by secondary modifiers, such as the various nutrients, may not prove to be nearly as relevant to the question simply because this is not the only mechanism through which modifiers may act. For example, nutrient effects on initiation may be less important than nutrient effects on the subsequent growth, development, and expression of the initiated cell. With respect to dietary protein level and AFB_1 hepatocarcinogenesis, we have just turned our attention to this latter question. Male weanling rats were administered 10 doses of AFB_1 over a 2-week period during which they were all fed the 20% casein diet. Afer a further week on the same diet without AFB_1, the group was subdivided, with half receiving the 5% casein diet and the other half continuing on the 20% casein diet. After receiving their diets for 12 weeks, they were killed and their livers examined for evidence of gamma glutamyl transferase foci (Kalengayi and Desmet 1978), which is a good indicator of early hepatocarcinogenesis. There is a striking difference in number of foci formed on these two levels of dietary protein when fed *after* the administration of AFB_1 is completed. Presumably, the difference involves dietary protein as a promotor or positive modifier of the carcinogenic process. This difference appears as great as that for adduct formation, leaving open the question of the relative importance of high dietary protein for each phase of carcinogenesis. It is impressive that the risk associated with protein for each phase is in the same direction (B. S. Appleton and T. C. Campbell, unpublished observation). Current studies are under way to gain more insight into the effect of protein on these two carcinogenic phases.

In conclusion, I must emphasize that this experimental model represents only one nutrient, one carcinogen, and one species. Whether other species and other carcinogens behave in a like manner needs further study. In spite of the incorrectness of extrapolating these data to other carcinogenic situations, we are impressed with the accumulating evidence in the literature that may indict high-protein intake on a much broader basis. Other experimental work, both with (Topping and Visek 1977) and without (Ross and Bras 1973, Tannenbaum and Silverstone 1949) experimental carcinogens, exhibit a similar effect of high protein. In addition, the impressive correlations cited in epidemiological studies (Gregor et al. 1969, Drasar and Irving 1973) indicate an association of certain cancers with protein level as impressive as that for total fat. Of course, these two dietary variables are cocorrelates, since diets high in animal products are also generally high in both nutrients. That raises the still larger question of which nutrient is the more important, total fat or protein. It may prove to be a moot point insofar as practical information is concerned.

This brings us to my initial question of whether there are any unifying themes that might begin to give perspective to the myriad nutrient effects on carcinogenesis. Could it be that, for practical purposes, it does not really make much difference which nutrient risk factor is the more important: high protein, high fat, low fiber, low vitamin A/carotene, low vitamin C, or low vitamin E? Perhaps they all are and perhaps by a variety of mechanisms. The unifying theme that may be emerging is that there may be a dietary lifestyle that would be consistent and comprehensive with all nutrients simultaneously, insofar as enhancement of cancer risk is concerned. Such a high-risk diet could be one that is simultaneously high in total fat and total protein but low in dietary fiber and vitamins A, E, and C. Moreover, this diet, in general, is the same one that presumably offers a higher risk for the cardiovascular diseases as well. I would certainly find it comforting to know that nature charted our course with a little more coordination than we researchers are sometimes able to comprehend.

ACKNOWLEDGMENTS

Research reported here was supported in part by NIH/NCI P01 CA 26755 and American Cancer Society Grant No. PDT-104.

REFERENCES

Adekunle, A. A., J. R. Hayes, and T. C. Campbell. 1977. Interrelationship of dietary protein level, aflatoxin B_1 metabolism, and hepatic microsomal expoxide hydrase activity. Life Sci. 21:1785–1792.

Allen-Hoffmann, B. L., and T. C. Campbell. 1977. The relationship between hepatic glutathione levels and the formation of aflatoxin B_1-DNA adducts as influenced by dietary protein intake. (Abstract) Fed. Proc. 36:1116.

Butler, W. H., and J. I. Clifford. 1965. Extraction of aflatoxin from rat liver. Nature 206:1045–1046.

Croy, R. G., and G. N. Wogan. 1981. Temporal patterns of covalent DNA adducts in rat liver after single and multiple doses of aflatoxin B_1. Cancer Res. 41:197–203.

Degan, G., and H-G. Neumann. 1978. The major metabolite of aflatoxin B_1 in the rat is a glutathione conjugate. Chem. Biol. Interact. 22:239–255.

deIongh, H., R. O. Vles, and J. G. van Pelt. 1964. Milk of mammals fed an aflatoxin-containing diet. Nature 202:466–467.

Doll, R., and R. Peto. 1981. Estimates of Cancer Risk from the Environment. Preliminary Report by Office of Technology Assessment. U.S. Congress, Washington, D.C.

Drasar, B. S., and D. Irving. 1973. Environmental factors and cancer of the colon and breast. Br. J. Cancer 27:167–172.

Garner, R. C. 1975. Reduction in binding of [^{14}C]aflatoxin B_1 to rat liver macromolecules by phenobarbitone pretreatment. Biochem. Pharmacol. 23:1553–1556.

Garner, R. C., E. C. Miller, and J. A. Miller. 1972. Liver microsomal metabolism of aflatoxin B_1 to a reactive derivative toxic to *Salmonella typhimurium* TA 1530. Cancer Res. 32:2058–2066.

Gregor, O., R. Toman, and F. Prusova. 1969. Gastrointestinal cancer and nutrition. Gut 10:1031–1034.

Guengerich, F. P. 1977. Separation and purification of multiple forms of microsomal cytochrome P-450. Activities of different forms of cytochrome P-450 towards several compounds of environmental interest. J. Biol. Chem. 252:3970–3979.

Kalengayi, M. M. R., and V. J. Desmet. 1978. Gamma-glutamyl transferase as oncofetal marker of experimental hepatocarcinogenesis in the rat. Scand. J. Immunol. 8:547–556.

LeBovit, C. 1977. The health food market, *in* National Food Situation. Economic Research Service, U.S. Department of Agriculture. NFS-161, pp. 17–18.

Lutz, W. K. 1979. In vivo covalent binding of organic chemicals to DNA as a quantitative indicator in the process of chemical carcinogenesis. Mutat. Res. 65:289–356.

Mabee, M., and J. R. Chipley. 1973. Tissue distribution and metabolism of aflatoxin B_1-^{14}C in broiler chickens. Appl. Microbiol. 25:763–769.

Madhavan, T. V., and C. Gopalan. 1968. The effect of dietary protein on carcinogenesis of aflatoxin. Arch. Pathol. 85:133–137.

Mainigi, K. C., and T. C. Campbell. 1981. Effects of low dietary protein and dietary aflatoxin on hepatic glutathione levels in F-344 rats. Toxicol. Appl. Pharmacol. (in press).

Margison, G. P., and P. Kleihues. 1975. Chemical carcinogenesis in the nervous system. Preferential accumulation of O^6-methylguanine in rat brain deoxyribonucleic acid during repetitive administration of N-methyl-N-nitrosourea. Biochem. J. 148:521–525.

Mgbodile, M. V. K., and T. C. Campbell. 1972. Effect of protein deprivation of male weanling rats on the kinetics of hepatic microsomal enzyme activity. J. Nutr. 102:53–60.

Mgbodile, M. V. K., M. Holscher, and R. A. Neal. 1975. A possible role for reduced glutathione in aflatoxin B_1 toxicity: Effect of pretreatment of rats with phenobarbital and 3-methylcholanthrene on aflatoxin toxicity. Toxicol. Appl. Pharmacol. 34:128–142.

Miller, J. A. 1970. Carcinogenesis by chemicals: An overview. G. H. A. Clowes Memorial Lecture. Cancer Res. 30:559–576.

Portman, R. S., and T. C. Campbell. 1970. In vitro inhibition of *E. coli* RNA polymerase transcription of rat liver chromatin by aflatoxin B_1. Biochem. Biophys. Res. Commun. 41:774–780.

Portman, R. S., K. M. Plowman, and T. C. Campbell. 1968. Aflatoxin metabolism by liver microsomal preparations of two different species. Biochem. Biophys. Res. Commun. 33:711–715.

Preston, R. S., J. R. Hayes, and T. C. Campbell. 1976. The effect of protein deficiency on the in vivo binding of aflatoxin B_1 to rat liver macromolecules. Life Sci. 19:1191–1198.

Ross, M. H., and G. Bras. 1973. Influence of protein under- and overnutrition on spontaneous tumor prevalence in the rat. J. Nutr. 103:944–963.

Rouiller, C. 1964. The morphology, biochemistry and physiology, *in* Experimental Toxic Injury of the Liver, C. Rouiller, ed. Academic Press, New York and London, pp. 335–476.

Swenson, D. H., J. A. Miller, and E. C. Miller. 1973. 2,3-Dihydro-2,3-dihydroxy-aflatoxin B_1: An acid hydrolysis product of an RNA-aflatoxin B_1 adduct formed by hamster and rat liver microsomes in vitro. Biochem. Biophys. Res. Commun. 53:1260–1267.

Tannenbaum, A., and H. Silverstone. 1949. The genesis and growth of tumors. IV. Effects of varying the proportion of protein (casein) in the diet. Cancer Res. 9:162–173.

Topping, D. C., and W. J. Visek. 1977. Nitrogen intake and tumorigenesis in rats injected with 1,2-dimethyl-hydrazine. J. Nutr. 106:1583–1590.

Woodcock, B. G., and G. C. Wood. 1971. Effect of protein-free diet on UDP-glucuronyl transferase and sulfotransferase activities in rat liver. Biochem. Pharmacol. 20:2703–2713.

Molecular Interrelations of Nutrition and Cancer,
edited by M. S. Arnott, J. van Eys, and Y.-M. Wang.
Raven Press, New York © 1982.

Alpha-Tocopherol as a Potential Modifier of Daunomycin Carcinogenicity in Sprague-Dawley Rats

Y.-M. Wang, S. K. Howell, J. C. Kimball, C. C. Tsai,* J. Sato, and C. A. Gleiser*

*Department of Pediatrics and *Division of Veterinary Medicine and Surgery, The University of Texas M. D. Anderson Hospital and Tumor Institute at Houston, Houston, Texas 77030*

Alpha-tocopherol (vitamin E) has long been accepted as a physiological antioxidant or free-radical scavenger. There are at least two ways that α-tocopherol is involved in the destruction of endogenously generated free radicals (see Machlin and Brin 1980); these reactions can be simplified as follows:

1. O_2 + tocopherol $\rightarrow$ tocopheroxide $\rightarrow$ α-tocopherylquinone
   (unstable)

   $$2. \ RO_2^{\cdot} + \text{tocopherol} \rightarrow \text{tocopherol radical} \xrightarrow{\overset{\text{GSSG GSH}}{\frown}} \text{tocopherol.}$$

The latter reaction depends upon glutathione redox enzymic reactions. A lesser known biological phenomenon related to α-tocopherol is its specific binding to the intranuclear nucleoprotein complex (Patnaik and Nair 1977). Subfractionation of this complex further reveals that α-tocopherol is predominantly associated with the fraction containing pheonol-soluble nonhistone proteins having a high affinity to DNA. It is mostly likely through this mechanism that the reduction in binding of benz(a)pyrene to nuclear macromolecules caused by α-tocopherol was seen (Harris et al. 1978, Matsuura et al. 1979). Furthermore, it has been suggested that α-tocopherol may serve as a corepressor of the biosynthesis of xanthine oxidase or creatine kinase (Olson 1974).

The anthracycline antibiotics daunomycin and Adriamycin have been extensively used since 1970 for the treatment of human cancers. The cumulative dose of these two agents frequently reaches 550 mg/m², a single dose usually being 60 mg/m². The major toxicity of the anthracycline antibiotics is cardiac, which limits the cumulative dosage. In addition, both drugs possess mutagenic and carcinogenic activities. The mechanism of the mutagenicity and carcinogenicity of the anthracyclines is unknown.

At least two schemes have been proposed for the interactions between the anthracyclines and DNA: by intercalation or by electrostatic interaction involving DNA phosphate groups and anthracycline amino groups (Pigram et al. 1972). Recently, free-radical generation has been demonstrated to be linked with the action of the anthracycline antibiotics (Sato et al. 1977, Bachur et al. 1977). Free-radical intermediates are formed through cellular electron-transport machinery, by the anthracyclines including xanthine oxidase, NADPH cyto-chrome P-450 reductase, and an as yet unidentified nuclear electron-transport system. The involvement of xanthine oxidase (Pan and Bachur 1980) is an interesting one. The wide distribution and the high content of this enzyme most probably make this particular reaction more important than the microso-mal reaction, and in addition the amount of α-tocopherol affects the activ-ity of xanthine oxidase (Catignani et al. 1974). An insufficient hepatocellular α-tocopherol concentration increases the activity of xanthine oxidase.

Sinha (1980) proposed a working model for the binding of the anthracycline antibiotics to nucleic acid, based upon his studies with synthetic polynucleotides. His results show that either a free-radical intermediate of the parent compound or its metabolites are reactive species that will induce covalent binding to DNA. We feel this may be one of the mechanisms for the induction of tumors in rats by daunomycin or Adriamycin. In addition, Umezawa and his collaborators (1978) suggested that the mutagenicity of daunomycin was the result of the amino moiety of the anthracycline glycosides.

Bertazzoli et al. (1971) reported a high incidence of mammary tumors in a relatively small group of Sprague-Dawley rats treated with single doses of Adria-mycin or daunomycin. These results were later confirmed by others (Marquardt et al. 1976, Bucciarelli 1981, Solcia et al. 1978, Wang et al. 1980a). Results obtained by Solcia et al. (1978) showed a great prevalence of fibroadenomas in Adriamycin-treated rats and adenocarcinomas in daunomycin-treated rats. The incidence of daunomycin-induced adenocarcinoma increased with the dose, whereas the frequency of Adriamycin-induced adenocarcinomas reached a pla-teau at 5 mg/kg. Bucciarelli (1981) reported that daunomycin (10 mg/kg) in-duced breast tumors in 18 of 28 female and 10 of 27 male Sprague-Dawley rats. The median induction time was about 80 days in both sexes. Adriamycin, however, induced tumors in 10 of 35 female rats, with a median induction time of 220 days. No tumors developed in 57 males. Table 1 summarizes the incidence of daunomycin-induced mammary tumors in female rats. When it was determined, the median induction time was 80 days or less, and the incidence was 40% to 50% at this time interval.

For more than a decade, numerous investigations, including our own, have been undertaken to explain the cellular damage, especially cardiotoxicity, of the anthracycline antibiotics. Their generation of hydrogen peroxide and reactive oxygen radicals in liver cells (Bachur et al. 1977) or cells without a microsomal system, such as the mammalian erythrocyte, has been suggested as one mecha-nism (Wang et al. 1980b). Treatment with α-tocopherol protects partially against Adriamycin-induced cardiac damage in animals, but does not reduce the cytotox-icity and antitumor activity of the anthracycline antibiotics (Myers et al. 1977,

TABLE 1. *Daunomycin-induced tumors in female Sprague-Dawley rats*

Dose (mg/kg)	No. rats	No. with tumor	Adeno-carcinoma	Fibro-adenoma	Other	Induction time, day (median)
5*	18	15	2	12	3	—
6.25†	7	6	1	6	—	—
10*	16	12	1	6	—	—
10‡	28	18	24	2	1	80
12.5†	65	37	37	14	—	80§

* Marquardt et al. (1976).
† Solcia et al. (1978).
‡ Bucciarelli (1981).
§ Estimated for adenocarcinoma.

Konings and Trieling 1977). These experiences suggested to us that the anthracycline antibiotic–induced cellular damage involves sequential oxidation of reduced cellular glutathione and other molecules in reduced form (Wang et al. 1980b). α-Tocopherol can effectively prevent the oxidation induced by Adriamycin.

In an attempt to explore the possibility that α-tocopherol can also ameliorate anthracycline-induced carcinogenicity, we initiated some preliminary studies. The objectives were: (1) to confirm the occurrence of daunomycin-induced mammary tumors in rats; (2) to determine if the protective effects of α-tocopherol against Adriamycin- or daunomycin-induced cellular damage could modify the appearance of such tumors; (3) to correlate results with the effect of α-tocopherol on intracellular reduced glutathione (GSH) and xanthine oxidase activity; and (4) to evaluate tissue distribution and metabolism of α-tocopherylacetate and daunomycin in rats, and to investigate the potential interaction between α-tocopherol and daunomycin.

We selected daunomycin as the investigative drug for two reasons: the shorter incubation time it requires to produce tumors and the higher incidence of mammary adenocarcinomas. Furthermore, we realized that daunomycin is more active in forming free radicals (Bachur et al. 1979). We propose three possible roles for α-tocopherol in reducing daunomycin-induced toxicities: (1) as a free-radical scavenger or a universal antioxidant; (2) as a reducer of the binding of daunomycin or its metabolities to nuclear macromolecules; and (3) as a suppressor at higher cellular concentrations of the biosynthesis of xanthine oxidase, thus reducing free-radical generation by daunomycin.

In late 1978 and early 1979, we injected daunomycin at either 10 mg/kg or 12.5 mg/kg into two sets of rats, doses equivalent to 60–75 mg/m². Albino, female Sprague-Dawley rats (Timco, Houston, Texas) were used in the first study arm. Thirty rats were given either α-tocopherylacetate (1.8 g/m²) i.p. or an equal volume of normal saline for 4 days prior to the daunomycin injection. On the fifth day, each of the 30 rats received 10 to 12.5 mg/kg daunomycin i.v. On days 14, 21, and 28 following daunomycin administration, each group of rats again received α-tocopherylacetate at similar dosages or equivalent volumes of saline according to their pre-daunomycin treatment selection. The dose and schedule of α-tocopherylacetate were largely borrowed from our previous cardiac toxicity study (Wang et al. 1980a). Twenty-two rats died prior to the planned date for necropsy and were excluded from analysis. One saline-treated rat had obvious tumor involvement. Nine rats served as saline control, while nine rats served as α-tocopherylacetate control animals. Each control group was treated similarly to previous study arms but did not receive any daunomycin.

Table 2 shows the incidence of mammary tumors in rats treated with daunomycin alone or the α-tocopherylacetate/daunomycin combination. This preliminary study demonstrated a delay or decrease in the formation of daunomycin-induced mammary tumors in rats pretreated with α-tocopherylacetate. The difference between α-tocopherylacetate pretreated and untreated rats was statistically significant ($X^2 = 3.841$, $p = 0.05$). All animals were killed by the 20th week after daunomycin injections. All tumors except two were mammary adenocarcinomas (Figures 1–3). Necropsies and histopathologic examinations were performed. There were no multiple tumors in any animal in this study. All tumors were either in inguinal or pectoral areas.

Mammary fat tissue levels of reduced glutathione, quantitated by the method of Crowley et al. (1975), failed to indicate a significant decrease of glutathione concentration 30 minutes (0.45 ± 0.07 μmol/g wet tissue) or 24 hours (0.41 ± 0.25 μmol/g wet tissue) after daunomycin treatment compared with the normal level (0.59 ± 0.42 μmol/g wet tissue). Whether there was a difference in GSH levels in mammary gland cells between the animals treated or not treated with α-tocopherylacetate prior to the daunomycin injection has yet to be explored. Xanthine oxidase activities were quantitated in the liver of animals 24 hours after the four consecutive daily α-tocopherylacetate injections. The treatment with α-tocopherylacetate significantly increased liver xanthine oxidase activity

TABLE 2. *Modification of daunomycin-induced tumors with high-dose vitamin E*

Treatment	No. rats* treated	No. rats examined	No. rats with mammary adenocarcinoma	No. rats with mammary fibroadenoma
10 mg/kg DM, Pretreated with				
Saline	15	12	6	0
Vitamin E	15	11	0	0
12.5 mg/kg DM, pretreated with				
Saline	15	10	3	2
Vitamin E	15	5	2	0
Control				
Saline	9	9	0	0
Vitamin E	9	9	0	0

DM, daunomycin.
* Rats were 48–65 days old and weighed 150–200 g.

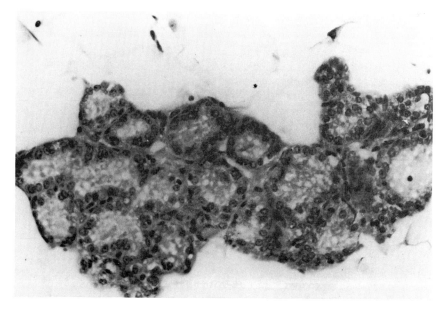

FIG. 1. Normal mammary gland in female SD rats. Glandular acini with normal epithelial lining. H & E, × 250.

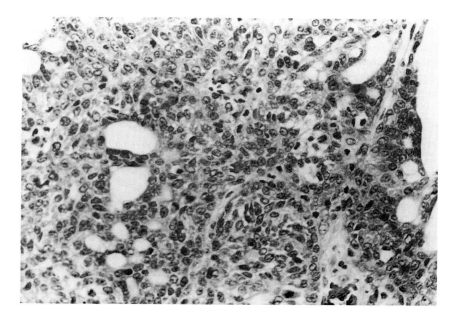

FIG. 2. Mammary adenocarcinoma induced in female SD rats by i.v. injections of daunomycin (10 mg/kg). Marked proliferation of glandular epithelium with loss of normal glandular structure; several mitotic figures. H & E, × 250.

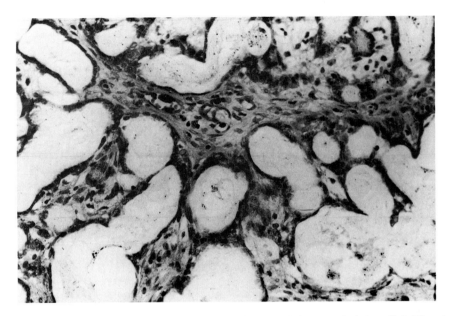

FIG. 3. Mammary fibroadenoma induced by i.v. injections of daunomycin (10 mg/kg). Dilated glands with modest proliferation of glandular epithelium and an increase in fibrous connective tissue stroma. H & E, × 250.

24 hours after the last α-tocopherylacetate injection (17.8 $\pm$ 1.8 μmol uric acid formed/hour/gram wet tissue, n = 3) compared with normal controls (14.7 $\pm$ 0.9 μmol uric acid/hour/gram wet tissue, n = 3). This result contradicts our hypothesis that was based upon the observation in vitamin E–deficient animals.

The distribution and the interaction between α-tocopherol and daunomycin were studied by following the radioactivity of either ^{14}C-tocopherylacetate (36 mCi/mol) or ^{3}H-daunomycin (2.9 Ci/mol) or both. Table 3 shows the distribution of ^{14}C-α-tocopherylacetate in animals treated with or without daunomycin. There were significant differences in spleen (p < 0.0005), heart (p < 0.05), mammary fat (p < 0.05), plasma (p < 0.0025), and erythrocytes (p < 0.05). Furthermore, the radioactive count of tritium was substantially decreased in the nuclear fraction in animals treated daily with α-tocopherylacetate for 4 days. Unfortunately, the radioactivity was not adequate to determine whether this activity was due to daunomycin or its metabolites.

To further confirm the observation of a decrease, two animals were given either α-tocopherylacetate (1.8 g/m² daily for 4 days) or the placebo (D-M Pharmaceuticals, Inc., Rockville, MD) at equal volumes for the same period of time. The animals were killed at day 5. Liver tissue was subjected to single-cell preparation following published methods (Sato et al. 1980). The cells were

TABLE 3. *Tissue distribution of ^{14}C-α-tocopherylacetate in the rat*

	^{14}C-αTA (μg/g wet tissue)	
	−DM	+DM
Spleen	4354* (488)†	1782 (288)
Liver	1826 (1113)	1862 (1238)
Kidney	454 (144)	362 (12)
Ovary	335 (274)	687 (131)
Lung	32 (5)	47 (27)
Heart	30 (6)	21 (1)
Mammary fat	20 (1)	32 (6)
Brain	20 (23)	9 (5)
Muscle	13 (11)	12 (3)
Plasma	13 (4)	29 (1)
Erythrocyte	6 (2)	14 (6)

* mean.
† standard deviation.

then incubated with ^{3}H-daunomycin for up to 2 hours, and the intracellular distribution of the daunomycin radioactivity was analyzed. The results obtained from the in vitro study support the observation of decreased tritium radioactivity in the nuclear fraction in vivo. α-Tocopherylacetate appears to modify the subcellular distribution of ^{3}H-daunomycin. To study the metabolic species of daunomycin further, radioactivity of the nuclear fraction was recovered, isolated, and injected into a high-pressure liquid chromatograph. Preliminary results show that radioactive profiles of the material eluted are different in the nuclear fractions from the two animals.

Unfortunately, we were not able to isolate fat-free mammary cells until very recently (Moon et al. 1969). Since tumors are located in this tissue, these studies must be extended to mammary cells.

Prior to our investigation of the pharmacokinetics and disposition of α-tocopherol and daunomycin, we initiated another study with younger and smaller female SD rats (125 g) to try to repeat our initial success of tumor "prevention" by α-tocopherol. The results were negative. The percentage of mammary tumors was substantially less than our original observation or those published by others. α-Tocopherylacetate did not show protective effects (Table 4), probably because of the younger age of the animals. The same batch of α-tocopherylacetate was used, but a different batch of daunomycin was used. Unfortunately, the purity of the drug was not analyzed.

In addition to repeating the early study with matched weight and age, we redesigned our study to follow the kinetics of daunomycin and α-tocopherol in vivo. We are exploring the possibility of injecting daunomycin directly into the mammary tissue (Figure 4). This approach should have two advantages: (1) increase the mammary tumor frequency in a given animal; (2) avoid unnecessary death due to daunomycin-induced kidney or cardiac toxicity in rats. Multiple

TABLE 4. *Modification of daunomycin-induced tumors with high-dose vitamin E*

Treatment	No. rats* treated	No. rats examined	No. rats with mammary tumor
1980			
10 mg/kg DM			
Saline	29	21	5
Vitamin E	39	27	9
1979 & 1980			
10–12.5 mg/kg DM			
Saline	59	43	16
Vitamin E	69	43	11

DM, daunomycin.
* Rats used in 1980 experiment were about 40 days old and weighed 125 g.

tumors have already appeared in some animals. The concentration injected was estimated by the peak daunomycin concentration detected in mammary tissue areas from daunomycin radioactivity.

Two other related activities were performed during our investigations of daunomycin-induced mammary tumors in SD rats. Serum was collected 16–21 weeks after a 10 mg/kg injection of daunomycin. Control samples were obtained from pair-animals of similar age. A persistently increased serum cholesterol level was seen in animals treated with daunomycin (from 74.5 mg/dl ± 11.1 to 365.4 mg/dl ± 121.2). These elevations could be seen up to 21 weeks after daunomycin injection and were significant at $p < 0.0025$. An equivalent increase was seen in animals treated with 300 mg/kg/day × 4 days α-tocopherylacetate plus daunomycin (337.7 mg/dl ± 149.8). This elevation was also seen in rats treated with Adriamycin (S. D. Morrison, personal communication). This in-

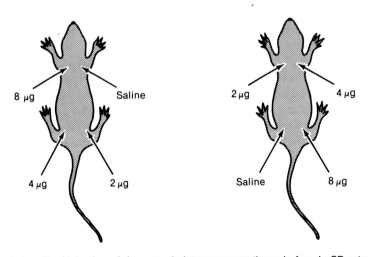

Fig. 4. Localized injection of daunomycin into mammary tissue in female SD rats.

crease appears to be species-related and has not been documented in humans (S. D. Morrison, personal communication). Whether this phenomenon relates to the etiology of tumor development has yet to be investigated. In addition, tissue peroxidase activity (Anderson et al. 1975, Duffy and Duffy 1977) was quantitated for possible tumor estrogen linkage. Enzyme activity in tumors (25.5 ± 6 μ/g wet tissue, n = 8) was not significantly different from normal tissues (2.06 ± 0.74 μ/g wet tissue, n = 6). [One unit (μ) was defined as the amount given at an initial rate of 1 absorbance unit/min. For method, see DeSombre and Lyttle (1978).] However, one tumor had substantial nonspecific peroxidase activity.

Jaffe (1946) first reported that diets enriched with wheat germ oil (a source of α-tocopherol) decreased the number of tumors induced by i.p. injections of 3-methylbenzanthracene. α-Tocopherol was later found to inhibit the formation of tumors induced by injection of methylcholanthrene (Harber and Wissler 1962), dibenzanthracene, and amino-fluorene (Hultin and Arrhenius 1965). Recently, dietary insufficiencies of vitamin E resulted in an increased incidence of tumors in animals treated with dimethylhydrazine (Cook and McNamara 1980) or 7, 12-dimethylbenz(a)anthracene (Lee and Chen 1979). In the literature thus far, no secondary malignancy has been linked to primary treatment with the anthracyclines. In monkeys, Sieber et al. (1980) reported one of ten healthy animals studied died of acute myeloblastic leukemia after treatment with Adriamycin at a cumulative dose of 324 mg/m². The induction time for cancer development was 29 months. Antineoplastic agents have been recognized as carcinogens for a number of years (Adamson and Sieber 1977, Schmahl and Habs 1978), and secondary malignancy in cancer patients treated with chemotherapeutic agents has been documented (Adamson and Sieber 1977). Malignancies induced by similar cytotoxic agents were also reported in patients treated for other diseases.

ACKNOWLEDGMENTS

This investigation was supported in part by grants from the National Cancer Institute CA-09070, and Hoffmann-La Roche, Inc., and a generous donation from Mr. and Mrs. Leland Anderson.

REFERENCES

Adamson, R. H., and S. M. Sieber. 1977. Antineoplastic agents as potential carcinogens, in Origins of Human Cancer, H. H. Hiatt, J. A. Watson, and J. A. Winsten, eds. Cold Spring Harbor Laboratory, Cold Spring Harbor, New York, pp. 429–443.
Anderson, W. A., Y.-H. Kang, and E. R. DeSombre. 1975. Endogenous peroxidase specific marker-enzyme for tissues displaying growth dependency on estrogen. J. Cell Biol. 64:668–681.
Bachur, N. R., S. L. Gordon, and M. V. Gee. 1977. Anthracycline antibiotics: Augmentation of microsomal electron transport and free radical formation. Mol. Pharmacol. 13:901–910.
Bachur, N. R., S. L. Gordon, M. V. Gee, and H. Kon. 1979. NADPH cytochrome P-450 reductase activation of quinone anticancer agents to free radicals. Proc. Natl. Acad. Sci. USA 76:954–957.

Bertazzoli, C., T. Chieli, and E. Solcia. 1971. Different incidence of breast carcinomas or fibroadeno-mas in daunomycin or Adriamycin treated rats. Experientia 27:1209–1210.

Bucciarelli, E. 1981. Mammary tumor induction in male and female Sprague-Dawley rats by Adria-mycin and daunomycin. JNCI 66:81–84.

Catignani, G. L., F. Chytil, and W. J. Darby. 1974. Vitamin E deficiency: Immunochemical evidence for increased accumulation of liver xanthine oxidase. Proc. Natl. Acad. Sci. USA 71:1966–1968.

Cook, M. G., and P. McNamara. 1980. Effect of dietary vitamin E on dimethylhydrazine-induced colonic tumors in mice. Cancer Res. 40:1327–1331.

Crowley, C., B. Gilham, and M. D. Thorn. 1975. Direct enzyme method for determinations of reduced glutathione in blood and other tissues. Biochem. Med. 13:287–292.

DeSombre, E. R., and C. R. Lyttle. 1978. Isolation and purification of rat mammary tumor peroxi-dase. Cancer Res. 38:4086–4096.

Duffy, M. J., and G. Duffy. 1977. Peroxidase activity as a possible marker for a functional oestradiol receptor in human breast tumors. Biochem. Soc. Trans. 5:1723–1739.

Harber, S. L., and R. W. Wissler. 1962. Effect of vitamin E on carcinogenicity of methylcholanthrene. Proc. Soc. Exp. Biol. Med. 111:774–775.

Harris, C. C., B. Conner, A. C. Frank, and C. A. Barrett. 1978. Inhibition of benzo(a)pyrene binding to DNA in cultured human bronchi, *in* Prevention and Detection of Cancer, part 1, vol. 2, H. E. Nieburgs, ed. Marcel Dekker, New York, pp. 1359–1364.

Howell, S. K., and Y.-M. Wang. 1981. High dose α-tocopherylacetate distribution and metabolism in Sprague-Dawley rats (abstract). Fed. Proc. 40:874.

Hultin, T., and E. Arrhenius. 1965. Effects of carcinogenic amines on amino acid incorporation by liver systems. III. Inhibition by aminofluorene treatment and its dependence on vitamin E. Cancer Res. 25:124–131.

Jaffe, W. G., 1946. The influence of wheat germ oil on the production of tumors in rats by methylcho-lanthrene. Exp. Med. Surg. 4:278–282.

Konings, A. W. T., and W. B. Trieling. 1977. The inhibition of DNA synthesis in vitamin-E-depleted lymphosarcoma cells by x-rays and cytostatics. Int. J. Radiat. Biol. 31:397–400.

Lee, J. L., and C. Chen. 1979. Enhancement of mammary tumorigenesis in rats by vitamin E deficiency (abstract). Proc. Am. Assoc. Cancer Res. 20:132.

Machlin, L. J. and M. Brin. 1980. Vitamin E, *in* Human Nutrition, A Comprehensive Treatise, vol. 3B, Nutrition and the Adult Micronutrients, R. B. Alfin-Slater and D. Kritchevsky, eds. Plenum Press, New York, pp. 245–266.

Marquardt, H., F. S. Philips, and S. S. Sternberg. 1976. Tumorigenicity in vivo and induction of malignant transformation and mutagenesis in cell cultures by Adriamycin and daunomycin. Cancer Res. 36:2065–2069.

Matsuura, T., H. Veyama, S. Nomi, and K. Veda. 1979. Effect of α-tocopherol on the binding of benzo(a)pyrene to nuclear macromolecules. J. Nutr. Sci. Vitaminol. 25:495–504.

Moon, R. C., D. H. Jones, and S. Young. 1969. Preparation of fat cell-free rat mammary gland. J. Histochem. Cytochem. 17:182–186.

Myers, C. E., W. McGuire, R. H. Liss, I. Ifrim, K. Grotzinger, and R. C. Young. 1977. Adriamycin: The role of lipid peroxidation in cardiac toxicity and tumor response. Science 197:165–166.

Olson, R. O. 1974. Creatine kinase and myofibrillar proteins in hereditary muscular dystrophy and vitamin E deficiency. Am. J. Clin. Nutr. 27:1117–1129.

Pan, S. S., and N. R. Bachur. 1980. Xanthine oxidase catalyzed reductive cleavage of anthracycline antibiotics and free radical formation. Mol. Pharmacol. 17:95–99.

Patniak, R. N., and P. P. Nair. 1977. Studies on the binding of d-α-tocopherol to rat liver nuclei. Arch. Biochem. Biophys. 178:333–341.

Pigram, W. J., W. Fuller, and L. D. Hamilton. 1972. Stereochemistry of intercalation: Interaction of daunomycin with DNA. Nature New Biol. 235:17–19.

Sato, J., Y.-M. Wang, and J. van Eys. 1980. Methylglyoxal formation with rat liver cells. J. Biol. Chem. 255:2046–2050.

Sato, S., M. Lwaizumi, K. Handa, and Y. Tamura. 1977. Electron spin resonance study on the mode of generation of free radicals of daunomycin, Adriamycin and carboquinone in NADPH-microsome system. Gann 68:603–608.

Schmahl, D., and M. Habs. 1978. Experimental carcinogenicity of antitumor drugs. Cancer Treat. Rev. 5:175–184.

Sieber, S. M., P. Correa, D. M. Young, D. W. Dalgard, and R. H. Adamson. 1980. Cardiotoxic and possible leukemogenic effects of Adriamycin in non-human primates. Pharmacology 20:9–14.

Sinha, B. K. 1980. Binding specificity of chemically and enzymatically activated anthracycline anticancer agents to nucleic acid. Chem. Biol. Interact. 30:67–77.

Solcia, E., L. Ballerini, O. Bellini, C. Sala, and C. Bertazzoli. 1978. Mammary tumors induced in rats bv Adriamvcin and daunomycin. Cancer Res. 38:1444–1446.

Umezawa, K., M. Sawamura, T. Matsushima, and T. Sugimura. 1978. Mutagenecity of actinomycin A and daunomycin derivatives. Cancer Res. 38:1782–1784.

Wang, Y.-M., J. C. Kimball, C. A. Gleiser, and E. Lantin. 1980a. Vitamin E and anthracycline antibiotics-induced cardiomyopathy and mammary carcinoma in animals (abstract). Fed. Proc. 39:788.

Wang, Y.-M., F. F. Madanat, J. Kimball, C. A. Gleiser, M. K. Ali, M. W. Kaufman, and J. van Eys. 1980b. Effect of vitamin E against Adriamycin-induced toxicity in rabbits. Cancer Res. 40:1022–1027.

Molecular Interrelations of Nutrition and Cancer,
edited by M. S. Arnott, J. van Eys, and Y.-M. Wang.
Raven Press, New York © 1982.

Endocrine Interactions in the Nutritional Modulation of Mammary Carcinogenesis in Rats

Adrianne E. Rogers, John D. Fernstrom, Keyou Ge,* Robert G. McConnell, Wendell W. Leavitt,† William C. Wetsel, Soon O. Yang, and Elise A. Camelio

*Department of Nutrition and Food Science, Massachusetts Institute of Technology, Cambridge, Massachusetts 02139, *Institute of Health, Chinese Academy of Medical Sciences, Beijing, China, and †the Worcester Foundation for Experimental Biology, Shrewsbury, Massachusetts*

Breast cancer incidence is higher in populations that ingest high-fat diets and in experimental animals fed similar diets (Carroll and Khor 1975, Reddy et al. 1980, Rogers and Wetsel 1981, Wetsel et al. 1981). Design of preventive dietary or other measures may be possible with understanding of the mechanisms by which dietary fat increases mammary carcinogenesis, by finding whether all fats are equally effective and defining more exactly what the significant amounts of dietary fat are and the influence of age on its effect.

EXPERIMENTAL STUDIES OF DIETARY FAT AND MAMMARY TUMORIGENESIS

Female rats fed high-fat (20–25% by weight) diets and treated with carcinogens for the mammary gland develop a higher incidence and a larger number of mammary tumors after a shorter latent period than rats fed low-fat (0.5–5%) diets (Carroll and Khor 1975, Reddy et al. 1980, Wetsel et al. 1981). Polyunsaturated fats are somewhat more effective than saturated fats in enhancing tumor development.

Enhanced tumor development in rats fed 20% corn oil or sunflower seed oil has been reported from several laboratories; significant but slightly less enhancement has occurred in rats fed 20% lard. Studies in rats fed beef tallow or coconut oil have showed no enhancement unless the diet was supplemented to make it adequate in essential fatty acids (Table 1). Although supplemented animals fed tallow or coconut oil had more tumors than animals fed the polyunsaturated oil supplement or the saturated fat alone, they tended to have fewer tumors and longer latent periods than rats fed the same total amount of fat as corn or sunflower seed oil. In another study, supplemented coconut oil increased tumor growth only slightly (Ip and Sinha 1981; see Table 2).

In experiments in which saturated fats have been fed without essential fatty

TABLE 1. *Dietary fat and mammary tumorigenesis in female Sprague-Dawley rats*

Dietary fat Type	% wt	Carcinogen	Tumor incidence (%)	Latent period (days)	Number tumors/ tumor-bearing rat	Reference
Corn oil*	0.5	DMBA,10 mg	71	76†	3	Gammal et al. 1967
Corn oil	20		96	56	5	
Coconut oil	20		76	70	3	
Sunflower seed oil‡	3	DMBA,5 mg	70	—	2	Hopkins and Carroll 1979, Carroll 1980
Sunflower seed oil	20		85–95	—	4–5	
Coconut oil	20		75	—	2	
Coconut oil + Oleate	17 3		75	—	2	
Beef tallow	20		70	—	2	
Lard	20		90	—	4	
Beef tallow + Sunflower seed oil	17 3		90	—	4	
Coconut oil + Sunflower seed oil	17 3		85	—	5	
Coconut oil + Linoleate	17 3		100	—	4	
Coconut oil + Fish oil	17 3		90	—	4	
Corn oil§	0.5	DMBA,5 mg	60	112//	—	Chan and Cohen 1974
Corn oil	20		70	74	—	
Linoleic acid #	2	DMBA,10 mg	43	189//	2	King et al. 1979
Corn oil	20		100	91	3	
Coconut oil + Linoleic acid	18 2		77	107	2	
Linoleic acid¶	2	DMBA,10 mg	45	—	6	Kollmorgen et al. 1981

TABLE 1. *Continued*

Dietary fat			Tumor incidence (%)	Latent period (days)	Number tumors/ tumor-bearing rat	Reference
Type	% wt	Carcinogen				
Corn oil	20		97	—	9	
Lard	5	NMU,25 mg/kg	70	96	—	Chan et al. 1977
Lard	20		95	82	—	
Lard	5	NMU,50 mg/kg	75	82	—	
Lard	20		95	68	—	
Corn oil	5	NMU,50 mg/kg	88	105	6	Chan and Dao 1981
Corn oil	25		100	83	10	
Corn oil**	5	DMBA,2.5 mg	68	110†	2	Wetsel et al. 1981
Corn oil	20		83	96	2	
Lard	5		57	117	2	
Lard	20		71	89	2	
Corn oil††	20		88	100	2	
Lard††	20		68	122	2	

* Diets, balanced for nutrient intake per calorie, were fed from weaning. In all experiments summarized in the table, carcinogens were given to rats between 50 and 60 days of age.
† Days to first palpable tumor.
‡ The rats were fed a natural ingredient diet until 1 week after DMBA treatment and then fed a purified diet with the specified fat content.
§The rats were fed a natural ingredient diet until 1 week after DMBA treatment and then fed the purified diet with the fat content balanced by weight, not calories, with carbohydrate.
// Days to 50% tumor incidence.
The diets were balanced by weight, not calories, with substitution of fat for sucrose and were fed from weaning. Tumor growth rate was measured also in this experiment and was found to be much lower in rats fed 2% linoleic acid (0.2 ± 0.2 [S.D.] mm/month) than in rats fed coconut oil (4.0 ± 0.6) or corn oil (7.2 ± 0.8). Regression of tumors occurred only in rats fed 2% linoleic acid.
¶ In this experiment, all rats were fed the 20% corn oil diet until 3 weeks after DMBA treatment and then the diet containing 2% linoleic acid was fed to the designated group. Diets were balanced by weight, not calories.
** Diets balanced by calories with substitution of fat for carbohydrate and fed from weaning.
†† Fed beginning 48 hours after DMBA treatment.

acid supplementation or in which total fat content has been below 2%, the presence of dietary deficiency must be suspected. A fat requirement has not been defined for the rat, but optimal growth and reproduction appear to require a dietary content of 5% or greater. The requirement for essential fatty acids is defined (National Academy of Sciences 1978, Rogers 1979). Mammary gland development and the hormonal milieu may be quite different in rats fed diets extremely low in fat than in normal rats or rats fed high-fat diets (Knazek et al. 1980).

Corn and sunflower seed oils influence tumorigenesis even if fed after carcinogen exposure (Carroll and Khor 1975, Wetsel et al. 1981) (Table 1). This suggests that corn oil, rather than acting during initiation, is a promoter of mammary tumorigenesis. However, in studies using lard we have found an effect if the fat was fed before and after carcinogen exposure, but no effect if it was fed

TABLE 2. *Selenium and mammary tumorigenesis in female Sprague-Dawley rats*

Selenium (mg/kg)	Fat	Carcinogen	Tumor incidence (%)	Latent period (days)	No. tumors/ tumor-bearing rat	Reference
0.5	—*	NMU, 50 mg/kg	95	—†	4	Thompson and Becci 1980
5.5	—		85	—	2	
0.01	—	NMU, 35 mg/kg	68	—	1	
1.0	—		68	—	1	
<0.02	Corn oil,		17	90‡	1	Ip and Sinha
0.1	1%	DMBA, 5 mg	12	100	1	1981, Ip 1981
<0.02	Corn oil,		44	88	2	
0.1	5%		33	88	2	
<0.02	Corn oil,		96	72	4	
0.1	25%		60	85	3	
<0.02	Corn oil, 1%		29	101	—	
0.1	Coconut oil, 24%		24	97	—	

* Natural product diet, fat content not given.
† Authors stated that high-selenium diet increased the latent period.
‡ Time to palpable tumor.

only after exposure (Wetsel et al. 1981) (Table 1). Therefore, lard appears to influence tumorigenesis at initiation and not to be effective at later stages. This finding emphasizes further the fact that dietary fats differ in their effects on tumorigenesis and that the differences may be both qualitative and quantitative. The effect of diets that contain amounts of fat between the 5% and 20% levels usually studied and the exact time periods during which they influence carcinogenesis are not known and represent areas in which research is needed.

There are several mechanisms by which dietary fat may act. It may alter the endocrine system, directly affect mammary gland growth, differentiation, and responses to hormonal or other influences, induce membrane abnormalities by changing their composition or increasing peroxidation, influence carcinogen metabolism or DNA repair processes, or have other effects in the complex series of events that results in tumor development.

INTERACTIONS OF HORMONES AND DIET IN MAMMARY TUMORIGENESIS

Induction of hormonal imbalances may be one pathway by which tumor development is influenced by dietary fat; two hormones, prolactin (PRL) and estrogen, have received the greatest attention to date.

Higher dietary fat content appears to be associated with increased incidence of breast cancer (Gray et al. 1979, Korenman 1980, Miller 1978). Might this apparent correlation be linked via circulating PRL levels? First, some data have been offered that support a connection between dietary fat and blood PRL: Hill and Wynder (1976, 1979) reported that the consumption of a high-fat diet is associated with elevated nocturnal levels of prolactin in plasmas of both male and female subjects, compared with those of subjects ingesting a diet of lower fat content. And second, at least some find subjects with mammary carcinoma to have elevated circulating levels of PRL (Malarkey et al. 1977).

While data of this nature in humans are suggestive at best, evidence pointing to an association between PRL and breast cancer and between dietary fat intake and PRL is more compelling from studies in rats. First, spontaneous tumor incidence is enhanced in rats (Welsch and Nagasawa 1977) and mice (Yanai and Nagasawa 1972) that have received pituitary isografts, suggesting that a pituitary factor is important in tumorigenesis. In addition, mammary cancers induced by 3-methylcholanthrene (3MC) (Dao and Sunderland 1959) or MRMT-1 implants (Harada 1976) regress if rats are hypophysectomized. That such effects are possibly attributable to PRL is suggested by such findings as: (1) the reduction in 3MC-induced tumorigenesis caused by ovariectomy is reversed by implantation of "mammotropic hormone"–producing tumors (Dao and Sunderland 1959, Kim and Furth 1960); (2) the reduction in dimethylbenzanthracene (DMBA)-tumorigenesis produced by combined ovariectomy-adrenalectomy is reversed by PRL but not growth hormone (GH) administration (Nagasawa and Yanai 1970, Leung and Sasaki 1975, Asselin et al. 1977), though in some cases both PRL and estrogen treatment are required or more effective; (3) MRMT-1 mammary tumor growth is enhanced by injections of pituitary homogenates or PRL alone (or by pituitary isografts) (Harada 1976); (4) injections of an anti-PRL serum reduce DMBA-induced mammary tumor proliferation (Butler and Pearson 1971). The connection between ovariectomy's reducing and PRL's restoring tumor growth is that estrogen secretion stimulates pituitary PRL secretion (Chen and Meites 1970). In the absence of ovaries, PRL secretion falls, and tumorigenesis by most routes is diminished. Of course, some also believe estrogens have a direct action on mammary tumorigenesis (e.g., Leung and Sasaki 1975, Asselin et al. 1977); this is discussed further below.

The notion that PRL is an essential element in mammary tumorigenesis, of course, is not proved conclusively from animal studies. One disparity involves timing. PRL promotes carcinogenesis if present in excess following tumor induction, but, if anything, suppresses induction if circulating levels are high before and during the time the initiator is administered (see Welsch and Nagasawa 1977, Meites 1972). Pituitary isografts implanted prior to induction by DMBA have a similar suppressing effect (Welsch et al. 1968), consistent with the findings with PRL itself. A second disparity relates to changes in plasma PRL that occur after treatments designed to induce tumorigenesis. If PRL is involved in induction or promotion, one hypothesis might be that plasma PRL would be elevated following treatment to induce tumor formation. This is found to occur transiently by some (e.g., Harada 1976, Kerdelhue and El Abed 1979), but not by other (Meites 1972) investigators. Clearly, more data are needed to resolve this question.

A related line of investigation that ties PRL to mammary carcinogenesis is the effects on tumor induction of neuropharmacologic agents that influence PRL secretion. Interesting results have been obtained in rats using a category of drug that modifies the secretion of dopamine (DA) from the median eminence. The control of pituitary PRL secretion is mediated largely by the hypothalamus, and especially by the median eminence. Unique neural elements reside within the median eminence, synthesize DA, and release it into the hypothalamohypophyseal portal circulation (see, for example, Fernstrom and Wurtman 1977). This "hormonal" DA interacts at the pituitary level to *suppress* PRL secretion. Thus, to *reduce* PRL secretion, one administers a drug that either stimulates DA production or release (e.g., dopa or pargyline) or acts directly as a DA agonist (e.g., bromocryptine). To *enhance* PRL secretion, one provides a drug that diminishes DA release (presumably reserpine) or directly blocks DA receptors (e.g., haloperidol) (see Fernstrom and Wurtman 1977).

With the aid of such neuropharmacologic agents, investigators have administered drugs to raise or lower serum PRL levels and studied whether such treatments modified the tumorigenic potential of chemical carcinogens. For example, dopa (Lu and Meites 1971), monoamine oxidase inhibitors (Lu and Meites 1971), LSD (Quadri and Meites 1971), and DA agonists (Pasteels et al. 1971) have been reported to suppress PRL secretion in rodents and also to reduce tumor growth and number (Yanai and Nagasawa 1972. Quadri et al. 1973a, 1973b, Brooks and Welsch 1974, Chan and Cohen 1974). This effect of DA agonists, like bromocryptine, is seen in rats following tumor induction with DMBA (Chan and Cohen 1974), and in mice studied for spontaneous tumor incidence (Yanai and Nagasawa 1972, Brooks and Welsch 1974). Consistent with this set of observations are the findings that (1) alpha-methyldopa both raises serum prolactin (Lu and Meites 1971, Wiggins et al. 1980) and increases DMBA-induced tumorigenesis (Quadri et al. 1973b); (2) reserpine, which also elevates serum PRL (e.g., Sved et al. 1979), increases tumor appearance and growth rate when administered after (but not before) DMBA (Welsch and Meites 1970); and (3) haloperidol, a DA antagonist (see Cooper et al. 1978), increases tumorigenesis in DMBA-treated rats (Quadri et al. 1973a).

The success in rats of the DA approach has led to trials of dopa and bromocryptine for controlling human breast cancer, unfortunately with only minimal success (Smithline et al. 1975). However, since only a fraction of human breast cancers are hormone dependent, perhaps more careful evaluation of patients is necessary to identify those whose cancers fit into this category and thus may be more likely to respond favorably to this form of therapy. Alternatively, despite the consistency of the data obtained in animals, perhaps too few data have yet been obtained to understand fully how or whether PRL is important in the induction or promotion process. In fact, very few data have been published on the effects of the above pharmacologic agents on blood PRL levels in DMBA-treated rats during the tumorigenic process. It is often difficult to conclude from published data if a particular drug treatment actually had an effect on blood PRL, since only single or occasional measurements have been made. This seems especially surprising, owing to the facts that (1) the natural history of blood PRL levels in the cycling female rat exhibits enormous variation (Saunders et al. 1976), and (2) the drugs employed to alter DA release often differ substantially in the extent and duration of their effect on blood PRL levels. Hence, it seems prudent to reexamine the relationship of serum PRL levels to breast cancer incidence in rats to obtain time profiles of blood hormone levels over extended periods associated with the induction and promotion phases of mammary carcinogenesis.

Finally, the associations in rats among dietary fat, serum PRL levels, and cancer incidence find some support in the work of Chan and associates (1975). They observed that the intake of high-fat diets by rats caused elevated circulating levels of PRL during proestrus-estrus. They also observed that the ingestion of such high-fat diets by DMBA-treated female rats was associated with enhanced tumor appearance and proliferation (Chan and Cohen 1974), an effect that could be abolished with bromocryptine treatment. This latter finding further suggested PRL is an important intermediary for DMBA (and presumably fat intake–related) tumorigenesis. However, many more data are needed to evaluate fully whether high-fat diets fed to DMBA-treated rats lead to sustained, or only transient, increases in serum PRL levels, and if bromocryptine treatment produces long-term, continuous suppression of serum PRL levels in animals showing beneficial effects from the drug.

Briefly, the induction or promotion of mammary cancer by DMBA, while appearing to be influenced to a great extent by PRL, seems also to be dependent on ovarian steroids. Estrogens have received the greatest attention, although some data are also available regarding progesterone (e.g., Dao and Sunderland 1959, Welsch et al. 1968).

The importance of sex steroids is suggested by the fact that ovariectomy alone or in combination with adrenalectomy generally reduces dramatically the ability of DMBA to induce cancer (Asselin et al. 1977, Welsch et al. 1968, Pearson et al. 1969, Sinha et al. 1973). Injections of estradiol will restore the ability of DMBA to induce mammary cancer in rats (Pearson et al. 1969). The mechanism of this effect is usually attributed to an indirect action on blood PRL, since ovariectomy reduces serum PRL (Sinha et al. 1973), and estrogen injections restore serum PRL levels to normal in ovariectomized rats (Pearson et al. 1969). In addition, estradiol implants into the median eminence have been shown to raise serum PRL and increase DMBA tumorigenesis (Nagasawa et al. 1969), and estrogen appears ineffective at restoring DMBA tumorigenesis in ovariectomized-adrenalectomized rats that have been hypophysectomized (Pearson et al. 1969). Despite this suggested link through PRL, other results infer an additional, direct role for estrogens in DMBA-induced tumorigenesis, perhaps at the mammary level (Leung and Sasaki 1975, Asselin et al. 1977). Of interest in the putative relationship of dietary fat to mammary tumorigenesis has been the finding that antiestrogenic compounds, administered to rats consuming high-fat diets, appear to diminish the incidence of cancer (Chan and Cohen 1974). This type of data is quite interesting, but much further work is required to assess the directness (and correctness) of the link between dietary fat and breast cancer via changes in serum estrogens. It seems an obvious necessity to determine, for example, whether the reported changes in serum PRL with high-fat intake account for or contribute to any estrogen-related alteration in tumorigenesis.

OTHER DIET-RELATED MODULATORS
OF MAMMARY TUMORIGENESIS

Other diet-induced effects that may be important include changes in cell turnover and differentiation and in membrane composition or peroxidation of membrane lipids.

DNA synthesis and differentiation in the rat mammary gland are correlated with susceptibility to carcinogenesis. In general, there is increased susceptibility with increased DNA synthesis and decreased susceptibility with increased differentiation (Russo and Russo 1980a, 1980b). The age effect is not seen if DMBA is administered locally rather than parenterally or intragastrically (Sinha and Dao 1980), but local administration results in a much greater exposure of the gland to carcinogen, which may overcome the effect of age.

Alternatively, the age dependence may rest on the state of DMBA metabolism in the liver and other tissues, possibly mediated by hormonal control. Age-related changes in hydrocarbon metabolism by mammary gland and liver cells and in DMBA binding by mammary gland (Greiner et al. 1980, Janss and Ben 1978) have been reported. Since dietary fat influences hepatic mixed function oxidases (Hammer and Wills 1980), its effect on carcinogenesis could operate through this mechanism rather than or in addition to influencing endocrine status.

The peroxide content of tissues and peroxidation damage to cell membranes arc postulated to play a role in carcinogenesis (Demopoulos et al. 1980). Diets high in unsaturated fat increase tissue peroxide content by increasing the degree of unsaturation of membrane lipids and rendering them susceptible to peroxidation; the diets themselves contain peroxidized lipids that may be absorbed but probably are rapidly destroyed (Demopoulos et al. 1980, Iritani et al. 1980).

There is no evidence that diets containing 20–25% fat by weight cause serious nutritional disturbances in rats. However, they may induce marginal abnormalities that may, in turn, be responsible for enhanced carcinogenesis. For example, high-fat diets may induce a relative deficiency of selenium, thereby reducing protection against endogenous peroxidation. DMBA mammary tumorigenesis was increased in rats fed a 25% corn oil, low-selenium diet compared to rats fed the same diet with an adequate selenium content or fed the low-selenium diet with a lower fat content (Ip 1981). A protective effect of selenium against mammary tumorigenesis has not been clearly demonstrated under conditions in which dietary fat is not high (Table 2).

Other nutritional questions to be considered in interpreting the dietary studies are the adequacy of the low-fat diets, as discussed above, and the possible effects of high-fat diets on weight gain and feed utilization. In most studies summarized in Table 1, the authors reported no effect on body weight or a relatively small effect, i.e., 10% difference or less between groups. It seems unlikely that a difference of that magnitude would induce the marked effects reported on tumor development. Hopkins and Carroll (1979) reported that differences in absorption of fats did not correlate with their effect on tumorigenesis, and we have not found differences in efficiency of utilization of diets to explain their influence on tumorigenesis (Rogers and Wetsel 1981, Wetsel et al. 1981).

Another nutrient-related effect on mammary carcinogenesis is suppression by vitamin A or synthetic retinoids (Moon et al. 1979, Welsch et al. 1980) (Table 3). There are no epidemiologic data to suggest a relationship between

TABLE 3. *Retinoids and mammary tumorigenesis in female Sprague-Dawley rats*

Retinoid	Carcinogen	% Mammary tumors	Reference
Retinyl acetate*			Grubbs et al. 1977
0	DMBA, 5 mg	32	
0	DMBA, 15 mg	65	
380	DMBA, 5 mg	33	
760		23	
380	DMBA, 15 mg	50	
760		37	
Retinyl methylether*			
380	DMBA, 5 mg	10	
760		10	
380	DMBA, 15 mg	50	
760		35	
Retinyl acetate†·‡			Welsch et al. 1980
328	NMU 5 mg/100 g	37	
0		73	
328	NMU 2.5 mg/100 g	10	
0		27	

* nM/kg diet added to natural ingredient diet beginning 1 week after DMBA (given at 50 days).

† mg/kg diet added to natural ingredient diet beginning 3 days after NMU (given at 50 and 57 days).

‡ The average number of tumors per tumor-bearing rat was decreased from 4 to 2 and from 2 to 1 in treated rats in the 2 experiments shown. The authors state that treatment had no effect on latent period.

vitamin A nutriture and breast cancer, and it is likely that the effect is pharmacological since it is expressed in rats given toxic doses of vitamin A. Like corn oil, retinoids exert their influences after carcinogen treatment. Retinyl acetate did not alter serum PRL (Welsch et al. 1980), but mammary gland development was inhibited (Moon et al. 1979). Retinyl acetate blocked carcinogen-induced DNA synthesis in the mammary gland (Mehta and Moon 1980). Detailed studies of hormonal effects or effects on cell division and morphology of the gland by retinoid treatment are needed. The many effects of vitamin A on composition of cell membranes and on enzyme activity (Lotan 1980) suggest that such studies would be fruitful.

Certain of the dietary effects on mammary carcinogenesis and their possible interactions with the endocrine system are discussed below in conjunction with results of studies in progress in our laboratories.

STUDIES IN PROGRESS OF MECHANISMS BY WHICH DIETARY FAT INFLUENCES MAMMARY CARCINOGENESIS

Fat and DMBA or Spontaneous Tumorigenesis

Many different fats have been studied in DMBA-treated female rats and shown to enhance tumorigenesis. We are evaluating hormonal status and mammary gland development in DMBA-treated rats fed corn oil, lard, beef tallow, or high erucic acid rapeseed oil (HEAR). The diets (Table 4) are adjusted to

TABLE 4. *Experimental diets* *

	g/100 g diet		Calories/100 g diet	
Component	5% Fat	20% Fat	5% Fat	20% Fat
Casein (vitamin-free)	19.9	22.7	80	91
Carbohydrate†	67.6	48.8	270	195
Corn oil‡	1.0	1.1	9	10
Test fat§	4.0	18.7	36	168
Minerals//	5.2	6.0	—	—
Vitamins#	2.3	2.7	6	9

* Each diet is incorporated into a 5% aqueous solution of agar.
† Equal parts sucrose, dextrose, and dextrin.
‡ Corn oil was present in all diets to assure adequate linoleic acid.
§ Corn oil, lard, tallow, rapeseed oil.
// Rogers-Harper salt mixture supplemented with manganese, zinc, fluoride, and chromium to meet current recommended dietary content for rats (NAS-NRC 1978, Rogers 1979).
Vitamins/kg of low-fat diet: vitamin A acetate, 32,475 I.U.; vitamin D_2, 3,248 I.U.; vitamin E, 169 mg; menadione, 1.1 mg; thiamine HCl, 8.7 mg; riboflavin, 4.3 mg; nicotinamide, 54.1 mg; pyridoxine HCl, 8.7 mg; calcium pantothenate, 21.7 mg; folic acid, 10.8 mg; inositol, 270.6 mg; choline chloride, 3,000 mg; vitamin B_{12}, 50 mg; and sucrose, 21 g.

give constant protein, vitamin, and mineral intake per calorie. DMBA mammary tumorigenesis is significantly increased in rats fed the diet containing 20% corn oil compared with rats fed 5% corn oil (Wetsel et al. 1981) (Table 1). The results are the same whether the high–corn oil diet is fed throughout the experiment or only beginning 48 hours after administration of DMBA.

When lard was fed in place of corn oil, tumorigenesis again was increased when the diet contained 20% fat throughout the experiment but not if rats were fed 20% fat beginning 48 hours after DMBA treatment (Table 1). There was no discernible effect of diet on tumor regression, which occurred in 45–55% of tumor-bearing rats in each group, or on reappearance of tumors that had regressed completely (25–50%).

Studies in progress show that not all fats increase DMBA mammary tumorigenesis, even if the diets are supplemented with essential fatty acids and selenium. Rats have been treated with 2.5 mg DMBA following the same protocol and fed the same diets (Table 4) with beef tallow or HEAR in place of corn oil or lard. The diet high in tallow has supported a slightly earlier appearance of tumors than the low-tallow diet, but changing the concentration of rapeseed oil has no effect (Table 5).

The 1.1% corn oil supplement we fed was lower than the 3% oil supplements in high-tallow diets that raised tumor incidence to the same level as occurred in rats fed 20% sunflower seed oil (Hopkins and Carroll 1979) (Table 1). It was similar to the 1% corn oil supplement in a high–coconut oil diet that did not increase DMBA tumorigenesis (Ip and Sinha 1980) (Table 2). These data suggest that the amount of polyunsaturated oil supplement is critical and that the effective content is greater than 1%. Linoleic acid content alone is not responsible for the effect, since 2% linoleic acid (equivalent to about 3.5%

TABLE 5. *DMBA mammary tumorigenesis in female Sprague-Dawley rats fed diets high in beef tallow or rapeseed oil**

Dietary fat†		Tumor incidence (%)	Days to palpable tumor
Type	% Weight		
Beef tallow	5	69	122
	20	71	109
HEAR	5	71	114
	20	63	110

* The experiment is in progress, and the results are preliminary. A concurrent group fed 5% or 20% corn oil in the diet is giving results consistent with earlier experiments; tumor latency is 130 days in rats fed 20% corn oil and 157 days in rats fed 5% corn oil.

† See Table 4. Diets designated 5% or 20% tallow or HEAR actually contain 4% or 18.7% of the fat plus 1% or 1.1% corn oil.

corn oil) did not increase DMBA tumorigenesis in rats fed 18% coconut oil to the level in rats fed 20% corn oil (King et al. 1979) (Table 1). HEAR contains 18% linoleic acid. (The oil was supplied and analyzed by E. R. Farnsworth, Animal Research Institute, Ottawa, Ontario.)

Rats subjected to the same dietary treatments (lard, corn oil) as the DMBA-treated rats but given no DMBA are being studied for development of spontaneous mammary tumors. At approximately 21 months, the tumor incidence is 35% and 20% in rats fed 20% or 5% corn oil, respectively, and 23% and 25% in rats fed 20% or 5% lard. Rats fed corn oil have developed tumors earlier than rats fed lard; the average latent periods are 416 days (20% corn oil), 379 days (5% corn oil), 460 days (20% lard), and 483 days (5% lard).

Effects of Dietary Fat on Sexual Maturation, Estrous Cycles, and Serum Hormone Content

Sexual maturation, measured by age at vaginal opening, was slightly accelerated by diets high in corn oil or lard but was delayed by tallow or erucic acid. The average changes in either direction were 1 day (Table 6). Frisch et al. (1975) reported acceleration by 2 days in rats fed a high-fat (25%) diet compared with rats fed 5% fat; first estrus also occurred earlier. The high-fat animals weighed less at onset of puberty than the low-fat animals, but both groups had reached the same caloric intake based on body weight, which was postulated to be the metabolic signal for puberty. Since estrus followed vaginal opening more quickly in rats fed the high-fat diet, the authors suggested that pituitary function was stimulated in them.

The duration of estrous cycles of tallow-fed rats in the current experiment

TABLE 6. *Age at vaginal opening in female Sprague-Dawley rats fed control or high-fat diets*

Dietary fat*			Age at vaginal opening (Days, $\overline{X} \pm$ S.E.)
Type	% wt	No. rats	
Corn oil	5	240	31 ± 0.2
Corn oil	20	75	30 ± 0.4
Lard	5	75	32 ± 0.4
Lard	20	75	31 ± 0.4
Corn oil	5	40	34 ± 0.6
Corn oil	20	20	33 ± 0.8
Beef tallow	5	110	32 ± 0.3
Beef tallow	20	55	33 ± 0.5
HEAR†	5	110	33 ± 0.4
HEAR	20	54	34 ± 0.5

* See Table 4. Lard, tallow, and erucic acid diets designated 5% or 20% actually contain 4% or 18.7% of the fat plus 1% or 1.1% corn oil.
† High erucic acid rapeseed oil.

has not been affected by the amount of fat or by DMBA. Irregular estrous cycles were occurring by age 30 weeks in 15–35% of rats fed corn oil or lard and in 30–100% of rats fed tallow or HEAR, but there was no apparent relationship to the amount of dietary fat or to DMBA treatment. More detailed analyses of duration and regularity of estrous cycles are in progress.

Weight and histologic evaluation of ovaries, pituitary, uterus, and adrenals show no consistent dietary effect.

Serum hormone content was measured in rats fed corn oil or lard and bled at estrus or diestrus II (Table 7). The studies were performed to look for large dietary effects over the diurnal and estrous cycles in preparation for more extensive studies. As discussed in the introduction, full evaluation of dietary or other effects on the endocrine system requires sampling at many points. Estradiol tended to be higher in serum of rats fed 20% corn oil than in any other group and to be higher in rats fed corn oil than in rats fed lard. In the high-fat groups there was a more consistent pattern than in rats fed low-fat diets of higher estradiol values at diestrus II than at estrus. Progesterone content was quite uniform in all groups and gave no suggestion of a dietary effect. Prolactin

TABLE 7. *Serum hormone content in rats fed diets containing 5% or 20% fat as corn oil or lard*

Dietary fat		Age (weeks)					
		10		15		21	
Type	% Weight	E	D	E	D	E	D
Estradiol* (pg/ml)							
Corn oil	5	29 ± 12	19 ± 3	49 ± 20	34 ± 12	64 ± 14	37 ± 13
	20	60 ± 16	73 ± 12	43 ± 11	72 ± 10	41 ± 12	64 ± 17
Lard	5	10 ± 5	14 ± 4	12 ± 5	35 ± 7	35 ± 12	17 ± 5
	20	9 ± 4	29 ± 12	26 ± 8	53 ± 13	25 ± 6	33 ± 7
Progesterone* (ng/ml)							
Corn oil	5	21 ± 2	22 ± 3	21 ± 2	18 ± 1	24 ± 2	30 ± 7
	20	19 ± 3	27 ± 6	22 ± 2	23 ± 3	24 ± 3	25 ± 2
Lard	5	23 ± 2	20 ± 3	25 ± 3	25 ± 2	29 ± 1	30 ± 3
	20	18 ± 2	19 ± 3	23 ± 2	30 ± 8	27 ± 3	39 ± 8
Prolactin* (ng/ml)							
Corn oil	5	555 ± 226	83 ± 28	338 ± 119	47 ± 14	—	—†
	20	586 ± 287	66 ± 25	250 ± 73	39 ± 13	—	—
Lard	5	680 ± 252	88 ± 25	156 ± 47	41 ± 15	—	—
	20	922 ± 304	68 ± 31	236 ± 74	100 ± 62	—	—

E, estrus; D, diestrus.
* Average ± S.E., 3–6 rats/group.
† Not measured.

was highly variable. The difference between the two times of the cycle was evident, but no effect of diet could be discerned. Growth hormone was measured in selected rats to ascertain whether it could be used to determine if the differences in PRL levels were the result of stress. Growth hormone is decreased in stressed male rats (Martin 1976) and episodic surges occur in female rats unrelated to stage of estrus (Saunders et al. 1976). We found no evidence of a relationship between serum content of PRL and growth hormone.

The preliminary results emphasize the need for detailed studies of serum hormone content in diet- and carcinogen-treated rats in evaluation of dietary and endocrine interactions.

Vitamin A-treated rats have been reported to have normal estrous cycles and serum PRL, and ovaries, adrenals, and pituitary of normal weight (Grubbs et al. 1977, Moon et al. 1979, Welsch et al. 1981). Again, more detailed studies are needed.

Dietary Fat, Mammary Gland DNA Synthesis, and Differentiation

Whole mounts of grossly normal mammary glands were prepared from DMBA-treated rats fed corn oil, lard, or tallow and necropsied when they bore mammary tumors. There was a small but consistent difference between dietary groups in that glands were somewhat more highly differentiated in rats fed the low-fat diets. Younger rats fed the 5% and 20% corn oil diets were then studied. If cycling, they were killed on day 2 of diestrus, 2 hours after intraperitoneal injection of 2.5 μCi [^{3}H]thymidine per gram body weight. Counts were made in autoradiographs of ^{3}H-labeled cells in the developing mammary glands. In rats examined at 35 days there was a greater shift in labeling, compared with 22-day-old rats, in rats fed 20% corn oil than in rats fed 5% corn oil (Table 8); no other significant differences were found. Whole mounts of mammary glands from the same rats again showed a slight but consistent increase in differentiation in rats fed the low-fat diet (Figure 1).

It appears, therefore, that the 20% corn oil diet retards differentiation slightly but does not cause significant alteration in DNA synthesis in the mammary gland in the time period during which initiation and early growth of tumors occur. Studies of the combined effect of dietary fat and carcinogen treatment are in progress. Retinyl acetate also had no effect on DNA synthesis in normal mammary glands, but inhibited the increase that followed NMU or DMBA treatment (Mehta and Moon 1980).

Kinetics of the cell cycle in the mammary gland change with differentiation induced by age or pregnancy; the terminal end buds and ducts, structures with most rapid epithelial cell turnover, decrease and disappear, whereas alveolar structures, with slower epithelial turnover, increase (Russo and Russo 1980b). These investigators have presented strong arguments in favor of a relationship between gland differentiation, i.e., the relative numbers of structures with different turnover times, and susceptibility to carcinogenesis. The degree of differentia-

TABLE 8. *DNA labeling index of terminal structures in the mammary glands of virgin Sprague-Dawley rats fed 20% or 5% corn oil in the diet*

Age (days)*	% Corn oil in diet	Terminal end bud ($\bar{X} \pm$ S.E.)	Terminal duct ($\bar{X} \pm$ S.E.)	Alveolar bud and lobule ($\bar{X} \pm$ S.E.)
22	(weanling rats)	17.8 ± 3.9	2.5 ± 0.3	6.7 ± 1.0
35	5	14.6 ± 0.2	2.1 ± 0.6	2.7 ± 1.6
	20	12.6 ± 0.0†	3.5 ± 0.0†	2.6 ± 0.0
55	5	not present	11.3 ± 3.0	8.0 ± 2.3
	20	not present	6.7 ± 2.4	5.5 ± 2.0
83–102	5	not present	1.0 ± 0.5	0.6 ± 0.3
	20	not present	0.5 ± 0.3	0.2 ± 0.05
142–147	5	not present	4.3 ± 0.7	4.3 ± 1.0
	20	not present	7.4 ± 3.5	5.2 ± 2.4

* 5 rats per group; studied on second day of diestrus after regular cycles established.
† Different from 5% corn oil, P < 0.05.

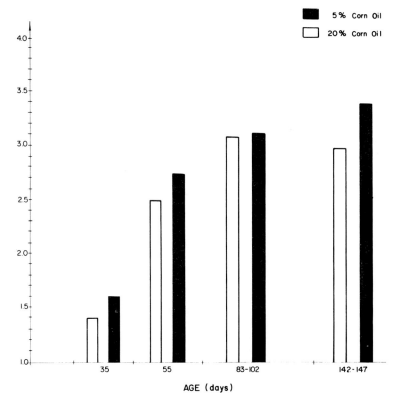

FIG. 1. Mammary gland differentiation in rats fed 5% or 20% corn oil. The glands were evaluated in whole mounts and graded 1–4 on the basis of ductal, acinar, and lobule development.

tion is, of course, hormonally induced, but the emphasis in this view is on local factors that control susceptibility to carcinogenesis. The Russos have shown that pregnancy confers long-term resistance to DMBA carcinogenesis. They attribute the resistance to persistent differences in structure and related differences in cell kinetics and the size of the proliferative compartment. These differences are postulated to govern carcinogen binding to DNA, subsequent DNA repair, and cell division required for expression of transformation (Russo and Russo 1980a). The evidence for the sequence of events is taken largely from studies in skin and liver, and confirmation requires studies in the mammary gland.

The argument presented raises questions about design of measures to prevent mammary tumorigenesis, since it implies that continuous dietary or other influence may be less important than one major differentiating effect such as pregnancy. However, epidemiologic evidence, while supporting the existence of an effect of pregnancy, indicates that it is weak relative to environmental effects, including diet.

CONCLUSIONS

High dietary fat content is correlated with a high incidence of breast cancer in humans and increased mammary tumorigenesis in rats. There are several mechanisms postulated to account for these observations, the most fully investigated being diet-induced changes in endocrine status. Studies to confirm and extend the results are needed, as are definition of the amount of fat necessary to increase tumorigenesis, the types of fat that are effective, and the time during which they must be fed to be effective.

Vitamin A and related compounds and selenium inhibit mammary tumorigenesis under certain experimental conditions. The mechanism by which they act is not known; there is some evidence that vitamin A inhibits both DNA synthesis and differentiation in the gland and that selenium is effective because of its antioxidant properties. Again, time and dose responses are not fully defined. Vitamin A appears to be effective only at toxic or near-toxic doses.

Design of dietary measures to reduce breast cancer incidence requires understanding and better definition of the effects of these and probably other nutrients in animal models of mammary tumorigenesis.

REFERENCES

Asselin, J., P. A. Kelly, M. G. Caron, and F. Labrie. 1977. Control of hormone receptor levels and growth of 7,12-dimethylbenz(a)anthracene-induced mammary tumors by estrogens, progesterone and prolactin. Endocrinology 101:666–671.

Brooks, C. L., and C. W. Welsch. 1974. Inhibition of mammary dysplasia in estrogen-treated C3H/Hed female mice by treatment with 2-bromo-a-ergocryptine (37836). Proc. Soc. Exp. Biol. Med. 145:484–487.

Butler, T. P., and O. H. Pearson. 1971. Regression of prolactin-dependent rat mammary carcinoma in response to antihormone treatment. Cancer Res. 31:817–820.

Carroll, K. K. 1980. Lipids and carcinogenesis. J. Environ. Pathol. Toxicol. 3:253–271.

Carroll, K. K., and H. T. Khor. 1975. Dietary fat in relation to tumorigenesis. Prog. Biochem. Pharmacol. 10:308–353.

Chan, P., and L. A. Cohen. 1974. Effect of dietary fat, antiestrogen and antiprolactin on the development of mammary tumors in rats. JNCI 52:25–30.

Chan, P. C., and T. L. Dao. 1981. Enhancement of mammary carcinogenesis by a high-fat diet in Fischer, Long-Evans and Sprague-Dawley rats. Cancer Res. 41:164–167.

Chan, P., F. Didato, and L. Cohen. 1975. High dietary fat, elevation of rat serum prolactin and mammary cancer. Proc. Soc. Exp. Biol. Med. 149:133–135.

Chan, P. C., J. F. Head, L. A. Cohen, and E. L. Wynder. 1977. Influence of dietary fat on the induction of mammary tumors by N-nitroso methylurea: Associated hormone changes and differences between Sprague-Dawley and F344 rats. JNCI 59:1279–1283.

Chen, C. L., and J. Meites. 1970. Effects of estrogen and progesterone on serum and pituitary prolactin levels in ovariectomized rats. Endocrinology 86:503–505.

Cooper, J. R., F. E. Bloom, and R. H. Roth. 1978. The Biochemical Basis of Neuropharmacology, 3rd ed. Oxford, New York, 327 pp.

Dao, T. L., and H. Sunderland. 1959. Mammary carcinogenesis by 3-methyl cholanthrene. I. Hormonal aspects of tumor induction and growth. JNCI 23:567–585.

Demopoulos, H. B., D. D. Pietronigro, E. S. Flamm, and M. L. Seligman. 1980. The possible role of free radical reactions in carcinogenesis. J. Environ. Pathol. Toxicol. 3:273–303.

Fernstrom, J. D., and R. J. Wurtman. 1977. Brain monoamines and reproductive function, *in* Reproductive Physiology II, R. O. Greep, ed. University Park Press, Baltimore, pp. 23–56.

Frisch, R. E., D. M. Hegsted, and K. Yoshinaga. 1975. Body weight and food intake at early estrus of rats on a high-fat diet. Proc. Natl. Acad. Sci. USA 72:4172–4176.

Gammal, E. B., K. K. Carroll, and E. R. Plunkett. 1967. Effects of dietary fat on mammary carcinogenesis by 7,12-dimethylbenz(α)anthracene in rats. Cancer Res. 28:384–385.

Gray, G. E., M. C. Pike, and B. E. Henderson. 1979. Breast-cancer incidence and mortality rates in different countries in relation to known risk factors and dietary practices. Br. J. Cancer 39:1–7.

Greiner, J. W., A. H. Bryan, L. B. Malan-Shibley, and D. H. Janss. 1980. Aryl hydrocarbon hydroxylase and epoxide hydratase activities: Age effects in mammary epithelial cells of Sprague-Dawley rats. JNCI 64:1127–1133.

Grubbs, C. J., R. C. Moon, M. B. Sporn, and D. L. Newton. 1977. Inhibition of mammary cancer by retinyl methyl ether. Cancer Res. 37:599–602.

Hammer, C. T., and E. D. Wills. 1980. Dependence of the rate of metabolism of benzo(a)pyrene on the fatty acid composition of the liver endoplasmic reticulum and on the dietary lipids. Nutrition and Cancer 2:113–118.

Harada, Y. 1976. Pituitary role in the growth of metastasizing MRMT-1 mammary carcinoma in rats. Cancer Res. 36:18–22.

Hill, P., and E. Wynder. 1976. Diet and prolactin release. Endocrinology 79:806–807.

Hill, P., and E. Wynder. 1979. Effect of a vegetarian diet and dexamethansone on plasma prolactin, testosterone and dehydroepiandrosterone in men and women. Cancer Lett. 7:273–282.

Hopkins, G. J., and K. K. Carroll. 1979. Relationship between amount and type of dietary fat in promotion of mammary carcinogenesis induced by 7,12-dimethylbenz(a)anthracene. JNCI 62:1009–1012.

Ip, C. 1981. Modification of mammary carcinogenesis and tissue peroxidation by selenium deficiency and dietary fat. Nutrition and Cancer 2:136–142.

Ip, C., and D. K. Sinha. 1981. Enhancement of mammary tumorigenesis by dietary selenium deficiency in rats with a high polyunsaturated fat intake. Cancer Res. 41:31–34.

Iritani, N., E. Fukuda, and Y. Kitamura. 1980. Effect of corn oil feeding on lipid peroxidation in rats. J. Nutr. 110:924–930.

Janss, D. H., and T. L. Ben. 1978. Age-related modification of 7,12-dimethylbenz[a]anthracene binding to rat mammary gland DNA. JNCI 60:173–177.

Kerdelhue, B., and A. E. Abed. 1979. Inhibition of preovulatory gonadotropin secretion and stimulation of prolactin secretion by 7,12-dimethylbenz(a)anthracene in Sprague-Dawley rats. Cancer Res. 39:4700–4705.

Kim, U., and J. Furth. 1960. Relation of mammary tumors to mammotropes. II. Hormone responsiveness of 3-methylcholanthrene induced mammary carcinomas (25622). Proc. Soc. Exp. Biol. Med. 103:643–645.

King, M. M., D. M. Bailey, D. D. Gibson, J. V. Pitha, and P. B. McCay. 1979. Incidence and growth of mammary tumors induced by 7,12-dimethylbenz[a]anthracene as related to the dietary content of fat and antioxidant. JNCI 63:657–663.

Knazek, R. A., S. C. Liu, J. S. Bodwin, and B. K. Vonderhaar. 1980. Requirement of essential fatty acids in the diet for development of the mouse mammary gland. JNCI 64:377–382.

Kollmorgen, G. M., M. M. King, J. F. Roszel, B. J. Daggs, and R. E. Longley. 1981. The influence of dietary fat and non-specific immunotherapy on carcinogen-induced rat mammary adenocarcinoma. Vet. Pathol. 18:82–91.

Korenman, S. G. 1980. The endocrinology of breast cancer. Cancer 46:874–878.

Leung, B. S., and G. H. Sasaki. 1975. On the mechanism of prolactin and estrogen action in 7,12 dimethylbenz(a)anthracene-induced mammary carcinoma in the rat. II. In vivo tumor responses and estrogen receptor. Endocrinology 97:564–572.

Lotan, R. 1980. Effects of vitamin A and its analogs (retinoids) on normal and neoplastic cells. Biochim. Biophys. Acta 605:33–91.

Lu, K., and J. Meites. 1971. Inhibition by L-dopa and monoamine oxidase inhibitors of pituitary prolactin release; stimulation by methyldopa and d-amphetamine (35604). Proc. Soc. Exp. Biol. Med. 137:480–483.

Malarkey, W. B., L. L. Schroeder, V. C. Stevens, A. G. James, and R. R. Lanese. 1977. Disordered nocturnal prolactin regulation in women with breast cancer. Cancer Res. 37:4650–4654.

Martin, J. B. 1976. Brain regulation of growth hormone secretion, in Frontiers in Neuroendocrinology, Vol. 4, L. Martini and W. F. Ganong, eds. Raven Press, New York, pp. 129–168.

Mehta, R. G., and R. C. Moon. 1980. Inhibition of DNA synthesis by retinyl acetate during chemically induced mammary carcinogenesis. Cancer Res. 40:1109–1111.

Meites, J. 1972. Relation of prolactin and estrogen to mammary tumorigenesis in the rat. JNCI 48:1217–1224.

Miller, A. B. 1978. An overview of hormone-associated cancers. Cancer Res. 38:3985–3990.

Moon, R. C., H. J. Thompson, P. J. Becci, C. J. Grubbs, R. J. Gander, D. L. Newton, J. M. Smith, S. L. Phillips, W. R. Henderson, L. T. Mullen, C. C. Brown, and M. B. Sporn. 1979. N-(4-hydroxyphenyl)retinamide, a new retinoid for prevention of breast cancer in the rat. Cancer Res. 39:1339–1346.

Nagasawa, H., C. L. Chen, and J. Meites. 1969. Effects of estrogen implant in median eminence on serum and pituitary prolactin levels in the rat. Proc. Soc. Exp. Biol. Med. 132:859–861.

Nagasawa, H., and R. Yanai. 1970. Effects of prolactin or growth hormone on growth of carcinogen-induced mammary tumors of adreno-ovarectomized rats. Int. J. Cancer 6:488–495.

National Academy of Sciences. The National Research Council. 1978. Nutrient Requirements of Laboratory Animals, No. 10, Ed. 3. National Academy of Sciences, Washington, D.C.

Pasteels, J. L., A. Danguy, M. Frerotte, and F. Ectors. 1971. Inhibition de la secretion de prolactine par l'ergocornine et la 2-Br-α-ergocryptine: action directe sur l'hypophyse en culture. Ann. Endocrinol. 32:188–192.

Pearson, O., O. Llerena, L. Llerena, A. Molina, and T. Butler. 1969. Prolactin-dependent rat mammary cancer: A model for man? Trans. Assoc. Am. Physicians 82:225–238.

Quadri, S. J., J. L. Clark, and J. Meites. 1973a. Effects of LSD, pargyline, and haloperidol on mammary tumor growth in rats. Proc. Soc. Exp. Biol. Med. 142:22–26.

Quadri, S. K., G. S. Kledzik, and J. Meites. 1973b. Effects of L-dopa and methyldopa on growth of mammary cancers in rats. Proc. Soc. Exp. Biol. Med. 142:759–761.

Quadri, S. K., and J. Meites. 1971. Induced decrease in serum prolactin in rats. Proc. Soc. Exp. Biol. Med. 137:1242–1243.

Reddy, B. S., L. A. Cohen, G. D. McCoy, P. Hill, J. H. Weisburger, and E. L. Wynder. 1980. Nutrition and its relationship to cancer. Adv. Cancer Res. 32:238–345.

Rogers, A. E. 1979. Nutrition, in The Laboratory Rat, H. J. Baker, J. R. Lindsey, and S. N. Weisbroth, eds. Academic Press, New York, pp. 123–152.

Rogers, A. E., and W. C. Wetsel. 1981. Mammary carcinogenesis in rats fed different amounts and types of fat. Cancer Res. 41:3735–3737.

Russo, J., and I. H. Russo. 1980a. Susceptibility of the mammary gland to carcinogenesis. Am. J. Pathol. 100:497–512.

Russo, J., and I. H. Russo. 1980b. Influence of differentiation and cell kinetics on the susceptibility of the rat mammary gland to carcinogenesis. Cancer Res. 40:2677–2687.

Saunders, A., L. C. Terry, J. Audet, P. Brazeau, and J. B. Martin. 1976. Dynamic studies of growth hormone and prolactin secretion in the female rat. Neuroendocrinology 21:193–203.

Sinha, D., D. Cooper, and T. L. Dao. 1973. The nature of estrogen and prolactin effect on mammary tumorigenesis. Cancer Res. 33:411–414.

Sinha, D. K., and T. L. Dao. 1980. Induction of mammary tumors in aging rats by 7,12-dimethylbenz[a]anthracene: Role of DNA synthesis during carcinogenesis. JNCI 64:519–521.

Smithline, F., L. Sherman, and H. D. Kolodny. 1975. Prolactin and breast cancer. N. Engl. J. Med. 292:784–792.

Sved, A. F., J. D. Fernstrom, and R. J. Wurtman. 1979. Tyrosine administration decreases serum prolactin levels in chronically-reserpinized rats. Life Sci. 25:1293–1300.

Thompson, H. J., and P. J. Becci. 1980. Selenium inhibition of N-methyl-N-nitrosourea-induced mammary carcinogenesis in the rat. JNCI 65:1299–1301.

Welsch, C. W., C. K. Brown, M. Goodrich-Smith, J. Chiusano, and R. C. Moon. 1980. Synergistic effect of chronic prolactin suppression and retinoid treatment in the prophylaxis of N-methyl-N-nitrosourea-induced mammary tumorigenesis in female Sprague-Dawley rats. Cancer Res. 40:3095–3098.

Welsch, C. W., J. A. Clemens, and J. Meites. 1968. Effects of multiple pituitary homografts or progesterone on 7,12-dimethylbenz(α)anthracene-induced mammary tumors in rats. JNCI 41:465–471.

Welsch, C. W., and J. Meites. 1970. Effects of reserpine on development of 7,12-dimethylbenzanthracene induced mammary tumors in female rats. Experientia 33:1133–1134.

Welsch, C. W., and H. Nagasawa. 1977. Prolactin and murine mammary tumorigenesis: A review. Cancer Res. 37:951–963.

Wetsel, W. C., A. E. Rogers, and P. M. Newberne. 1981. Detection and Prevention of Cancer (in press).

Wiggins, J. F., A. F. Sved, and J. D. Fernstrom. 1980. Effects of alpha-methyldopa and its metabolites on prolactin release: In vivo and in vitro studies. J. Pharmacol. Exp. Therap. 212:304–308.

Yanai, R., and H. Nagasawa. 1972. Inhibition of mammary tumorigenesis by ergot alkaloids and promotion of mammary tumorigenesis by pituitary isografts in adreno-ovariectomized mice. JNCI 48:715–719.

Molecular Interrelations of Nutrition and Cancer,
edited by M. S. Arnott, J. van Eys, and Y.-M. Wang.
Raven Press, New York © 1982.

The Chemopreventive Role of Selenium in Carcinogenesis

A. Clark Griffin

The University of Texas Science Park, Smithville, Texas 78957

The major objective of this chapter will be to discuss the role that selenium (Se) may have in the origin or genesis of tumors. Since knowledge of this trace or micronutrient has evolved through a prolonged period of considerable controversy, it will require some degree of sorting of the facts and fiction to attain this stated goal.

As most are now aware, Se compounds possess a high degree of toxicity and have been associated with a number of diseases or syndromes in animals, especially in areas where the Se exposure may be excessively high. Contrastingly, there are dozens of well-established Se-deficiency diseases in a variety of animals that respond to the administration of this element in one or more of its chemical forms. Recently, it has been reported that a cardiomyopathy occurs in children living in some areas within China that are markedly deficient in Se (Chen et al. 1981). This syndrome, called Keshan disease, responds to Se administration. Interestingly, other cardiomyopathies have been reported in other parts of the world, including Finland and even regions within the U.S.A.

These are rather remarkable nutritional findings. However, since this monograph is concerned with cancer, we may only note in passing that any major progress in the alleviation of cardiovascular problems may in the long run result in an older age population that will live to develop one or more cancers. The good news is that prevention of heart diseases via Se intervention may also prevent or delay carcinogenesis, the major theme and purpose of this presentation. The bottom line of this brief introduction is simply to inform you that Se is becoming increasingly recognized as an important trace nutrient required by cells of all higher forms as well as many lower forms of life.

The role of Se in cancer may be considered from three, and I believe fundamentally different, aspects. The first involves those reports that Se may be a causative factor of cancer. The second relates to studies claiming Se compounds may have some chemotherapeutic value in the treatment of certain established tumors, that is, these compounds will slow or even inhibit tumor growth. The third area concerns the role that Se may have in the inhibition of carcinogenesis, the basis for the possible chemopreventive effects attributed to this element. It is with this area that most of this chapter will be concerned. However, I will comment briefly on the first two mentioned aspects.

There have been scattered reports in the literature that Se administration may cause hepatic tumors in rodents. These studies are controversial but nevertheless provided the background that resulted in Se's being listed as a carcinogen according to the Delaney criteria. Se has since been removed from this select category, and this implication of carcinogenicity may be dealt with by a quotation that appeared in the I.A.R.C. monograph on the *Evaluation of Carcinogenic Risk of Chemicals to Man* (Vol. 9, 1975, page 245): "the available data provide no suggestion that selenium is carcinogenic in man." Likewise, Se compounds have not shown any remarkable effectiveness in the treatment of established tumors. Reference should be made to the recent report of Greeder and Milner (1980) that i.p. administration of various forms of Se inhibited the growth of Ehrlich ascites tumor.

INHIBITION OF CARCINOGENESIS BY SELENIUM IN ANIMAL MODEL SYSTEMS

There are increasing numbers of reports in the literature that Se administration will inhibit or greatly delay the appearance of tumors in a spectrum of animal model systems, and these are summarized in Table 1.

Clayton and Baumann in 1949 were among the first to report Se may be involved in carcinogenesis. Albino rats were maintained on semisynthetic diets and were given 0.064% 3′methyl-4-dimethyl aminoazobenzene (3′MeDAB) in the diet for 2 weeks. At that time, the animals were changed to the dye-free diet supplemented with 5 ppm Se (sodium selenite) for 4 weeks. Finally, the

TABLE 1. *Chemoprevention of experimental carcinogenesis by selenium compounds*

Chemopreventive compound	System	Species	Carcinogen	Reference
Sodium selenite	Colon	Rat	1,2 Dimethylhydrazine	Jacobs et al. 1977
" "			Methylazomymethanol	Jacobs et al. 1977
" "	Hepatic	Rat	3′Methyl-4-dimethylamino azobenzene	Clayton and Baumann 1949
" "		Rat	2-Acetylaminofluorene	Marshall et al. 1978
" "		Rat	3′Methyl-4-dimethylamino azobenzene	Griffin and Jacobs 1977
Selenium	Skin	Mouse	Benzo(a)pyrenephorbol ester	Wilt et al. 1979
Selenide	Skin	Mouse	DMBA	Shamberger 1970
H_2SeO_3	Colon	Rat	Azoxymethane (high-fat diet)	Soullier et al. 1981
Selenite	Trachea	Rat	1-Methyl-1-nitrosourea	Thompson and Becci 1979

animals were placed back on the dye-containing diet for an additional 4 weeks and in a few more weeks the study was terminated. In two studies, these investigators reported an approximate 50% reduction in the liver tumor incidence with added Se during the intermediate period compared with the control animals that received the basal diet. Shamberger (1970) also showed that sodium selenite inhibited chemical carcinogenesis.

Our laboratory showed during 1977–79 that administration of 5–6 ppm Se (sodium selenite) in the drinking water reduced the number of colon tumors appearing in rats given 20 weekly s.c. injections of dimethylhydrazine. Similar results were also observed in hepatic tumor formation in rats fed diets containing the hepatocarcinogens 3'MeDAB or 2-acetylaminofluorene (Griffin 1979, Griffin and Jacobs 1977, Marshall et al. 1979, Jacobs et al. 1977).

Wilt et al. (1979) indicated that Se must be present during the initiation phase for inhibition of papilloma formation to occur in mice exposed to an initiation application of dimethylbenz(a)anthracene (DMBA) followed by multiple application of the promoting phorbol compounds. Also of note is the recent report of Soullier et al. (1981) that rats on a high-fat diet and treated with azoxymethane, a regimen that ordinarily causes a very high incidence of intestinal cancer, exhibited a marked reduction in the number of tumors, especially in the proximal half of the colon, when the animals were given 8 ppm H_2SeO_3 in the drinking water.

Of equal interest and importance are those findings involving the chemoprevention of mammary carcinogenesis by Se compounds (Table 2). Schrauzer and co-workers (Schrauzer and Ishmael 1974, Schrauzer 1976, Schrauzer and White 1978) for several years have maintained that administration of Se (SeO_2) would result in a marked reduction in the number of spontaneously appearing tumors in C3H mice. These findings were confirmed last year by Medina and Shepherd (1980). As early as 1972, Harr et al. had reported that sodium selenite would inhibit or delay the number of mammary tumors that appeared in female rats given diets containing 2-acetylaminofluorene, and Thompson and Becci (1979, 1980) reported similar findings in that sodium selenite inhibited mammary carcinogenesis in rats given methylnitrosourea. To add to this story, Thompson

TABLE 2. *Chemoprevention of mammary carcinogenesis by selenium compounds*

Species	Carcinogen	Compound	Reference
Mouse	Spontaneous	SeO_2	Schrauzer and Ishmael 1974
			Schrauzer and White 1978
			Medina and Shepherd 1980
Rat	2-Acetylaminofluorene	Sodium selenite	Harr et al. 1972
Rat	Methylnitrosourea	" "	Thompson and Becci 1979, 1980
Mouse	7,12-Dimethylbenzanthracene	SeO_2	Medina and Shepherd 1981
Rat	" "	Sodium selenite	Thompson and Tagliaferro 1980

and Tagliaferro (1980) recently showed that mammary tumors induced in rats by application of 7,12-DMBA were inhibited by the addition of sodium selenite to the diet.

Medina and Shepherd (1981) showed that selenium administered as SeO_2 in the drinking water (6 ppm) inhibited mammary tumor formation in DMBA-treated (C57B1xDBA/2f) F_1, C3H/StW$_1$, and BALB/c female mice. They also reported that Se inhibited DMBA-induced ductal alveolar hyperplasias in (C57B1xDBA/2f) F_1 and BALB/c mice and mammary tumor virus-induced alveolar hyperplasias in BALB/cf C3H mice. Their studies indicated that supplemental Se *did not alter the growth of established mammary tumors.* These findings may be best summarized by quoting Drs. Medina and Shepherd: "These results demonstrated that supplemental selenium inhibits both chemical and viral-induced mammary tumorigenesis, and secondly, that the development of preneoplastic lesions, an early stage in mammary tumorigenesis, is very sensitive to selenium-mediated inhibition" (Medina and Shepherd 1981).

The discussion thus far has been concerned with the generalized concept that Se may inhibit carcinogenesis in an increasing number of animal model systems. I have omitted most of the actual experimental conditions, carcinogen involved, mode of administration, time factors, and the actual final evaluations of each of these studies. Each of these studies is referenced for further detailed studies you may wish to consider (see also Griffin 1979). There are many studies in different laboratories involving varying approaches that lead to the conclusion that Se may have an important bearing on the induction of cancer and may be applicable to cancer prevention in selected human populations.

What are the basic mechanisms that may be involved? I will first review briefly what is known about the physiological, biochemical, toxicological, and nutritional roles of selenium and, second, how it may be applied to the findings on inhibition of carcinogenesis.

BIOLOGICAL ASPECTS OF SELENIUM

A brief summary of some of the established plus the reasonably speculated roles of Se in biological systems are shown in Table 3. Some additional biological functions of Se are shown in Table 4. The first listed in Table 3 are the selenium-dependent enzymes (for review see Stadtman 1980). Se is specifically required as a component of several enzymes, perhaps the most important being glutathione peroxidase (GP) in view of its wide distribution in mammalian cells. Most of the other selenoprotein enzymes have been found in microbial systems. However, their function and properties have been well established. Other selenoproteins have also been isolated, as shown in Table 3. Chen and Stadtman (1980) reported the existence of Se-containing transfer RNAs from microbial species, one of them having L-proline acceptor activity.

At this time, the best-established physiological role of Se concerns its presence in the enzyme GP. The enzyme is widely distributed in mammalian tissues. I

TABLE 3. *Biological role of selenium*

Selenium-dependent enzymes
  Glutathione peroxidase in red blood cells kidney, heart, liver
  Formate dehydrogenase
  Clostridial glycine reductase
  Nicotinic acid hydroxylase
  Xanthine dehydrogenase
Miscellaneous selenoproteins
  Heart muscle
  Testis of some species
  Fetal calf serum
Other
  Selenium-containing transfer RNAs (possible regulatory role)

---

wish to refer briefly to the studies indicating the essentiality of Se in animals first noted by Schwarz and Foltz (1957). They reported that liver necrosis in rats was prevented by vitamin E and "factor 3," an organic form of Se. The complex interrelationships between vitamin E and Se have been reviewed by Hoekstra (1974), and the antioxidant properties of Se were further elucidated by Hoekstra and co-workers with the discovery that erythrocyte GP is a selenoenzyme. GP contains 4 atoms per mole of protein of 88,000 daltons, or approximately one Se per protein subunit of 22,000. In brief, this Se-dependent enzyme breaks down lipid hydroperoxides and other peroxides that may cause oxidant damage to cellular membranes (Hoekstra 1975). Lipid content and, more specifically, the unsaturated lipids of the diet have been implicated in carcinogenesis.

It is of interest to refer again to the report of Soullier et al. (1981) that extradietary Se prevented or delayed colon carcinogenesis in rats maintained on a high-fat diet and exposed to dimethylhydrazine. Since erythrocyte glutathione peroxidase is an easily measurable enzyme, it is possible to correlate Se intake, blood levels of Se, etc., with the activity of this enzyme in animal or human studies, and a number of elaborate studies of this have been completed or are in progress (see Griffin and Layne 1980). The results will add greatly to our knowledge of Se requirements and the role that this nutrient may have in a number of problems related to carcinogenesis.

TABLE 4. *Postulated biological functions of selenium*

Enzyme function
Oxidation-reduction
Protection of membranes-oxidant damage
Essential nutrient, growth
Reproduction
Regulatory role, initiation of protein synthesis
Immunological functions, antibody formation
Detoxification reactions

ROLE OF SELENIUM IN CANCER PREVENTION

Admittedly, we do not have any precise explanations of the mechanisms that account for the inhibition of carcinogenesis attributed to Se compounds (Griffin 1979, 1980). A few postulated or speculated roles are shown in Table 5. The true role of Se in cancer chemoprevention must await further studies.

Finally, while the evidence for the Se inhibition of carcinogenesis in animal model systems has been amply demonstrated, the application in the reduction of tumors in humans still awaits well-planned and controlled studies. There are some reports of an inverse relation between "environmental selenium" and the incidence of several forms of cancer, which await further verification. Also, there are advocates of enhancing the dietary intake of Se for all individuals. I am opposed to this and can only recommend Se supplementation when it is established that intakes of Se are insufficient as evident from carefully conducted studies of actual Se intake, blood or tissue levels of Se, and the levels of blood glutathionine peroxidase, or other established functions of Se. Certainly, the Se deficiency syndrome in China resulting in cardiomyopathies calls for Se enhancement of the diet. There are numerous cases in animal nutrition in which Se supplementation is indicated and commonly practiced.

If it is established that exposure to carcinogens creates extra demand for available Se, a strong basis for the Se supplementation for select populations who may fall into the higher cancer risk groups would be provided. For the present, it appears that the average person requires a daily intake of 150–200 μg of Se. Considering the ubiquitous distribution of this element in our environment, including food and water, it appears that this nutritional requirement is usually met. We do not know yet whether we would benefit from additional Se in terms of protection from cancer, cardiovascular disorders, or a host of other diseases, resulting in a longer and better life. It is of interest to note that a group of workers from New Jersey (Bogden et al. 1981) reported that tobaccos from countries with a high incidence of lung cancer had a mean Se concentration of 0.16 μg/g while in the tobaccos from the low incidence coun-

TABLE 5. *Some postulated roles of selenium in cancer chemoprevention*

Enhances detoxification of carcinogens
  Ring hydroxylation, glucuronide conjugation
  (Marshall and Griffin 1981)
Exposure to carcinogens increases body requirement for
  selenium (?)
Protects against oxidants involved in fat metabolism
Affects carcinogen-DNA binding, DNA repair
Has combined effects with other compounds such as reti-
  noids, antioxidants, protease inhibitors, other dietary fac-
  tors

---

tries it was significantly higher, 0.49 μg/g. Draw your own conclusions. Mine would be to give up smoking.

ACKNOWLEDGMENT

Some of the findings reported herein were supported by grants from the Robert A. Welch Foundation, Houston, Texas, the American Cancer Society, and Mr. T. K. Dixon, Jr. I wish to acknowledge the major contributions to these studies of many colleagues including Drs. Milton Marshall, Maryce Jacobs, A. H. Daoud, Helen Layne, Jerry Goodman, Marilyn Arnott, and Thomas Matney.

REFERENCES

Bogden, D., F. W. Kemp, M. Buse, S. Thind, D. B. Louria, J. Forgacs, G. Llanos, and I. M. Terrones. 1981. Composition of tobaccos from countries with high and low incidences of lung cancer. I. Selenium, polonium-210, alternaria, tar, and nicotine. JNCI 66:27–31.

Chen, C. S., and T. C. Stadtman. 1980. Selenium-containing tRNAs from *Clostridium*—sticklandii: Cochromatography of one species with L-prolyl-tRNA. Proc. Natl. Acad. Sci. USA 77:1403–1407.

Chen, X., G. Yang, J. Chen, Z. Wen, and K. Ge. 1981. Relation of selenium deficiency to the occurrence of Keshan disease, *in:* Selenium in Biology and Medicine, 2nd International Symposium, Lubbock, Tx., May 14–16, 1980. AVI Press, Westport, Connecticut (in press).

Clayton, C. C., and C. A. Baumann. 1949. Diet and azo tumors: Effect of diet during a period when the dye is not fed. Cancer Res. 9:575–582.

Greeder, G. A., and J. A. Milner. 1980. Factors influencing the inhibitory effect of selenium on mice innoculated with Ehrlich ascites tumor cells. Science 209:825–827.

Griffin, A. C. 1979. Role of selenium in the chemoprevention of cancer. Adv. Cancer Res. 29:419–441.

Griffin, A. C. 1980. Cancer chemoprevention (guest editorial). J. Cancer Res. Clin. Oncol. 98:1–7.

Griffin, A. C., and M. M. Jacobs. 1977. Effects of selenium on azo dye hepatocarcinogenesis. Cancer Lett. 3:177–181.

Griffin, A. C., and H. W. Layne. 1981. Selenium chemoprevention of cancer in animals and possible human implications, *in* Selenium in Biology and Medicine, 2nd International Symposium, Lubbock, Tx., May 14–16, 1980. AVI Press, Westport, Connecticut (in press).

Harr, J. R., J. H. Exon, P. D. Whanger, and P. H. Weswig. 1972. Effect of dietary selenium on N-2 fluorenylacetamide (FAA)-induced cancer in vitamin E supplemented, selenium depleted rats. Clin. Toxicol. 5:187–194.

Hoekstra, W. G. 1974. Biochemical role of selenium, *in* Trace Element Metabolism in Animals, Ed. 2, W. G. Hoekstra, J. W. Suttie, H. E. Ganther, and W. Mentz, eds. University Park Press, Baltimore, p. 61.

Hoekstra, W. G. 1975. Biochemical function of selenium and its relation to vitamin E. Fed. Proc. 34:2083–2089.

Jacobs, M. M., B. Jansson, and A. C. Griffin. 1977. Inhibitory effects of selenium on 1,2-dimethylhydrazine and methylazoxymethanol acetate induction of colon tumors. Cancer Lett. 2:133–138.

Marshall, M. V. and A. C. Griffin. 1981. Chemoprevention: A new field with much promise, *in* Prevention of Occupational Cancer, C. Shaw, ed. CRC Press, Inc., Boca Raton (in press).

Marshall, M. V., M. S. Arnott, M. M. Jacobs, and A. C. Griffin. 1978. Selenium effects on the carcinogenicity and metabolism of 2-acetylaminofluorene. Cancer Lett. 7:331–338.

Medina, D., and F. Shepherd. 1980. Selenium-mediated inhibition of mouse mammary tumorigenesis. Cancer Lett. 8:241–245.

Medina, D., and F. Shepherd. 1981. Selenium-mediated inhibition of 7,12-dimethylbenzanthracene-induced mouse mammary tumorigenesis. Carcinogenesis (in press).

Schrauzer, G. N. 1976. Selenium and cancer: A review. Bioinorg. Chem. 5:275–281.

Schrauzer, G. N., and D. Ishmael. 1974. Effects of selenium and arsenic on the genesis of spontaneous mammary tumors in inbred C3H mice. Ann. Clin. Lab. Sci. 4:441–447.

Schrauzer, G. N., and D. N. White. 1978. Selenium in human nutrition: Dietary intakes and effect of supplementation. Bioinorg. Chem. 8:303–318.

Schwarz, K., and C. M. Foltz. 1957. Selenium as an integral part of factor 3 against dietary necrotic liver degeneration. J. Am. Chem. Soc. 79:3292–3293.

Shamberger, R. J. 1970. Relationship of selenium to cancer. I. Inhibitory effect of selenium on carcinogenesis. JNCI 44:931–936.

Soullier, B. K., P. S. Wilson, and N. D. Nigro. 1981. Effect of selenium on azoxymethane-induced intestinal cancer in rats fed high fat diet. Cancer Lett. 12:343–348.

Stadtman, T. C. 1980. Selenium-dependent enzymes. Annu. Rev. Biochem. 49:93–110.

Thompson, H. J., and P. J. Becci. 1979. Effect of graded dietary levels of selenium on tracheal carcinomas induced by 1-methyl-1-nitrosourea. Cancer Lett. 7:215–219.

Thompson, H. J., and P. J. Becci. 1980. Selenium inhibition of N-methyl-N-nitrosourea-induced mammary carcinogenesis in the rat. JNCI 65:1299–1302.

Thompson, H. J., and A. R. Tagliaferro. 1980. Effect of selenium on 7,12-dimethylbenz(a)anthracene-induced mammary tumorigenesis. Fed. Proc. 39:1117.

Wilt, S., M. Pereira, and D. Couri. 1979. Selenium effect on initiation and promotion of tumors by benzl(a)pyrene and 12-0-tetradecanolylphorbol (abstract). Proc. Am. Assoc. Cancer Res. 20:21.

Molecular Interrelations of Nutrition and Cancer,
edited by M. S. Arnott, J. van Eys, and Y.-M. Wang.
Raven Press, New York © 1982.

Retinoid-Binding Proteins and Human Cancer

Frank Chytil and David E. Ong

*Department of Biochemistry, Vanderbilt University School of Medicine,
Nashville, Tennessee 37232*

The necessity of vitamin A, a nutritional component, for the maintenance of most if not all epithelial tissue was pointed out most strikingly in the elegant histopathological studies of Wolbach and Howe on the Vitamin A–deficient rat (Wolbach and Howe 1925). In many tissues, replacement of the normal columnar and transitional epithelium by squamous, frequently keratinizing epithelial cells that multiplied rapidly was observed. As illustration, the following is taken from their report:

In the epithelium of the bladder, ureters, and pelvis of the kidney the original epithelium becomes replaced by keratinizing epithelium which develops as in other locations from underlying nests of cells. In the kidneys, the apices of the pyramids become covered by a thick layer of keratinizing epithelium, while the epithelium of the pelvis, ureters, and bladder show the most remarkable pictures encountered in this study. In these latter locations there is evidence of very rapid growth of the epithelium: in some instances keratinization ceased. Mitotic figures are to be found in every field of a 3 mm immersion objective and frequently there are two to four mitoses per field. In the bladder invaginations and dermoid cyst-like formations occur. In ureter, pelvis, and bladder epithelial downgrowth resulting in the incorporation of blood vessels is frequent. The behaviours indicate growth power suggestive of neoplastic potentiality.

These dramatic changes are fully reversed by restoring a normal diet containing vitamin A (Wolbach and Howe 1933). These early studies have been continually reaffirmed through the years and laid the foundation for the continuing interest and research on possible effects of vitamin A on cancers.

EVIDENCE THAT VITAMIN A CAN INFLUENCE CANCER

There is a fairly extensive literature on the effect of vitamin A on cancer, dating from soon after the discovery of the vitamin in 1919. As early as 1922 an attempt was made to modify vitamin A intake for the treatment of patients suffering from cancer, without success (Wyard 1922). The phenotypic similarity of the metaplasia caused by vitamin A deficiency to some "spontaneous" neoplasms observed in epithelial tissues has certainly been a spur to research in this area.

Two compounds of the vitamin A family (retinoids) are of particular interest.

All-*trans* retinol, provided in the diet, is able to maintain all physiological functions requiring vitamin A, such as vision, reproduction, growth, and differentiation. Retinoic acid (vitamin A acid), a natural metabolite of retinol, can maintain growth and proper differentiation of most tissues, but cannot substitute for retinol in vision and maintenance of reproductive capacity in male or female rodents. There is a considerable body of evidence that suggests that these two compounds and analogs of these compounds can influence the development of some epithelial tumors. In particular, retinol, esters, and ethers of the alcohol: retinoic acid and various synthetic analogs of the acid have shown promise as prophylactic or therapeutic agents against spontaneous and chemically induced tumors. These findings have been reviewed recently (Sporn et al. 1976, Mayer et al. 1978). Since, as mentioned, vitamin A is necessary for the control of proliferation and the direction of differentiation of many epithelial tissues (Wolbach and Howe 1925, 1933), its ability to act on some tumors of such tissues is perhaps not surprising.

Conversely, lack of vitamin A has been reported to cause a significantly greater incidence of carcinogen-induced epithelial metaplasia and tumors, including bladder tumors in rat (Cohen et al. 1976), papillomas of mouse skin (Davies 1967), rat salivary gland neoplasia (Rowe et al. 1970), and rat lung tumors (Nettesheim and Williams 1976). Also, it has been reported that human smokers with a history of low vitamin A intake had a significantly higher incidence of pulmonary carcinomas than smokers with higher vitamin A intake (Bjelke 1975). However, vitamin A–deficient rats developed significantly fewer colon adenocarcinomas than normal rats when both were challenged with N-methyl-N'-nitrosoguanidine (Narisawa et al. 1976). Consequently, the experimental evidence suggests that vitamin A deficiency may permit a higher incidence of some tumors in some test systems, but may inhibit development of other types of cancers in other test systems. This presents the simple point that vitamin A therapy or prophylaxis cannot be expected to be successful for all types of malignancy in epithelial tissue.

DISCOVERY OF INTRACELLULAR BINDING PROTEINS FOR RETINOIDS

Efforts to unravel molecular mechanisms involved in vitamin A action in differentiation of epithelia as well as in its effects on malignant growth have produced little success at this point. The field of mechanism of action of vitamin A on the cellular level was, in the past, dominated by the search for an active form of vitamin A other than retinol (DeLuca 1979) and by the experiments implicating retinol in glycoprotein synthesis (DeLuca et al. 1979, Wolf et al. 1979). Demonstration of a cellular binding protein for retinol added a new element that had to be considered in the mechanism of retinoid action (Bashor et al. 1973). This was soon followed by discovery of a cellular binding protein for retinoic acid (Ong and Chytil 1975a, Sani and Hill 1976). This discussion

TABLE 1. *Nomenclature of the cellular retinol and retinoic acid–binding protein*

Most frequently used term	Abbreviation	Synonyms
Cellular retinol-binding protein	CRBP	Intracellular retinol-binding protein Cytosol retinol-binding protein Cytosol retinol receptor
Cellular retinoic acid– binding protein	CRABP	Retinoic acid–binding protein (RABP) Retinoic–acid receptor

will concentrate on these now well-characterized and intensively studied intracellular binding proteins. The first is cellular retinol-binding protein (CRBP); the second is cellular retinoic acid-binding protein (CRABP). The nomenclature is still not unified. Table 1 shows the alternate names for these two proteins. Review of the recent literature indicates that most of the journals have accepted the nomenclature used in this article.

Both binding proteins have been purified to homogeneity from rat tissues. Table 2 shows some of the properties of the proteins. CRBP binds retinol with high specificity and affinity, but does not bind retinal or retinoic acid. CRABP has high affinity for retinoic acid but does not bind retinol or retinal. The proteins are different from the well-known serum retinol–binding protein, known as RBP (Smith and Goodman 1979). Both proteins are present in most fetal tissues, but their tissue distribution differs in adult animals (Ong and Chytil 1976a). The levels of these proteins change differently during perinatal development, showing that they are not regulated in a synchronous manner and that they are not interchangeable in function (Ong and Chytil 1976a).

Most evidence has been generated by characterizing these proteins from rats. However, it appears that generally the characteristics of these binding proteins in human tissues are similar to those for rats, having similar size and binding

TABLE 2. *Characteristics of the cellular retinol-(CRBP) and retinoic acid-binding protein (CRABP) from rat*

Property	CRBP	CRABP
Molecular weight	14,600	14,600
Subunits	No	No
Preferred ligand (in vitro)	Retinol	Retinoic acid
K_d (app.)	1.6×10^{-8} M	4.2×10^{-9} M
ϵ	50,200 (350 nm)	50,000 (350 nm)
Ligand (in vivo)	Retinol	Not known

Reproduced from Chytil and Ong (1979) with permission of *Federation Proceedings.*
ϵ, The molar absorption coefficient.

specificity, although different immunochemical properties (Ong and Chytil 1981). The discovery of intracellular retinoid–binding proteins has offered an opportunity to evaluate the involvement of these binding proteins in cancer. It is customary to call the very wide variety of malignant tumors by the single term "cancer." That this leads to oversimplification is evident. Because of the diversity of malignant growth it can be expected *a priori* that the metabolism of vitamin A, in the wide sense of that word, will not be identical in the different cancers studied. The results for the binding proteins appear not to be an exception.

PRESENCE OF RETINOID-BINDING PROTEINS IN HUMAN CANCER

This chapter will review the present status of detection and quantitation of the intracellular binding proteins in human cancers. The detection and quantitation of the proteins is most often accomplished by sucrose gradient centrifugation (see Figure 1). The sensitivity of detection depends on the specific activity of the tritiated retinol or retinoic acid used. The purity of the radioactive ligands is also important. Because the specific activity of the available radioactive compounds varies, the "absence" of these proteins should always be taken with caution. A prime example that the method of detection is crucial is the fact that improvement of the sensitivity of the method can lead to detection in tissues previously thought to lack it (Huber et al. 1978, Küng et al. 1980). Information about the presence of binding proteins in various human tissues is still somewhat limited. Table 3 shows the occurrence of these proteins in normal human tissues examined thus far.

Since the first detection of CRABP in human lung and breast carcinomas (Ong et al. 1975), considerable effort has been given in various laboratories to detecting and quantitating this protein, as well as CRBP in human carcinomas, as summarized in Table 4. In some carcinomas, the presence of a binding protein has been noted, whereas it may be detectable at lower levels or not at all in adjacent normal tissue. An example is shown in Figure 1 and Table 5. Malignancy of organs that contain a binding protein in the normal state, such as the uterus (Chytil et al. 1975), may bring about an elevation of the level of binding protein (Palan and Romney 1980). The effect of malignancy on the quantity of the particular binding protein is diversified even when the organ of tumor origin is the same. This is emphasized by the data shown in Table 6, all samples being primary breast carcinomas. Such a diversified effect may be a reflection of tumor type. At this point it seems safe to say that each tumor must be evaluated individually for binding-protein content.

Some evidence of the binding specificity of cellular binding proteins of human tumor origin is available. It appears that the binding specificity of human breast tumor CRABP is very similar to CRABP of rat (as well as CRABP of human uterus). The similarity of the ability of various retinoid analogs to bind to rat and human CRABP and their ability to reverse metaplasia or inhibit tumor growth has been noted (Chytil and Ong 1976). It was therefore suggested that the action of retinoic acid may well be mediated by this cellular protein. Previ-

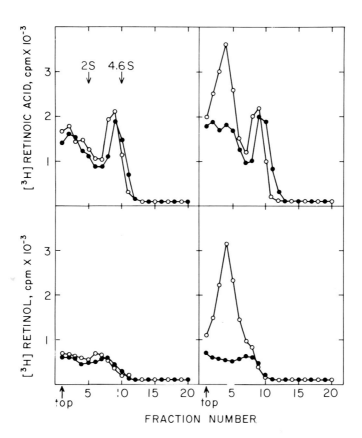

FIG. 1. Detection of CRABP and CRBP in epidermoid carcinoma of the oral cavity. After incubation with ³H-labeled retinoic acid or ³H-labeled retinol, aliquots of extracts of tumor tissue (right panels) or adjacent tissue (left panels) were submitted to sucrose gradient centrifugation. Fractions were collected and radioactivity determined for each fraction. Incubations were done with radioactive ligand alone (O) or in the presence of a 100-fold excess of unlabeled ligand (●) to demonstrate specific binding, revealed as a peak in the 2S region of the gradient (Ong et al. 1982).

TABLE 3. *Retinoids in human normal tissue*

Tissue of origin	CRBP	CRABP	Reference
Uterus	+	+	Chytil et al. (1975)
Lung	+	−	Bashor et al. (1973), Ong et al. (1975)
Breast	+	−	Ong et al. (1975)
			Palan and Romney (1980)
Testis	+	+	Ahluwalia et al. (1978)
Breast	ND	+	Küng et al. (1980)
Liver	+	−	Ong (unpublished)
Kidney	+	+	Ong (unpublished)

+, present; −, absent; ND, not determined.

TABLE 4. *Detection of CRBP and CRABP in human carcinomas*

Tissue of origin	CRBP	CRABP	Reference
Breast	−	+	Ong et al. (1975)
Lung	−	+	Ong et al. (1975)
Kidney	+	+	Chytil and Ong (1978)
Breast	+	+	Huber et al. (1978)
			Chytil and Ong (1978)
			Palan and Romney (1980)
Liver	+	+	Muto et al. (1979)
Cervix	+	+	Palan and Romney (1980)
Endometrium	+	+	Palan and Romney (1980)
Ovary	+	+	Palan and Romney (1980)
Colon	ND	+	Sani et al. (1980)
Oral cavity	+	+	Ong et al. (1981)

+, present; −, absent; ND, not determined.

ously, the binding affinity of CRBP for analogs of retinol brought a similar conclusion (Ong and Chytil 1975b). Consequently, evaluating analogs of retinol and retinoic acid for their ability to bind to CRABP or CRBP may be a useful preliminary step in identifying those with potential growth and antitumor activity (Chytil and Ong 1976). Further work on experimental tumors led to the proposition that the CRABP may be a required, although not necessarily sufficient, condition for tumors to be sensitive to treatment with retinoic acid (Ong and Chytil 1976b). And, as corollary to this point, screening tumors for the presence of binding proteins may indicate which patients could be considered candidates for treatment by such compounds (Chytil and Ong 1976). Indirect evidence in this respect is now available from the screening of various cell lines for the binding proteins (Lotan et al. 1980). The studies on experimental tumors and tissue cultures have been reviewed recently (Chytil and Ong 1978, Lotan 1980).

TABLE 5. *Quantitation of binding proteins in samples of human epidermoid carcinomas of the oral cavity and adjacent, grossly normal tissue*

Patient	CRBP Tumor (pmol/g)	CRBP Adjacent tissue (pmol/g)	CRABP Tumor (pmol/g)	CRABP Adjacent tissue (pmol/g)
A	65	B.D.	270	60
B*	175	B.D.	210	95
C	100	B.D.	190	B.D.
D	40	B.D.	180	220
E	65	10	320	290
F	45	B.D.	140	B.D.

B.D., Below detection level by method of Ong et al. 1982.
  * Secondary tumor from lymph node of this patient had levels of 180 pmol/g, CRABP; 120 pmol/g, CRBP.

TABLE 6. *Quantitation of retinoid-binding proteins in human primary breast cancers*

Patient	CRABP (pmol/g)	CRBP (pmol/g)
A	530	455
B	340	235
C	275	135
D	465	95
E	130	B.D.
F	1370	B.D.

B.D., below detection (Ong, Juing, and Toft, unpublished data).

Because the function of these proteins in cellular differentiation has not yet been elucidated, we are left primarily with speculation. For example, the fact that vitamin A deficiency can have opposite effects on growth of tumors, together with the variation in appearance of the binding proteins, offers the suggestion, in analogy with variable breast cancer estrogen dependence and occurrence of tumor estrogen receptors (Jensen et al. 1971), that some tumors may actually require vitamin A for growth. If so, indiscriminate use of retinoids in cancer therapy is not advisable.

Of course it is obvious that alterations of vitamin A metabolism, as reflected by the appearance or disappearance of the cellular vitamin A–binding proteins, is not the only defect of the malignant cell. Morphological as well as biochemical studies strongly implicated alterations of nuclear metabolism in malignancy. It has been hypothesized that CRBP interacts with the nucleus (Bashor et al. 1973). Indeed, evidence is available that this protein delivers retinol specifically into the nucleus (Takase et al. 1979). Retinoic acid, as shown first by Prutkin and Bogart (1970), also appears to localize in the nucleus, perhaps in association with its binding protein (Wiggert et al. 1977). Thus, in order to elucidate the mechanism by which the binding proteins mediate proper differentiation and rate of proliferation in the normal cell, but in some malignant cells inhibit growth and induce differentiation (Strickland and Mahdavi 1978), alterations in the nucleus of the malignant cells should be examined.

SUMMARY

The levels of CRPB and CRABP are frequently altered in human tumors compared to normal tissue. The alterations in level are not uniform but may reflect the type of tumor. In tumors affected by retinoids, the action may well be mediated by these binding proteins. The actual effect of the retinoid, either tumor regression or stimulation, may also prove to be related to tumor type.

ACKNOWLEDGMENTS

The work of the authors was supported by USPHS grants HD-05384, HD-09195 from the National Institute for Child and Human Development, HL-14214 from the National Heart, Lung and Blood Institute, and grant CA-20850 from the National Cancer Institute.

REFERENCES

Ahluwalia, G. S., S. K. Soni, and B. S. Ahluwalia. 1978. Retinol-binding proteins in human testis cytosol. J. Nutr. 108:1121–1127.

Bashor, M. M., D. O. Toft, and F. Chytil. 1973. In vitro binding of retinol to rat-tissue components. Proc. Natl. Acad. Sci. USA 70:3483–3487.

Bjelke, E. 1975. Dietary vitamin A and human lung cancer. Int. J. Cancer 15:561–565.

Chytil, F., and D. E. Ong. 1976. Mediation of retinoic acid-induced growth and anti-tumor activity. Nature 260:49–51.

Chytil, F., and D. E. Ong. 1978. Cellular vitamin A binding protein. Vitam. Horm. 36:1–32.

Chytil, F., and D. E. Ong. 1979. Cellular retinol and retinoic acid binding proteins in vitamin A action. Fed. Proc. 38:2510–2513.

Chytil, F., D. L. Page, and D. E. Ong. 1975. Presence of cellular retinol and retinoic acid binding proteins in human uterus. Int. J. Vitam. Nutr. Res. 45:293–298.

Cohen, S. M., J. F. Wittenberg, and G. T. Bryant. 1976. Effect of avitaminosis A and hypervitaminosis A on bladder carcinogenicity of N-(4-(5-nitro-2-furyl-2-thiazolyl)formamide. Cancer Res. 36:2334–2339.

Davies, D. E. 1967. Effect of vitamin A on 7,12-dimethylbenz(a)anthracene-induced papillomas in rhino mouse skin. Cancer Res. 27:237–241.

DeLuca, H. F. 1979. Retinoic acid metabolism. Fed. Proc. 38:2519–2523.

DeLuca, L. M., P. V. Bhat, W. Sasak, and S. Adamo. 1979. Biosynthesis of phosphoryl and glycosyl phosphoryl derivatives of vitamin A in biological membranes. Fed. Proc. 38:2535–2539.

Huber, P. R., E. Geyer, W. Kung, A. Matter, J. Torhorst, and U. Eppenberger. 1978. Retinoic acid binding protein in human breast cancer and dysplasia. JNCI 61:1375–1378.

Jensen, E. V., G. E. Bloc, S. Smith, K. Kyser, and E. R. DeSombre. 1971. Estrogen receptors and breast cancer response to adrenalectomy. Natl. Cancer Inst. Monogr. 34:55–70.

Küng, W. M., E. Geyer, U. Eppenberger, and P. R. Huber. 1980. Quantitative estimation of cellular retinoic acid binding protein activity in normal, dysplastic and neoplastic human breast tissue. Cancer Res. 40:4265–4269.

Lotan, R. 1980. Effects of vitamin A and its analogs (retinoids) on normal and neoplastic cells. Biochim. Biophys. Acta 609:33–91.

Lotan, R., D. Ong, and F. Chytil. 1980. Comparison of the level of cellular retinoid-binding proteins and susceptibility to retinoid-induced growth inhibition of various neoplastic cell lines. JNCI 64:1259–1262.

Mayer, H., W. Bollag, R. Hanni, and R. Ruegg. 1978. Retinoids, a new class of compounds with prophylactic and therapeutic activities in oncology and dermatology. Experientia 34:1105–1246.

Muto, Y., M. Omori, and K. Sugawara. 1979. Demonstration of novel cellular retinol-binding protein, F-type, in hepatocellular carcinoma. Gann 70:215–222.

Narisawa, T., B. S. Reddy, C.-Q. Wong, and J. H. Weisburger. 1976. Effect of vitamin A deficiency on rat colon carcinogenesis by N-methyl-N'-nitro-N-nitrosoguanidine. Cancer Res. 36:1379–1383.

Nettesheim, P., and M. L. Williams. 1976. The influence of vitamin A on the susceptibility of the rat lung to 3-methylcholanthrene. Int. J. Cancer 17:351–357.

Ong, D. E., and F. Chytil. 1975a. Retinoic acid binding protein in rat tissue. J. Biol. Chem. 250:6113–6116.

Ong, D. E., and F. Chytil. 1975b. Specificity of cellular retinol-binding protein for compounds with vitamin A activity. Nature 255:74–75.

Ong, D. E., and F. Chytil. 1976a. Changes in levels of cellular retinol and retinoic acid binding proteins of liver and lung during perinatal development. Proc. Natl. Acad. Sci. USA 73:3976–3978.

Ong, D. E., and F. Chytil. 1976b. Presence of retinol and retinoic acid binding proteins in experimental tumors. Cancer Lett. 2:25–30.

Ong, D. E., and F. Chytil. 1981. Immunochemical studies on cellular vitamin A binding proteins. Ann. N.Y. Acad. Sci. 359:415–417.

Ong, D. E., W. J. Goodwin, R. H. Jesse, and A. C. Griffin. 1982. Presence of cellular retinol and retinoic acid binding proteins in epidermoid carcinoma of the oral cavity and oropharynx. Cancer (in press).

Ong, D. E., D. L. Page, and F. Chytil. 1975. Retinoic acid binding protein: Occurrence in human tumors. Science 190:60–61.

Palan, P. R., and S. L. Romney. 1980. Cellular binding proteins for vitamin A in human carcinomas and in normal tissues. Cancer Res. 40:4221–4224.

Prutkin, L., and B. Bogart. 1970. The uptake of labeled vitamin A acid in kerato-acanthoma. J. Invest. Dermatol. 55:249–255.

Rowe, N. H., F. C. Grammer, F. R. Watson, and N. H. Nickerson. 1970. A study of environmental influence upon salivary gland neoplasia in rats. Cancer 26:436–444.

Sani, B. P., S. M. Condon, R. W. Brockman, L. H. Weiland, and A. J. Schutt. 1980. Retinoic acid binding protein in experimental and human tumors. Cancer 45:1199–1206.

Sani, B. P., and D. L. Hill. 1976. A retinoic acid binding protein from chick embryo skin. Cancer Res. 36:409–413.

Smith, J. E., and D. S. Goodman. 1979. Retinol binding protein and the regulation of vitamin A transport. Fed. Proc. 38:2504–2509.

Sporn, M. B., N. M. Dunlop, D. L. Newton, and J. M. Smith. 1976. Prevention of chemical carcinogenesis by vitamin A and its synthetic analogs (retinoids). Fed. Proc. 35:1332–1338.

Strickland, S., and V. Mahdavi. 1978. The induction of differentiation in teratocarcinoma stem cells by retinoic acid. Cell 15:393–403.

Takase, S., D. E. Ong, and F. Chytil. 1979. Cellular retinol-binding protein allows specific interaction of retinol with the nucleus in vitro. Proc. Natl. Acad. Sci. USA 76:2204–2208.

Wiggert, B., P. Russell, M. Lewis, and G. Chader. 1977. Differential binding to soluble nuclear receptors and effects on cell viability of retinol and retinoic acid in cultured retinoblastoma cells. Biochem. Biophys. Res. Commun. 79:218–226.

Wolbach, S. B., and P. R. Howe. 1925. Tissue changes following deprivation of fat-soluble A vitamin. J. Exp. Med. 43:753–777.

Wolbach, S. B., and P. R. Howe. 1933. Epithelial repair in recovery from vitamin A deficiency. J. Exp. Med. 57:511–526.

Wolf, G., T. C. Kiorpes, S. Masushuge, J. B. Schreiber, and M. J. Smith. 1979. Recent evidence for the participation of vitamin A in glycoprotein synthesis. Fed. Proc. 38:2540–2543.

Wyard, S. 1922. The treatment of malignant disease by diet free from fat-soluble vitamin A. Lancet 202:840.

Molecular Interrelations of Nutrition and Cancer,
edited by M. S. Arnott, J. van Eys, and Y.-M. Wang.
Raven Press, New York © 1982.

The Effect of Dietary Retinoids on Experimentally Induced Carcinogenesis in the Rat Bladder

R. M. Hicks, J. Chowaniec, J. A. Turton, E. D. Massey,* and A. Harvey

School of Pathology, Middlesex Hospital Medical School, London W1P 7LD, England

Carcinogenesis in the urinary bladder, as in many other epithelial tissues, involves a multistage process of initiation, promotion, and propagation (Hicks and Chowaniec 1978, Hicks et al. 1978, Hicks 1980). In man, clinically observable bladder cancer is undoubtedly preceded for many years by foci of dysplasia and preneoplastic change in the epithelial lining (the urothelium), which, being symptom free, usually remain undetected. Bladder cancer is characteristically a multifocal disease, and although it may start as an individual papillary growth, in the course of time new tumors will arise with increasing frequency at disparate sites throughout the urothelium of first the bladder, then the urethra, ureters, and kidney calyx.

Recently, epidemiological observations have indicated that vitamin A deficiency in human populations carries with it an increased risk of cancer (Bjelke 1975, Wald et al. 1980), but the use of excess naturally occurring vitamin A as an anticancer agent in experimental animal models has produced equivocal results (Sporn et al. 1976). Natural vitamin A (retinol and all *trans*-retinoic acid, retinyl palmitate, etc.) cannot be advocated for cancer therapy because at high doses these compounds are toxic at a systemic level. Various synthetic analogs have been developed in the hope of finding a derivative that is less toxic and yet retains its biological activity (Sporn 1978). Some of these synthetic retinoids have been shown experimentally to modulate the development of preneoplastic lesions in many different tissues, including the urothelium lining the urinary bladder. In particular, Sporn and Moon and their colleagues found that, in the short term, the development of neoplastic lesions in the bladder in rats and mice could be delayed or even halted by retinoids (Becci et al. 1979a, 1979b, 1981, Grubbs et al. 1977, Sporn et al. 1977, Squire et al. 1977, Thompson et al. 1981). These observations have exciting implications (Sporn et al. 1979) and suggest an improved clinical therapy regime might be developed for patients presenting with bladder cancer. For therapy to be effective against a multifocal

---

* Current address: Group Research and Development Centre, British-American Tobacco Company Ltd., Regent's Park Road, Southampton SO9 1PE

recurrent disease such as bladder cancer, it is probable that long-term, high-level dosing with retinoids will be required. It is thus imperative to determine how well long-term dosing with individual retinoids can be tolerated and to investigate their systemic, as well as their anticancer, effects in whole animals.

The effects in F344 rats of life-time dosing with two retinoids, namely 13-*cis*-retinoic acid (CRA) and N-ethyl-retinamide (NER), have been assessed from survival rates, skeletal development, and various other physiological parameters. At the same time the course of development of bladder cancer has been investigated in rats treated with the specific bladder carcinogen N-butyl-N-butanol nitrosamine (BBN) and subsequently maintained on a retinoid-containing or on a placebo diet. A summary of some of the results obtained is presented here, and various aspects of the work will be treated in greater detail in other, subsequent publications.

MATERIALS AND METHODS

Animals: Maintenance and Measurements

Female SPF F344 rats (Bantin and Kingman Ltd., Grimston, Hull) approximately 100 g at the start of the experiment, were fed *ad libitum* on a basic ground diet (rat and mouse No. 1, BP Nutrition Ltd., Witham, Essex), with free access to drinking water from the main supply. Animals were randomly distributed into 23 groups (Table 1), numerically coded by ear punches, and housed 6 or 8 to a cage. They were observed daily for signs of ill health; those that became ill and whose condition did not improve were killed *in extremis* and subjected to postmortem examination. All animals were weighed individually at weekly intervals, and diet and water consumption determinations were carried out weekly.

Urine was collected as 16-hour overnight samples from rats housed individually in metabolic cages (Forth-Tech Services Ltd., Mayfield, Midlothian) with access to water but not to food. Urine volume and the presence of crystals were recorded and the samples examined by N-Labstix (Ames Company, Stoke Poges, Slough) for pH and content of protein, glucose, ketones, blood, and nitrite. Life table estimates of percent survivors were constructed according to the method of Peto et al. (1977).

Treatment Groups

The experimental design is set out in Table 1. Four experimental protocols were used. In groups A to D, pairs of animals were killed by CO_2 anesthesia at weekly intervals for 4 weeks after the administration of the final dose of carcinogen, fortnightly for 8 weeks, and thereafter monthly, in order to determine how 13-*cis*-retinoic acid (CRA) affected the histology, ultrastructure, and rate of development of urothelial carcinomas in the carcinogen-treated animals. In groups E to H, the experimental design was similar, but N-ethyl-retinamide

TABLE 1. *Experimental design*

Experiment	Group	Total weight (mg) of carcinogen (BBN) administered	Diet after carcinogen or vehicle administration (mg retinoid/kg diet)
1. CRA	A	1,200	Placebo-CRA
Animals killed	B	1,200	240 CRA
sequentially	C	Vehicle	240 CRA
	D	Vehicle	Placebo-CRA
2. NER	E	600	Placebo-NER
Animals killed	F	600	654 NER
sequentially	G	Vehicle	654 NER
	H	Vehicle	Placebo-NER
3. NER	J	1,200	Placebo-NER
Animals killed at	K	1,200	654 NER
1 or 2 years	L	Vehicle	Placebo-NER
	M	Vehicle	654 NER
	N	1,200	327 NER
	P	Vehicle	327 NER
	Q	0.9% NaCl	Basic diet
	R	600	Placebo-NER
	S	600	654 NER
	T	300	Placebo-NER
	U	300	654 NER
4. CRA	V	Nil	Basic diet
Animals killed at	W	Nil	Placebo-CRA
18 months	X	Nil	240 CRA
	Y	Nil	480 CRA

Abbreviations: BBN, N-butyl-N-(4-hydroxybutyl) nitrosamine; CRA, 13-cis-retinoic acid; NER, N-ethyl-retinamide.

(NER) was used instead of CRA. Furthermore, half the dose level of carcinogen and approximately 2.7 times the dietary level of retinoid (in mg/kg) was used (Table 1). In groups J to U, in order to compare tumor prevalance in placebo-versus NER-fed animals, half the animals were killed at 1 year after the administration of the final dose of carcinogen, and the survivors at 2 years; three dose levels of carcinogen and two of NER were employed. In groups V to Y, the animals received no carcinogen. They were fed CRA to study the long-term effects of retinoid ingestion at a high dose level; all were killed at 18 months.

Animals in groups A to U not treated with carcinogen were administered alcoholic (vehicle) or NaCl solutions as a control. All were fed the basic diet before and during the administration of carcinogen, vehicle, or NaCl solution, and were given retinoid, placebo, or basic diet (see Table 1) at 24 hours after the administration of the final dose of carcinogen or control solution.

Retinoids

Both CRA and NER were supplied by the National Cancer Institute through the courtesy of Dr. M. Sporn. CRA was in the form of a stable gelatinized beadlet protected by antioxidants; placebo beadlets containing no retinoid were supplied as a control. Beadlets were blended into the ground basic diet using a commercial mixing machine (Model A120, Hobart Manufacturing Co. Ltd., London) to give the appropriate concentration of beadlets for the required retinoid dose level, about 1 mM. NER (327 or 654 mg, equivalent to 1 mM and 2 mM) was dissolved in 50 ml of a 1:3 (v/v) ethanol: trioctanoin mixture to which 0.05 ml each of Tenox 20 and DL-α-tocopherol were added. Trioctanoin (Fluka Flowachem Ltd., Glossop, Derbyshire), Tenox 20 (Eastman Kodak Ltd., Kirby, Liverpool) and DL-α-tocopherol (Sigma Chemical Co. Ltd., Poole, Dorset) were gifts from the NCI. The control solution for the NER was prepared as described above, but without NER. The NER or placebo-NER solutions were incorporated into 1 kg of ground diet with the mixing machine. All diets were prepared fresh each week, stored at 4°C, and presented to the animals in feeding pots designed to minimize and collect spillage.

Carcinogen

N-butyl-N-(4-hydroxybutyl) nitrosamine (BBN) was synthesized by IIT Research Institute, Chicago, and supplied through NCI by courtesy of Dr. R. Moon. It was diluted with ethanol:water (30:70, v/v) and administered via gastric intubation to rats lightly anesthetized with CO_2. Control animals received the ethanol:water solution (vehicle) or a 0.9% NaCl solution. Each rat received 12 0.5-ml doses of carcinogen, vehicle, or NaCl solution over a 6-week period. The carcinogen was administered to give a total dose of 300, 600, or 1,200 mg BBN per animal (Table 1).

POSTMORTEM PROCEDURES AND TISSUE PREPARATION

Animals were killed by CO_2 overdose in a randomized predetermined sequence, and the bladders were exposed, inflated, and bathed with buffered formalin fixative and removed. Organs from some control groups were removed and weighed, and some body measurements were taken. Samples of major organs and all tissues appearing abnormal were taken for histologic examination. The internal surface of the urinary bladder was examined under a dissecting microscope and the position and approximate size of any exophytic lesion noted. The dimensions of the lesions were measured in three directions and the volumes of the exophytic growths subsequently calculated from known formulas. The bladders were then cut into three zones, a posterior area including the ureteric and urethral openings, a median area, and an anterior, dome area. These zones were further divided into two or three segments and wax embedded separately for histological examination. For ultrastructural studies, in bladders of normal macroscopic appearance, each zone was sliced into four serial strips and processed either for histologic examination or for transmission or scanning electron microscopy. In tumor-bearing bladders, an area from every tumor was prepared for each type of microscopy. Tissues were prepared for electron microscopy by embedding in Spurr resin and thin sections were examined in a JEOL 100B or Philips 200 transmission electron microscope. Other tissue was critical-point dried and examined in a JEOL 35 scanning electron microscope. At postmortem examination, each rat was assigned a random histology number and the pathological assessment was carried out "blind." Urothelial carcinoma was diagnosed and assessed according to the World Health Organization grading and staging of human bladder tumors (Mostofi et al. 1973).

RESULTS

Consumption of Retinoids and Their Effects on Body Weights, Organ Weights, and Urine Values

Both NER and CRA were palatable; although the diet consumption by the CRA-fed animals was slightly lower than by the respective placebo-fed controls (Table 2), this was not the case for the NER-fed animals (Table 3). The body weight increases of all groups of animals fed the two retinoids were satisfactory (Figures 1 and 2). Nevertheless, significant reductions in body weights were evident in the NER-fed and in the high-dose CRA-fed animals after maintenance on the retinoid-containing diets for 6 months (Figures 1 and 2), but no sign of weight reduction was observed after the lower dose of CRA.

The weights of various organs taken at postmortem were recorded on a relative basis (organ weight in g/kg body weight) in the NER trial at 1 and 2 years. In rats fed 654 mg NER/kg diet for 1 year, there was no effect on the relative weights of the femur, liver, lungs, adrenal gland, uterine horn, pituitary gland, or skin, but the weights of the stomach, heart, kidney, and brain were significantly

TABLE 2. *Diet consumption* by female F344 rats fed 13-cis-retinoic acid*

Period (age of rats, weeks)	No. consumption determined	Diet† Mean diet consumption (g/rat/day) ± SD			
		BD	BD + placebo CRA	BD + 240 mg/kg CRA	BD + 480 mg/kg CRA
6–27	13	11.0 ± 1.1	11.8 ± 1.0	11.0 ± 1.2	10.9 ± 0.9
28–43	14	13.5 ± 1.0	13.6 ± 1.1	12.8 ± 1.2	11.6 ± 1.4
44–59	14	10.7 ± 1.3	11.2 ± 1.1	10.6 ± 1.3	10.0 ± 0.8
60–75	11	9.0 ± 1.0	8.6 ± 0.6	7.8 ± 0.8	7.6 ± 0.9

* Diet consumption determinations were 7-day ones and in most cases were done weekly. Each determination for each dietary group was calculated initially from three cages containing five or six rats. Results show the mean of 11 to 14 determinations over 15- or 21-week periods.
† All animals were fed BD until 5.3 weeks of age when the 3 treatment groups were fed retinoid or placebo diets.
Abbreviations: CRA, 13-cis-retinoic-acid; BD, basic diet.

TABLE 3. *Diet consumption* by female F344 rats fed N-ethyl-retinamide*

Period (age of rats, weeks)	No. consumption determined	Diet† Mean diet consumption (g/rat/day) ± SD			
		BD	BD + placebo NER	BD + 327 mg/kg NER	BD + 654 mg/kg NER
17–32	14	11.1 ± 1.7	11.3 ± 1.4	11.4 ± 2.4	10.8 ± 1.8
33–48	16	10.4 ± 0.7	11.3 ± 0.8	10.4 ± 0.4	10.2 ± 0.6
49–64	14	12.0 ± 1.0	11.5 ± 0.7	11.6 ± 0.6	11.8 ± 0.8
65–80	15	10.7 ± 1.6	9.6 ± 1.5	10.0 ± 1.6	11.6 ± 2.0
81–96	9	11.6 ± 0.8	10.6 ± 0.5	10.4 ± 1.0	11.3 ± 0.6
97–114	14	13.3 ± 1.3	12.2 ± 1.7	12.3 ± 1.0	13.2 ± 2.1

* Diet consumption determinations were 3-day ones from 17 to 35 weeks and 7-day ones from 36 to 114 weeks, and in most cases were done weekly. Each determination for each dietary group was calculated initially from eight cages containing six to eight rats. Results show the mean of 9 to 16 determinations over 15- or 17-week periods.

† All animals were fed BD until 16.7 weeks of age, when the three treatment groups were fed retinoid or placebo diets.

Abbreviations: NER, N-ethyl-retinamide; BD, basic diet.

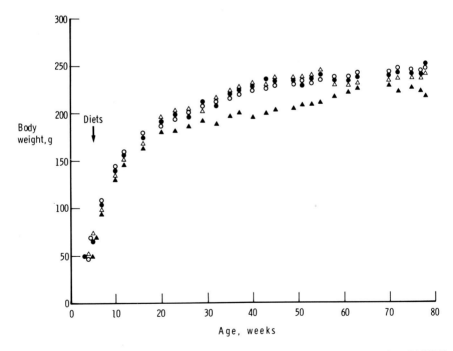

FIG. 1. Mean body weights of female F344 rats fed diets containing 13-cis-retinoic acid (CRA) from 5 to 78 weeks of age. ○, basic diet; ●, placebo CRA diet; △, CRA at 240 mg/kg diet; ▲, CRA at 480 mg/kg diet. All animals were fed basic diets until 5.3 weeks of age (↓), when the three treatment groups were fed retinoid or placebo diets.

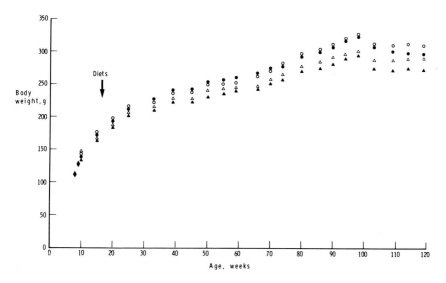

FIG. 2. Mean body weights of female F344 rats fed diets containing N-ethyl-retinamide (NER) from 16 to 120 weeks of age. ○, basic diet; ●, placebo NER diet; △, NER at 327 mg/kg diet; ▲, NER at 654 mg/kg diet; ◆, mean body weight of rats in all groups. All animals were fed basic diet until 16.7 weeks of age (↓), when the three treatment groups were fed retinoid or placebo diets. Rats were distributed into treatment groups at 10 weeks of age.

increased, and the spleen significantly decreased. However, after feeding NER at 654 mg/kg diet for 2 years there were no significant effects on the weights of any of these organs in comparison with the placebo-fed controls. Feeding NER for 1 or 2 years had no effect on the length of the tail, hind limb, or femur, but the length of the body was reduced in NER-fed animals at 1 year (Table 4). Furthermore, the width of the shaft of the femur was significantly reduced in NER-fed animals at 1 and 2 years in comparison with placebo-fed controls (Table 4). This effect on bone remodeling was confirmed independently by another investigator; x-ray examination and sectional measurements of the femur revealed the reduction in shaft diameter to be associated with a reduction in the diameter of the medullary cavity rather than a thinning of the compact bone (Darby et al. 1981). Indeed, the relative weights of the femur were similar in placebo-fed and NER-fed animals. There were no fractures of the femur in the 14 animals examined at 1 year on the NER diet and none in 19 animals examined at 2 years. Neither were fractures seen in 8 rats fed CRA at 240 mg/kg diet, nor in 10 rats fed CRA at 480 mg/kg diet, killed at 18 months, although the diameters of the femurs of these animals also were significantly reduced.

Analysis of 16-hour overnight urine samples 1 year after dosing with 1,200 mg BBN demonstrated increased levels of protein and blood in an increased volume of urine. These effects, attributable to tumor development in the bladders, were not prevented by feeding NER at 654 mg or CRA at 240 mg/kg diet,

TABLE 4. *Measurements* of the body and femur of female F344 rats fed N-ethyl-retinamide for 1 year*

Body measurement	Diet†		
	BD	BD + placebo NER	BD + 654 mg/ kg NER
Body weight (g)	275.2 ± 28.4	276.4 ± 33.4	251.0 ± 9.6‡
Body length (cm)	21.54 ± 0.62	21.53 ± 0.55	21.10 ± 0.32‡
Tail length (cm)	17.56 ± 0.78	17.66 ± 0.61	16.91 ± 1.23
Hind limb length (cm)	10.65 ± 0.16	10.62 ± 0.16	10.65 ± 0.12
Femur weight (g/kg body weight)	2.292 ± 0.146	2.203 ± 0.174	2.201 ± 0.088
Femur length (cm)	3.329 ± 0.092	3.292 ± 0.083	3.296 ± 0.053
Femur diameter (mm)	2.99 ± 0.122	3.02 ± 0.163	2.68 ± 0.121§

* Mean and SD; 14 rats per group.
† All animals were fed basic diet until 16.7 weeks of age, when the two treatment groups were fed retinoid or placebo diets.
‡ $p < 0.02$. Differences in body measurements between placebo-fed and NER-fed rats were examined using Student's t test.
§ $p < 0.001$.
Abbreviations: NER, N-ethyl-retinamide; BD, basic diet.

nor did the retinoids alone affect urinary protein or blood values. Neither carcinogen dosing nor retinoid feeding affected values for urinary pH, glucose, ketones, nitrite, or the presence of crystals in samples tested at 1 year by comparison with the appropriate placebo-fed controls.

Effect of Retinoids on Survival of Control and Carcinogen-Treated Rats, Based on Life Table Estimates

In the control group on normal diet, very few rats died before 70 weeks. Inclusion of 327 mg/kg or 654 mg/kg of NER (1 mM and 2 mM, respectively) or the vehicle (placebo) in the diet did not significantly alter survivorship, nor was there a statistically significant trend towards an increased survivorship with increasing dose of NER (Figure 3). In rats treated with CRA, mortality followed a similar course.

In all groups receiving the highest, 1,200-mg, dose of BBN, there was a relatively high, early mortality irrespective of retinoid treatment. Postmortem examination revealed that in these groups more than 90% of the deaths were caused by bladder tumors; thus the life tables indicate both the rate and extent of risk of death due to bladder tumors (Figures 4 and 5). The few animals whose cause of death was diagnosed to be other causes were omitted from these life tables.

As shown in Figure 4, from 50 weeks onwards, NER treatment did not significantly affect the rate of death due to bladder tumors since the parallel slopes of the survival curves indicate that rats became moribund or died at the same rate, irrespective of treatment. However, the separation of the parallel

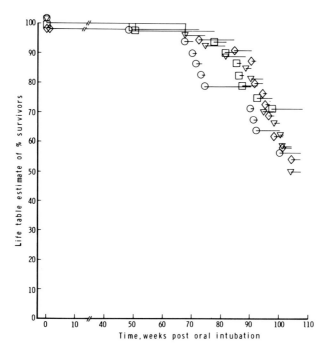

FIG. 3. Life tables for control groups given alcoholic (BBN vehicle) or NaCl solution and subsequently fed retinoid, placebo, or basic diet. ○ saline + basic diet, ◇ alcohol + placebo diet, ▽ alcohol + 1 mM NER, □ alcohol + 2 mM NER. The number of rats still alive after the 1-year kills (56 weeks) and at 70, 80, 90, 100 weeks were: ○ 26, 24, 21, 19, and 15; ◇ 27, 27, 26, 24, and 16; ▽ 27, 26, 25, 22, and 16; □ 26, 26, 25, 21, and 19.

life tables over the period of maximum death rate demonstrates that there was a time shift of the survival curves for rats fed the low and high doses of NER by 7 and 5 weeks, respectively, relative to that of BBN-placebo–treated controls. A similar shift of about 5 weeks is also evident after 1 year in rats pretreated with 1,200 mg BBN and fed CRA at about 1 mM in the diet (Figure 5), although in this experiment, the small numbers of animals that died (as opposed to those sequentially killed) permits only cautious interpretation of the life tables. The shifts in survival curves for both NER- and CRA-treated rats indicate that at any time after 1 year, the estimated chance of surviving the following week was greater for retinoid-fed rats than for placebo-fed, BBN-treated controls. For example, at 55 weeks survivors in the placebo-fed groups had a 53–54% estimated chance of surviving the following week, whereas those treated with CRA or the high dose or low dose of NER had estimated survival probabilities of 71%, 72%, or 81%, respectively. By 88 weeks, however, all rats that had received 1,200 mg BBN were dead except for one fed the lower dose of NER.

After 600 mg BBN, deaths due to bladder tumors did not occur until after the time of the 1-year interim kills, and the death rate due to bladder tumors

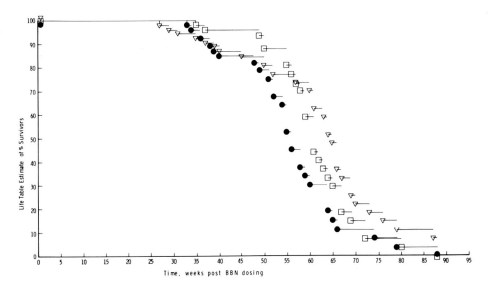

FIG. 4. Life tables for groups given 1,200 mg BBN and subsequently fed placebo or N-ethyl-retinamide in the diet. Deaths due to bladder tumors. ● BBN + placebo, ▽ BBN + 1mM NER, □ BBN + 2 mM NER. The numbers of rats still alive at 40 weeks, after the 1-year kills (55 weeks) and at 65, 75, and 85 weeks were: ● 45, 14, 4, 2, and 1; ▽ 46, 21, 13, 5, and 3; □ 52, 22, 8, 2, and 1.

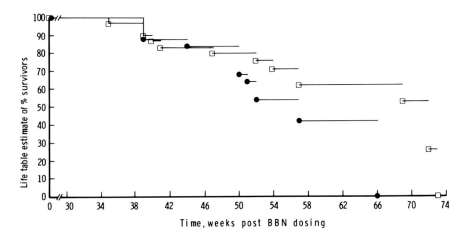

FIG. 5. Life tables for groups given 1,200 mg BBN and subsequently fed placebo or 13-cis-retinoic acid in the diet. Deaths due to bladder tumors. ● BBN + placebo, □ BBN + 1 mM CRA. The numbers of rats still alive at 40, 50, 60, and 70 weeks were: ● 27, 16, 7, and 1; □ 29, 21, 13, and 8.

remained fairly constant, i.e., linear, until the time of the terminal, 2-year kills (Figure 6). The start of the linear death rate was at 55 weeks, compared with about 48 weeks in rats given 1,200 mg BBN. Again, inclusion of NER in the diet did not affect the rate of death but did shift the life table along the time axis by about 10 weeks, indicating a consistently increased chance of surviving the following week for NER-treated animals at any time studied. In these two groups treated with 600 mg BBN, 10–15% of the rats died from other causes, and these animals were excluded from the life tables. Only three rats treated with BBN alone survived to 2 years, compared with six of those additionally treated with NER.

After 300 mg BBN, tumors developed later in the life-span of the animals and approximately 50% of deaths were attributed to other causes, even though bladder tumors were present in some animals. If life tables are constructed

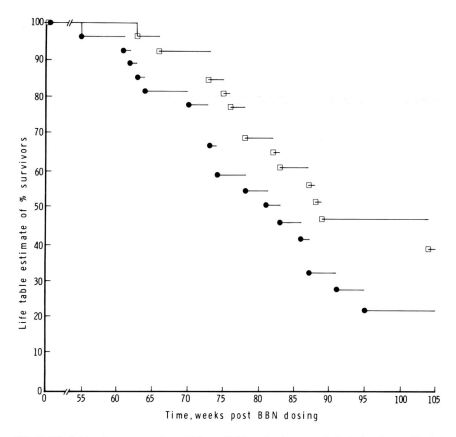

FIG. 6. Life tables for groups given 600 mg BBN and subsequently fed placebo or N-ethyl-retinamide in the diet. Deaths due to bladder tumors. ● BBN + placebo, □ BBN + 2 mM NER. The number of rats still alive after the 1-year kills (55 weeks) and at 65, 75, 85, and 95 weeks were: ● 26, 22, 15, 10, and 4; □ 26, 25, 21, 13, and 10.

for deaths due to bladder tumors only, the numbers of animals involved are too small to demonstrate unequivocally a difference due to administration of the NER (Figure 7). However, a consistent trend towards decreased rate of death in NER-fed rats is apparent after 75 weeks. A similar trend is also evident from the life tables of deaths due to all causes including bladder tumors (Figure 8). Eight rats treated with 300 mg BBN alone survived to 2 years, compared with 13 rats additionally fed the higher dose of NER.

The Effect of Retinoids on Bladder Cancer Development in BBN-Treated Animals

BBN is a specific organotropic bladder carcinogen for the rat. Repeated intragastric dosing elicited a rapid proliferative response in the urothelium (Figure

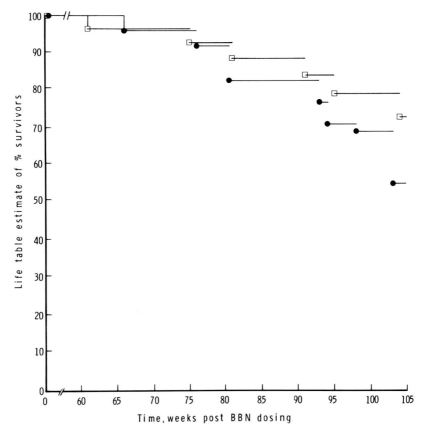

FIG. 7. Life tables for groups given 300 mg BBN and subsequently fed placebo or N-ethyl-retinamide in the diet. Deaths due to bladder tumors. ● BBN + placebo, □ BBN + 2 mM NER. The number of rats still alive after the 1-year kills (55 weeks) and at 70, 80, 90, and 100 weeks were: ● 26, 23, 20, 17, and 9; □ 27, 25, 24, 20, and 15.

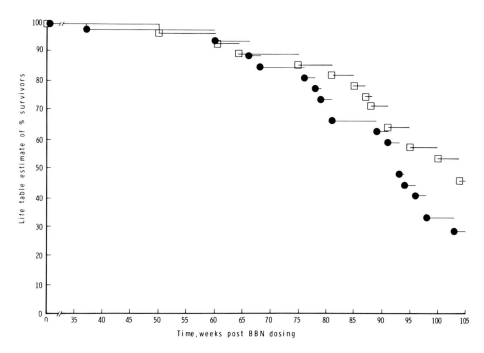

FIG. 8. Life tables for groups illustrated in Figure 7, but deaths from all causes considered. Key and legend as for Figure 7.

9), which was most marked in the dome and became progressively less towards the trigone. After completion of the BBN treatment in placebo-fed animals, these hyperplastic lesions apparently remained static for a period of months, but then increased in size and complexity to produce macroscopically visible, rapidly growing tumors (Figure 10). The length of the latent period before rapid tumor growth commenced was inversely related to the dose of BBN used, being 2–3 months after 1,200 mg, 4–6 months after 600 mg, and about 12–14 months after 300 mg BBN. This underlies the dose-related times at which linear death rates were established, i.e., at about 12, 14, and 18 months, respectively, by which time some tumor volumes were so large they killed the animals.

In those animals in groups J to U killed 1 year after dosing with BBN, no significant effect of NER on bladder carcinogenesis could be detected when the response was measured in terms of the number of tumor-bearing animals. However, if the response was recorded as the total volume of exophytic tumor present in the bladder at autopsy, after either 600 or 1,200 mg BBN there was a significantly lower mean tumor volume in animals fed NER than in those fed placebo (Figure 11). In animals pretreated with 1,200 mg BBN, the reduction in tumor volume was greater in animals fed the lower dose of NER than in those receiving the higher dose. After 300 mg BBN, no differential response could be detected between the placebo-fed and NER-fed groups at 12 months, for at that time the hyperplastic urothelium was often still in the

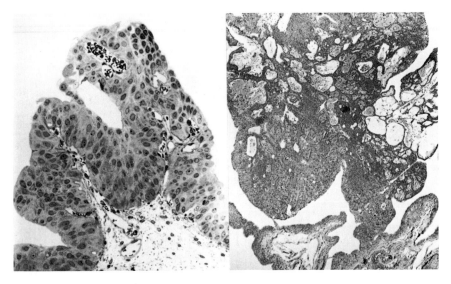

FIG. 9. Part of the bladder from a rat 5 weeks after termination of dosing with 1,200 mg BBN. The urothelium is hyperplastic, mildly dysplastic, and well vascularized. × 145.

FIG. 10. A large, well-vascularized, papillary, transitional cell carcinoma, attached to the bladder wall by a small pedicle, in a rat dosed 50 weeks previously with 1,200 mg BBN. × 23.

latent period before the start of rapid tumor growth, and only a few animals, both placebo- and NER-fed, had developed measurable tumors.

At 2 years, nearly all animals given 1,200 or 600 mg BBN were dead, mainly as a result of their bladder tumors, irrespective of the presence or absence of NER in the diet, and thus no comparison of tumor size could be made. Although a few animals survived in the 300 mg BBN-treated groups, the numbers were too small for a statistically significant comparison of tumor volumes to be made.

The reduction in tumor volume seen 12 months after 600 mg BBN in animals fed the higher dose of NER was reflected by a constant and significant reduction in tumor volume after 20 weeks in the sequentially killed pairs of animals given the same doses of carcinogen and NER (Figure 12). However, as the tumors became progressively larger, the difference in the mean volume between groups tended to decrease. Thus, the difference between the placebo-fed and NER-fed animals for weeks 0–56 was significant, $p < 0.01$, and overall, from 0–84 weeks, $p < 0.01$, but for 57–84 weeks, $p < 0.05$.

Following a 1,200-mg dose of BBN, there was no significant difference in the mean total tumor volume found between pairs of placebo-fed and CRA-fed animals killed sequentially in groups A to D after 36 weeks. In this trial, however, using the highest dose of BBN, random deaths from bladder tumors started earlier than in the sequentially killed animals that had only received 600 mg BBN, and therefore the average tumor size in the population remaining

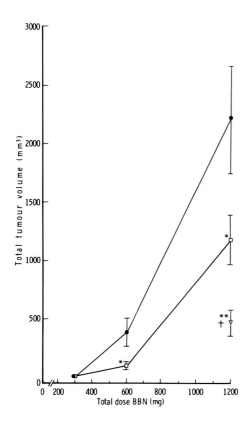

FIG. 11. Mean total bladder tumor volume per rat, related to dose of BBN and the presence or absence of N-ethyl-retinamide in the diet, at 1 year. ●, BBN + placebo; ▽, BBN + 1 mM NER; □, BBN + 2 mM NER. * p < 0.05 when tested against ●; ** p < 0.01 when tested against ●; † p < 0.05 when tested against □. (p Values estimated according to Peto and Peto 1972.) Data from 23–27 rats per group.

available for sampling was inevitably affected, i.e., lowered. This would be particularly true of the BBN-placebo group in which animals started to die earlier than those fed CRA and would tend to mask any effect of the CRA on the volumes. A similar effect is seen in the 600 mg BBN, NER trial from 57 weeks.

The Effects of NER on the Growth Rate of Bladder Tumors

In BBN-dosed animals, the reduction in mean tumor volume observed at 12 months in the NER-fed groups could theoretically have resulted either from a delay in the onset of tumor growth or from a retardation of the rate of tumor growth. It was therefore important to determine the growth rate of the BBN-induced tumors, but the size and fragility of the rat bladder does not permit repeated observations of single tumors to be made over a period of many months. Examination of the bladders of sequentially killed animals showed, however, that a single tumor always appeared first, usually in the dome, and at every time interval one tumor, also in the dome, was constantly larger than all the others at up to 60 weeks or longer. Based on this observation, the assumption was made that the largest tumor seen at autopsy was also the one that

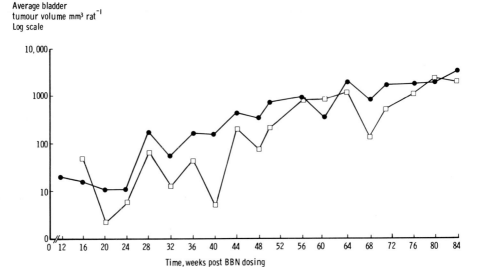

FIG. 12. Variation in average total bladder tumor volume with time, in pairs of rats given 600 mg BBN and subsequently fed placebo or N-ethyl-retinamide in the diet. ● BBN + placebo, □ BBN + 2mM NER. Weeks 0 to 56, ● vs □, $p < 0.01$; 57 to 84, ● vs □, $p < 0.05$; 0 to 84, ● vs □, $p < 0.01$. (p Values estimated according to Peto and Peto 1972.)

had developed first and grown at the expense of other neoplasms in the bladder. The volume of this largest tumor was recorded for sequentially killed pairs of placebo- or NER-fed animals given 600 mg BBN.

The variation in the logarithm of the volume of the largest tumor versus time is shown in Figure 13. The regression lines indicate that in both the placebo-fed and NER-fed animals, the theoretical growth of the tumor was exponential and, since the slopes of the lines were parallel (no significant difference between the regression coefficients), that the NER neither accelerated nor decelerated the tumor growth rate. However, the lines were not superimposed but were separated by 8 to 10 weeks on the time axis. Similar parallel regression lines, again demonstrating a separation of 8 to 10 weeks, can be constructed from the data shown in Figure 12, where total bladder tumor volumes in pairs of sequentially killed rats from the two groups are compared. This suggests that in these experiments, the primary effect of the NER on the response of the bladder to 600 mg BBN was to extend by 8 to 10 weeks the latent period before exponential tumor growth was established.

Effect of Retinoids on Histology and Ultrastructure of BBN-treated Animals

Lifetime dosing with retinoids had no effect on the histology or ultrastructure of the normal urothelium (Figure 14). The doses used were not cytotoxic and the urothelium remained normal and healthy by all criteria.

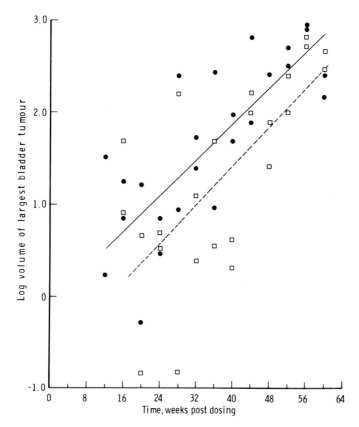

FIG. 13. Correlation between logarithm of volume of the largest bladder tumor, y, and time after BBN dosing, x, in rats given 600 mg BBN and then fed placebo or N-ethyl-retinamide in the diet. ● BBN + placebo, r = 0.80, p < 0.001; □ BBN + 2 mM NER, r = 0.69, p < 0.001. For the fitted regression lines, ● y = 0.081 + 0.046x; □ y = −0.626 + 0.052x. ● vs □, p < 0.02 (Peto and Peto 1972).

In rats treated with BBN and maintained on a placebo diet, the early urothelial hyperplasias were either flat or small, exophytic and polypoidal. After a latent period that varied inversely with the dose of carcinogen used, the BBN-induced lesions in the placebo-fed animals progressed rapidly in size and complexity to produce both papillary and nodular lesions that were well vascularized, the majority of which were benign. However, as time progressed many exophytic growths were also associated with invasive cords of cells that extended into the submucosa (Figure 15), and in some the degree of dysplasia and growth pattern of the urothelium merited classification as carcinoma according to the WHO/UICC system. The tumors were predominantly transitional in cell type, but focal areas of squamous metaplasia were observed in the developing tumors from 5 weeks and 16 weeks after completion of dosing with 1,200 and 600 mg BBN, respectively.

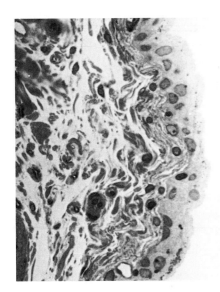 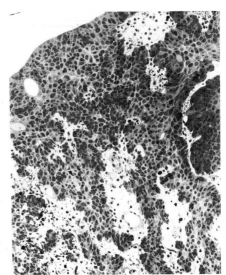

FIG. 14. Normally differentiated urothelium from a rat maintained for over a year on a diet containing 2 mM NER. No evidence of toxic damage to the bladder can be seen. × 275.

FIG. 15. Invasive cords of neoplastic urothelium extending from a nodular lesion into the bladder wall of a rat dosed 22 weeks previously with 1,200 mg BBN. In this transitional cell carcinoma there was considerable cell atypia but no squamous metaplasia. × 135.

In sequentially killed animals given 1,200 or 600 mg BBN large areas of the urinary face of the bladder were examined by scanning electron microscopy for the presence of pleiomorphic microvilli, which are generally accepted to be indicators of neoplastic transformation in the urothelium (Arai et al. 1974, Hicks et al. 1974, Hicks 1976, 1977, Hicks and Wakefield 1976, Hodges et al. 1976, Jacobs et al. 1976, Newman and Hicks 1977, Friedell et al. 1977). In general, the early nodules and proliferative lesions were covered by urothelial cells with an immature surface differentiation pattern. Pleiomorphic microvilli were not seen before 9 weeks after cessation of carcinogen treatment in the group given the highest dose of 1,200 mg BBN. Their development heralded or coincided with the commencement of rapid, visible tumor growth. Characteristic histological and subcellular markers of this rapid growth phase were also identified at the urothelial-mesenchymal interface of developing tumors. The start of visible tumor growth was characterized by the extension of numerous cytoplasmic processes and large multicellular processes of the urothelium into the submucosa (Figures 16 and 17). These features were not seen in the persistent hyperplasias found during the latent period after carcinogen dosing and before visible tumor growth commenced.

Histopathological assessment of the bladders of rats killed sequentially between 0 and 52 weeks after dosing with 600 mg BBN and fed placebo or NER-contain-

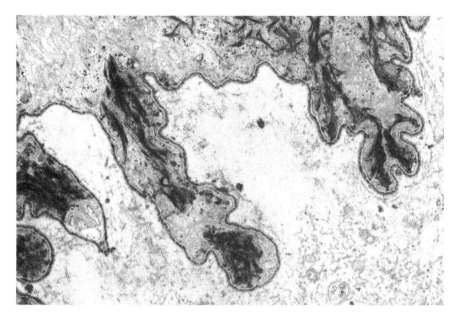

FIG. 16. Small, pseudopodia-like extensions of the urothelium into the submucosa at the base of a BBN-induced transitional cell carcinoma. The processes, which contain excessive amounts of tonofibrils, are still limited by basal lamina but the submucosa is edematous and contains remnants of destroyed collagen. Electron micrograph, × 11,750.

ing diet revealed that far more placebo-fed rats were afflicted by virtually all categories of proliferative lesions than those given NER. This trend was most readily detected in the dome, which was the area with the maximum number of lesions (Figure 18). Although the total number of bladder areas (domes, medians, and trigones, from 0 to 52 weeks) containing P1 carcinomata of grade I, i.e., well-differentiated histology, was the same in both placebo-fed and NER-fed rats (Figure 19), the cumulative incidence of areas with more poorly differentiated, grade II carcinomata was greater at any time in placebo-fed than in NER-fed animals (Figure 20).

Again, the curves illustrate a shift along the time axis of the response of the NER-fed animals by comparison with the placebo-fed group. Conversely, when the presence of normal urothelium was assessed in the dome, median, and trigone areas of the bladders, more areas containing normal urothelium were found in the NER-treated than in the placebo-fed animals. Thus, the NER appeared to have produced a better differentiated urothelium, irrespective of growth pattern, and to have decreased the degree of involvement by hyperplastic and neoplastic lesions. However, because of the delay in tumor development introduced by the NER treatment, the histology reflected the reduced tumor volumes in the NER- versus placebo-fed group. Thus, when the regression lines for the total number of bladder areas involved by proliferative lesions were

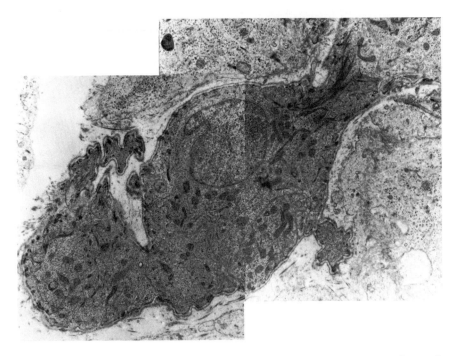

FIG. 17. A large, multicellular process (at higher magnification four separate cells can be distinguished) projecting from the urothelium into the submucosa at the base of a BBN-induced transitional cell carcinoma of the rat bladder. The basal lamina is missing from the urothelium adjacent to the neck of this process. Electron micrograph collage, × 6,750.

plotted against time, they showed quite clearly that after NER the degree of involvement at any time was less than in placebo-fed animals (Figure 21). Again, the separation of the regression lines on the time axis indicates that it took an average of approximately 7 weeks longer for the NER-fed animals to reach the same degree of urothelial involvement as the placebo-fed animals.

In the sequentially killed pairs of animals given CRA after 1,200 mg BBN, again the proliferative response of the urothelium to the carcinogen was not prevented, but the length of the latent period was extended. The appearance of microvilli on the surface of the neoplastic urothelium and of changes at the urothelial-mesenchymal interface was delayed by about the same length of time as the delay in the start of rapid tumor growth. Once tumor growth commenced, the ultrastructure of the lesions reflected the histopathological observations. The retinoid delayed, but did not prevent, the development of morphological features found in the rapidly growing tumors in the placebo-fed BBN-treated animals.

Similarly, electron microscopic examination of the bladders from sequentially killed animals on the NER trial confirmed the ultrastructure to be related to the size of the tumor rather than to the presence or absence of NER in the

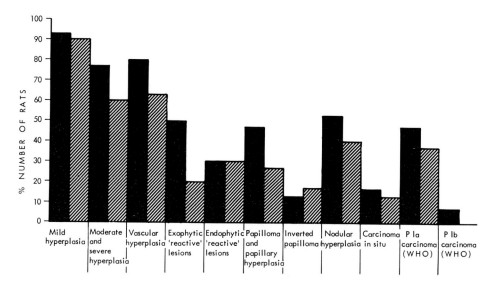

FIG. 18. Percentage of rats with proliferative urothelial lesions in the dome killed sequentially between 0 and 52 weeks after receiving 600 mg BBN and then placebo or N-ethyl-retinamide in the diet. ■ 600 mg BBN + placebo; ▨ 600 mg BBN + 2 mM NER. Difference in percent incidence between treatment groups, when all categories of proliferative lesions are combined: ■ vs ▨, p < 0.01 (X² test)

diet. The larger tumors had more frequent alterations of the basal lamina, more and larger multicellular processes projecting into the submucosa, and proportionately more cells with microvilli on their luminal surface than did small tumors. In general the same markers of malignancy were seen in both the placebo-fed and the NER-fed animals pretreated with BBN. Because the mean total tumor volume was reduced by the NER, the incidence and severity of subcellular changes in these animals were consequently reduced at every time. Although

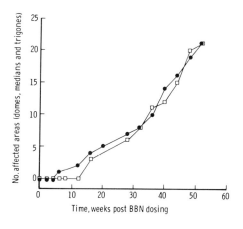

FIG. 19. Cumulative incidence of bladder areas (domes, medians, and trigones) containing well-differentiated, i.e. grade I, superficial (Pla or Plb) carcinomata in rats given 600 mg BBN and then fed placebo or N-ethyl-retinamide in the diet, from 0 to 52 weeks. ● BBN + placebo; □ BBN + 2 mM NER.

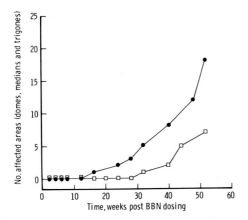

FIG. 20. Cumulative incidence of bladder areas (domes, medians, and trigones) containing moderately differentiated, i.e. grade II, superficial (PIa or PIb) carcinomata in rats given 600 mg BBN and then fed placebo or N-ethyl-retinamide in the diet, from 0 to 56 weeks. ● BBN + placebo; □ BBN + 2 mM NER. Difference in incidence of total number of areas affected: ● vs □, $p < 0.02$ (χ^2 test).

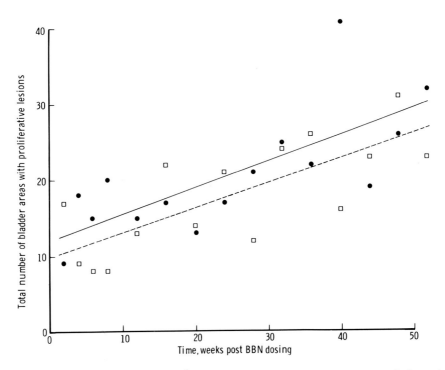

FIG. 21. Correlation of the total number of bladder areas (domes, medians, and trigones) containing proliferative urothelial lesions, y, with time after BBN dosing, x, in rats given 600 mg BBN and then fed placebo or N-ethyl-retinamide in the diet. ● BBN + placebo, r = 0.71, $p < 0.001$; □ BBN + 2 mM NER, r = 0.73, $p < 0.001$. For the fitted regression lines: ● y = 12.185 + 0.342 x; □ y − 9.784 + 0.331 x.

many bizarre alterations in subcellular organelles were observed, particularly in the larger tumors, these all appeared to be related to the stage in development of the tumor and were not influenced by the presence or absence of retinoids in the diet. For example, neither retinoid prevented the eventual development of squamous metaplasia in the BBN-induced urothelial tumors. The subcellular features of large, fast-growing tumors in retinoid-treated animals were indistinguishable from comparable tumors in placebo-fed controls, and alterations in morphological criteria could be explained by the several weeks' delay, induced by retinoid treatment, before tumor growth commenced.

DISCUSSION

Previous demonstrations of retinoid inhibition of bladder cancer development in rodents pretreated with high doses of either N-methyl-N-nitrosourea (MNU) or BBN have involved assessment of the carcinogenic response at a single time some months after the animals were placed on a retinoid-containing diet. Thus, Becci et al. (1979a, 1981), Grubbs et al. (1977), and Thompson et al. (1981) terminated their experiments 6 months after start of carcinogen dosing or after about 4½ months on the retinoid diet; Sporn et al. (1977), Squire et al. (1977), and Murasaki et al. (1980) killed the animals 9 months after starting the carcinogen or after about 8 months on the retinoid; Tannenbaum et al. (1979) killed the animals after 9 months and Becci et al. (1979b) after 9 to 11 months on retinoid. In all these experiments, most of which were testing CRA as the anticarcinogen, the inhibition of bladder carcinogenesis was not complete but there was a consistent reduction in the incidence of papillomas and carcinomas found at autopsy, and overall the differentiation of the tumors and the rest of the urothelium was better in the retinoid-fed than in the placebo-fed groups.

The results reported here with BBN-treated F344 rats maintained for up to 2 years on a diet containing either NER or CRA confirm these previous observations and give some additional information. Thus, there was a significant reduction in the mean total tumor volume of animals killed 12 months after BBN treatment if they had been maintained on an NER-containing diet as opposed to a placebo diet. This was coupled with better differentiation of the urothelium in the NER-fed animals by comparison with the placebo-fed group, irrespective of the method used to assess normal differentiation. Interestingly, far from the anticarcinogenic effect of the retinoid being overwhelmed by the highest dose of carcinogen, the reduction in tumor volume was readily seen after both 1,200 and 600 mg BBN, but was undetectable 12 months after the lowest dose of 300 mg BBN. Similarly, Becci et al. (1979b), using even higher doses of the carcinogen, found 4½-month treatment with CRA to be more effective against 2,400 and 1,800 mg BBN than it was against 1,200 mg in preventing the incidence of transitional cell carcinomas.

The reduction in tumor volume in our experiments did not increase with the dose of NER, and a greater effect was achieved by the lower dose than by the higher dose. At present we have no explanation for this anomalous result; it was not apparently the result of tissue damage by the higher dose since there was no visible histological or subcellular urothelial damage produced by either dose of NER alone. By contrast, Thompson et al. (1981) reported the reduction in carcinogenic response of male mice to BBN to be directly related to the dose of NER used.

In view of the consistent reports of anticarcinogenic activity by retinoids, the poor long-term survival of our retinoid-treated animals over the lifetime experiments was both unexpected and disappointing, but data from animals killed sequentially enable these observations to be reconciled. The immediate effect on the urothelium of the 6-week treatment with BBN is to produce areas of flat, papillary and polypoidal hyperplasia in the urothelia of all animals. These neoplastically transformed urothelia remain quiescent for a period of time that is inversely proportional to the dose of BBN used. During this period, the hyperplasias produced by the BBN treatment do not regress but persist without visibly increasing in thickness or complexity. At the end of the latent period the urothelia visibly enter a period of growth and tumors develop rapidly from the areas of hyperplasia. It has recently been demonstrated that after treatment with the bladder carcinogen 2-acetylaminofluorene (AAF), the incidence of bladder cancer could be accurately predicted from the presence of persistent urothelial hyperplasia 9 months previously; the bladder cancer incidence curve could be accurately superimposed on that for persistent hyperplasia if the 9 months delay on the time axis was removed (Littlefield et al. 1979). In our experiments with CRA and NER, all sequentially collected data, whether death prediction from life-table data, theoretical growth rate of the largest tumor, or quantitative analysis of normal and abnormal areas of urothelium, indicate the anticarcinogenic action of the retinoids was entirely attributable to an increase in the latent period before the neoplastically transformed urothelial hyperplasias commenced to grow rapidly into tumors. There was no evidence to suggest that these retinoids had any ability to reduce the growth rate of the tumor once the visible linear growth phase had been reached.

Figure 22 shows hypothetical growth curves for bladder cancer in which the latent periods L1 and L2 before tumor growth is established are inversely related to the doses of carcinogen, D1 and D2. In our animals, death from bladder cancer was related to tumor size, and it is assumed for these hypothetical curves that death results when a critical tumor volume, V, is reached. If inclusion of a retinoid in the diet increases the latent period by n weeks, but as indicated by our results, does not affect the growth rate of the tumor, the growth curve for the tumor in the retinoid-fed groups will be parallel to that in the placebo-fed groups but be shifted along the time axis by the time n. Providing the animals are killed at any time between L + n and the time the placebo-fed animals reached the critical volume V, a consistent inhibitory effect of the retinoid will be observed, since the tumors in the retinoid-fed group will be n weeks behind those of the placebo fed animals in terms of size, histology, and subcellular

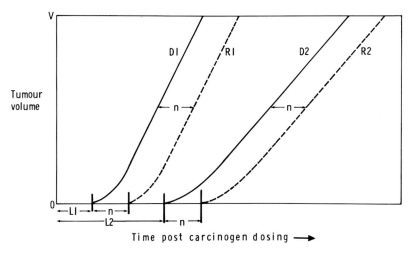

FIG. 22. D1 and D2 are theoretical exponential growth curves, volume versus time, of tumors resulting from exposure to a high dose and a lower dose, respectively, of a carcinogen. It is assumed that a critical tumor volume, V, kills the animal. L1 and L2 are the latent periods, inversely related to the carcinogen dose, before tumor growth commences. If retinoid treatment extends the latent period by the time n but does not alter the rate of tumor growth, then the tumor growth curves R1 and R2 in retinoid-fed animals will be parallel to those of D1 and D2 but separated by n on the time axis.

change. If, however, animals treated with the carcinogen dose D1 are sampled during the period of time L1 to L1 + n, or the D2-treated animals between L2 and L2 + n, the inhibition of tumor growth may appear to be complete because the retinoid-fed group will still be in the prolonged latent period before the persistent hyperplasias have started to grow into tumors.

It follows from this that the anticarcinogenic efficacy of the retinoid can only be assessed from the differential response between the retinoid- and placebo-fed animals at a single time, if the time-related response to the dose of carcinogen used is also accurately known. If very low doses of carcinogen are used, the latent period may be long and tumors may not appear until late in the animal's life-span, by which time other competing causes of death such as other age-related neoplasms may mask any retinoid effect. This was our experience following the dose of 300 mg BBN in our experiments. In practice, then, it is easier to detect the anticarcinogenic effect of the retinoid after a high dose than after a low dose of carcinogen, provided the animals are killed during the period when the linear growth phase has been established for tumors both in the placebo-fed and in the retinoid-fed groups and deaths due to bladder tumors or other causes have not become predominant.

The anticarcinogenic actions of NER and CRA, both reported previously and in our own laboratories, can be entirely accounted for by an increase of a few weeks, 7 to 10 in our experiments, before the hyperplasias start to grow into overt tumors. A comparable delay in the development of MNU-induced rat mammary cancers by another retinoid, 4-hydroxyphenylretinamide, has also been reported (Moon et al. 1979). A parallel can be drawn with the sex-related difference in response of the mouse bladder to BBN, observed by Bertram and Craig (1972). For a time it was believed that BBN was only carcinogenic for male and not for female mice, because male mice develop bladder cancer several weeks earlier than females given the same dose. However, sequentially killed animals showed that for any given dose of BBN, the curves of tumor incidence versus time were parallel in the two sexes and simply separated along the time axis by about 9 weeks. Following castration of the male or supplementation of testosterone for females the time difference was removed and the tumor incidence curves could be superimposed. It would appear that either absence of the male sex hormone or the presence of retinoids prolongs the latent period before the start of the linear phase of tumor growth. Retinoids appear to work completely independently of the sex hormones, since they are equally effective in both male and female rats.

The molecular mechanisms by which retinoids delay the start of tumor growth in the bladder or any other organ are not yet understood. The original rationale for using retinoids for the chemoprevention of cancer was based on the known requirement of all epithelial tissues for vitamin A to maintain normal differentiation; since neoplastic growth is always associated with aberrations of cell differentiation, it seemed possible that vitamin A or its analogues might, concomitant with maintaining and reinforcing normal cell differentiation, actually oppose tumor progression (Sporn et al. 1976).

Retinoids were subsequently shown to antagonize the effect of diterpene promoters in multistage skin carcinogenesis models in vitro (Verma and Boutwell 1977, Slaga et al. 1980), and it has been customary for some time to regard retinoids as "antipromoting" agents. However, in the in vivo bladder cancer models discussed here, the animals were pretreated over a period of 6 weeks with BBN, a complete carcinogen that demonstrably both initiated and promoted neoplastic change in numerous urothelial cells, since multiple bladder cancers subsequently developed in all animals surviving the duration of the experiment. In this model, carcinogenic treatment terminated before the animals were exposed to either NER or CRA and the retinoids could not have acted either as antiinitiators or antipromoters, but only at a later stage of progression of the neoplastically transformed, hyperplastic but quiescent urothelium.

There is evidence that another retinoid, ethyl all-*trans*-9-(4-methoxy-2,3,6-trimethylphenyl)-3,7-dimethyl-2,4,6,8-nonatetraenoate (AR) has a greater anticarcinogenic effect in BBN-treated rats if applied before rather than after the carcinogen treatment (Murasaki et al. 1980), and it also prevented DNA damage in the urothelial cells by one of the major urinary metabolites of BBN (Miyata et al. 1980). This indicates that retinoids may be capable of opposing initiation as well as progression of tumor growth in the bladder. However, if the use of retinoids as chemotherapeutic agents for the treatment of bladder cancer in man is envisaged, it is their ability to delay tumor growth in already neoplastically transformed urothelia that is likely to prove their most useful attribute.

It is now of great importance to determine whether retinoids act directly on the urothelium or indirectly on as yet unidentified systemic factors. Even a delay in tumor development of as little as 7 to 10 weeks in the rat could equate to an extra 5 or 6 years of symptom-free life for the human bladder cancer patient if he could tolerate the same level of retinoids as can the rat. Unfortunately, both CRA and NER, though less toxic than naturally occurring vitamin A, are still toxic at high doses at the systemic level. Rats will tolerate much higher doses of CRA than will man, and these doses do not produce the same symptoms of retinoid toxicity as are seen in man treated with much lower doses. Nevertheless, in our animals weight gain was depressed and bone remodeling was affected, with the long bones thinning. It is known that alteration of the polar-terminal group of the retinoid molecule can modify its activity, toxicity, metabolism, and tissue distribution (Sporn et al. 1979), and many other new analogs are now under investigation as anticarcinogenic agents for specific organs in animal models.

ACKNOWLEDGMENTS

This project has been funded with federal funds from the Department of Health and Human Services under contract number NO1 CP75938. The contents of this publication do not necessarily reflect the views or policies of the Department of Health and Human Services, nor does mention of trade names, commercial products, or organizations imply endorsement by the U.S. Government.

We are indebted to J. Gwynne for her expert animal husbandry, to H. Ogbolu for assistance in preparing material for histology, and to R. Wright for much technical assistance. We would also like to thank Dr. M. Sporn and Dr. R. Moon for advice and helpful discussion of the work.

REFERENCES

Arai, M., T. Kani, S. Sugihara, K. Matsumura, Y. Miyata, Y. Shinohara, and N. Ito. 1974. Scanning and transmission electron microscopy of changes in the urinary bladder in rats with N-butyl-N-(4-hydroxybutyl) nitrosamine. Gann 65:529–540.

Becci, P. J., H. J. Thompson, C. J. Grubbs, R. A. Squire, C. C. Brown, M. B. Sporn, and R. C. Moon. 1979a. Inhibitory effect of 13-cis-retinoic acid on urinary bladder carcinogenesis induced in C57BL/6 mice by N-butyl-N(4-hydroxybutyl) nitrosamine. Cancer Res. 38:4463–4466.

Becci, P. J., H. J. Thompson, C. J. Grubbs, C. C. Brown, and R. C. Moon. 1979b. Effect of delay in administration of 13-cis-retinoic acid on the inhibition of urinary bladder carcinogenesis in the rat. Cancer Res. 39:3141–3144.

Becci, P. J., H. J. Thompson, J. M. Strum, C. C. Brown, M. B. Sporn, and R. C. Moon. 1981. N-butyl-N-(4-hydroxybutyl) nitrosamine-induced urinary bladder cancer in C57BL/6 × DBA2-F_1 mice, a useful model for study of chemoprevention of cancer with retinoids. Cancer Res. 41:927–932.

Bertram, J. S., and A. W. Craig. 1972. Specific induction of bladder cancer in mice by butyl-(4-hydroxybutyl) nitrosamine and the effects of hormonal modifications on the sex difference in response. Eur. J. Cancer 8:587–594.

Bjelke, E. 1975. Dietary vitamin A and human lung cancer. Int. J. Cancer 15:561–565.

Darby, A. J., N. E. Frater, M. D. Hershey, J. A. Turton, and R. M. Hicks. 1981. Effects of N-ethyl-retinamide on bone remodelling in the rat. A role for retinoid therapy in osteoporosis? *in* Proceedings of the Third International Workshop on Bone Histomorphometry (in press).

Friedell, G. H., J. B. Jacobs, G. K. Nagy, and S. M. Cohen. 1977. The pathogenesis of bladder cancer. Am. J. Pathol. 89:431–442.

Grubbs, C. J., R. C. Moon, R. A. Squire, G. M. Farrow, S. E. Stinson, D. G. Goodman, C. C. Brown, and M. B. Sporn. 1977. 13-Cis-retinoic acid: Inhibition of bladder carcinogenesis induced in rats by N-butyl-N-(4-hydroxybutyl) nitrosamine. Science 198:743–744.

Hicks, R. M. 1976. Changes in differentiation of the urinary bladder during benign and neoplastic hyperplasia, *in* Progress in Differentiation Research, N. Muller-Berat, ed. North-Holland Pub. Co., Amsterdam, pp. 339–353.

Hicks, R. M. 1977. Morphological markers of early neoplastic change in the urinary bladder. Cancer Res. 37:2822–2823.

Hicks, R. M. 1980. Multistage carcinogenesis in the urinary bladder. Br. Med. Bull. 36:39–46.

Hicks, R. M., and J. Chowaniec. 1978. Experimental induction, histology and ultrastructure of hyperplasia and neoplasia of the urinary bladder epithelium. Int. Rev. Exp. Pathol. 18:199–280.

Hicks, R. M., J. Chowaniec, and J. St. J. Wakefield. 1978. The experimental induction of bladder tumours by a 2-stage system, *in* Carcinogenesis, vol. 2, Mechanisms of Tumor Promotion and Co-carcinogenesis, T. J. Slaga, A. Sivak, and R. K. Boutwell, eds. Raven Press, New York, pp. 475–489.

Hicks, R. M., B. Ketterer, and R. C. Warren. 1974. The ultrastructure and chemistry of the luminal plasma membrane of the mammalian urinary bladder: A structure with low permeability to water and ions. Phil. Trans. Roy. Soc. B 268:23–38.

Hicks, R. M., and J. St. J. Wakefield. 1976. Membrane changes during urothelial hyperplasia and neoplasia. Cancer Res. 36:2502–2507.

Hodges, G. M., R. M. Hicks, and G. Spacey. 1976. Scanning electron microscopy of cell-surface changes in methylnitrosourea (MNU)-treated rat bladders in vivo and in vitro. Differentiation 6:143–150.

Jacobs, J. B., M. Arai, S. M. Cohen, and G. H. Friedell. 1976. Early lesions in experimental bladder cancer: Scanning electron microscopy of cell-surface markers. Cancer Res. 30:2512–2517.

Littlefield, N. A., D. L. Greenman, J. H. Farmer, and W. G. Sheldon. 1979. Effects of continuous and discontinued exposure to 2-AAF on urinary bladder hyperplasia and neoplasia. J. Environ. Pathol. Toxicol. 3:35–54.

Miyata, Y., T. Nakatsuka, M. Arai, G. Murasaki, K. Nakanishi, and N. Ito. 1980. Inhibition by an aromatic retinoid of DNA damage induced by the bladder carcinogen N-butyl-N-(3-carboxypropyl)-nitrosamine. Gann 71:341–348.

Moon, R. C., H. J. Thompson, P. J. Becci, C. J. Grubbs, R. J. Gander, D. L. Newton, J. M. Smith, S. L. Phillips, W. R. Henderson, L. T. Mullen, C. C. Brown, and M. B. Sporn. 1979. N-(4-hydroxyphenyl)-retinamide, a new retinoid for prevention of breast cancer in the rat. Cancer Res. 39:1339–1346.

Mostofi, F. K., L. H. Sobin and H. Torloni, eds. 1973. International Histological Classification of Tumours No. 10. Histological Typing of Urinary Bladder Tumours. World Health Organization, Geneva, pp. 9–36.

Murasaki, G., Y. Miyata, K. Babaya, M. Arai, S. Fukushima, and N. Ito. 1980. Inhibitory effect of an aromatic retinoic acid analog on urinary bladder carcinogenesis in rats treated with N-butyl-N-(4-hydroxybutyl) nitrosamine. Gann 71:333–340.

Newman, J., and R. M. Hicks. 1977. Detection of neoplastic and preneoplastic urothelia by combined scanning and transmission electron microscopy of urinary surface of human and rat bladder. Histopathology 1:125–135.

Peto, R., M. C. Pike, P. Armitage, N. E. Breslow, D. R. Cox, S. V. Howard, N. Mantel, K. McPherson, J. Peto, and P. G. Smith. 1977. Design and analysis of randomized clinical trials requiring prolonged observation of each patient. II analyses and examples. Br. J. Cancer 35:1–39.

Peto, R., and J. Peto. 1972. Asymptotically efficient rank invariant test procedures (with discussion). J. R. Statist. Soc. A 135:185–206.

Slaga, T. J., A. J. P. Klein-Szanto, S. M. Fischer, C. E. Weeks, K. Nelson, and S. Major. 1980.

Studies on the mechanism of action of anti-tumor promoting agents: Their specificity in two-stage promotion. Proc. Natl. Acad. Sci. USA 77:2251–2254.

Sporn, M. B. 1978. Pharmacological prevention of carcinogenesis by retinoids, *in* Carcinogenesis, vol. 2. Mechanisms of Tumor Promotion and Co-carcinogenesis, T. J. Slaga, A. Sivak and R. K. Boutwell, eds. Raven Press, New York, pp. 545–551.

Sporn, M. B., N. M. Dunlop, D. L. Newton, and J. M. Smith. 1976. Prevention of chemical carcinogenesis by vitamin A and its synthetic analogs (retinoids). Fed. Proc. 35:1332–1338.

Sporn, M. B., D. L. Newton, J. M. Smith, N. Acton, A. E. Jacobson, and A. Brossi. 1979. Retinoids and cancer prevention: The importance of the terminal group to the retinoid molecule in modifying activity and toxicity, *in* Carcinogens: Identification and Mechanisms of Action, A. C. Griffin and C. R. Shaw, eds. Raven Press, New York, pp. 441–453.

Sporn, M. B., R. A. Squire, C. C. Brown, J. M. Smith, M. L. Wenk, and S. Springer. 1977. 13-Cis-retinoic acid: Inhibition of bladder carcinogenesis in the rat. Science 195:487–489.

Squire, R. A., M. B. Sporn, C. C. Brown, J. M. Smith, M. L. Wenk, and S. Springer. 1977. Histopathological evaluation of the inhibition of rat bladder carcinogenesis by 13-cis-retinoic acid. Cancer Res. 37:2930–2936.

Tannenbaum, M., S. Tannenbaum, B. N. Richelo, and P. W. Trown. 1979. Effects of 13-cis- and all-*trans*-retinoic acid on the development of bladder cancer in rats: An ultrastructural study, *in* Scanning Electron Microscopy, 1979, III. SEM Inc., AMF O'Hare, Illinois, pp. 673–676.

Thompson, H. J., P. J. Becci, C. J. Grubbs, Y. F. Shealy, E. J. Stanek, C. C. Brown, M. B. Sporn, and R. C. Moon. 1981. Inhibition of urinary bladder cancer by N-(ethyl)-all-*trans*-retinamide and N-(2-hydroxyethyl)-all-*trans*-retinamide in rats and mice. Cancer Res. 41:933–936.

Verma, A. K. and R. C. Boutwell. 1977. Vitamin A acid (retinoic acid), a potent inhibitor of 12-0-tetradecanoyl-phorbol-13-acetate induced ornithine decarboxylase activity in mouse epidermis. Cancer Res. 37:2196–2201.

Wald, N., M. Idle, J. Boreham, and A. Bailey. 1980. Low serum-vitamin A and subseqent risk of cancer. Lancet 2:813–815.

Molecular Interrelations of Nutrition and Cancer,
edited by M. S. Arnott, J. van Eys, and Y.-M. Wang.
Raven Press, New York © 1982.

Nutrition, Basic Science, and Past Mistakes

Jan van Eys

*Department of Pediatrics, The University of Texas M. D. Anderson Hospital and Tumor
Institute at Houston, Houston, Texas 77030*

Nutrition is an uneasy science. In almost all other biomedical sciences the image held by the public is largely determined by the scientists themselves. Until recently, the integrity of a given field was entirely the responsibility of the scientist. The rigor of the scientific approach was entirely for the scientific community to judge. (There is a disturbing trend, however, to use the public forum to manipulate political opinion; but the scientists themselves are to blame, not the public.)

Nutrition as a science is different. The public already has an opinion about what nutrition means, and political opinion is heavily swayed by nutritional considerations. The public opinion is so pervasive that the dictionary sanctions that view. Webster's New Collegiate Dictionary (1975) defines nutrition as: "The act or process of nourishing or being nourished; the sum of the processes by which an animal or plant takes in and utilizes food substances." While the second part of that definition implies that nutrition is a science, it does not explicitly define it as one. A nutritionist is called: "A specialist in the study of nutrition." Again, no definition lists a nutritionist as a scientist.

A medical dictionary does not help. Nutrition is defined in Dorland's Illustrated Medical Dictionary as follows:

1. The sum of the processes involved in taking in nutriments and assimilating and utilizing them.
2. Nutriment.

A nutritionist is called: "A specialist in food and nutrition." Nutriment is: "Nourishment, nutritious material, food." The science of nutrition is defined as nutriology, a word hardly ever used by anyone. Even that word has a dual meaning: "The science of nutrition; the study of foods and their use in diet and therapy." One cannot get away from the concept of food. It is in fact very revealing that while the term science is not used in nutrition, it is used in the definition of dietetics: "The science or study and regulation of the diet."

There is thus a profound misconception built into the language about nutrition as a science. This is the more true because people do not think about words in terms of definitions but in terms of concepts. And concepts are far more complex than definitions ever seem to imply. Concepts are broadened by needs, feelings, beliefs. The concept that nutrition embodies all that is basic about protection of the helpless, support of the downtrodden, self-control, and self-help in times of illness is all prevailing. The scientific evidence is readily misjudged or at best prejudged. This can best be illustrated by the preamble and declaration of purpose of the Child Nutrition Act of 1966:

In recognition of the demonstrated relationship between food and good nutrition and the capacity of children to develop and learn, based on the years of cumulative successful experience under the National School Lunch Program with its significant contributions in the field of applied nutrition research, it is hereby declared to be the policy of Congress that these efforts shall be extended, expanded, and strengthened . . . as a measure to safeguard the health and well being of the nation's children. . . .

Little more evidence needs to be added to prove the point that the public concept of nutrition is very different from that of the scientific approach in other biomedical fields.[1] It might be added here that there is no provision for research in the school lunch program act alluded to. Such research as was done was post hoc evaluation of data, rather than prospective hypothesis testing, as good research ought to be.

In a symposium on the translation of scientific and nutrition findings to social policy, held at the 63rd annual meeting of the Federation of American Societies for Experimental Biology, Orlans (1979) summarized his own paper, and through that the problem, very succinctly:

Knowledge of the nation's health and nutritional status is dated, uncertain, incomplete and complex, whereas politicians demand simplicity and administrators, practicability; and everyone wants more and better information. Rational policy, the unicorn intellectuals hunt, should combine clarity, realism, and conviction, which calls for a touch of passion. Attempts to reconcile these contradictory elements can lead to dangerous political pressures on research: the simplification, exaggeration, and over-generalization of findings: and excessive expectations for humdrum programs that often bear little resemblance to their glorified goals.

Having thus stated the problem and the past mistakes, how can we avoid such a cycle again? There is a general problem in biomedical research of great expectations and overemphasis on so-called relevance. In purely clinical research aimed at developing a therapeutic modality, there has long been the concept of phase I, II, III, and IV research. If we utilize the description of such an approach as it is used for drug development in cancer chemotherapy we get a sequence, defined in Table 1, for phase I through III (Carter and Goldin 1977). Before phase I, the applicability of the research to a specific therapeutic problem is not yet conceived, let alone perceived. Beyond phase III is phase IV, wherein the general applicability and potential for safe and effective noncontrolled use is evaluated.

---

[1] There is an additional complication that the economic impact of the poultry and livestock industries is so great that the nutrition of a healthy chicken or other domestic animal is subject to many of the same pressures as human nutrition.

TABLE 1. *Clinical trials of new drugs developed by the National Cancer Institute*

Phase	Activities
I. Clinical pharmacology	Establish maximum tolerated dose at schedule(s) tested
	Establish toxicity parameters and determine if toxicity is predictable, treatable, and/or reversible
	Pharmacologic evaluation
	Antitumor activity not required
II. Screening for clinical activity	Treat 20–30 patients who can be evaluated with measurable disease in each of a range of "signal" tumor types
	Evaluate on the basis of objective response rate and characteristics of pharmacology, mechanism of action, and cell-cycle sensitivity
III. Trial for recommendations of general use	Controlled clinical trials
	Combination studies

Reproduced from Carter and Goldin (1977), with permission of the authors.

Nutrition research has, by definition, potential medical applicability. As already discussed, this can create excessive expectation and a dilution, if not destruction, of scientific rigor. It is useful to look upon research that is potentially relevant to medicine in the same division of phases I through IV. There is a prephase I wherein the research is not yet definable in its biomedical applicability. In the context of this discussion, one would say that the research cannot yet be called nutritional research. As an example, the discovery of coenzyme A as the carrier of "active acetate" was not phase I nutritional research until pantothenic acid was found to be an integral component of the molecule (Lipmann et al. 1947). Table 2 summarizes the description of the conceptual division of biomedical research, with nutrition as paradigm in the phases I through III, in an analogy to phases I through III for drug development (see Table 1). In contrast to clinical trials for drugs, there is no requirement that humans be the main experimental animals. However, in drug research, animal data are also gathered to establish suggested human dosages and are therefore an integral part of phase I studies.

In basic biomedical research, phase I research deals only with the understanding of the relationship between nutritional principles and metabolism and with the consequences of nutritional manipulation. In contrast to clinical research, in which phase I research is quantitatively limited, in basic research, phase I research is the most frequent. Phase II research is like the clinical research center setting: research about nutrition is done in the clinical setting. In phase III research, in the more general clinical setting, research with nutrition is executed.

TABLE 2. *Biomedical research phases with nutrition as an example*

Phase	Activities
I. Basic research	Research in areas relevant to nutrition Establishment of consequences of nutritional manipulation (experimental deficiency disease) Metabolic role of nutrients Clinical relevance is not required (research in nutrition)
II. Research on applicability	Research on nutritional concepts in clinical settings Evaluation for relevance of nutritional concepts in disease (research about nutrition)
III. Research in nutritional medicine	Research utilizing nutritional principles in treating and understanding disease (research with nutrition)

Beyond phase III lies phase IV, in which general applicability is tested. It is in that arena where public policy and basic research meet. Between phase III and IV research in drug development and phase III and IV research in nutrition stands the same watchdog agency: the Food and Drug Administration.

There is some misconception that most phase I research in nutrition has in fact already been done, and that little new can be discovered. The decade and a half between the 1930s and middle 1940s was an era of unprecedented discoveries wherein chemistry became the approach to the science of nutrition (Jukes 1979). The application of the nutrition of lactic acid bacteria to the solution of the narrower human nutrition questions made the application of biochemical thought to nutrition more rigorous and general (Snell 1979). This sequence of development is also clearly reflected in the history of the *Journal of Nutrition* (Krehl 1978).

There was still a concept of great simplicity in the nutritional research of that era. One disease, one nutrient, one function was a dominant concept in the thoughts of the public and dietitians alike. Whittling with Occam's razor beyond a true likeness made many biochemists think likewise. Yet, even if such an old-fashioned concept of nutrition were valid, nutritional research has far from exhausted areas of discovery. The elucidation of the action of vitamins D (Schnoes and deLuca 1980) and K (Suttie 1980) has clearly demonstrated that. Furthermore, the recent prominence of nutrition in the Federation Meetings, to which many citations in this paper refer, makes it clear that scientists are still excited about these developments. It is therefore not true that nutrition is a spent science at the phase I level, even if the conceptual view of nutrition of the 1930s were to be maintained. But the science of nutrition is more than that; it always was more than that.

The nutritional analogy to genetics, one metabolic function, one nutrient, one deficiency disease, served well as a research-directing model. But function is more complex than that. In biology we are rarely interested in the function of an isolated area of metabolism. We are interested in the integrated function of the whole cell. Ultimately, we are interested in health, part of which, though by no means all, is absence of disease. There is a presumed promise that humans can live long lives without disease, followed by sudden death of old age because of multisystem collapse (Fries 1980). That is extreme, and again, a typical example of exaggerated expectations. It is multisystem integration that is the question at hand. Even in integrated systems such as immunity, single nutrients play such a unique role in a complex sequence of regulated events that the deficiency of any one can interrupt the sequence (Biesel et al. 1981). The research by Good and colleagues has produced the prime example, of zinc and T cell function, which is summarized in this monograph.

It is therefore little wonder that nutrition and cancer are a tempting and enticing juxtaposition of scientific inquiry. By definition such research is at the phase II level in that the relevance of the nutritional research is accepted. However, the impetus for this juxtaposition came from the cancer side. The revised National Cancer Act of 1974 states that:

In carrying out the National Cancer Program, the Director of the National Cancer Institute shall: collect, analyze and disseminate information respecting nutrition programs for cancer patients and the relationship between nutrition and cancer, useful in the prevention, diagnosis and treatment of cancer.

Out of that mandate, the Diet, Nutrition and Cancer Program of the National Cancer Institute was born (Gori 1975). Again, the public and nonscientists used the definition of nutrition that does not allow rigorous scientific approaches. It is no wonder that the Diet, Nutrition and Cancer Program had a very stormy history with much infighting, charges of internal overstepping of authority, and eventually subjugation of the program to the therapeutic approach that typifies the cancer program. In oncology parlance, phase III research was being done without proper phase I background.

The fact that humans and all the animal systems that serve as models for human disease have complex nutritional requirements provides the possibility for a magnificent experiment in nature. That experiment is far more useful than the genetic experiments in nature that have taught us so much about functional systems. It is better because nutrition can be manipulated, at the whole animal level, and even more readily at the cellular level.

It remains a mystery why nutrition as a discipline keeps repeating past mistakes, and keeps falling into the same trap. It is a permanent puzzle why the discipline of nutrition allows outsiders to define its own being. Many biochemists, biologists, and molecular biologists are engaged in nutrition research, but would never admit it. Others, who are so engaged and are willing to call themselves nutritionists, especially those working in areas with overt relevance to human disease, are constantly trying to improve the image of nutrition. During a workshop on physician education in cancer nutrition, this was a recurring theme, prompting the following statement (in Sherlock and Aker 1980):

We seem to spend all of our time defending ourselves rather than going back to the laboratories and being good scientists. I have only heard nutritionists say we have a bad image. It is more our thinking poorly of ourselves that others thinking poorly of us.

Such lack of self image and assertiveness can cost dearly. A specific example can be cited. Riley wrote an interesting short review about the enzyme L-asparaginase as a cancer chemotherapeutic agent (Riley 1980). The discovery that the systemic depletion of asparagine would result in tumor regression in mouse systems was rapidly promoted to clinical application with disappointing results. According to Riley, the discrepancy is partially explained by the presence of the LDH virus in the model tumors, which magnifies the overall amino acid pool disturbances that asparagine depletion causes. If that virus is absent, the tumor is far less sensitive (Figure 1). The research on asparaginase was most promising because the question could have been *why* it worked (a phase I or II question), not *whether* it worked in humans (a phase III research problem). We again did phase III research before phase I or II research was properly completed. The conceptual confusion had far-reaching consequences. As Riley (1980) observed:

The asparginase studies that have been carried out to date constitute a promising but somewhat primitive prototype of what can be a highly imaginative approach to an extremely complex problem. To allow the imperfect trials at the clinical level to suppress a promising and rational concept that functioned remarkably well under the controlled conditions of the laboratory is scientifically short-sighted.

Unfortunately, the understandable disappointment of clinical oncologists has diffused in an unfiltered fashion to peer review groups and to the funding agencies, with the usual consequences that occur when a subject falls from grace or is no longer fashionable.

It is not totally true that the concept of amino acid deprivation has died, but it is almost entirely transferred to cancer therapy as the guiding research concept. A workshop was held by the National Cancer Institute entitled "Amino Acid Imbalance in the Treatment of Cancer" (Hanka 1979). Amino acid analogues are being revived as antineoplastic agents, such as diazo norleucine (Burchenal 1979). It should be remembered that much of chemotherapy is therapy based on nutritional principles (van Eys 1979). Therefore, nutrition scientists should speak up and keep in front of their scientific peers, the medical community, and the general population the maxim: since no disease is ever controlled by cure, *why* the treatment works is the important observation, not *that* it works. The scientist should ask the questions, not the physician. There is a basic error to which all of us are prone: confusing immediately visible results with conceptual advances (van Eys 1980).

Nutrition as a concept is one of the greatest achievements of modern western man. The political and humanistic applications are among the best evidence of the good in man, and the remaining disproportion in food among populations of this world is one major piece of evidence of the worst in man. Many of

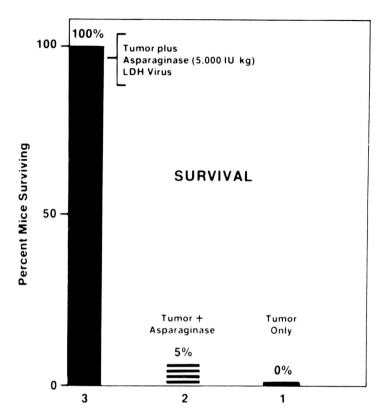

FIG. 1. Comparative survival of mice 30 days following implantation of an asparagine-dependent leukemia, following: 1, no treatment; 2, asparaginase (5,000 IU/kg); 3, asparaginase in the presence of the LDH virus. (Reproduced from Riley (1980) with permission of the publishers.)

the choices we can now make for populations, or for patients with cancer, could only have been achieved by careful and rigorous science. A historical example may be in order. Dr. McCollum, who laid the groundwork for nutritional research as a biochemical discipline, wrote (McCollum 1953):

It was such considerations that led me to conclude that the only promising course lay in the use of the simplest possible diets in the chemical sense, and of employing small animals . . . and to make an effort to solve the problem of what, in chemical terms constitutes the minimum quota of chemical substances on which an animal can function normally.

However, the idea of using the vermin rat as a study object for improving the nutrition of the cow struck the powers that controlled funding as totally irrational. McCollum persisted and the practical consequences of his discoveries are rewards that arise naturally from the scientific rigor of his approach to problems and not because they represented the end goal of his research (Herriott 1980). Good research has a habit of proving itself. Our past and continually repeated mistakes should have taught us to have faith in that axiom. Basic scientists should learn from their clinical colleagues that phase III research cannot be done profitably until phase I research is completed.

This conference has shown that excellent, imaginative, and profitable phase I and II research is ongoing in nutrition. Let the data speak for themselves and their applicability to the practical cancer problem will prove itself naturally.

REFERENCES

Beisel, W. A., R. Edelman, K. Nauss, and R. M. Suskind. 1981. Single nutrient effects on immunologic functions. JAMA 245:53–58.

Burchenal, J. H. 1979. Antitumor effects of azaserine and DON. Cancer Treat. Rep. 63:1031–1032.

Carter, S. K., and A. Goldin. 1977. Experimental models and their clinical correlations. Natl. Cancer Inst. Monogr. 45:63–74.

Child Nutrition Act of 1966, Public Law 89–642, 80 Stat. 885, October 11, 1966, Section 2.

Dorland's Illustrated Medical Dictionary, ed. 25, s.v. "nutrition," "nutritionist," "nutriment," "nutriology."

Fries, J. F. 1980. Aging, natural death, and the compression of morbidity. N. Engl. J. Med. 303:130–135.

Gori, G. B. 1975. The diet, nutrition, and cancer program of the NCI National Cancer Program. Cancer Res. 35:3545–3547.

Hanka, L. J. 1979. Introduction: Possibilities for biochemically rational chemotherapy for some malignancies with depleting enzymes and antimetabolites of specific amino acids. Cancer Treat. Rep. 63:1009–1011.

Herriott, R. M. 1980. Life and contributions of Elmer V. McCollum. Fed. Proc. 39:2713–2715.

Jukes, T. H. 1979. Living history: Nutritional discoveries of the 1930s. Introductory remark. Fed. Proc. 38:2679–2680.

Krehl, W. A. 1978. An era of nutritional growth and maturation. Highlights of the *Journal of Nutrition* during the editorship of George R. Cowgill, 1939–1959, *in* The American Institute of Nutrition, A History of the First 50 Years, 1928–1978, and The Proceedings of a Symposium Commemorating the 50th Anniversary of the *Journal of Nutrition,* F. W. Hill, ed. Bethesda, The American Institute of Nutrition, pp. 8–12.

Lipmann, F., N. O. Kaplan, G. D. Novelli, L. C. Tuttle, and B. M. Quirard. 1947. Coenzyme for acetylation, a pantothenic acid derivative. J. Biol. Chem. 17:869–870.

McCollum, E. V. 1953. My early experiences in the study of foods and nutrition. Ann. Rev. Biochem. 22:1–16.

National School Lunch Act, Public Law 79–396, 60 Stat. 230, June 4, 1946, and as amended subsequently.

Orlans, H. 1979. On knowledge, policy, practice and fate. Fed. Proc. 38:2553–2556.

Riley, V. 1980. Whatever happened to the asparaginase concept of amino acid deprivation therapy. Nutrition and Cancer 2:4–8.

Schnoes, H. K. and H. F. deLuca. 1980. Recent progress in vitamin D metabolism and the chemistry of vitamin D metabolites. Fed. Proc. 39:2723–2729.

Sherlock, P., and S. Aker, 1980. Working group III: Content, faculty, and development of cancer nutrition education programs at the graduate level. Nutrition and Cancer 2:48–51.

Snell, E. E. 1979. Lactic acid bacteria and identification of B vitamins. Some historical notes, 1937–1940. Fed. Proc. 38:2690–2693.

Suttie, J. W. 1980. The metabolic role of vitamin K. Fed. Proc. 39:2730–2735.

van Eys, J. 1979. Nutritional therapy in childhood malignancies—A historical perspective, *in* Nutrition and Cancer, J. van Eys, M. S. Seelig, and B. L. Nichols, Jr., eds. S. P. Medical and Scientific Books, New York, pp. 91–110.

van Eys, J. 1980. Basic research versus clinical research—Where is the problem? Cancer Bulletin 32:222–226, 1980.

Webster's New Collegiate Dictionary. 1975. s.v. "nutrition," "nutritionist."

Author Index

Author Index

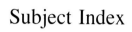

Subject Index

Subject Index

S